Preventing Mental, Emotional, and Behavioral Disorders Among Young People

Progress and Possibilities

Committee on the Prevention of Mental Disorders and Substance Abuse
Among Children, Youth, and Young Adults:
Research Advances and Promising Interventions

Mary Ellen O'Connell, Thomas Boat, and Kenneth E. Warner, *Editors*

Board on Children, Youth, and Families
Division of Behavioral and Social Sciences and Education

NATIONAL RESEARCH COUNCIL *AND*
INSTITUTE OF MEDICINE
OF THE NATIONAL ACADEMIES

THE NATIONAL ACADEMIES PRESS
Washington, D.C.
www.nap.edu

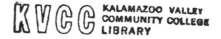

THE NATIONAL ACADEMIES PRESS 500 Fifth Street, N.W. Washington, DC 20001

NOTICE: The project that is the subject of this report was approved by the Governing Board of the National Research Council, whose members are drawn from the councils of the National Academy of Sciences, the National Academy of Engineering, and the Institute of Medicine. The members of the committee responsible for the report were chosen for their special competences and with regard for appropriate balance.

This study was supported by Grant No. NO1-OD-4-2139, Task Order #181 between the National Academy of Sciences and the Department of Health and Human Services. Any opinions, findings, conclusions, or recommendations expressed in this publication are those of the author(s) and do not necessarily reflect the views of the organizations or agencies that provided support for the project.

Library of Congress Cataloging-in-Publication Data

Preventing mental, emotional, and behavioral disorders among young people : progress and possibilities / Committee on Prevention of Mental Disorders and Substance Abuse Among Children, Youth, and Young Adults: Research Advances and Promising Interventions ; Mary Ellen O'Connell, Thomas Boat, and Kenneth E. Warner, editors ; Board on Children, Youth, and Families, Division of Behavioral and Social Sciences and Education.
   p. cm.
  Rev. ed. of: Reducing risks for mental disorders. 1994.
  Includes bibliographical references and index.
  ISBN 978-0-309-12674-8 (hardcover) — ISBN 978-0-309-12675-5 (pdf) 1. Mental illness—Prevention—Research—Government policy—United States. 2. Mental health promotion—Research—Government policy—United States. 3. Mental illness—United States—Prevention. 4. Mental health promotion—United States. I. O'Connell, Mary Ellen. II. Boat, Thomas F. III. Warner, Kenneth E., 1947- IV. Institute of Medicine (U.S.). Committee on Prevention of Mental Disorders and Substance Abuse Among Children, Youth, and Young Adults: Research Advances and Promising Interventions. V. National Research Council (U.S.). Board on Children, Youth, and Families. VI. Reducing risks for mental disorders.
  RA790.6.R44 2009
  362.196'890072—dc22

2009003378

Additional copies of this report are available from National Academies Press, 500 Fifth Street, N.W., Lockbox 285, Washington, DC 20055; (800) 624-6242 or (202) 334-3313 (in the Washington metropolitan area); Internet, http://www.nap.edu.

Suggested citation: National Research Council and Institute of Medicine. (2009). *Preventing Mental, Emotional, and Behavioral Disorders Among Young People: Progress and Possibilities*. Committee on the Prevention of Mental Disorders and Substance Abuse Among Children, Youth, and Young Adults: Research Advances and Promising Interventions. Mary Ellen O'Connell, Thomas Boat, and Kenneth E. Warner, Editors. Board on Children, Youth, and Families, Division of Behavioral and Social Sciences and Education. Washington, DC: The National Academies Press.

First Printing, August 2009
Second Printing, July 2010

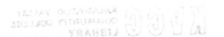

THE NATIONAL ACADEMIES
Advisers to the Nation on Science, Engineering, and Medicine

The **National Academy of Sciences** is a private, nonprofit, self-perpetuating society of distinguished scholars engaged in scientific and engineering research, dedicated to the furtherance of science and technology and to their use for the general welfare. Upon the authority of the charter granted to it by the Congress in 1863, the Academy has a mandate that requires it to advise the federal government on scientific and technical matters. Dr. Ralph J. Cicerone is president of the National Academy of Sciences.

The **National Academy of Engineering** was established in 1964, under the charter of the National Academy of Sciences, as a parallel organization of outstanding engineers. It is autonomous in its administration and in the selection of its members, sharing with the National Academy of Sciences the responsibility for advising the federal government. The National Academy of Engineering also sponsors engineering programs aimed at meeting national needs, encourages education and research, and recognizes the superior achievements of engineers. Dr. Charles M. Vest is president of the National Academy of Engineering.

The **Institute of Medicine** was established in 1970 by the National Academy of Sciences to secure the services of eminent members of appropriate professions in the examination of policy matters pertaining to the health of the public. The Institute acts under the responsibility given to the National Academy of Sciences by its congressional charter to be an adviser to the federal government and, upon its own initiative, to identify issues of medical care, research, and education. Dr. Harvey V. Fineberg is president of the Institute of Medicine.

The **National Research Council** was organized by the National Academy of Sciences in 1916 to associate the broad community of science and technology with the Academy's purposes of furthering knowledge and advising the federal government. Functioning in accordance with general policies determined by the Academy, the Council has become the principal operating agency of both the National Academy of Sciences and the National Academy of Engineering in providing services to the government, the public, and the scientific and engineering communities. The Council is administered jointly by both Academies and the Institute of Medicine. Dr. Ralph J. Cicerone and Dr. Charles M. Vest are chair and vice chair, respectively, of the National Research Council.

www.national-academies.org

Acknowledgments

This report is the work of the Committee on the Prevention of Mental Disorders and Substance Abuse Among Children, Youth, and Young Adults: Research Advances and Promising Interventions, a project of the National Research Council (NRC) and the Institute of Medicine (IOM). The expertise and hard work of the committee were advanced by the support of our sponsors, the contributions of able consultants and staff, and the input of outside experts. The majority of funding for this project was provided by the Center for Mental Health Services of the Substance Abuse and Mental Health Services Administration (SAMHSA), with supplementary funding from the National Institute of Mental Health (NIMH), the National Institute on Drug Abuse (NIDA), and the National Institute on Alcohol Abuse and Alcoholism (NIAAA). The guidance and support of Anne Mathews-Younes and Paul Brounstein, SAMHSA; Robert Heinssen, NIMH; Elizabeth Robertson, NIDA; and Vivian Faden, NIAAA, were much appreciated.

Throughout this process, the committee benefited from presentations or written input by individuals with a range of perspectives (see Appendix B). The committee is thankful for the useful contributions of these many individuals. We would like to thank those who wrote papers that were invaluable to the committee's discussions: Tom Dishion, University of Oregon; Daniel Eisenberg, University of Michigan; Pauline E. Ginsberg, Utica College; Mark Greenberg, Pennsylvania State University; J. David Hawkins, University of Washington; Kamilah Neighbors, University of Michigan; Ron Prinz, University of South Carolina; Anne W. Riley, Johns Hopkins University; Herbert Severson, Oregon Research Institute; Brian

Smith, University of Washington; Hill Walker, Oregon Research Institute; and Hirokazu Yoshikawa, Harvard University. We are also thankful to those who assisted committee members with literature searches, background research, or analyses, including Mark Alter, Columbia University; Christine Cody, Oregon Research Institute; Alaatin Erkanli, Duke University Medical Center; Erika Hinds, University of Oregon; Armando Pina, Arizona State University; and Joan Twohey-Jacobs, University of La Verne. We also thank Casey Family Programs for their travel support.

This report has been reviewed in draft form by individuals chosen for their diverse perspectives and technical expertise, in accordance with procedures approved by the Report Review Committee of the NRC. The purpose of this independent review is to provide candid and critical comments that will assist the institution in making its published report as sound as possible and to ensure that the report meets institutional standards for objectivity, evidence, and responsiveness to the study charge. The review comments and draft manuscript remain confidential to protect the integrity of the deliberative process.

We thank the following individuals for their review of this report: Sherry Glied, Mailman School of Public Health, Columbia University; Larry A. Green, University of Colorado Health Science Center, Denver, CO; Mark T. Greenberg, Prevention Research Center, Pennsylvania State University; Deborah Gross, Department of Psychiatry and Behavioral Sciences, Johns Hopkins University, School of Nursing and School of Medicine; Peter S. Jensen, President's Office, The REACH Institute (REsource for Advancing Children's Health), New York; Sheppard G. Kellam, Center for Integrating Education and Prevention Research in Schools, American Institutes for Research; Bruce G. Link, Mailman School of Public Health, Columbia University; Patricia J. Mrazek, independent consultant; Estelle B. Richman, Secretary's Office, Pennsylvania Department of Public Welfare; and Huda Y. Zoghbi, Departments of Pediatrics, Molecular and Human Genetics, Neurology, and Neuroscience, Baylor College of Medicine.

Although the reviewers listed above have provided many constructive comments and suggestions, they were not asked to endorse the conclusions or recommendations nor did they see the final draft of the report before its release. The review of this report was overseen by Floyd E. Bloom, Professor Emeritus, Department of Molecular and Integrative Neuroscience, Scripps Research Institute, and Richard G. Frank, Department of Health Care Policy, Harvard University Medical School. Appointed by the NRC, they were responsible for making certain that an independent examination of this report was carried out in accordance with institutional procedures and that all review comments were carefully considered. Responsibility for the final content of this report rests entirely with the authoring committee and the institution.

The committee appreciates the support provided by members of the Board on Children, Youth, and Families, under the leadership of Bernard Guyer, and we are grateful for the leadership and support of Rosemary Chalk, director of the Board on Children, Youth, and Families.

Finally, numerous National Academies' staff played meaningful roles that contributed to the production of this report. Ann Page, with the IOM Board on Health Care Services, provided useful guidance and suggestions during the launch of the study. Bridget Kelly, who initially joined the team as a policy fellow, was convinced to stay on to assist with innumerable analytic and writing tasks that were consistently handled with the utmost competence. Along with Bridget, Margaret Hilton served as a reviewer of project abstracts, and Hope Hare helped set up an abstract database. Wendy Keenan was an asset to the team from the very first day by helping with a range of research, analysis, contracting, and logistical challenges. In addition, Matthew Von Hendy and Bill McLeod, research librarians, provided invaluable assistance with literature searches and references. Jay Labov provided a very insightful review of an earlier draft of the neuroscience chapter. A final thanks is due to Mary Ann Kasper, who managed numerous administrative details during our multiple meetings, workshops, and conference calls.

Kenneth E. Warner, *Chair*
Thomas F. Boat, *Vice Chair*
Mary Ellen O'Connell, *Study Director*
Committee on the Prevention of Mental
Disorders and Substance Abuse Among
Children, Youth, and Young Adults:
Research Advances and Promising Interventions

Contents

*Only Appendix A is printed in this volume. The other appendixes are available online. Go to http://www.nap.edu and search for *Preventing Mental, Emotional, and Behavioral Disorders Among Young People.*

Preface

This report calls on the nation—its leaders, its mental health research and service provision agencies, its schools, its primary care medical systems, its community-based organizations, its child welfare and criminal justice systems—to make prevention of mental, emotional, and behavioral disorders and the promotion of mental health of young people a very high priority. By all realistic measures, no such priority exists today. The report therefore urges action at the highest levels to ensure that public health decision makers and the public understand the nature and magnitude of this problem; that research to prevent it is carefully coordinated and well funded; and that institutions and communities have the resources and the responsibility to promote the implementation of prevention interventions that can address shortfalls in the public response.

Mental, emotional, and behavioral disorders incur high psychosocial and economic costs for the young people who experience them, for their families, and for the society in which they live, study, and will work. Yet there is a significant imbalance in the nation's efforts to address such disorders. People await their emergence and then attempt to treat them, to cure them if possible, or to limit the damage they cause if not. This happens with any number of expensive interventions, ranging from psychiatric care to incarceration. Myopically, we devote minimal attention to preventing future disorders or the environmental exposures that increase risk.

This report builds on a highly valued predecessor, the 1994 Institute of Medicine (IOM) report entitled *Reducing Risks for Mental Disorders: Frontiers for Preventive Intervention Research*. That report provided the basis for understanding prevention science, elucidating its then-existing research base, and contemplating where it should go in the future. This report documents that an increasing number of mental, emotional, and behavioral problems in young people are in fact preventable. The proverbial ounce of prevention will indeed be worth a pound of cure: effectively applying the evidence-based prevention interventions at hand could potentially save billions of dollars in associated costs by avoiding or tempering these disorders in many individuals. Furthermore, devoting significantly greater resources to research on even more effective prevention and promotion efforts, and then reliably implementing the findings of such research, could substantially diminish the human and economic toll. This could be done, but as Hadorn[1] has observed, the basic tendency is to focus on "the rule of rescue . . . the powerful human proclivity to rescue endangered life." As a society, we suffer from a collective health care myopia: we have not yet figured out how to balance rescue—which is after-the-fact treatment—with the less dramatic but often far more cost-effective and socially desirable prevention of the onset of a problem.

The very definition of prevention is itself a problem. The authors of the 1994 IOM report emphasized the need for clear definitions to guide the field. The authors proposed a new typology of prevention: *universal interventions*, which address the population at large, *selective interventions*, which target groups or individuals with an elevated risk, and *indicated interventions*, which target individuals with early symptoms or behaviors that are precursors for disorder but are not yet diagnosable. In essence, this typology of prevention was proposed as a set of interventions to target individuals and populations that do not currently have a disorder, with variations in exactly who is targeted. Yet ardent proponents of prevention, including members of the 1994 IOM committee, do not wish to exclude the prevention of disease relapse or disability from their conception of prevention.

While acknowledging the legitimacy of this perspective, our committee thinks that the disproportionate emphasis on treatment of existing conditions needs to be corrected. We propose a new emphasis on true prevention, which for the purposes of this report we define as occurring prior to the onset of disorder, as well as mental health promotion, discussed immediately below. We do not disparage society's emphasis on treatment and indeed think that in the domain of mental health, far more resources should be devoted to the effort. Rather, we want to highlight the critical need for a more proactive, preventive focus on mental health.

The primary charge for this committee is prevention, but we add to our focus the emerging field of mental health promotion, an important

---

[1]Hadorn, D.C. (1991, May 1). Setting health care priorities in Oregon: Cost-effectiveness meets the rule of rescue. *Journal of the American Medical Association, 265*(17), 2218-2225.

and largely ignored approach toward building healthy development in all young people. Prevention emphasizes the avoidance of risk factors; promotion strives to promote supportive family, school, and community environments and to identify and imbue in young people protective factors, which are traits that enhance well-being and provide the tools to avoid adverse emotions and behaviors. While research on promotion is limited, emerging interest and involvement in it and the potential it holds for enhancing health warrant its inclusion in the consideration of how the nation can improve its collective well-being.

The committee's focus on young people and the stigma associated with the term "mental disorder" led us to adopt the term "mental, emotional, and behavioral disorders" to encompass both disorders diagnosable using *Diagnostic and Statistical Manual of Mental Disorders, 4th Edition* (DSM-IV) criteria and the problem behaviors associated with them, such as violence, aggression, and antisocial behavior. Many mental, emotional, and behavioral disorders of youth exist on a continuum and exert significant costs on the young people themselves, the people affected by them, and society at large. The term "mental, emotional, and behavioral disorders" encompasses mental illness and substance abuse, while including a somewhat broader range of concerns associated with problem behaviors and conditions in youth.

One factor lurks in the background of every discussion of the risks for mental, emotional, and behavioral disorders and antisocial behavior: poverty. Poverty in the United States often entails a range of material hardships, such as overcrowding, frequent moves (which often mean changes of school), poor schools, limited health care, unsafe and stressful environments, and sometimes lack of adequate food. All of these imperil cognitive, emotional, and behavioral development. Although not the focus of this report, there is evidence that changes in social policy that reduce exposure to these risks are at least as important for preventing mental, emotional, and behavioral disorders in young people as other preventive interventions. We are persuaded that the future mental health of the nation depends crucially on how, collectively, the costly legacy of poverty is dealt with.

As chairs of the committee that has produced this report, we have benefited immensely from the commitment, energy, and effort of two groups of people. We are grateful to the committee members, who demonstrated devotion to the subject of this report and to the arduous task of developing it. All committee members contributed to the writing of the report, and the "think tank" nature of our innumerable meetings, conference calls, and e-mail exchanges played enormously important roles in shaping both the structure and content of the report. We are deeply indebted, as well, to the National Academies' staff, who performed at a consistently high level all of the myriad tasks that are essential to compiling a large and complex report such as this one. One staff member is particularly deserving of mention: Mary Ellen O'Connell, the study director, is the consummate Jill of all trades. From the inception of the study to the crossing of the final *t*, she directed all aspects of the committee's work with insight and across-the-board competence. We admire her incredible work ethic and express our jealousy at her apparent ability to work without sleep.

> Kenneth E. Warner, *Chair*
> Thomas F. Boat, *Vice Chair*
> Committee on the Prevention of Mental
> Disorders and Substance Abuse Among
> Children, Youth, and Young Adults:
> Research Advances and Promising Interventions

Acronyms

ABCD	Assuring Better Child Health and Development
ABFM	American Board of Family Medicine
ACF	Administration for Children and Families of the U.S. Department of Health and Human Services
ACGME	Accreditation Council for Graduate Medical Education
ADAMHA	Alcohol, Drug Abuse, and Mental Health Administration, the predecessor to the Substance Abuse and Mental Health Services Administration
ADHD	attention deficit hyperactivity disorder
AHRQ	Agency for Healthcare Research and Quality of the U.S. Department of Health and Human Services
AILS	American Indian Life Skills Program
AIM	awareness, intervention, and methodology
AMERSA	Association for Medical Education and Research in Substance Abuse
ASPE	Office of the Assistant Secretary for Planning and Evaluation of the U.S. Department of Health and Human Services
ATP	Adolescent Transitions Program
AUD	alcohol use disorder
CAPT	Regional Centers for the Application of Prevention Technologies of the Substance Abuse and Mental Health Services Administration
CBA	cost-benefit analysis
CBPR	community-based participatory research

CBT	cognitive-behavioral therapy
CD	conduct disorder
CDC	Centers for Disease Control and Prevention of the U.S. Department of Health and Human Services
CDISC	Computerized Diagnostic Interview Schedule for Children
CEA	cost-effectiveness analysis
CHAMP	Chicago HIV Adolescent Mental Health Program, renamed the Collaborative HIV Adolescent Mental Health Program when expanded beyond Chicago
CHAMP-SA	Collaborative HIV Adolescent Mental Health Program, South Africa
CMHS	Center for Mental Health Services of the Substance Abuse and Mental Health Services Administration
CMS	Centers for Medicare and Medicaid Services of the U.S. Department of Health and Human Services
CPC	Child-Parent Centers
CRISP	Computer Retrieval of Information on Scientific Projects of the National Institutes of Health
CSAP	Center for Substance Abuse Prevention of the Substance Abuse and Mental Health Services Administration
CTC	Communities That Care
DALY	disability-adjusted life year
DBD	disruptive behavior disorders
DHA	docosahexaenoic acid
DSM-IV	*Diagnostic and Statistical Manual of Mental Disorders*, 4th Edition
ED	U.S. Department of Education
EIFC	Early Intervention Foster Care
EPA	eicosapentaenoic acid
EPSDT	Early and Periodic Screening, Diagnostic, and Treatment
ESOL	English for Speakers of Other Languages
FY	fiscal year
GBG	Good Behavior Game
GSMS	Great Smoky Mountains Study
HFA	Healthy Families America
HFNY	Healthy Families New York
HHS	U.S. Department of Health and Human Services

HRSA   Health Resources and Services Administration of the U.S.
            Department of Health and Human Services

ICD-9   *International Statistical Classification of Diseases and
            Related Health Problems,* 9th Edition
IDEA   Individuals with Disabilities Education Act
IES   Institute of Education Sciences of the U.S. Department of
            Education
IOM   Institute of Medicine

LIFT   Linking Interests of Families and Teachers project
LST   Life Skills Training Program

MCHB   Maternal and Child Health Bureau of the U.S. Department of
            Health and Human Services
MDE   major depressive episode
MEB   mental, emotional, and behavioral
MI   motivational interviewing
MPP   Midwestern Prevention Program
MTF   Monitoring the Future
MTFC   multidimensional treatment foster care

NAMHC   National Advisory Mental Health Council
NASHP   National Academy of State Health Policy
NBP   New Beginnings Program
NCAST   Nursing Child Assessment Satellite Training
NCLB   No Child Left Behind Act of 2001
NCS   National Comorbidity Survey
NCS-R   National Comorbidity Survey-Replication
NECON   New England Coalition for Health Promotion and Disease
            Prevention
NFP   Nurse-Family Partnership
NHANES   National Health and Nutrition Examination Survey
NHIS   National Health Interview Survey
NIAAA   National Institute on Alcohol Abuse and Alcoholism
NICHD   National Institute of Child Health and Human Development
NIDA   National Institute on Drug Abuse
NIH   National Institutes of Health of the U.S. Department of
            Health and Human Services
NIJ   National Institute of Justice of the U.S. Department of Justice
NIMH   National Institute of Mental Health
NRC   National Research Council

NREPP   National Registry of Evidence-Based Programs and Practices
             of the Substance Abuse and Mental Health Services
             Administration
NSDUH   National Survey on Drug Use and Health

ODD   oppositional defiant disorder
OJJDP   Office of Juvenile Justice and Delinquency Prevention of the
             U.S. Department of Justice

PALS   Positive Attitudes Toward Learning in Schools
PATHS   Promoting Alternative Thinking Strategies
POP   Penn Optimism Program
PPN   Promising Practices Network
PPP   Penn Prevention Program
PROSPER   PROmoting School-community-university Partnerships to
             Enhance Resilience
PRP   Penn Resiliency Program
PSMG   Prevention Science and Methodology Group
PTC   Parenting Through Change
PTSD   posttraumatic stress disorder
PUP   Prohibition of Youth Possession, Use, or Purchase of Tobacco

QALY   quality-adjusted life year

SAMHSA   Substance Abuse and Mental Health Services Administration
             of the U.S. Department of Health and Human Services
SBD   sleep-related breathing disorder
SCHIP   State Children's Health Insurance Program
SDB   sleep-disordered breathing
SDFS   Safe and Drug-Free Schools Program of the U.S. Department
             of Education
SEL   social and emotional learning
SFP   Strengthening Families Program
SPR   Society for Prevention Research
SSDP   Seattle Social Development Program
SS/HS   Safe Schools Healthy Students Program of the U.S.
             Departments of Health and Human Services, Education,
             and Justice

TANF   Temporary Assistance for Needy Families
TLFB   Timeline Follow Back Interview
TPRCs   Transdisciplinary Prevention Research Centers of the
             National Institute on Drug Abuse

Triple P   Positive Parenting Program

USPHS   U.S. Public Health Service

WHO   World Health Organization
WIC   Special Supplemental Nutrition Program for Women, Infants,
             and Children
WISC-R   Wechsler Intelligence Scale for Children, Revised

YRBSS   Youth Risk Behavior Surveillance System

Glossary

Adaptation: The modification of evidence-based interventions that have been developed for a single ethnic, linguistic, and/or cultural group for use with other groups.

Adoption: The selection and incorporation of a prevention program into a service system.

Alcohol abuse: The consumption of alcohol despite negative consequences.

Alcohol dependence: The persistent consumption of alcohol despite negative consequences, often with a physiological dependence characterized by tolerance and/or symptoms of withdrawal.

Alcohol use disorder: An inclusive term referring to either alcohol abuse or alcohol dependence.

Comorbidity: The presence of one or more disorders in addition to a primary disorder.

Confound: A variable in an experiment or trial that may be related to observed effects and therefore may limit the ability to make inferences about causal effects of the experimental variables.

Cost-benefit analysis: A method of economic analysis in which costs and outcomes of an intervention are both valued in monetary units, permitting a direct comparison of the benefits produced by the intervention with its costs.

Cost-effectiveness analysis: A method of economic analysis in which outcomes of an intervention are measured in nonmonetary terms. The outcomes and costs are compared with both the costs and the same outcome measure for competing interventions or an established standard to determine if the outcomes are achieved at a reasonable monetary cost.

Cross-sectional study: A study to estimate the relationship between an outcome of interest and specified variables by comparing groups that differ on those variables at a single point in time.

Developmental competence: The ability to accomplish a broad range of appropriate social, emotional, cognitive, and behavioral tasks at various developmental stages, including adaptations to the demands of different social and cultural contexts and attaining a positive sense of identity, efficacy, and well-being.

Developmental competencies: Social, emotional, cognitive, and behavioral tasks that are appropriate at various developmental stages and in various social and cultural contexts.

Developmental neuroscience: The study of the anatomical and functional development of the nervous system in humans and animal models. This encompasses the fields of molecular and behavioral genetics, molecular and cellular neurobiology, biochemistry, physiology, pharmacology, pathology, and systems-level neuroscience and applies methods ranging from molecular biology to imaging to functional studies of cognition and behavior.

Dissemination: The distribution of program information with the aim of encouraging program adoption in real-world service systems or communities.

Dissemination trial: A trial designed to experimentally test approaches and strategies to influence providers, communities, or organizations to adopt evidence-based prevention programs in real-world service settings.

DSM-IV: The current edition of the *Diagnostic and Statistical Manual of Mental Disorders*, a handbook published by the American Psychiatric Association describing different categories of mental disorders and the criteria for diagnosing them.

Effect size: A statistical measure of the strength of the relationship between two variables.

Effectiveness: The impact of a program under conditions that are likely to occur in a real-world implementation.

Effectiveness trial: A trial designed to test whether an intervention can achieve effects when delivered by a natural service delivery system (i.e., similar to the institutions or communities that are ultimately intended to implement the intervention). The emphasis is on demonstrating positive outcomes in a real-world setting using nonresearch staff to deliver the intervention.

Efficacy: The impact of a program under ideal research conditions.

Efficacy trial: A trial designed to test whether a new or significantly modified intervention has effects when it is delivered in a research environment by research staff under optimal conditions. Efficacy trials can take place in research or real-world settings but are typically delivered by trained research staff under the direction and control of the research team, using resources beyond what might be available in the natural course of service delivery. A trial is also considered an efficacy trial if an intervention is being tested by research staff with a new population or in an amended form.

Encouragement designs: Trial designs that randomize individuals to different modalities of recruitment, incentives, or persuasion messages to influence their choice to participate in one or another intervention condition.

Epidemiology: The study of factors that influence the health and illness of populations.

Epigenetics: Alterations in gene expression through mechanisms other than modifications in the genetic sequence.

Etiology: The cause of a disease or condition.

Externalizing: Problems or disorders that are primarily behavioral (e.g., conduct disorder, oppositional defiant disorder).

Fidelity: The degree to which an intervention is delivered as designed.

Genotype: An individual's genetic makeup.

Iatrogenic effect: An adverse effect caused by an intervention.

ICD-9: The current *International Statistical Classification of Diseases and Related Health Problems*, a classification system published by the World Health Organization and used to code disease as well as signs, symptoms, abnormal findings, complaints, social circumstances, and external causes of injury or disease.

Implementation: The process of introducing and using interventions in real-world service settings, including how interventions or programs are adopted, sustained, and taken to scale.

Implementation trial: A trial designed to experimentally test approaches and strategies for successful utilization of evidence-based prevention programs in real-world service settings.

Incidence: The number, proportion, or rate of occurrence of new cases of a disorder in a population within a specified period of time.

Indicated prevention: Preventive interventions that are targeted to high-risk individuals who are identified as having minimal but detectable signs or symptoms that foreshadow mental, emotional, or behavioral disorder, as well as biological markers that indicate a predisposition in a person for such a disorder but who does not meet diagnostic criteria at the time of the intervention.

Internalizing: Problems or disorders that are primarily emotional (e.g., anxiety, depression).

Longitudinal study: A study that involves repeated observations of targeted outcomes over a long period of time.

Main effect: The effect of an independent variable averaged over all levels of other variables in an experiment.

Mediator: A variable factor that explains how an effect occurs (i.e., the causal pathway between an intervention and an outcome).

Mental, emotional, and behavioral disorders: A diagnosable mental or substance use disorder.

Mental, emotional, and behavioral problems: Difficulties that may be early signs or symptoms of mental disorders but are not frequent or severe enough to meet the criteria for a diagnosis.

Mental health promotion: Interventions that aim to enhance the ability to achieve developmentally appropriate tasks (developmental competencies) and a positive sense of self-esteem, mastery, well-being, and social inclusion and to strengthen the ability to cope with adversity.

Mental illness: A condition that meets DSM-IV diagnostic criteria.

Meta-analysis: A statistical analysis that combines the results of several studies that address the same research question.

Moderator: A variable factor that influences how an intervention or mediator exerts its effect.

Natural experimental design: A naturally occurring opportunity to observe the effects of defined variables that approximates the properties of a controlled experiment.

Neural systems: Functionally integrated circuits in the nervous system that operate in the context of genetic and environmental influences to produce complex behaviors.

Nonexperimental studies: Observational research designs that do not include an experimental manipulation of variables by the researchers.

Odds ratio: The ratio of the odds of an outcome occurring in an experimental group to the odds of it occurring in a control group, a measure of the size of the effect of an intervention.

Pathogenesis: The mechanisms by which etiological factors cause a disease or disorder.

Pathophysiology: The disturbance of normal functions that are the result of a disease or disorder.

Phenotype: An individual's observed physical or behavioral characteristics.

Polymorphism: A variation in genetic sequence.

Premorbid: A sign or symptom that occurs before the development of disease.

Pre-post studies: Nonrandomized studies that evaluate an intervention on the basis of the changes that occur in the same subject from a baseline (the "pre" measurement) to after the intervention period (the "post" measurement).

Prevalence: The total number of cases of a disorder in a population.

Prevention: Interventions that occur prior to the onset of a disorder that are intended to prevent or reduce risk for the disorder.

Prevention research: The study of theory and practice related to the prevention of social, physical, and mental health problems, including etiology, methodology, epidemiology, and intervention.

Prevention science: A multidisciplinary field devoted to the scientific study of the theory, research, and practice related to the prevention of social, physical, and mental health problems, including etiology, epidemiology, and intervention.

Preventionist: A practitioner who delivers prevention interventions.

Problem behaviors: Behaviors with negative effects that are often signs or symptoms of mental, emotional, or behavioral disorders that may not be frequent or severe enough to meet the criteria for a diagnosis (e.g., aggressiveness, early alcohol use) but have substantial personal, family, and societal costs.

Prodrome: An early, nonspecific set of symptoms that indicate the onset of disease before specific, diagnosable symptoms occur.

Protective factor: A characteristic at the biological, psychological, family, or community (including peers and culture) level that is associated with a lower likelihood of problem outcomes or that reduces the negative impact of a risk factor on problem outcomes.

Psychiatric disorder: A condition that meets DSM-IV diagnostic criteria.

Psychopathology: Behaviors and experiences that are indicative of mental, emotional, or behavioral disorder or impairment.

Qualitative data: Research information that is descriptive but not measured or quantified for statistical analysis.

Qualitative review: A review of research evidence relevant to a research question that does not include new statistical analysis.

Quantitative data: Research information that is measured for statistical analysis.

Quasi-experimental studies: Experimental designs in which subjects are not randomly assigned to experimental and control groups.

Randomized studies: Experimental designs that randomly assign subjects (individuals, families, classrooms, schools, communities) into equivalent groups that are exposed to different interventions in order to compare outcomes with the goal of inferring causal effects.

Replication: The reproduction of a trial or experiment by an independent researcher.

Research funders: For purposes of this report, federal agencies and foundations that fund research on mental health promotion or prevention of mental, emotional, or behavioral disorders.

Resilience: The ability to recover from or adapt to adverse events, life changes, and life stressors.

Retrospective study: A study that looks back at the histories of a group that currently has a disorder or characteristic in comparison to a similar group without that disorder or characteristic to determine what factors may be associated with the disorder or characteristic.

Risk factor: A characteristic at the biological, psychological, family, community, or cultural level that precedes and is associated with a higher likelihood of problem outcomes.

Selective prevention: Preventive interventions that are targeted to individuals or to a subgroup of the population whose risk of developing mental, emotional, or behavioral disorders is significantly higher than average. The risk may be imminent or it may be a lifetime risk. Risk groups may be identified on the basis of biological, psychological, or social risk factors that are known to be associated with the onset of a disorder. Those risk factors may be at the individual level for nonbehavioral characteristics (e.g., biological characteristics such as low birth weight), at the family level (e.g., children with a family history of substance abuse but who do not have any history of use), or at the community/population level (e.g., schools or neighborhoods in high-poverty areas).

Substance abuse: The use of alcohol or drugs despite negative consequences.

Substance dependence: The persistent use of alcohol or drugs despite negative consequences, often with a physiological dependence characterized by tolerance and/or symptoms of withdrawal.

Substance use disorder: An inclusive term referring to either substance abuse or substance dependence.

Systematic review: A literature review that tries to identify, appraise, select, and synthesize all high-quality research evidence relevant to a research question.

Taxonomy: A system of names and classifications.

Translational research (type 1): The transfer of basic science discoveries into clinical research as well as the influence of clinical research findings on basic science research questions.

Translational research (type 2): The study of the real-world effectiveness and implementation of programs for which efficacy has been previously demonstrated.

Treatment: Interventions targeted to individuals who are identified as currently suffering from a diagnosable disorder that are intended to cure the disorder or reduce the symptoms or effects of the disorder, including the prevention of disability, relapse, and/or comorbidity.

Universal prevention: Preventive interventions that are targeted to the general public or a whole population group that has not been identified on the basis of individual risk. The intervention is desirable for everyone in that group.

Wait-list designs: Research designs that provide the new intervention first to the experimental group and later to those who were initially assigned to the control group.

Young people: For purposes of this report, children, youth, and young adults (to age 25).

Summary

Several decades of research have shown that the promise and potential lifetime benefits of preventing mental, emotional, and behavioral (MEB) disorders are greatest by focusing on young people and that early interventions can be effective in delaying or preventing the onset of such disorders. National priorities that build on this evidence base should include (1) assurance that individuals who are at risk receive the best available evidence-based interventions prior to the onset of a disorder and (2) the promotion of positive MEB development for all children, youth, and young adults.

A number of promotion and prevention programs are now available that should be considered for broad implementation. Although individuals who are already affected by a MEB disorder should receive the best evidence-based treatment available, interventions before the disorder occurs offer the greatest opportunity to avoid the substantial costs to individuals, families, and society that these disorders entail.

Most MEB disorders have their roots in childhood and youth. Among adults reporting a MEB disorder during their lifetime, more than half report the onset as occurring in childhood or adolescence. In any given year, the percentage of young people with these disorders is estimated to be between 14 and 20 percent. MEB issues among young people—including both diagnosable disorders and other problem behaviors, such as early drug or alcohol use, antisocial or aggressive behavior, and violence—have enormous personal, family, and societal costs. The annual quantifiable cost of such disorders among young people was estimated in 2007 to be $247 billion. In addition, MEB disorders among young people interfere with their abil-

1

ity to accomplish normal developmental tasks, such as establishing healthy interpersonal relationships, succeeding in school, and transitioning to the workforce. These disorders also affect the lives of their family members.

A 1994 report by the Institute of Medicine (IOM), *Reducing Risks for Mental Disorders: Frontiers for Preventive Intervention Research,* highlighted the promise of prevention. In response to a subsequently burgeoning research base and an increasing understanding of the developmental pathways that lead to MEB problems, the Substance Abuse and Mental Health Services Administration, the National Institute of Mental Health, the National Institute on Drug Abuse, and the National Institute on Alcohol Abuse and Alcoholism requested a study from the National Academies to review the research base and program experience since that time, focusing on young people. The Committee on the Prevention of Mental Disorders and Substance Abuse Among Children, Youth, and Young Adults was formed under the auspices of the Board on Children, Youth, and Families to conduct this review (see Box S-1 for the complete charge).

The 1994 IOM report reaffirmed a clear distinction between prevention and treatment. The current committee supports this distinction. The prevention of disability, relapse, or comorbidity among those with currently existing disorders are characteristics and expectations of good treatment. Although treatment has preventive aspects, it is still treatment, not prevention. The strength of prevention research using this concept of prevention, coupled with the need for focused research on risks prior to the onset of illness, warrants the field's continued use of a typology focused on interventions for those who do not have an existing disorder. Interventions classified as *universal* (population-based), *selective* (directed to at-risk groups or individuals), or *indicated* (targeting individuals with biological markers, early symptoms, or problematic behaviors predicting a high level of risk) are important complementary elements of prevention. Going beyond the 1994 IOM report, we strongly recommend the inclusion of mental health promotion in the spectrum of mental health interventions.

The volume and quality of research since 1994 have increased dramatically. Clear evidence is available to identify many factors that place certain young people or groups of young people at greater risk for developing MEB disorders, as well as other factors that serve a protective role. Box S-2 summarizes key advances since 1994.

A number of specific preventive interventions can modify risk and promote protective factors that are linked to important determinants of mental, emotional, and behavioral health, especially in such areas as family functioning, early childhood experiences, and social skills. Interventions are also available to reduce the incidence of common disorders or problem behaviors, such as depression, substance use, and conduct disorder. Some interventions reduce multiple disorders and problem behaviors as well as

---

BOX S-1
Committee Charge

- Review promising areas of research that contribute to the prevention of mental disorders, substance abuse, and problem behaviors among children, youth, and young adults (to age 25), focusing in particular on genetics, neurobiology, and psychosocial research as well as the field of prevention science.
- Highlight areas of key advances and persistent challenges since the publication of the 1994 IOM report *Reducing Risks for Mental Disorders: Frontiers for Preventive Intervention Research.*
- Examine the research base within a developmental framework throughout the life span, with an emphasis on prevention and promotion opportunities that can improve the mental health and behavior of children, youth, and young adults.
- Review the current scope of federal efforts in the prevention of mental disorders and substance abuse and the promotion of mental health among at-risk populations, including children of parents with substance abuse or mental health disorders, abused and neglected children, children in foster care, children whose parents are absent or incarcerated, and children exposed to violence and other trauma, spanning the continuum from research to policy and services.
- Recommend areas of emphasis for future federal policies and programs of research support that would strengthen a developmental approach to a prevention research agenda as well as opportunities to foster public- and private-sector collaboration in prevention and promotion efforts for children, youth, and young adults, particularly in educational, child welfare, and primary care settings.
- Prepare a final report that will provide a state-of-the-art review of prevention research.

---

increase healthy functioning. While the evidence on the costs and benefits of interventions is limited, it suggests that many are likely to have benefits that exceed costs.

In addition, a number of interventions have demonstrated efficacy to reduce risk for children exposed to serious adversities, such as maternal depression and family disruption. Like family adversities, poverty is a powerful risk factor, and its reduction would have far-reaching effects for multiple negative mental, emotional, and behavioral outcomes. Numerous policies and programs target poverty as a risk factor by giving priority to low-income children and their families and by promoting resources for healthy functioning of those living in poverty through, for example, early childhood education programs, programs to strengthen families and schools, and efforts to reduce neighborhood violence.

The 1994 IOM report expressed hope that identification of the genetic

---

BOX S-2
Key Areas of Progress Since 1994

- Evidence that MEB disorders are common and begin early in life.
- Evidence that the greatest prevention opportunity is among young people.
- Evidence of multiyear effects of multiple preventive interventions on reducing substance abuse, conduct disorder, antisocial behavior, aggression, and child maltreatment.
- Evidence that the incidence of depression among pregnant women and adolescents can be reduced.
- Evidence that school-based violence prevention can reduce the base rate of aggressive problems in an average school by one-quarter to one-third.
- Promising evidence regarding potential indicated preventive interventions targeting schizophrenia.
- Evidence that improving family functioning and positive parenting serves as a mediator of positive outcomes and can moderate poverty-related risk.
- Emerging evidence that school-based preventive interventions aimed at improving social and emotional outcomes can also improve academic outcomes.
- Evidence that interventions that target families dealing with such adversities as parental depression and divorce demonstrate efficacy in reducing risk for depression among children and increasing effective parenting.
- Evidence from some preventive interventions that benefits exceed costs, with the available evidence strongest for early childhood interventions.
- Evidence of interactions between modifiable environmental factors and the expression of genes linked to behavior.
- Greater understanding of the biological processes that underlie both normal brain function and the pathophysiology of MEB disorders.
- Emerging opportunities for the integration of genetics and neuroscience research with prevention research.
- Advances in implementation science, including recognition of implementation complexity and the importance of relevance to the community.

---

determinants of mental illnesses was on the horizon. It is now recognized that most disorders are not caused by a small number of genes and that this area of research is highly complex. An emerging area of research involves the influence of the environment on the expression of a specific gene or set of genes, the importance of epigenetic modification of gene expression by experience, and direct injury to neural systems that give rise to illness. This exciting new knowledge has the potential to inform future preventive interventions.

The future of prevention requires combined efforts to (1) apply existing knowledge in ways that are meaningful to families and communities and (2) pursue a rigorous research agenda that is aimed at improving both the quality and implementation of interventions across diverse communities.

PUTTING KNOWLEDGE INTO PRACTICE

No concerted federal presence or clear national leadership currently exists to advance the use of prevention and promotion approaches to benefit the mental health of the nation's young people. Infusing a prevention focus into the public consciousness requires development of a shared public vision and attention at a higher national level than currently exists.

> **Recommendation:** The federal government should make the healthy mental, emotional, and behavioral development of young people a national priority, establish public goals for the prevention of specific MEB disorders and for the promotion of healthy development among young people, and provide needed research and service resources to achieve these aims. (13-1)

Mental, emotional, and behavioral disorders among young people burden not only traditional mental health and substance abuse programs, but also multiple other service systems that support young people and their families—most notably the education, child welfare, primary medical care, and juvenile justice systems. According to one estimate, more than a quarter of total service costs for children who have these disorders are incurred in the school and juvenile justice systems. Similarly, a quarter of pediatric primary care visits address behavioral issues. The cost savings of prevention programs likewise are experienced in a range of service systems. A national-level response therefore requires the creation of a designated entity with the authority to establish common prevention goals, to direct relevant federal resources, and to influence the investment of state, local, or private resources toward these goals as well as coordination and leadership across and within multiple federal agencies.

> **Recommendation:** The White House should create an ongoing mechanism involving federal agencies, stakeholders (including professional associations), and key researchers to develop and implement a strategic approach to the promotion of mental, emotional, and behavioral health and the prevention of MEB disorders and related problem behaviors in young people. The U.S. Departments of Health and Human Services, Education, and Justice should be accountable for coordinating and aligning their resources, programs, and initiatives with this strategic approach and for encouraging their state and local counterparts to do the same. (13-2)

Federal resources should support the continued evaluation and refinement of programs to increase understanding of what works for whom and when. The braiding of programmatic funding from service agencies, such as the Substance Abuse and Mental Health Services Administration, with evaluation funding from research agencies, such as the National Institute of Mental Health, would advance these efforts. Establishment of an ongoing national monitoring system that is capable of regular reporting on the incidence and prevalence of specific disorders, as well as the rates of exposure to key risk and protective factors, is needed to assess performance compared with national goals.

Determining what is "evidence-based" is an important component of ensuring that these efforts have a positive impact on the lives of young people. Priority should be given to programs that have been tested and replicated in real-world environments, that have reasonable cost, and that are supported by tools that will help to implement key elements of the programs with fidelity. Federal and state agencies should not endorse programs that lack empirical evidence solely on the basis of general community endorsement. In turn, states and communities need to consider the relevance of available models to their own needs, priorities, and cultural contexts. They should evaluate programs and systems that they adopt, so as to continue to build the prevention knowledge base. Programs should also engage in and document the results of quality improvement efforts to continuously enhance program outcomes.

> **Recommendation:** States and communities should develop networked systems to apply resources to the promotion of mental health and prevention of MEB disorders among their young people. These systems should involve individuals, families, schools, justice systems, health care systems, and relevant community-based programs. Such approaches should build on available evidence-based programs and involve local evaluators to assess the implementation process of individual programs or policies and to measure community-wide outcomes. (13-3)

Concurrently, concerted attention should be paid to developing a workforce that has the knowledge base and skill sets necessary to research, implement, and disseminate relevant interventions in diverse community contexts and cultures. Training and certification programs for the next generation of professionals working with young people should include the latest knowledge of the early trajectories of disorders and of prevention approaches in a life-course framework. Box S-3 provides a list of other specific recommendations relevant to putting knowledge into practice.

BOX S-3
Recommendations: Putting Knowledge into Practice

Funding and Implementation

- Congress should establish a set-aside for prevention services and innovation in the Community Mental Health Services Block Grant, similar to the set-aside in the Substance Abuse Prevention and Treatment Block Grant. (12-1)
- The U.S. Departments of Health and Human Services, Education, and Justice should braid funding of research and practice so that the impact of programs and practices that are being funded by service agencies (e.g., the Substance Abuse and Mental Health Services Administration, the Office of Safe and Drug Free Schools, the Office of Juvenile Justice and Delinquency Prevention) are experimentally evaluated through research funded by other agencies (e.g., the National Institutes of Health, the Institute of Education Sciences, the National Institute of Justice). This should include developing appropriate infrastructure through which evidence-based programs and practices can be delivered and evaluated. (12-2)
- The U.S. Departments of Health and Human Services, Education, and Justice should fund states, counties, and local communities to implement and continuously improve evidence-based approaches to mental health promotion and prevention of MEB disorders in systems of care that work with young people and their families. (12-3)
- The U.S. Departments of Health and Human Services, Education, and Justice should develop strategies to identify communities with significant community-level risk factors and target resources to these communities. (8-2)
- Researchers and community organizations should form partnerships to develop evaluations of (1) adaptation of existing interventions in response to community-specific cultural characteristics; (2) preventive interventions designed based on research principles in response to community concerns; and (3) preventive interventions that have been developed in the community, have demonstrated feasibility of implementation and acceptability in that community, but lack experimental evidence of effectiveness. (11-4)
  (Also in Box S-5, Recommendations for Researchers)
- Federal and state agencies should prioritize the use of evidence-based programs and promote the rigorous evaluation of prevention and promotion programs in a variety of settings in order to increase the knowledge base of what works, for whom, and under what conditions. The definition of evidence-based should be determined by applying established scientific criteria. (12-4)

Data Collection and Monitoring

- The U.S. Department of Health and Human Services should be required to provide (1) annual data on the prevalence of MEB disorders in young people, using an accepted current taxonomy (e.g., the *Diagnostic and Statistical Manual of Mental Disorders*, the *International Statistical Classification of Diseases*) and (2) data that can provide indicators and trends for key risk and protective factors that serve as significant predictors for MEB disorders. (2-1)

continued

BOX S-3 Continued

- The Substance Abuse and Mental Health Services Administration should expand its current data collection to include measures of service use across multiple agencies that work with vulnerable populations of young people. (2-2)

Workforce Development
- Training programs for relevant health (including mental health), education, and social work professionals should include prevention of MEB disorders and promotion of mental, emotional, and behavioral health. National certifying and accrediting bodies for training should set relevant standards using available evidence on identifying and managing risks and preclinical symptoms of MEB disorders. (12-6)
- The U.S. Departments of Health and Human Services, Education, and Justice should convene a national conference on training in prevention and promotion to (1) set guidelines for model prevention research and practice training programs and (2) contribute to the development of training standards for certifying trainees and accrediting prevention training programs in specific disciplines, such as health (including mental health), education, and social work. (12-7)
- Once guidelines have been developed, the U.S. Departments of Health and Human Services, Education, and Justice should set aside funds for competitive prevention training grants to support development and dissemination of model interdisciplinary training programs. Training should span creation, implementation, and evaluation of effective preventive interventions. (12-8)

NOTE: The first number refers to the chapter in which the recommendation appears; the second number references its order of appearance in the chapter.

CONTINUING A COURSE OF RIGOROUS RESEARCH

The National Institutes of Health (NIH) fund research related to the prevention of MEB disorders through multiple centers and institutes. A significant body of research now points to common trajectories across multiple disorders and highlights the potential for interventions to affect multiple disorders. However, no definition of prevention is shared across agencies, no NIH-wide planning or accounting of prevention spending exists, and there are no common research priorities. In addition, most NIH research centers address single disorders. The ability of prevention research to approach issues from a comprehensive developmental perspective would be aided by cross-institute dialogue and by coordinated funding for interventions that address co-occurring outcomes, common risk and protective factors, and shared developmental pathways.

Recommendation: The National Institutes of Health, with input from other funders of prevention research, should develop a comprehensive 10-year research plan targeting the promotion of mental health and prevention of both single and comorbid MEB disorders. This plan should consider current needs, opportunities for cross-disciplinary and multi-institute research, support for the necessary research infrastructure, and establishment of a mechanism for assessing and reporting progress against 10-year goals. (13-5)

Continued investment in research can lead to interventions that will mitigate risks and strengthen protective factors prior to the onset of disorders and that will help to set young people on an appropriate developmental course. Substantial evidence has shown that the incidence of many disorders and problem behaviors can be reduced significantly, thereby justifying the need for dedicated efforts to refine these approaches.

Recommendation: Research funders[1] should establish parity between research on preventive interventions and treatment interventions. (13-4)

The report makes a number of specific recommendations aimed at identifying areas of focus for future research in a 10-year plan that will inform future federal, state, and local initiatives (see Box S-4). The following focus areas should serve as the research priorities for both federal agencies and foundations, and they should stimulate prevention partnerships:

- **Approaches to screening in conjunction with intervention.** Screening can take place at multiple levels, including the level of the population to identify communities at risk (e.g., high-poverty neighborhoods), the level of groups to identify those at risk (e.g., children with depressed parents), and the level of individuals to identify those who have either behavioral symptoms or biological markers indicating the likelihood of developing a disorder (e.g., young children who exhibit highly aggressive behavior). However, screening without community acceptance and sufficient service capacity to respond to identified needs is of limited value. Models are needed that partner screening with implementation of evidence-based interventions.
- **Implementation.** Implementation has only recently been identified as an area of research in its own right. The effectiveness of state

---

[1]The term "research funders" is used throughout the recommendations to refer to federal agencies and foundations that fund research on mental health promotion or prevention of MEB disorders.

BOX S-4
Recommendations: Continuing a
Course of Rigorous Research

Overall
- Research funders* should fund preventive intervention research on (1) risk and protective factors for specific disorders; (2) risk and protective factors that lead to multiple mental, emotional, and behavioral problems and disorders; and (3) promotion of individual, family, school, and community competencies. (4-3)
- Research funders should invest in studies that (1) aim to replicate findings from earlier trials, (2) evaluate long-term outcomes of preventive interventions across multiple outcomes (e.g., disorders, academic outcomes), and (3) test the extent to which each prevention program is effective in different race, ethnic, gender, and developmental groups. (10-1)
- The National Institutes of Health and other federal agencies should increase funding for research on prevention and promotion strategies that reduce multiple MEB disorders and that strengthen accomplishment of age-appropriate developmental tasks. High priority should be given to increasing collaboration and joint funding across institutes and across federal agencies that are responsible for separate but developmentally related outcomes (e.g., mental health, substance use, school success, contact with justice). (12-5)
- Research funders should strongly support research to improve the effectiveness of current interventions and the creation of new, more effective interventions with the goal of wide-scale implementation of these interventions. (7-2)

Screening Linked to Interventions
- Research funders should support a rigorous research agenda to develop and test community-based partnership models involving systems such as education (including preschool), primary care, and behavioral health to screen for risks and early mental, emotional, and behavioral problems and assess implementation of evidence-based preventive responses to identified needs. (8-1)

Implementation
- The National Institutes of Health should be charged with developing methodologies to address major gaps in current prevention science approaches, including the study of dissemination and implementation of successful interventions. (10-2)
- Research funders should fund research and evaluation on (1) dissemination strategies designed to identify effective approaches to implementation of evidence-based programs, (2) the effectiveness of programs when implemented by communities, and (3) identification of core elements of evidence-based programs, dissemination, and institutionalization strategies that might facilitate implementation. (11-1)
- Research funders should fund research on state- or community-wide implementation of interventions to promote mental, emotional, or behavioral health

or prevent MEB disorders that meet established scientific standards of effectiveness. (11-2)

Adaptation
- Research funders should prioritize the evaluation and implementation of programs to promote mental, emotional, or behavioral health or prevent MEB disorders in ethnic minority communities. Priorities should include the testing and adoption of culturally appropriate adaptations of evidence-based interventions developed in one culture to determine if they work in other cultures and encouragement of adoption when they do. (11-3)

Neuroscience Linkages
- Research funders, led by the National Institutes of Health, should dedicate more resources to formulating and testing hypotheses of the effects of genetic, environmental, and epigenetic influences on brain development across the developmental span of childhood, with a special focus on pregnancy, infancy, and early childhood. (5-1)
- The National Institutes of Health should lead efforts to study the feasibility and ethics of using individually identified genetic and other neurobiological risk factors to target preventive interventions for MEB disorders. (5-4)
- Research funders, led by the National Institutes of Health, should dedicate resources to support collaborations between prevention scientists and basic and clinical developmental neuroscientists. Such collaborations should include both basic science approaches and evaluations of the effects of prevention trials on neurobiological outcomes, as well as the use of animal models to identify and test causal mechanisms and theories of pathogenesis. (5-2)
- Research funders, led by the National Institutes of Health, should fund research consortia to develop multidisciplinary teams with expertise in developmental neuroscience, developmental psychopathology, and preventive intervention science to foster translational research studies leading to more effective prevention efforts. (5-3)

Economic Analyses
- The National Institutes of Health, in consultation with government agencies, private-sector organizations, and key researchers, should develop outcome measures and guidelines for economic analyses of prevention and promotion interventions. The guidelines should be widely disseminated to relevant government agencies and foundations and to prevention researchers. (9-1).
- Funders of intervention research should incorporate guidelines and measures related to economic analysis in their program announcements and provide supplemental funding for projects that include economic analyses. Once available, supplemental funding should also be provided for projects with protocols that incorporate recommended outcome measures. (9-2)

continued

BOX S-4 Continued

Competencies
- Research funders, led by the National Institutes of Health, should increase funding for research on the etiology and development of competencies and healthy functioning of young people, as well as how healthy functioning protects against the development of MEB disorders. (4-1)
- The National Institutes of Health should develop measures of developmental competencies and positive mental health across developmental stages that are comparable to measures used for MEB disorders. These measures should be developed in consultation with leading research and other key stakeholders and routinely used in mental health promotion intervention studies. (4-2)

Technology
- Research funders should support research on the effectiveness of mass media and Internet interventions, including approaches to reducing stigma. (7-3)

Other Research Gaps
- Research funders should address significant research gaps, such as preventive interventions with adolescents and young adults, in certain high-risk groups (e.g., children with chronic diseases, children in foster care), and in primary care settings; interventions to address poverty; approaches that combine interventions at multiple developmental phases; and approaches that integrate individual, family, school, and community-level interventions. (7-4)

NOTE: The term "research funders" is used to refer to federal agencies and foundations who fund research on mental health promotion or prevention of MEB disorders.

and community-level implementation processes and approaches is one of the frontiers of future prevention research.

- **Analysis of adaptation.** Little research has addressed factors that either facilitate or impede the transfer or adaptation of evidence-based interventions that have been developed for a single setting to a range of other ethnic, linguistic, and cultural groups. Additional research is needed to ensure the availability of interventions that are culturally relevant and that have been informed by the nation's many ethnic, linguistic, and cultural environments.
- **Linkages with neuroscience.** Environment and experience have powerful effects on modifying brain structure and function, including influences on the expression of genes and their protein products that can dictate or alter the course of development. Cross-disciplinary collaborations that formulate and test hypotheses concerning the

roles and interactions among multiple genetic and epigenetic influences on brain development may lead to strategies to tailor preventive interventions to specific individuals or groups of individuals at greatest risk.

- **Economic analyses.** The challenges of conducting economic analyses and the relative novelty of this type of analysis in the prevention field suggest the need for guidelines for conducting economic analyses (cost-effectiveness and cost-benefit analyses) as well as provision of incentives to encourage their inclusion in study designs. Evidence of the economic benefits of preventive interventions will make them more valuable to communities as they decide about the distribution of limited resources.

- **Competencies.** Competencies related to age-appropriate developmental tasks in the family, school, peer group, and community play an important role in mental health. The etiology and development of competencies need to be better understood. Methods to assess the relative value and effects of different types of competencies on development of and protection from disorders require attention.

- **Use of technology.** The Internet, mass media, and other current technologies (e.g., CD-ROMs) represent potential mechanisms to reach large segments of the population. Research in this area should be conducted to determine whether such media can be used effectively to promote mental health or to prevent disorders.

- **Other research gaps.** Despite dramatic increases in prevention research, significant gaps remain regarding populations and settings to be targeted.

Given the modest effect sizes of some interventions, research funders are encouraged to support research to improve the breadth of the application and effectiveness of current evidence-based interventions and to develop new, more effective interventions. They should also direct researchers to measure outcomes over time, ideally across developmental periods, analyze multiple outcomes (including the effects on multiple disorders), and assess iatrogenic effects. Researchers in turn are encouraged to design interventions and evaluations that respond to these concerns (see Box S-5).

Finally, the gap is substantial between what is known and what is actually being done. The nation is now well positioned to equip young people with the skills, interests, assets, and health habits needed to live healthy, happy, and productive lives in caring relationships that strengthen the social fabric. This can be achieved by refining the science and by developing the infrastructure and large-scale collaborative systems that allow the equitable delivery of population-based preventive approaches. We call on the nation to build on the extensive research now available by implement-

---

BOX S-5
Recommendations for Researchers

- Research and interventions on the prevention of MEB disorders should focus on interventions that occur before the onset of disorder but should be broadened to include promotion of mental, emotional, and behavioral health. (3-1)
- Prevention researchers should broaden the range of outcomes included in evaluations of prevention programs and policies to include relevant MEB disorders and related problems, as well as common positive outcomes, such as accomplishment of age-appropriate developmental tasks (e.g., school, social, and work outcomes). They should also adequately explore and report on potential iatrogenic effects. (7-1)
- Researchers should include analysis of the costs and cost-effectiveness (and whenever possible cost-benefit) of interventions in evaluations of effectiveness studies (in contrast to efficacy trials). (9-3)
- Researchers and community organizations should form partnerships to develop evaluations of (1) adaptation of existing interventions in response to community-specific cultural characteristics; (2) preventive interventions designed based on research principles in response to community concerns; and (3) preventive interventions that have been developed in the community, have demonstrated feasibility of implementation and acceptability in that community, but lack experimental evidence of effectiveness. (11-4)

---

ing evidence-based preventive interventions, testing their effectiveness in specific communities, disseminating principles in support of prevention, addressing gaps in the available research, and monitoring progress at the national, state, and local levels.

1

Introduction

Mental, emotional, and behavioral (MEB) disorders—such as depression, conduct disorder, and substance abuse—among children, youth, and young adults create an enormous burden for them, their families, and the nation. They threaten the future health and well-being of young people. Between 14 and 20 percent of young people experience an MEB disorder at a given point in time. A survey of adults reported that half of all lifetime cases of diagnosable mental illness began by age 14 and three-fourths by age 24 (Kessler, Berglund, et al., 2005). A review of three longitudinal studies concluded that close to 40 percent of young people have had at least one psychiatric disorder by the time they are 16 (Jaffee, Harrington, et al., 2005). Furthermore, about one in five (21.3 percent) adolescents ages 12-17 received treatment or counseling for MEB disorders in 2006 (Substance Abuse and Mental Health Services Administration, 2007b). Signs of potential MEB disorders are often apparent at a very young age. Parents often report concerns before age 5, and there are indications that the expulsion rate of children from preschool for behavioral concerns is higher than similar expulsion rates of children from grades K-12 (Gilliam and Sharar, 2006). But mental health costs are often hidden from national accounting methods because a major portion of these costs do not take place in mental health care settings, accruing instead to such systems as education, justice, and physical health care. By the same token, the savings that can accrue from prevention are likely to most benefit these systems.

Early onset of MEB disorders is predictive of lower school achievement, an increased burden on the child welfare system, and greater demands on the juvenile justice system (Institute of Medicine, 2006b). One study estimated that more than one-quarter of the total costs for mental health treatment services among adolescents were incurred in the education and juvenile justice systems (Costello, Copeland, et al., 2007). One estimate puts the total annual economic costs in 2007 at roughly $247 billion (Eisenberg and Neighbors, 2007). In addition, youth with emotional and behavioral problems are at greatly increased risk of psychiatric and substance abuse problems (Gregory, Caspi, et al., 2007). The earlier young people start drinking, the more likely they are to have serious alcohol dependence as adults (Grant and Dawson, 1997; Gruber, DiClemente, et al., 1996). Early aggressive behavior greatly increases the risk of conduct disorder, drug use, and other externalizing behaviors, while environmental and individual-level protective factors (Kellam, Ling, et al., 1998) and preventive interventions can reduce these risks.

The good news, as this report documents, is that research has identified multiple factors that contribute to the development of MEB disorders, and interventions have been developed to successfully intervene with these factors. Through the application of policies, programs, and practices aimed at eliminating risks and increasing strengths, there is great potential to reduce the number of new cases of MEB disorders and significantly improve the lives of young people.

A variety of factors—including individual competencies, family resources, school quality, and community-level characteristics—can increase or decrease the risk that a young person will develop an MEB disorder or related problem behaviors, such as early substance use, risky sexual behavior, or violence. These factors tend to have a cumulative effect: A greater number of risk factors (and for some, a longer exposure, such as from parental mental illness) increases the likelihood of negative outcomes, and a greater number of protective factors (e.g., resources within an individual, family strengths, access to mentors, and good education) decreases the likelihood of negative outcomes. This report makes the case that preventing the development of MEB disorders and related problems among young people, reducing risks, and promoting positive mental health should be high priorities for the nation.

Families, policy makers, practitioners, and scientists share a conceptual commitment to the well-being of young people—that is not a new idea. However, a solid body of accumulated research now shows that it is possible to positively impact young people's lives and prevent many MEB disorders. In addition, a consensus is emerging around the need to promote positive aspects of emotional development. While additional research is needed, the efficacy of a wide range of preventive interventions has been established, particularly ones that reduce risk factors or enhance protective factors. Less research had been conducted to empirically evaluate strategies to implement relevant policies on prevention, to widely and effectively adopt preventive interventions, to develop culturally relevant interventions, or to build the infrastructure for prevention, so that effective practices are available to every family and young person who could benefit from them.

CORE CONCEPTS

Several core concepts underlie the ability to adopt prevention and promotion as national priorities. The committee views these concepts as essential elements that must be embraced by families, policy makers, service systems, and scientists in order to continue to make progress in this area. They also shed light on why not enough attention has been directed to prevention or promotion to date.

Prevention requires a paradigm shift. Prevention of MEB disorders inherently involves a way of thinking that goes beyond the traditional disease model, in which one waits for an illness to occur and then provides evidence-based treatment. Prevention focuses on the question, "What will be good for the child 5, 10, or more years from now?" and tries to mobilize resources to put these things in place. A growing body of prevention research points to the need for the national dialogue on mental health and substance abuse issues to embrace the healthy development of young people and at the same time to respond early and effectively to the needs of those with MEB disorders.

Mental health and physical health are inseparable. The prevention of MEB disorders and physical disorders and the promotion of mental health and physical health are inseparable. Young people who grow up in good physical health are more likely to also have good mental health. Similarly, good mental health often contributes to maintenance of good physical health. In their calculations of the burden of disease and injury in the United States in 1996 (the latest data available), Michaud, McKenna, and colleagues (2006) show that in children ages 5-14, 15 percent of disability-adjusted life years (DALYs) lost to illness are caused by mental illness. In youth ages 15-24, almost two-thirds of DALYs lost are due to mental illness, to substance abuse, or to homicide, suicide, or motor vehicle accidents, all of which have a strong association with mental illness and substance abuse. Furthermore, MEB disorders increase the risk for communicable and noncommunicable diseases and contribute to both intentional and unintentional injuries, so the percentage may be even higher (Prince, Patel, et al., 2007). Almost one-quarter (24 percent) of pediatric primary care office visits involve behavioral and mental health problems (Cooper, Valleley, et al., 2006).

Conversely, young people with special health care needs or chronic physical health problems are at greater risk for MEB disorders (Kuehn, 2008; Wolraich, Drotar, et al., 2008). Associations have been demonstrated between MEB disorders and a number of chronic diseases. For example, one study showed that 16 percent of asthmatic youth ages 11-17 demonstrated criteria for anxiety and depressive disorders (McCauly, Katon, et al., 2007). Health professionals in both sectors contribute to the maintenance of good physical and good mental health.

Successful prevention is inherently interdisciplinary. The prevention of MEB disorders is inherently interdisciplinary and draws on a variety of different strategies. For example, strategies at multiple levels have led to effective tobacco control and reductions in underage drinking. These include broad interventions that address policy or regulation (product taxation, purchase and use age minimums, advertising restrictions), interventions that address community behaviors (blue laws, smoke-free workplaces), interventions within the legal system (fines for underage sales, lawsuits against manufacturers), and individually focused interventions both within and independent of the health care system (parents educating their children about smoking and drinking).

Mental, emotional, and behavioral disorders are developmental. The health status of young people has a significant influence on the trajectory of health into adulthood (National Research Council and Institute of Medicine, 2004a). While research suggests that the earliest years of life are one of the most opportune times to affect change (National Research Council and Institute of Medicine, 2000), other developmental periods (e.g., early adolescence) or settings (e.g., schools) in young people's lives also provide opportunities for intervention (National Research Council and Institute of Medicine, 2001, 2002). Children develop in the context of their families (or, for some, the institutions that replace their families), their schools, and their communities.

Coordinated community-level systems are needed to support young people. Supporting the development of children requires that infrastructure be in place in one or more systems—public health, health care, education, community agencies—to support and finance culturally appropriate preventive interventions at multiple levels. Similarly, the benefits or savings of prevention may occur in a system (e.g., education, justice) other than the one that paid for the prevention activity (e.g., health), requiring a broad, community-wide perspective. For example, an outcome of a family-based preventive intervention delivered by the health care system may be children who are more successful academically or have fewer legal difficulties. Sharing costs and benefits of interventions across agencies and programs would likely create new opportunities for broad advances.

INTERVENTION RATIONALE

The past decade and a half has witnessed an explosion in knowledge regarding how to help young people experience healthy development. The evidence that these efforts can have a positive impact on the trajectory of their lives makes a compelling case for them. However, there have been strong pressures by some public interest groups against many types of preventive interventions. Objections have been particularly strong related to mandatory screening of children to identify those at high risk and therefore presumably in need of prevention or treatment, as well as to screening done with passive consent. Concerns have also been raised about the reliability of screenings conducted to identify suicide risk, as well as the effectiveness of preventive interventions designed to reduce suicide (Institute of Medicine, 2002).

Public views about mental health treatment and prevention often differ; this is certainly true in the United States. Insurance and government-funded programs typically support treatment but do so less for many kinds of prevention. A fundamental difference between some forms of prevention and treatment is that treatment is typically based on a one-on-one relationship between a person seeking care and a provider of care, whereas prevention can be on an individual (e.g., early child health screenings), group (e.g., a classroom behavior management program), or population (e.g., antidrug advertising campaigns or citywide antibullying programs) basis. In the case of prevention, the public sector, in the shape of a legislative body or a school system, sometimes takes it on itself to intervene in the lives of individuals in the interest of the common good. Public resistance may result when this public intervention infringes on individual rights. For example, the predominant view in the United States is that parenting—unless it results in abuse or neglect—is a private matter not subject to government intervention.

Both the practical public health context and various philosophical contexts provide strong justification for taking a preventive approach to the emotional and behavioral problems of youth. First, public health's core focus is preventing rather than treating disease. The primary concern is the health of the population, rather than the treatment of individual diseases. Public health recognizes the importance of identifying and then intervening with known risk factors. In a public health context, population health is understood to result from the interaction of a range of factors beyond the individual. In the case of children, youth, and young adults, a public health model would call for the involvement of families, schools, health and other child service systems, neighborhoods, and communities to address the interwoven factors that affect mental health. Behavioral health could learn from public health in endorsing a population health perspective.

From a philosophical perspective, promoting the general welfare and protecting society's most vulnerable individuals are part of the nation's foundation, codified in the founding documents of the nation. Government has an obligation to ensure the health, safety, and welfare of its citizens. Thus, government has a responsibility to address unmet mental health needs, particularly for children.

Second, economics suggests that the public sector should intervene when one person's action or behavior adversely impacts others (i.e., negative externalities). Young people who suffer from MEB disorders impose costs on society beyond those that they suffer themselves: the costs of health and other care; disruptions of work, school, or family; the costs to the criminal justice system and other service systems for actions resulting from MEB disorders; and, in the case of young people, the costs of special education or other remedial services. Preventing MEB disorders and promoting mental health thus benefits not only the individuals who would have directly experienced these problems and their families, but also society as a whole. Similarly, the basic human suffering that individuals with MEB disorders and their families experience calls for public preventive intervention, as there are strategies available that can avoid some of that suffering.

Third, a political science perspective calls on government to intervene in areas in which shared interests require shared solutions—such issues as public education, global warming, national defense, and others for which wider societal action is needed. Political science considers inequities when considering how and when society should be involved in the affairs of its citizens. The distribution of the burden imposed by preventable MEB disorders is one such inequity warranting collective decision making to include population-level issues that affect communities as a whole. Finally, the basic ethical principles of justice, beneficence, and fidelity call for reasonable actions to protect the nation's young people and promote their well-being.

Collectively, these different perspectives provide a strong rationale for government to employ its resources to prevent a large future burden of MEB disorders that, directly or indirectly, affects all of society. The case is particularly compelling in the instance of preventable disorders among young people. Government, communities, and families should be called on to make changes with documented benefit in their lives.

STUDY BACKGROUND

In 1994, in response to a congressional request, the Institute of Medicine (IOM) published *Reducing Risks for Mental Disorders: Frontiers for Preventive Intervention Research*, a landmark assessment of research related to prevention of mental disorders (referred to throughout as the 1994 IOM report). The report acknowledged incremental progress since the nation was first called to pay attention to mental illness and its prevention by President John F. Kennedy in the early 1960s. The report provided a new definition of mental illness prevention and a conceptual framework that emphasized the reduction of risks for mental disorders. And it proposed a focused research agenda, with recommendations on how to develop effective intervention programs, create a cadre of prevention researchers, and improve coordination among federal agencies.

Numerous other reports and activities have emerged since the 1994 IOM report, drawing more attention to the need for research, prevention, and treatment of mental disorders (see Box 1-1 for a timeline of key events), including the New Freedom Commission on Mental Health report (2003), reports of the National Advisory Mental Health Council's Workgroup on Child and Adolescent Mental Health Intervention Development and Deployment (2001) of the National Institute of Mental Health, and reports from the surgeon general on children's mental health (U.S. Public Health Service, 2000), violence (U.S. Public Health Service, 2001c), and suicide prevention (U.S. Public Health Service, 1999b, 2001b). The *Surgeon General's Call to Action to Prevent and Reduce Underage Drinking* (U.S. Public Health Service, 2007) similarly called for concerted national action to address this significant concern affecting young people. Mental health and substance abuse professional and consumer organizations have taken steps to embrace prevention without abandoning the need for treatment.

At the same time, the growth in research-based evidence and new government mandates related to program accountability have prompted focused attention on specific preventive interventions. The Government Performance and Results Act of 1993 launched a trend toward requiring federal programs to provide evidence of effectiveness (U.S. Office of Management and Budget, 2003). The Safe and Drug Free Schools Act of 1990 specified "principles of effectiveness," and the No Child Left Behind Act of 2001 called for school districts to implement evidence-based programming (Hallfors and Godette, 2002). More recently, the Consolidated Appropriations Act of 2008 created a new grant program to support "evidence based home visitation programs" that meet "high evidentiary standards" as well as a new wellness program in the mental health programs of regional and national significance that would require grantees to "evaluate the success of the program based on their ability to provide evidence-based services."

The number of preventive interventions tested using randomized controlled trials (RCTs), an approach generally considered to be the "gold standard" and strongly recommended by the 1994 IOM report, has increased substantially since that time. Figure 1-1 illustrates the number of published RCTs (between 1980 and 2007) based on a search of articles related to preventive interventions for MEB disorders with young people included

BOX 1-1
Timeline of Recent Prevention-Related Events

1994   The Institute of Medicine (IOM) published *Reducing Risks for Mental Disorders: Frontiers for Preventive Intervention Research*, which presented a focused research agenda, with recommendations on how to develop effective intervention programs, create a cadre of prevention researchers, and improve coordination among federal agencies.

1996   The Center for the Study and Prevention of Violence at the University of Colorado at Boulder, with funding from the U.S. Department of Justice, designed and launched a national violence prevention initiative called *Blueprints for Violence Prevention* to identify effective violence prevention programs.

1997   As part of a model programs initiative, the Center for Substance Abuse Prevention of the Substance Abuse and Mental Health Services Administration (SAMHSA) created the National Registry of Effective Prevention Programs.

The National Institute on Drug Abuse (NIDA) released *Preventing Drug Use Among Children and Adolescents: A Research-Based Guide for Parent, Educators, and Community Leaders*, which includes examples of research-based drug abuse prevention programs.

1998   The National Research Council (NRC) and IOM held a workshop on adolescent decision making and its implications for prevention programs; the workshop report summarized issues raised related to the design and implementation of prevention programs for youth.

The National Advisory Mental Health Council's Workgroup on Mental Disorder Prevention Research of the National Institute of Mental Health (NIMH) released *Priorities for Prevention Research at NIMH*.

The Promising Practices Network (PPN) was launched by a partnership between four state-level intermediary organizations with the goal of encouraging a shift toward results-oriented policy and practice by providing easier access to evidence-based information via the Internet. The site, which is now administered by RAND, provides information about "what works" to improve the lives of children, youth, and families. Programs are reviewed and assigned to one of the evidence level categories (proven, promising, proven/promising, and screened).

1999   *Mental Health: A Report of the Surgeon General* was issued to address mental health and mental illness across the life span, focusing attention on the role of mental health, including prevention of disorders, in the lives of individuals, communities, and the nation.

The Safe and Drug Free Schools Act created a new interagency program (U.S. Department of Education, U.S. Department of Health and Human Services, and Office of Juvenile Justice and Delinquency Prevention) to prevent violence and substance abuse among the nation's youth, schools, and communities. The act specifies "principles of effectiveness."

The Surgeon General's Call to Action to Prevent Suicide proposed "a nationwide, collaborative effort to reduce suicidal behaviors, and to prevent premature death due to suicide across the life" by using AIM (awareness, intervention, and methodology) as an approach to address suicide.

The American Academy of Pediatrics' Task Force on Violence published *The Role of the Pediatrician in Youth Violence Prevention in Clinical Practice and at the Community Level.*

2000   The Society for Prevention Research (SPR) released the first edition of its flagship journal, *Prevention Science*, as an interdisciplinary forum designed to disseminate new developments in the theory, research, and practice of prevention. (SPR was created in 1991 to advance science-based prevention programs and policies through empirical research.)

Report of the Surgeon General's Conference on Children's Mental Health: A National Action Agenda was released, which introduces a "blueprint for addressing children's mental health in the United States" based on a conference sponsored by the U.S. Departments of Health and Human Services, Education, and Justice.

The World Federation for Mental Health, the Clifford Beers Foundation, and the Carter Center Mental Health Program organized the First World Conference on the Promotion of Mental Health and Prevention of Mental and Behavioral Disorders.

2001   *Youth Violence: A Report of the Surgeon General* reviewed the factors that protect youth from perpetrating violence and identified effective research-based preventive strategies.

The Coalition for Evidence-Based Policy was established to promote government policy making based on rigorous evidence of program effectiveness.

Mental Health: Culture, Race, and Ethnicity (a supplement to *Mental Health: A Report of the Surgeon General*) was released by the Office of the Surgeon General.

The National Advisory Mental Health Council's Workgroup on Child and Adolescent Mental Health Intervention Development and Deployment released *Blueprint for Change: Research on Child and Adolescent Mental Health.*

The American Psychological Association released a special issue of *Prevention and Treatment*, with 13 commentaries on the 1998 report *Priorities for Prevention Research at NIMH.*

Child Trends published two reports on mental health and emotional well-being, *Background for Community-Level Work on Mental Health and Externalizing Disorders in Adolescence: Reviewing the Literature on*

continued

BOX 1-1 Continued

Contributing Factors and *Background for Community-Level Work on Emotional Well-Being in Adolescence: Reviewing the Literature on Contributing Factors*, as part of its series of "what works" in youth development.

2002   The IOM published *Reducing Suicide: A National Imperative*, which includes consensus statements on the scientific literature on the causes of and risk factors for suicide and illuminates contentious issues and gaps in the knowledge base that should guide prevention efforts and intervention.

The What Works Clearinghouse was established by the U.S. Department of Education's Institute of Education Sciences to provide educators, policy makers, researchers, and the public with a central and trusted source of scientific evidence for what works in education, including programs aimed at character education.

The President's New Freedom Commission on Mental Health was established to identify policies that could be implemented by federal, state, and local governments to maximize the utility of existing resources, improve coordination of treatments and services, and promote successful community integration for adults with a serious mental illness and children with a serious emotional disturbance.

2003   The President's New Freedom Commission on Mental Health released *Achieving the Promise: Transforming Mental Health Care in America*, recommending a wholesale transformation of the nation's mental health care system that involves consumers and providers, policy makers at all levels of government, and the public and private sectors.

NIDA released a second edition of *Preventing Drug Use Among Children and Adolescents: A Research-Based Guide for Parents, Educators, and Community Leaders*.

NIMH released *Breaking Ground, Breaking Through: The Strategic Plan for Mood Disorders Research*, which included a section titled "Treatment, Prevention, and Services: Improving Outcomes."

The Congressional Mental Health Caucus was established to "discuss awareness and find solutions in a bipartisan manner on improving mental health care and its delivery to every American."

2004   The NRC and IOM published *Reducing Underage Drinking: A Collective Responsibility*, which explored the ways in which different individuals and groups contribute to the problem of underage drinking and how they can be enlisted to prevent it.

SPR issued *Standards of Evidence: Criteria for Efficacy, Effectiveness and Dissemination*.

The New England Regional Conference on Evidence-Based Programs for the Promotion of Mental Health and Prevention of Mental and Substance

Abuse Disorders was sponsored by the New England Coalition for Health Promotion and Disease Prevention (NECON), with funding support from the Center for Mental Health Services (CMHS) in SAMHSA.

NIMH and NIDA sponsored a two-day meeting to consider research on the prevention of depression in children and adolescents and to consider new opportunities to develop further the empirical base for additional preventive approaches. Following the meeting, some of the participants prepared articles for a special issue of the *American Journal of Preventive Medicine* (Volume 31, Issue 6, Supplement 1, pp. 99-188, December 2006).

The National Council for Suicide Prevention issued the *National Strategy for Suicide Prevention* to promote broad collaboration in prevention activities.

2006 The World Federation of Mental Health established an Office for the Promotion of Mental Health and Prevention of Mental Disorders.

2007 SAMHSA launched a new, expanded website to review mental health and substance abuse programs and practices. The system is renamed the National Registry of Evidence-Based Programs and Practices (NREPP).

The surgeon general released *The Surgeon General's Call to Action to Prevent and Reduce Underage Drinking.*

The American Psychological Association hosted a congressional briefing entitled "Children's Mental Health: Key Challenges, Strategies, and Effective Solutions," with a focus on prevention.

Psychiatric Annals published a series of articles on prevention in the field of psychiatry. This issue provided a survey of the recent literature on prevention topics for practicing clinical psychiatrists, such as prevention psychiatry, suicide prevention, prodromal states and early intervention in psychosis, alcohol and drug abuse prevention, adverse childhood events as risk factors, becoming a preventionist, and a resident's perspective on prevention in psychiatry.

The Carter Center convened its annual Rosalynn Carter Mental Health Policy Symposium, with a focus on prevention.

The National Co-Morbidity Study provided additional data confirming that half of all lifetime diagnosable mental illness begins by age 14.

SAMHSA released a report to Congress, *Promotion and Prevention in Mental Health: Strengthening Parenting and Enhancing Child Resilience.*

2008 Congress included a requirement in the FY 2008 budget of the U.S. Department of Health and Human Services to implement an evidence-based wellness and prevention initiative in the mental health program of regional and national significance and an evidence-based home visitation program within the child abuse and neglect program.

Mental Health America launched an Inaugural Promotion and Prevention Summit.

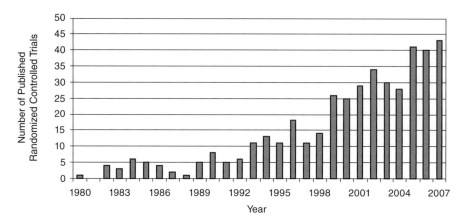

FIGURE 1-1 Growth in randomized controlled trials.

in Medline and Psychinfo.[1] Although there may be some published (and clearly unpublished) RCTs that were not identified by this search, the overall trend is unlikely to be affected. While not all of the articles report successful interventions or interventions that have a major impact on outcomes, the evidence base available now is significantly advanced beyond what was available at the time of the 1994 IOM report.[2] Similarly, other types of evaluations that provide meaningful insights into mental health promotion and the prevention of MEB disorders have also been conducted. Although RCTs remain the gold standard, they are not always feasible, and other designs can make important contributions.

Some federal programs have directed that resources be used only for programs with evidence of effectiveness, and numerous efforts have emerged to identify and share model programs or best practices. The Substance Abuse and Mental Health Services Administration, the U.S. Department of Justice, and the U.S. Department of Education have each launched a mechanism to identify and disseminate information about interventions, including many preventive interventions. Numerous federal and state organizations have published guides or lists of "model" or "effective" programs (National

---

[1]The search, modeled on the approach used by the Cochrane Collaboration, identified articles that self-identified as an RCT or included such terms as "random," "control," and "double" or "single blind" to describe their design. The abstracts of articles identified by the database search were then reviewed to eliminate those that were not an RCT, did not address the prevention of emotional and behavioral disorders, or were not targeted at young people.

[2]The committee notes that it typically takes years for the results of an RCT to appear in a journal. As a result, the year of publication may not correspond to the year in which the RCT took place.

Institute on Drug Abuse, 1997; National Institute on Alcohol Abuse and Alcoholism, 2002; Maryland Governor's Office of Crime Control and Prevention, 2003). However, there is wide variation in the evidence criteria used to identify and classify programs as well as the terminology used to describe them (research-based, evidence-based, model, promising, etc.). Impressive advances have been made in the development and documentation of efficacious interventions that successfully reduce an array of risk factors or enhance protective factors for MEB disorders and substance abuse. Increasingly, there is evidence that some of these interventions can be effectively implemented in community settings. And there is a relatively young but growing body of evidence that some interventions are cost-effective.

Despite these substantial developments, translating existing knowledge into widespread reductions in the incidence and prevalence of MEB disorders of young people remains a challenge. Prevention science and practice still lack empirically tested strategies for widespread dissemination of evidence-based interventions and an infrastructure of schools, family service organizations, or health care providers to reliably deliver evidence-based interventions.

The astonishing number of young people with MEB disorders has placed extraordinary demands on the education, child welfare, and justice systems as children and youth with unmet needs enter those systems. As well, it has sparked interest in preventive approaches that may help stem the tide. Many interventions have been demonstrated to be efficacious (i.e., tested in a research environment), and several have been demonstrated to be effective (i.e., tested in the real world). However, implementation of any intervention on a large scale and demonstration that it reliably improves mental health outcomes remain a daunting challenge. Similarly, a shared public vision about prevention of MEB disorders or promotion of mental health, which prioritizes the healthy development of young people and places prevention of MEB disorders on equal footing with physical health disorders, is seriously lacking. Collective attention to the fact that the vast majority of MEB disorders begins in youth will require transformation in multiple systems that work with young people.

THE COMMITTEE'S CHARGE

Recognizing significant changes in the policy and research contexts and substantial increases in the availability of prevention research, the Substance Abuse and Mental Health Services Administration, the National Institute of Mental Health, the National Institute on Drug Abuse, and the National Institute on Alcohol Abuse and Alcoholism requested that the Board on Children, Youth, and Families of the National Research Council and Institute of Medicine provide an update on progress since release of

---

BOX 1-2
Committee Charge

- Review promising areas of research that contribute to the prevention of mental disorders, substance abuse, and problem behaviors among children, youth, and young adults (to age 25), focusing in particular on genetics, neurobiology, and psychosocial research as well as the field of prevention science.
- Highlight areas of key advances and persistent challenges since the publication of the 1994 IOM report *Reducing Risks for Mental Disorders: Frontiers for Preventive Intervention Research.*
- Examine the research base within a developmental framework throughout the life span, with an emphasis on prevention and promotion opportunities that can improve the mental health and behavior of children, youth, and young adults.
- Review the current scope of federal efforts in the prevention of mental disorders and substance abuse and the promotion of mental health among at-risk populations, including children of parents with substance abuse or mental health disorders, abused and neglected children, children in foster care, children whose parents are absent or incarcerated, and children exposed to violence and other trauma, spanning the continuum from research to policy and services.
- Recommend areas of emphasis for future federal policies and programs of research support that would strengthen a developmental approach to a prevention research agenda as well as opportunities to foster public- and private-sector collaboration in prevention and promotion efforts for children, youth, and young adults, particularly in educational, child welfare, and primary care settings.
- Prepare a final report that will provide a state-of-the-art review of prevention research.

---

the 1994 IOM report, *Reducing Risks for Mental Disorders: Frontiers for Preventive Intervention Research,* with special attention to the research base and program experience with younger populations since that time (see Box 1-2 for the complete charge). The committee was asked to focus on populations through age 25. As mentioned above, most MEB disorders have their origins before this age, and most individuals have adopted adult roles by age 25 (Furstenberg, Kennedy, et al., 2003). In this way, this report differs from the 1994 IOM report, which included the entire life span.

Terminology

The committee's charge references "mental disorders, substance abuse, and problem behaviors." "Mental disorders" are defined by a cluster of symptoms, often including emotional or behavioral symptoms, codified in the *Diagnostic and Statistical Manual of Mental Disorders* (DSM) or the *International Classification of Diseases* (ICD). They include a variety of conditions, such as schizophrenia, depression, conduct disorder, attention deficit hyperactivity disorder, and anxiety disorder. Although the DSM and ICD criteria are widely used for diagnostic purposes, federal agencies have adopted alternative terminology, such as "mental and behavioral disorders,"[3] "emotional, behavioral and mental disorders,"[4] and "mental, emotional, and behavioral disorders"[5] to communicate information about the range of disorders experienced by young people. The National Association of School Psychologists has identified children with "emotional and behavioral disorders"[6] as needing focused attention in the education system. Similarly, health care professionals are seeing significant numbers of children as a result of parental concerns regarding their behavior.

The committee debated the term to use for purposes of this report, weighing the potential implications for the DSM and the ICD, the stigma often associated with the term "mental disorders," and the perspectives of the multiple audiences at whom the report is aimed—including researchers; service providers in the education, health, and social service systems; and parents themselves. Although "mental disorders" is the accepted term among many in diagnostic roles, less stigmatizing terminology is likely to resonate with others, including parents and school personnel. In the end, the committee decided to use "mental, emotional, and behavioral (MEB) disorders" based on its comprehensiveness, relevance to multiple audiences, and reduced stigma. More specific terminology is used when the discussion refers to a specific disorder.

Substance abuse and dependence are mental disorders included in the DSM and diagnosed when symptoms and impairment reach a high level. However, substance use, including underage drinking, is a problem behavior of significant public health concern even when the symptoms are not severe enough to be considered a substance use disorder. Such problem behaviors as early substance use, violence, and aggression are often signs or symptoms of mental disorders, although they may not be frequent or severe enough to meet diagnostic criteria. Nonetheless, intervention when these signs or symptoms are apparent, or actions to prevent them from occurring in the first place, can alter the course toward disorder and, as this report outlines, are an important component of prevention in this area. The committee could not thoroughly consider the complete range of behaviors (e.g., truancy, unprotected sex, reckless driving) that might be considered

---

[3]See http://mentalhealth.samhsa.gov/publications/allpubs/svp05-0151/.

[4]See http://www.mchlibrary.info/knowledgepaths/kp_mental_conditions.html.

[5]See http://mentalhealth.samhsa.gov/publications/allpubs/CA-0006/default.asp.

[6]See http://www.nasponline.org/about_nasp/pospaper_sebd.aspx.

problem behaviors among young people. Prevention of substance use is included in the report given the inclusion of substance abuse in our charge; discussion of other problem behaviors is intended to illustrate the synergy in risk factors and approaches to prevention.

Similarly, for ease of reading, the committee has adopted the term "young people" throughout the report when referring to "children, youth, and young adults" as a group. When the discussion of a particular topic or preventive approach applies to a specific developmental phase (e.g., childhood, adolescence), the relevant descriptor (e.g., children) is used instead.

Scope of the Study

In general, prevention research is focused on the factors empirically demonstrated to be associated with MEB disorders, either as risk factors, protective factors, or constructive interventions to reduce them; risk factors often represent risks for multiple disorders or problem behaviors. In addition, relatively few studies to date measure the incidence of actual MEB disorders as an outcome. The committee's review focuses on the developmental processes and factors that modify mental, emotional, and behavioral outcomes, rather than on individual disorders. When evidence is available related to the prevention of specific disorders (e.g., depression, schizophrenia, substance abuse), as opposed to risks for disorders, we have presented it as well. Over the long term, studies to address risk factors and improve the lives of children as well as studies to demonstrate the effects of interventions on the actual incidence of disorders are needed.

Given the extensive work already done by the IOM and others on smoking prevention, substance abuse was interpreted to mean primarily prevention of alcohol and drug use, with a focus on the trajectories and mechanisms they share with other mental, emotional, or behavioral problems. We do not provide a comprehensive epidemiological review of use of various substances by this population. Lessons from smoking are drawn on when appropriate.

The committee considers problem behaviors, such as risky sexual behavior and violence, to be integrally related to future mental, emotional, and behavioral problems among young people, with common trajectories and risk factors associated with both. HIV preventive interventions aimed at reducing risky sexual behavior as well as interventions designed to prevent violence are included in our review.

The committee was not asked to consider the status of treatment. Although we recognize that there are significant issues related to the quality and accessibility of treatment for young people (Burns, Costello, et al., 1995; Masi and Cooper, 2006), this was outside our charge. Still, given our charge to focus on promotion and prevention, we have articulated distinctions among what is considered promotion, prevention, and treatment. However, as discussed in more detail later in the report, there is no bright line separating promotion from prevention or prevention from treatment. We hope that readers of the report will appreciate that mental health promotion, prevention of mental health disorders, and treatment lie on a continuum, with each aspect of the continuum warranting attention. We also hope that the distinctions we draw among them will help guide policy, research, and funding decisions to ensure that progress in the areas of mental health promotion and prevention can accelerate. Unlike the 1994 IOM report, the committee has embraced mental health promotion as an integral component of the continuum that warrants attention.

The committee also recognizes that the term "prevention" applies to multiple fields of health. However, for simplicity, as used in this report, the term refers to prevention of mental, emotional, and behavioral problems rather than prevention of other sources of illness and disability.

The committee met five times during the course of the study and commissioned a series of papers on evidence related to early childhood, school-based, family-based, community-based, and culturally specific interventions, intervention cost-effectiveness, and aspects of screening and assessment. At the beginning of our deliberations, the committee heard from a variety of professional and other organizations actively involved in children's mental health issues. We convened a full-day workshop to hear from experts representing a variety of methodological issues, prevention approaches, and policy considerations. The workshop also included a panel to discuss recent developments in epigenetics and developmental neuroscience and a series of presentations on issues specific to youthful alcohol use (see Appendix B for a list of public meetings and presenters[7]). In addition to an assessment of the evidence by leading experts at the workshop, the committee reviewed available meta-analyses and systematic reviews regarding prevention and promotion and key literature since 1994 related to our charge.

ORGANIZATION OF THE REPORT

The remainder of this report is organized in three parts. Part I provides contextual and background information, beginning with a description of the available epidemiological literature on the prevalence and incidence of MEB disorders (Chapter 2). It then moves to a discussion of the scope of prevention, including the definitions of the various types of prevention and discussion of recent developments and definitions of mental health promotion (Chapter 3). The next two chapters outline perspectives on the

---

[7]This appendix is available only online. Go to http://www.nap.edu and search for *Preventing Mental, Emotional, and Behavioral Disorders Among Young People.*

developmental pathways that may lead to disorder and provide an empirical and theoretical basis for preventive interventions. The first presents available research on risk and protective factors related to prevention and promotion in a developmental context (Chapter 4). The second focuses on research related to genetics and developmental neuroscience, highlighting developmental plasticity and the important findings from research on epigenetics and gene–environment interactions that present potential intervention opportunities (Chapter 5).

Part II includes two chapters that present the evidence related to interventions aimed at individual, family, and community-level factors associated with mental, emotional, and behavioral outcomes (Chapter 6) and those that either target a specific disorder or are directed at overall promotion of health (Chapter 7). Given the potential relevance of population, group, and individual screening for the targeting of interventions, the next chapter discusses issues and opportunities related to screening (Chapter 8). The costs associated with MEB disorders and the available evidence on the benefits and costs of interventions discussed in Chapters 6 and 7 are discussed in the next chapter (Chapter 9). The last chapter in Part II outlines how methodologies have improved since the 1994 IOM report, methodological and statistical approaches to strengthen inferences, and the advantages of randomized and other designs. It also introduces methodological challenges for the next decade (Chapter 10).

Part III includes chapters that outline the frontiers for prevention science. It begins with a discussion of implementation; although there is an emerging implementation science, neither research nor practice related to implementation has kept pace with the available evidence, and this represents an important area of needed focus for prevention science (Chapter 11). Infrastructure issues, particularly systems concerns, and lack of funding and training are discussed next (Chapter 12). This part closes with a chapter that provides summative observations about the future of prevention (Chapter 13).

Part I:

Overview and Background

2

The Nature and Extent of the Problem

Epidemiology, the basic science of public health (Rothman and Greenland, 1998), provides vital information about diseases that threaten the health and well-being of the population. Epidemiology provides basic information that can be used to identify where and what kind of prevention is needed and to monitor the success (or failure) of preventive interventions. In order to be of use in the prevention of mental, emotional, and behavioral (MEB) disorders, epidemiology must provide information about which individuals are suffering from or at risk for mental, emotional, or behavioral problems, at what ages or developmental stages, and must be able to assess whether interventions have reduced the prevalence of a disorder.

National surveys of adults have shown the extent of the problem. In the early 1990s, the National Comorbidity Survey (NCS) of mental illness in the United States showed that more than one in four (26.2 percent) adults had a mental disorder in the 12 months up to the time of the survey (Kessler, Anthony, et al., 1997). The NCS-Replication (NCS-R) a decade later reported this figure as close to one-third (Kessler, Chiu, et al., 2005). In these and other surveys, roughly half of all affected adults recalled that their mental disorders started by their mid-teens, and three-quarters by their mid-20s (Kessler, Berglund, et al., 2005). However, studies of young people themselves are needed to establish accurately when MEB disorders first occur and what their consequences are in terms of chronicity, impaired functioning, and impact on their ability to reach developmental milestones, such as graduating from school, finding work, and forming adult relationships. The NCS-R includes a sample of over 10,000 adolescents ages 13 and older, but the findings are not yet available.

MEB disorders in young people are a public health concern for several reasons: (1) they cause suffering to individuals and their families; (2) they limit the ability to reach normal goals for social and educational achievement; (3) they increase the risk of further psychopathology, functional impairment, and suboptimal functioning throughout life; and (4) they impose heavy costs to society because of the resultant need for extra care, the social disruption that they can cause, and the risk that affected young people will underperform as adults. The significant economic costs of treating disorders warrant an increased focus on preventing them (Smit, Cuijpers, et al., 2006). However, support for prevention programs depends on knowing the size of the problem and its societal burden and on being able to monitor reductions in that burden when prevention programs are put in place. The United States is significantly behind other countries in supporting the necessary information-gathering programs.

In this chapter, we review the evidence available from epidemiological studies to answer the following questions:

- What kind of research methods and data are needed to answer questions about areas of high priority for prevention?
- How prevalent are MEB disorders of major public health concern?
- Is prevalence increasing or decreasing?
- How many new cases are there (incidence)?
- Is incidence increasing or decreasing?
- At what age do diagnosable disorders first occur (onset)?
- What is known about factors affecting prevalence, incidence, and age of onset?
- Are rates of these factors increasing or decreasing?
- Are some groups at particularly high risk for specific disorders?

Chapters 4 and 5 provide additional information related to the factors that affect the prevalence of disorders and define high-risk groups. A closely related set of questions deals with the cost to society of the harm caused by MEB disorders and the cost-effectiveness of prevention. These are addressed in Chapter 9.

RESEARCH METHODS AND DATA

The prevention of disease is a challenge for the whole community, not just for clinicians and their patients. Prevention is, by definition, an intervention that occurs before it is known who will develop a disorder and who will not. It follows that epidemiological information about whole communities (or representative samples of whole communities) is usually needed to answer questions about prevalence (the total number of cases in a given period of time) and incidence (the number of new cases in a population). In addition, many young people have more than one MEB disorder (Angold, Costello, and Erkanli, 1999). This comorbidity can increase the severity of a disorder (Kessler, Chiu, et al., 2005). Rates of comorbidity cannot be determined using clinic-based data, because cases seen in treatment settings are different in many ways from untreated cases (Berkson, 1946). Population-level information is needed to determine which diseases are of public health concern. It needs to encompass a wide range of disorders, including their rates of occurrence and co-occurrence and the burden they cause to individuals, their families, and the social organizations and agencies in which individuals live their lives.

The standard method of finding out how many cases of a disease exist in the community is to carry out a randomized survey of the general population. The size of a sample needed to provide precise answers to questions about the prevalence of an emotional or behavioral disorder depends on how common or rare it is. The less common the disorder, the larger the sample needed to provide a reliable prevalence estimate. For example, if a disorder occurs in 1 child in 10,000, researchers would need a population sample of at least 1 million children to find approximately 100 cases.

If a disorder produces such a high level of disability that every case comes to the attention of doctors, schools, or other agencies, then agency records can sometimes be used to estimate prevalence and even incidence. This method has been used by the Centers for Disease Control and Prevention (CDC) to estimate the prevalence of autism. In some countries, databases of inpatient and outpatient treatment are maintained and can be used to estimate treated prevalence. But many MEB disorders rarely come to the attention of doctors or teachers. Studies in the United States show that fewer than one in eight children with an MEB disorder is currently receiving treatment in the mental health or substance abuse systems, and only about one in four has ever received treatment (Burns, Costello, et al., 1995; Farmer, Burns, et al., 2003; Kataoka, Zhang, and Wells, 2002). To estimate the full burden of MEB disorders among children and adolescents, it is usually necessary to interview large community-based samples of parents and their children.

As mentioned earlier, there have been two recent surveys of mental illness in representative samples of the U.S. adult population: the NCS (Kessler, 1994), a follow-up of the same participants (NCS-2) (Kessler, Gruber, et al., 2007), and a second sample (NCS-R) a decade later (Kessler, Chiu, et al., 2005). The NCS included no one younger than 15. The NCS-R includes a sample of 10,000 adolescents (ages 13-17), but the data on this sample are not yet published. Although the United States supports several national surveys of health and drug abuse, these include very little on child and adolescent mental illness, and so there are almost no national prevalence and incidence estimates.

Table 2-1 is a summary of various nationally representative studies, sponsored by federal agencies, that have made some effort to produce estimates of the prevalence of MEB disorders of youth and, in some cases, the need for or use of mental health services. There is a dramatic contrast between the richness of the data on drug use and abuse from the National Health and Nutrition Examination Survey (NHANES), the National Survey on Drug Use and Health (NSDUH), and Monitoring the Future (MTF), and the paucity and lack of continuity of measures of MEB disorders. MTF has been collecting information on drug use and abuse since 1975, and NSDUH since 1988. However, the latter added some mental health questions only in 1994, and the results have not yet been published. NHANES used selected modules of a diagnostic interview for about five years, but since 2004 has limited its relevant data collection to a screener for depression for two years (2005, 2006) and some questions about conduct disorder since 1999. For three years, the National Health Interview Survey (NHIS) included the Strengths and Difficulties Questionnaire (Goodman and Gotlib, 1999), a 25-item parent report that produces symptom scales but not diagnoses. The current NHIS includes only three to five mental health questions. The new National Children's Study, which will begin recruiting participants in 2009, offers a wonderful opportunity for nationally representative, longitudinal data collection on the development of MEB disorders, the need for services, and the role of prevention and treatment in their course. No plans have been published for the data to be collected beyond the first few months, so it is unknown whether this opportunity will be realized.

Given the limitations of national surveys, conclusions about prevalence and incidence of MEB disorders among young people have to be drawn from (1) national surveys from other countries and (2) local population surveys in the United States. Despite being the best available data, both of these also have limitations. In the first case, rates can be very different in different countries, so that extrapolation to the United States is difficult. For example, using the same diagnostic interview (Development and Well-Being Assessment) with 8- to 10-year-olds in three different countries produced rates of conduct disorder in Norway that were much lower than those found in the United Kingdom (Heiervang, Stormark, et al., 2007) or the United States (see below). Within the United States, local surveys also show variation in rates. For example, in a set of studies using identical methods, the prevalence of disruptive behavior disorders was lowest in Puerto Rican youth living in Puerto Rico, higher in mainland Hispanic and white youth, and highest in mainland African Americans, even after controlling for a range of risk factors (Bird, Canino, et al., 2001).

TABLE 2-1 Review of National Surveys Providing Information About Emotional and Behavioral Disorders in Youth

Survey and Agency	Relevant Information Collected	Design and Comments
National Health Interview Survey (NHIS) Agency: National Center for Health Statistics (CDC)	Adult respondent is asked whether a doctor has ever told the respondents that the child has mental retardation, developmental delay, ADHD, or autism, or if a school or health professional has said that the child had a learning disability. In 2001, 2002, and 2003, ~10,000 adults completed 25-item Strengths and Difficulties Questionnaire (SDQ) for children ages 4-17. From 2007 on, 3-5 mental health questions asked (depending on child's age and sex). No diagnostic information.	Cross-sectional household interview survey. Sampling and interviewing continuous throughout each year. Multistage area probability design. Oversampling of both blacks and Hispanics. Sample size ~43,000 households (~106,000 persons) annually. For children, information provided by a responsible adult family member.
National Health and Nutrition Examination Survey (NHANES) Agency: National Center for Health Statistics (CDC)	Age/topic/method/dates: 12+/Depression screener/(CAPI)/2005, 2006 12-19/Alcohol use/(ACASI)/1999 on 12-19/Conduct disorders/(ACASI)/1999 on 12+/Drug use/(ACASI)/1999 on 12-19/Tobacco use/(ACASI)/1999 on 8-19/Eating disorders/(CDISC)/2000-2004 8-19/Depression/(CDISC)/2000-2004 8-19/Panic and anxiety/(CDISC)/1999-2004 8-15/ADHD/(parent CDISC)/2000-2004 8-15/Conduct disorders/(parent CDISC)/2000-2004 8-15/Depression/(parent CDISC)/2000-2004 8-15/Eating disorders/(parent CDISC)/2000-2004 8-11/Elimination disorders/(parent CDISC)/2000-2004 No data yet published.	Examines a nationally representative sample of about 5,000 persons each year. 15 counties are visited each year.

continued

TABLE 2-1 Continued

Survey and Agency	Relevant Information Collected	Design and Comments
	CAPI = computer-assisted personal interview ACASI = audio computer-assisted self-interview CDISC = computerized diagnostic interview schedule for children	
Youth Risk Behavior Surveillance System (YRBSS) Agency: National Center for Chronic Disease Prevention and Health Promotion (CDC)	Covers tobacco use, unhealthy dietary behaviors, inadequate physical activity, alcohol and other drug use, sexual behaviors that contribute to unintended pregnancy and sexually transmitted diseases, including HIV infection, behaviors that contribute to unintentional injuries and violence. No MEB disorders included.	Since 1990, monitors health risk behaviors using self-report questionnaires administered in school.
National Survey on Drug Use and Health (NSDUH) Agency: Office of Applied Studies, Substance Abuse and Mental Health Services Administration	Designed to produce drug and alcohol use incidence and prevalence estimates and report the consequences and patterns of use and abuse in the general U.S. civilian population ages 12 and older. Since 1994, questions added on mental health and access to care. Treatment for youth ages 12-17 is defined as receiving treatment or counseling for problems with behaviors or emotions from specific mental health or other health professionals in school, home, or from other outpatient or inpatient settings in the past year. A module on lifetime and past year prevalence of major depressive episode (MDE), severity of the MDE as measured by role impairments, and treatment for depression was administered to adults ages 18 or older and youth ages 12-17, from 2004 to 2006; 8.5% of youth had an episode of MDE in the past 12 months (see http://oas.samhsa.gov/2k8/youthDepress/youthDepress.pdf).	Running since 1988 (formerly National Household Survey on Drug Abuse). Extensive data on drug use, including age at first use, lifetime, annual, and past-month usage for alcohol, marijuana, cocaine (including crack), hallucinogens, heroin, inhalants, tobacco, pain relievers, tranquilizers, stimulants, and sedatives; substance abuse treatment history and DSM-IV diagnoses.

Monitoring the Future (MTF) Agency: National Institute on Drug Abuse	Has been collecting self-report anonymous data on drug use since 1975. Is able to show rise and fall of use of different drugs.	Ongoing study of the behaviors, attitudes, and values of U.S. secondary school students, college students, and young adults. Each year, ~50,000 8th, 10th, and 12th grade students are surveyed (12th graders since 1975 and 8th and 10th graders since 1991). Annual follow-up questionnaires mailed to a sample of each graduating class for several years.
National Survey of Children's Health Agency: Maternal and Child Health Bureau of the Health Resources and Services Administration	Questions asked for ADHD, depression, anxiety, oppositional defiant disorder, behavioral or conduct problems, autism, developmental delay, Tourette syndrome: Has a doctor or other health care provider ever told you that selected child (SC) had...? Does SC currently have...? Would you describe his/her ... as mild, moderate, or severe? In case of ADHD, a fourth question is asked: Is SC currently taking medication for ADD or ADHD? Results not yet published.	One-time survey (2007-2008) of ~86,000 children ages 0-17. Data collected from responsible adult by telephone.
National Children's Study Agency: National Institute for Child Health and Human Development	No information yet collected. So far, there is no planned collection of information on emotional or behavioral disorders.	Will examine the effects of environmental influences on the health and development of ~100,000 children across the United States from before birth until age 21. Congress authorized the National Children's Study with the Children's Health Act of 2000. Will take place in 105 representative counties around the United States. 1,000 mothers and their children will be recruited from each site and followed for 20 years.

Precise estimates of the size of the problem of MEB disorders of youth in the United States, or changes in the problem over time, require nationally representative population surveys that make valid and reliable diagnoses. However, as discussed below, the consensus from a large number of recent studies with smaller samples or from other countries provides a ballpark estimate.

PREVALENCE OF MENTAL, EMOTIONAL, AND BEHAVIORAL DISORDERS

Clinical psychiatry has mapped out a range of MEB disorders and related problems seen in children and adolescents. These are listed in the two main taxonomies of disease, the section on mental and behavioral disorders in the *International Statistical Classification of Diseases and Related Health Problems* (ICD) (World Health Organization, 1993) and the *Diagnostic and Statistical Manual of Mental Disorders*, 4th Edition (DSM-IV) (American Psychiatric Association, 1994). Some other major public health problems, like crime and violence, are subsumed within the diagnostic criteria for conduct disorder. The disorders examined in this chapter are those in the American Psychiatric Association's DSM-IV. The DSM-IV includes abuse of and dependence on alcohol and illicit drugs, as well as dependence on tobacco.

This section reviews current epidemiological information about the more common MEB disorders up to age 25: conduct disorder and oppositional defiant disorder, often combined as disruptive behavior disorders; attention deficit hyperactivity disorder (ADHD); anxiety disorders, including posttraumatic stress disorder; depression; and drug abuse and dependence. Disorders of low population frequency, with little reliable epidemiological data but considerable societal burden—such as autism spectrum disorders and pervasive developmental disorders, schizophrenia, bipolar disorder, eating disorders, and obsessive compulsive disorder—are discussed when information is available. More specific information may be available when the adolescent version of the NCS is published.

Table 2-2 presents the results of a meta-analysis of data on the prevalence of MEB disorders in young people from more than 50 community surveys from around the world, published in the past 15 years (updated from Costello, Mustillo, et al., 2004). The analysis controlled for sample size, number of prior months that subjects were asked about in reporting their symptoms, and age of participants. Not all studies report on all diagnoses. The table includes the 16 diagnoses or diagnostic groupings that were reported by at least 8 studies (number of studies shown in parentheses).

Figure 2-1 illustrates with a box-and-whisker plot the range of estimates from these surveys for each diagnosis. The ends of the "whiskers" for each

TABLE 2-2 Prevalence Estimates of Mental, Emotional, and Behavioral Disorders in Young People

Diagnosis or Diagnostic Group (N of studies contributing to estimate)	Prevalence (%)	Standard Error (%)	Lower 95%	Upper 95%
One or more disorders (44)	17.0	1.3	14.4	19.6
Unipolar depression (31)	5.2	0.7	4.0	7.0
Any anxiety disorder (29)	8.0	1.0	6.2	10.3
Generalized anxiety disorder (17)	1.3	0.3	0.9	2.0
Separation anxiety disorder (17)	4.1	0.9	2.6	9.4
Social phobia (15)	4.2	1.1	2.4	7.3
Specific phobia (13)	3.7	1.3	1.7	7.7
Panic (12)	0.7	0.2	0.3	1.5
Posttraumatic stress disorder (7)	0.6	0.2	0.3	1.1
Attention deficit hyperactivity disorder (34)	4.5	0.7	3.3	6.2
Any disruptive behavior disorder (23)	6.1	0.5	5.4	7.3
Conduct disorder (28)	3.5	0.5	2.7	4.7
Oppositional defiant disorder (21)	2.8	0.4	2.1	3.7
Substance use disorder (12)	10.3	2.2	6.3	16.2
Alcohol use disorder (9)	4.3	1.4	2.1	8.9

NOTE: The prevalence estimates from each study were transformed to logit scale and their standard errors computed using the available information about the sample size and prevalences. Using weights inversely proportional to estimated variances, weighted linear regression models were fit in SAS, using PROC GENMOD with study as a fixed effect (class variable). The overall estimate (on the logit scale) and its standard error were then used to recompute the overall prevalence and its standard error using the delta method.

SOURCE: Based on a meta-analysis for the committee by Alaattin Erkanli, Department of Biostatistics, Duke University. A list of the data sets used in the meta-analysis is in Appendix D, which is available online.

diagnosis show the highest and lowest estimates, and the upper and lower bounds of the box show the interquartile range of the estimates—that is, the 75th and 25th percentiles of the range of estimates. It shows estimates only for diagnoses reported by at least eight studies (number of studies shown in parentheses). The mean estimate for any diagnosis was 17.0 percent (standard error, SE, 1.3 percent) and the median 17.5 percent. The most common diagnostic group was substance abuse or dependence, including nicotine dependence (10.3 percent, SE 2.2 percent). Anxiety disorders were common (8.0 percent, SE 0.1 percent), followed by depressive disorders (5.2 percent, SE 0.07 percent) and ADHD (4.5 percent, SE 0.07 percent).

Some disorders, notably anxiety disorders, have a much wider range of estimates than others. The range of estimates for specific phobias was particularly broad. It is also noticeable that the top 25 percent of the range

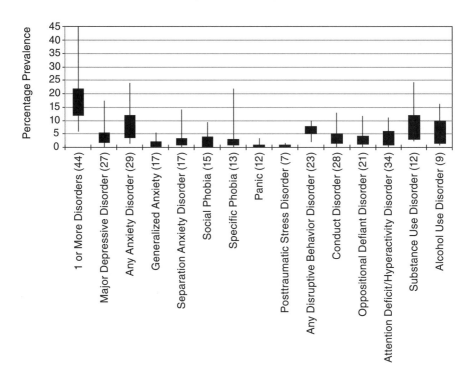

FIGURE 2-1 Ranges in data on the prevalence of mental, emotional, and behavioral disorders among young people.
NOTE: Lines represent the range of estimates from different studies. Boxes represent the interquartile range.
SOURCE: Based on a meta-analysis for the committee by Alaattin Erkanli, Department of Biostatistics, Duke University. A list of the data sets used in the meta-analysis is in Appendix B, which is available online.

of estimates is generally much wider than the lowest 25 percent range, indicating that a few studies tend to generate much higher estimates than do the majority. Several factors contribute to the variability in prevalence estimates: (1) changes in the taxonomy or definitions and criteria used for disorders in different versions of the DSM and the ICD, (2) the evolution of assessment tools over the past few decades, and (3) differences in the populations sampled and the inclusion and exclusion criteria used. For example, since different disorders have different onset ages (see the section on incidence below), samples with different age ranges will show different prevalence rates for many disorders. A fourth factor is that, in surveys of young people (but rarely in surveys of adults), it is normal to collect information from several informants: mothers, fathers, teachers, and children themselves. Each informant brings a unique view of the child, so the number and nature of informants affect the prevalence estimate.

Missing from both Table 2-2 and Figure 2-1 are some rare but often severe disorders; for example, schizophrenia, bipolar disorder, and pervasive developmental disorders. The reason is that studies to date have not been large or numerous enough to capture these rare disorders with any hope of accuracy. For example, the two studies that included schizophrenia had rates of 6 per 1,000 and 7 per 1,000, respectively (Wittchen, Essau, et al., 1992; Costello, Angold, et al., 1996). The three available estimates for adolescent bipolar disorder (two from the same study) fell between 1 and 3 per 1,000 (Lewinsohn, Rohde, et al., 1998; Costello, Angold, et al., 1996), although prevalence increases in young adulthood (Wittchen, Nelson, and Lachner, 1998). No population-based estimates are available for prepubertal bipolar disorder.

Despite the variability across studies, it is possible to draw some general observations about prevalence. The mean (17 percent) and median (17.5 percent) estimates for one or more MEB disorders were very close, with 50 percent of studies producing estimates between 12 and 22 percent, suggesting that this estimate is fairly reliable. The rank ordering of prevalence estimates for the different disorders was remarkably consistent across the individual studies. Of the diagnoses included in Figure 2-1, the lowest prevalence rates came from studies of younger children, especially those from Scandinavia, while the highest rates were reported from studies of young adults (ages 19-24). However, from the point of view of prevention, it should be noted that a review of studies of preschool children concluded that almost 20 percent of 2- to 5-year-olds had at least one DSM-IV disorder in the past three months (Egger and Angold, 2006), the same rate as seen in older children, adolescents, and young adults.

Within studies, after controlling for risk exposures that are often confounded with race/ethnicity, such as poverty (Costello, Compton, et al., 2003), parental incarceration (Phillips, Erkanli, et al., 2006), or migrant status (Bengi-Arslan, Verhulst, et al., 1997), similarities across different racial/ethnic groups are much more noticeable than are differences (Costello, Keeler, and Angold, 2001; Loeber, Farrington, et al., 2003). Disruptive behavior disorders (conduct disorder, oppositional defiant disorder), ADHD (Rutter, Caspi, and Moffitt, 2003), and substance use disorders (Wittchen, Nelson, and Lachner, 1998) tend to be more common in boys than girls, while the opposite is true of emotional disorders (depression, anxiety disorders). About half of the children with a diagnosis have a disorder that causes significant functional impairment—that is, a disorder that impedes their ability to function and develop appropriately in human relationships or in cognitive, social, or emotional development (Angold, Erkanli, et al., 2002; Costello, Angold, et al., 1996).

As noted earlier, no representative population surveys of rates of the full range of MEB disorders in children in the United States have been published, although results from a survey of 13- to 17-year-olds in the NCS will be published in 2009. The NSDUH, a household survey from the Substance Abuse and Mental Health Services Administration, includes adolescents ages 12 and over. In 2005 and 2006 it included a module on major depressive episodes and found that 8.8 percent (2005) and 7.9 percent (2006) of youth reported such an episode in the past 12 months.[1] NHANES has also begun to include selected modules addressing MEB disorders in young people, but no data have yet been published. In addition, more work is needed to expand epidemiological studies to include representative samples of all racial/ethnic groups in the United States, to control for socioeconomic confounds in such studies, and to develop international collaborations that provide comparisons among nations using comparable measures (see Heiervang, Goodman, and Goodman, 2008).

Cumulative Prevalence

Several longitudinal studies have calculated the proportion of the population that has received at least one diagnosis of a MEB disorder across repeated assessments, from childhood through adolescence and into early adulthood (Costello, Mustillo, et al., 2004). Jaffee and colleagues compared three such studies and found that between 37 and 39 percent of youth in the three studies had received one or more diagnoses between ages 9 and 16 (Jaffee, Harrington, et al., 2005). In later follow-ups of these studies, the cumulative prevalence rose to between 40 and 50 percent by age 21 (Arseneault, Moffitt, et al., 2000; Costello, Angold, et al., 1996). This is similar to a 46.4 percent lifetime prevalence rate based on retrospective data from the NCS of adults (Kessler, Berglund, et al., 2005). In the one study for which cumulative data are available by diagnosis (Costello, Angold, et al., 1996), rates of reporting one or more episodes of a disorder by age 21 were 16.4 percent for disruptive behavior disorders, 14.5 percent for anxiety disorders, and 10.4 percent for depressive disorders.

Comorbidity

Many children have more than one MEB disorder. Figure 2-2 summarizes the data from a meta-analysis of comorbidity among the major classes of disorder, after controlling for comorbidity between the comorbid condi-

---

[1]See http://oas.samhsa.gov/NSDUH/2k6nsduh/tabs/Sect6peTabs1to41.htm#Tab6.27B.

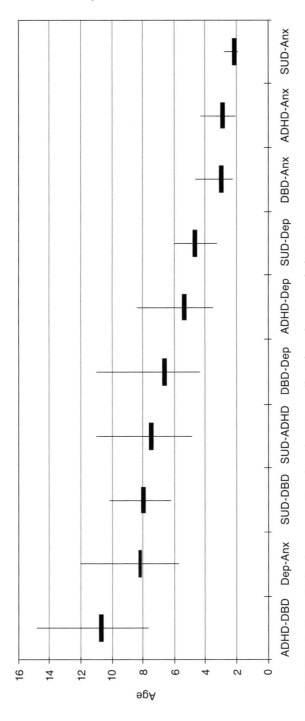

FIGURE 2-2 Comorbidity between major disorders (controlling for other comorbidities).
NOTE: ADHD = attention deficit hyperactivity disorder; Anx = anxiety; DBD = conduct disorder/oppositional defiant disorder; Dep = depression; SUD = substance use disorder. Bars represent odds ratios; lines represent 95 percent confidence intervals.
SOURCE: Adapted from Angold, Costello, and Erkanli (1999) and Armstrong and Costello (2002).

tion and other disorders. For example, it adjusts the comorbidity between anxiety and depression for comorbidity between anxiety and ADHD and depression and ADHD. As the figure demonstrates, comorbidity is widespread, and there are clear patterns; there is greater comorbidity among disruptive behavior disorders, ADHD, and substance abuse disorders, on one hand, and among the emotional disorders (anxiety and depression), than between emotional and disruptive behavioral disorders, on the other. Comorbidity remains high from early childhood (Egger, Erkanli, et al., 2006) through adolescence (Roberts, Roberts, and Xing, 2007) and into adulthood (Kessler, Chiu, et al., 2005).

In summary, there is consistent evidence from multiple recent studies that early MEB disorders should be considered as commonplace as a fractured limb: not inevitable but not at all unusual. The prevalence of these disorders is the same in young people as it is in adults. An implication for prevention is that universal programs will not be wasted on large numbers of risk-free children.

IS PREVALENCE INCREASING OR DECREASING?

Repeated surveys are needed to tell whether rates of any disorder are going up or down. For adults, a second NCS has recently been completed, and should provide some information for the population ages 18 and older. The one area of problem behavior in which data on trends in young people are available is alcohol and other drug use and abuse. Three national surveys—NSDUH, the Youth Risk Behavior Surveillance System, and MTF—regularly measure alcohol and drug use and abuse in young people. All restrict their data collection to adolescents (12 and over for NSDUH, 8th, 10th, and 12th grade students for MTF). MTF tends to produce slightly higher estimates than NSDUH; however, they are remarkably consistent in their reports of trends, which show a clear reduction in use across nearly all categories between 2002 and 2007 (see http://oas.samhsa. gov/NSDUH/2k6NSDUH/2k6results.cfm#Tab9-1).

Reviews or meta-analyses have used cross-sectional studies conducted at different periods, together with the small longitudinal data sets available, to put together a picture over time (Collishaw, Maughan, et al., 2004; Costello, Foley, and Angold, 2006). Evidence of this sort has produced two fairly clear conclusions: there has been an increase in disruptive behavior symptoms over the past few decades (Collishaw, Maughan, et al., 2004), whereas there is no evidence for a similar increase in child or adolescent depression (Costello, Erkanli, and Angold, 2006). The question of whether the prevalence of autism has increased (Fombonne, 2005) is fraught with problems of broadening of the diagnostic category, heightened public awareness, and more attention from clinicians (Schechter and Grether, 2008). The same is true of

ADHD and juvenile onset bipolar disorder (Moreno, Laje, et al., 2007). It is certainly the case that more young people are being given these diagnoses.

INCIDENCE OF MENTAL, EMOTIONAL, AND BEHAVIORAL DISORDERS

To estimate the incidence, or number of new cases, in a given period of time, it is necessary to make repeated estimates in the *same* representative population sample, excluding those who had the disorder at the previous assessment. The same lack of basic data from repeated, representative sampling hampers the ability to answer questions about incidence. However, in this case, some of the small community-based longitudinal studies can provide data about incidence of the more common disorders. For example, data on 1,420 youth ages 9-21, over a 14-year period, from the Great Smoky Mountains Study (GSMS), a community study from the southeastern United States, shows a mean annual incidence rate of any disorder of around 3.5 percent in this age group. Of the 55 percent of youth in this community sample who had MEB disorders in one or more years of assessment, more than half (57.2 percent) had a diagnosis at two or more assessments, indicating that, in the majority of cases, the disorder was not confined to a single episode (Costello, Angold, et al., 1996).

A related issue relevant to prevention is the age at onset of child and adolescent emotional or behavioral disorders. In the NCS and NCS-R studies of adults, which ask people with a lifetime history of mental illness to remember their age at the first episode, half of all adults report onset in childhood or adolescence; the NCS-R found that in a population sample ages 18 and older, "half of all lifetime cases start by age 14 years and three fourths by age 24 years" (p. 593). Similarly, as noted earlier, in the GSMS, 55 percent of participants had been diagnosed with at least one MEB disorder by age 21 (see also Kim-Cohen, Caspi, et al., 2003).

Age at Onset

Figure 2-3 shows the age at onset of the first symptom in youth from the GSMS sample who would eventually receive a diagnosis by age 21, as well as the age at onset of the full-blown disorder. Disruptive behavioral disorders and ADHD had the earliest onset, followed by emotional disorders (anxiety and depressive disorders). Although many adolescents began using alcohol and other illicit drugs in their early teens, they tended not to meet criteria for abuse or dependence until their late teens.

Epidemiological findings like these raise questions of the utmost importance for prevention. If at least half of those who will have an MEB disorder during their lives have onset in childhood, then prevention resources need

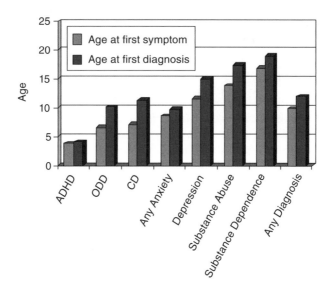

FIGURE 2-3 Age at onset of first symptom and of full psychiatric disorder, by age 21: Data from Great Smoky Mountains Study.
NOTE: First symptom = age at first symptom in youth who at some point received this diagnosis. First diagnosis = age when subject reported the minimum number of symptoms for this diagnosis.
SOURCE: Costello, Angold, et al. (1996).

to be focused on this period of life. In addition to universal prevention programs, Figure 2-3 suggests that there may be a window of opportunity lasting two to four years between the first symptom and the full-blown disorder, when preventive programs might be able to reduce the rate of onset of specific disorders. Recently developed measures (Egger and Angold, 2006) now make it possible to identify children with symptoms of several disorders at an early stage. In addition, developmentally informed interventions that aim at known antecedent risk factors during childhood and early adolescence can provide important opportunities for prevention.

Is Incidence Increasing or Decreasing?

To determine whether the number of new cases is rising or falling over time, it is important to distinguish between incident (new) cases and newly referred or treated cases. For example, according to one survey of clinical referrals, the number of children and adolescents in the United States treated for bipolar disorder increased 40-fold from 1994 to 2003, to about

1 percent of the population under age 20 (Moreno, Laje, et al., 2007). In contrast, the three studies that have assessed rates of mental illness across time in the general population found a prevalence of bipolar disorder of between 1 and 3 per 1,000 children, with no increase over the past two decades (Lewinsohn, Rohde, et al., 1998; Costello, Angold, et al., 1996). The reason for this discrepancy between epidemiological and clinical data may arise from the increased use of psychopharmacological treatments for children. The availability of a treatment may encourage clinicians to make a diagnosis and parents to seek professional help. Thus, the advent of a new drug or greater willingness of parents to bring their children for treatment can greatly increase the number of children seen by professionals, while the baseline prevalence of the disease in the population may remain unchanged.

In order to find out whether population incidence and prevalence are changing we need several longitudinal studies covering different time periods, so that new case rates can be calculated for different historical periods. National surveys like MTF make it possible to chart, for example, the rise and fall of alcohol and cocaine use by adolescents (Banken, 2004). Data like these are not available for other MEB disorders. Although a variety of federal agencies are making efforts to monitor mental, emotional, or behavioral problems, with the exception of substance use disorders, these efforts have not yet produced the repeated estimates over time necessary to plot the rise and fall of disease prevalence and the effects of interventions.

FACTORS AFFECTING PREVALENCE AND INCIDENCE

In the language of infectious disease epidemiology, it is possible to talk about various pathogens as "causes" of disease. Epidemiology invented the term "risk factors" in the 1950s when the Framingham Heart Study showed that cardiovascular disease did not have a single cause but many different factors contributing to increased risk, no single factor being either necessary or sufficient. MEB disorders seem to have more in common with chronic diseases like cardiovascular disease than with infectious diseases, in having multiple risk factors.

A mountain of research on environmental risk and protective factors for MEB disorders in young people has identified a large number of predictors, from internal (e.g., intellectual ability, brain development) to familial, educational, communal, and national (see also Chapter 4). Several theorists have developed multilevel risk models that predict complex interactions among the various levels of risk and protection. As with the prevalence and incidence of disorders, the prevalence and incidence of risk factors vary across the nation and at different developmental stages. To take a single example, data from the 2000 decennial census show that the proportion of families living in poverty in 2004 varied from 5.3 percent in Minnesota to 17.6 percent in Mississippi.

In order to focus prevention efforts most effectively, it is essential to know when vulnerability to an emotional or behavioral disorder increases simply with an increasing number of risk factors, irrespective of their nature, and when increased risk follows specific risk exposures. (Of course, both may occur at the same time.) We illustrate how both aspects of risk come into play with data from over 6,000 assessments of 1,420 youth from the GSMS. On one hand, there was a clear relationship between total risk exposure, using a list of over 80 risk factors, and MEB disorders. Rates of nearly all of these disorders were three or more times higher in the highest risk group than in the lowest risk group, irrespective of the type of risk.

On the other hand, when the question of specific risk factors for specific disorders was examined in the same data set, both general and disease-specific risk factors emerged (Shanahan and Hofer, 2005). Parental unemployment and maternal depression were associated with increased risk for most MEB disorders, but the analyses revealed "signature sets" of factors associated only with certain diagnoses. For example, while sexual abuse, poor parental supervision, and deviant peers were risk factors for both conduct disorder and oppositional defiant disorder, parental depression and loss of close relations and friends were specific to conduct disorder in these analyses. In the emotional disorders, parental depression was a specific risk for depression but was not associated with any anxiety disorders, whereas parental drug use and unemployment were associated with anxiety disorders but not with depression (see also Chapter 4).

The role of individual differences in genetic makeup has been the focus of intensive study in recent decades (see Chapter 5). Twin and adoption studies have identified a genetic component of risk for most child and adolescent psychiatric[2] disorders (Rutter, Silberg, et al., 1999a, 1999b), and genetic research in psychiatry began with the hypothesis that genes "cause" mental illness (Kendler, 2005). However, with the exception of a number of rare disorders, such as Williams syndrome, Turner syndrome, fragile X syndrome, and velocardiofacial syndrome (Davies, Isles, and Wilkinson, 2001; Inoue and Lupski, 2003; Thapar and Stergiakouli, 2008) so far no unequivocal candidate genes for specific mental, emotional, or behavioral disorders in children or adults have survived the test of replication in multiple studies (Joober, Sengupta, and Boksa, 2005; Thapar and Stergiakouli, 2008). There are some indications that variations in specific genes may contribute to such disorders as depression (Levinson, 2006; Lopez-Leon, Janssens, et al., 2008).

---

[2]The term "psychiatric" rather than "mental, emotional, or behavioral" is used here as that is the term used by the authors.

Current efforts focus on the search for genes that influence underlying processes, such as threat appraisal or risk aversion, that may be common to more than one mental, emotional, or behavioral disorder. More recently, genetic approaches are also being used to map out the role of environmental factors in the etiology of MEB disorders in people with different genetic profiles; that is, the extent to which (1) a disorder occurs in the presence of a given risk factor only in those with a specific genetic trait or (2) genetic effects on environmental exposure increase risk of a disorder.

As discussed in Chapter 5, continued research may make it possible to identify and target the most genetically vulnerable children for prevention interventions. Also, identifying gene variants that are associated with MEB disorders may eventually lead to prevention approaches based on modifying components of the pathways from genes to behaviors. However, the focus of prevention for the foreseeable future will still be on psychosocial interventions that change environmental risk factors. Research on signature sets of risk factors suggests that it may also be possible to target prevention efforts for some disorders to youth with high levels of signature risk for that disorder, potentially including both environmental and genetic factors. There is also an argument to be made for paying attention to risk factors, like maternal depression or family disruption, that affect multiple types of MEB disorders (see Chapter 4).

Are Rates of Causal Factors Increasing or Decreasing?

There is, of course, no simple answer to this question. National surveys and databases can be helpful in monitoring some of the epidemiological factors thought to be associated with emotional or behavioral disorders. For example:

- Low birth weight and other perinatal hazards may be increasing in the United States because of the increasing number of births from in vitro fertilization, the increasing age of women at first birth, and other factors. The proportion of newborns under 2,500 grams rose by more than 20 percent between 1980 and 2005.[3]
- Family poverty fell in the 1990s but has been level since then (according to the 2000 U.S. census).
- Divorce rates have fallen since their peak in the 1980s (U.S. census).
- Single-parent households have risen steadily, especially since the 1970s (U.S. census).

---

[3]See http://www.cdc.gov/media/pressrel/r061121.htm?s_cid=mediarel_r061121_x.

However, unless these changes can be linked with outcomes in specific data sets, the causal links remain very weak. Countries that maintain national databases on illness, crime, and household structure are beginning to use record linkage to monitor changes in risk exposure, but this is not possible in the United States.

High Risk of Some Sociodemographic Groups for Specific Disorders

It appears that boys are more vulnerable to disorders with early onset, such as developmental disabilities, autism, disruptive behavior disorders, and ADHD (Rutter, Caspi, and Moffit, 2003). After puberty, several divergences appear. Depression and anxiety increase markedly in girls but not in boys (Rutter, Caspi, and Moffitt, 2003). Substance abuse develops faster in boys than girls, and behavioral disorders remain higher in boys (Rutter, Caspi, and Moffitt, 2003). However, sex differences can vary depending on how a disorder or its consequences are defined. For example, the DSM-IV diagnosis "conduct disorder" is not much more common in boys than girls, but boys are increasingly more likely than girls to be arrested, charged with an offense, convicted, and incarcerated (Copeland, Miller-Johnson, et al., 2007). Similarly, conduct disorder is equally common in African American and Hispanic youth, controlling for socioeconomic status and rural/urban residence (Angold, Erkanli, et al., 2002), but arrests, criminal charges, and convictions are more common in African American youth (U.S. Public Health Service, 2001c). Even in urban settings, after controlling for socioeconomic status, delinquency rates were similar in three urban and African American samples (Loeber, Wei, et al., 1999), perhaps due to the tendency for poor African American youth to be concentrated in urban ghettos (Sampson, Raudenbush, and Earls, 1997).

CONCLUSIONS AND RECOMMENDATIONS

Epidemiology provides the basic information needed to establish the size and community burden of MEB disorders and to track the effectiveness (and cost-effectiveness) of large-scale preventive interventions. To carry out this task, a nation needs to be able to monitor the changing rates of risk exposure and illness in the population as a whole, at different developmental stages, and also in minority groups that may have different patterns of risk. Based on an amalgam of small surveys, about one in five or six young people has one or more recent MEB disorders. Retrospective studies of adults show that half or more had their first episode as a child, adolescent, or young adult. The first symptoms of most disorders precede onset of the full-blown condition by several years, so the opportunity exists for preventive intervention.

Conclusion: Mental, emotional, and behavioral disorders are as common among young people as among adults. The majority of adults with a mental, emotional, or behavioral disorder first experienced a disorder while young, and first symptoms precede the full-blown disorder, providing an opportunity for prevention and early intervention.

As discussed in more detail in Chapter 9, MEB disorders impose a heavy national burden of disability. Early emotional and behavioral problems predict school failure, unplanned pregnancy, and crime. MEB disorders are not well tracked by the mortality statistics that are among the few monitoring tools available in the United States. Other tools are needed, including regular household surveys and surveys of institutions, such as hospitals and prisons, where rates of mental illness are high. The United States supports several household and school-based surveys suitable for this purpose. Although these provide very detailed coverage of drug use and abuse, they have many limitations in the area of mental illness, particularly for younger populations, and they are sketchy in their measurement of risk. Data specific to the United States come from a patchwork of small, local studies.

Conclusion: Although the United States collects rich data related to drug use and abuse, systematic data related to the prevalence and incidence of mental, emotional, and behavioral disorders in young people are sparse.

It is notable that the Foundation for Child Development's annual Child Well-Being Index,[4] which has been charting trends in child well-being since 1975, because data are not available, includes only one measure related to MEB disorders: the teenage suicide rate. Similarly, given the limitations of available data, the only national indicators related to MEB disorders reported by the federal Forum on Child and Family Statistics[5] are alcohol and drug use and the percentage of children ages 4-17 reported by their parent as having serious emotional or behavioral difficulties.[6] The forum is planning to add an indicator related to adolescent depression using data collected in NSDUH.

Recommendation 2-1: The U.S. Department of Health and Human Services should be required to provide (1) annual data on the prevalence of

---

[4]See http://www.soc.duke.edu/~cwi/.

[5]See http://www.childstats.gov/americaschildren/index.asp.

[6]The indicator is based on a parental response to one question from the Strengths and Difficulties Questionnaire and does not provide information about any diagnosis.

MEB disorders in young people, using an accepted current taxonomy (e.g., the *Diagnostic and Statistical Manual of Mental Disorders*, the *International Statistical Classification of Diseases*) and (2) data that can provide indicators and trends for key risk and protective factors that serve as significant predictors for such disorders.

Methods for collecting such data should:

- be capable of providing reliable prevalence estimates for minority populations and high-risk groups (e.g., incarcerated youth, foster children, immigrant children, youth with chronic diseases, children with developmental delays);
- be capable of providing accurate estimates at the level of individual states, ideally with unique identifiers that would facilitate the use of data by local communities and potential linkage with other state databases, such as those created as part of the No Child Left Behind Act of 2001; and
- include measurement of identified risk and protective factors, either directly or by building links to appropriate databases (e.g., parental death, foster care placement, divorce, incarceration).

As illustrated in Table 2-1, multiple agencies of the U.S. Department of Health and Human Services (HHS) administer surveys that collect data related to MEB disorders. The Centers for Disease Control and Prevention, which has public health surveillance and prevention within its mandate and administers several major surveys potentially relevant to this task, is one possible lead agency for the collection of prevalence and incidence data. Similarly, the Substance Abuse and Mental Health Services Administration is the lead federal agency charged with "building resilience and facilitating recovery" in relation to substance abuse and mental disorders. It has recently expanded its population survey, NSDUH, beyond substance abuse, making it another potential option. However, while a specific agency may need to be identified to provide data on the prevalence and incidence of disorders, inclusion of data related to risk and protective factors is likely to require the involvement and input of multiple HHS agencies, making this a departmental responsibility. The Office of Disease Prevention and Health Promotion and the Office of the Assistant Secretary for Planning and Evaluation, both in the Office of the Secretary, would potentially be able to serve a coordinating function.

Young people with MEB disorders tend to receive care from a wide range of service providers and agencies, including the child welfare, education, and juvenile justice systems, as well as primary medical and specialty mental health care providers. Very little is known about the adequacy of this patchwork of care. Under its statutory mandate, the Substance Abuse and Mental Health Services Administration (SAMHSA) must provide national data on mental health and substance abuse treatment services and on persons with mental and substance use disorders. This mandate includes the determination of the national incidence and prevalence of the various forms of mental disorder and substance abuse, as well as characteristics of treatment programs.

SAMHSA has focused much of its efforts on specialty providers and services supported through state substance abuse and mental health agencies. However, nontraditional settings, such as jails, prisons, schools, and general hospitals, are becoming increasingly important as sites of care for youth with MEB disorders. Exclusion of other settings in which young people often receive care provides a misleading and incomplete picture of service use.

Recommendation 2-2: The Substance Abuse and Mental Health Services Administration should expand its current data collection to include measures of service use across multiple agencies that work with vulnerable populations of young people.

The Centers for Medicare and Medicaid Services (CMS) and programs funded by CMS collect information on use of Medicaid-funded services for prevention and treatment. These data could provide a rich set of information on trends in utilization of services across various health care providers. Analysis of these data in conjunction with the above prevalence and service use data, with appropriate privacy protections, could provide additional insights.

3

Defining the Scope of Prevention

This chapter provides a framework for the report by addressing the conceptual and definitional issues that are fundamental to understanding the scientific study of prevention. Discussed first are issues in defining the domain of prevention research. While the boundaries between prevention and other concerns, especially treatment, are sometimes difficult to draw, making these distinctions is critical for establishing the scope of the committee's work.

In this report, prevention is seen as distinct from treatment, but complementary in a common goal of reducing the burden of mental, emotional, and behavioral (MEB) disorders on the healthy development of children and young people. By contrast, health promotion, which some consider as separate from prevention, is viewed by the committee as so closely related that it should be considered a component of prevention. Prevention and health promotion both focus on changing common influences on the development of children and adolescents in order to aid them in functioning well in meeting life's tasks and challenges and remaining free of cognitive, emotional, and behavioral problems that would impair their functioning.

ISSUES IN DEFINING PREVENTION

Definitional issues have been much discussed since the earliest efforts to bring preventive approaches to the field of mental health and substance abuse. *Reducing Risks for Mental Disorders: Frontiers for Preventive Intervention Research*, the 1994 Institute of Medicine (IOM) report, included an extensive discussion of alternative approaches, including consideration of the implications of alternative definitions for prevention research and practice. The report argued that "without a system for classifying specific interventions, there is no way to obtain accurate information on the type or extent of current activities, . . . and no way to ensure that prevention researchers, practitioners, and policy makers are speaking the same language" (Institute of Medicine, 1994, p. 24).

Early Frameworks

Preventive approaches to MEB disorders have been proposed as a complementary approach to the treatment services that have long been society's dominant approach to reducing their burden on the population. Treatment services, regardless of their variation in content, share the common features that people are identified (either by themselves or by others) as currently suffering from a recognizable disorder, and they enter treatment with the expectation of receiving some form of relief from the disorder. Prevention is a complementary approach in which services are offered to the general population or to people who are identified as being at risk for a disorder, and they receive services with the expectation that the likelihood of a future disorder will be reduced.

Developing definitions that clearly discriminate different types of prevention from each other and prevention from treatment is fraught with difficulty. Caplan's (1964) application of the concepts of primary, secondary, and tertiary prevention, which are common in a public health context, had an important influence in developing early prevention models. Cowen (1977, 1980) later found that much of what was labeled as primary prevention did not meet any rigorous standards for such a definition. He suggested two criteria for primary prevention efforts: (1) that they be intentionally designed to reduce dysfunction or promote health before the onset of disorder and (2) that they be population focused, targeted either to the whole population or to subgroups with known vulnerabilities.

From a developmental perspective, however, many MEB disorders are risk factors for later disorders or disability, so all treatment could potentially be labeled as prevention. Gordon (1983) noted that distinctions between prevention and treatment are often based more on historical than on rational or scientific reasons. He reserved the term "prevention" for services for those individuals who were identified as not "suffering from any discomfort or disability from the disease or disorder to be prevented." Thus the category of tertiary prevention proposed by Caplan (1964), which referred to the prevention of disability for those suffering from disorders, was excluded.

Gordon (1983) proposed an alternative threefold classification of prevention based on the costs and benefits of delivering the intervention to the targeted population. *Universal prevention* includes strategies that can be offered to the full population, based on the evidence that it is likely to provide some benefit to all (reduce the probability of disorder), which clearly outweighs the costs and risks of negative consequences. *Selective prevention* refers to strategies that are targeted to subpopulations identified as being at elevated risk for a disorder. *Indicated prevention* includes strategies that are targeted to individuals who are identified (or individually screened) as having an increased vulnerability for a disorder based on some individual assessment but who are currently asymptomatic. Selective and indicated prevention strategies might involve more intensive interventions and thus involve greater cost to the participants, since their risk and thus potential benefit from participation would be greater.

The 1994 IOM Framework

The 1994 IOM report *Reducing Risks for Mental Disorders: Frontiers for Preventive Intervention Research* emphasized the importance of putting prevention into a broader context, which includes not only treatment but also maintenance interventions when continued care is indicated (Institute of Medicine, 1994). Treatment was distinguished by two features: "(1) case identification and (2) standard treatment for the known disorder, which includes interventions to reduce the likelihood of future co-occurring disorders" (Institute of Medicine, 1994, p. 23). The features of maintenance were "(1) the patient's compliance with long-term treatment to reduce relapse and recurrence and (2) the provision of after-care services to the patient, including rehabilitation" (Institute of Medicine, 1994, p. 24).

The term "prevention" was reserved for interventions designed to reduce the occurrence of new cases. While noting that neither the Gordon framework (universal, selective, and indicated prevention) nor the public health framework (primary, secondary, and tertiary prevention) was specifically developed for mental health, a modified version of the Gordon approach was adopted. The defining feature for classifying preventive interventions was the population that was targeted. Similar to that of Gordon, the 1994 IOM report's rationale for targeting a type of intervention either universally or to a high-risk subgroup was that the potential benefit was substantially higher than the cost and the risk of negative effects. The concepts of universal and selective prevention were essentially the same as in Gordon's system. The concept of indicated prevention was modified to include interventions targeted to high-risk individuals who do not meet diagnostic criteria for a disorder but who have detectable markers that warn of its onset.

The 1994 IOM report acknowledged that some people in the groups targeted for universal, selective, or indicated preventive interventions may have mental disorders when the intervention begins. However, if they are selected into the intervention on the basis of being in a high-risk group (selective) or for having early symptoms (indicated), then the intervention is considered preventive. The report also acknowledged that good treatment should often include preventive elements to reduce the likelihood of relapse or of disability, but it emphasized that interventions selected on the basis of an existing disorder should be considered treatment rather than prevention.

Recent Definitional Debates

A significant modification of the classification system developed in the 1994 IOM report was proposed by the National Advisory Mental Health Council (NAMHC) Workgroup on Mental Disorders Prevention Research (1998). This report argued that the IOM system was too narrow because it excluded "all individuals with full-blown disorder" (National Advisory Mental Health Council Workgroup on Mental Disorders Prevention Research, 1998, p. 16). The workgroup recommended expanding the definition of preventive intervention research to include (National Advisory Mental Health Council Workgroup on Mental Disorders Prevention Research, 1998, p. 18):

> trials involving participants who (1) have no current symptoms of mental disorder and were never symptomatic; (2) have current sub-clinical symptoms; (3) have a currently diagnosed disorder and/or were previously symptomatic—for them the emphasis is on prevention of relapse or recurrence; or (4) have a currently diagnosed disorder, with the emphasis on prevention of comorbidity or disability.

Despite the broadening of the definition of prevention, the report specifically stated that the expanded research agenda "does not represent a decreased commitment to preventing mental disorders in people currently without symptoms or those who have never been mentally ill" (National Advisory Mental Health Council Workgroup on Mental Disorders Prevention Research, 1998, p. 20).

Comments on the report proposed that the broadened definition had several problems. One concern was that it failed to make distinctions between prevention and treatment, and therefore all treatment could essentially be considered prevention (Greenberg and Weissberg, 2001). Another concern was that the potential relabeling of treatment studies as prevention could dilute resources for prevention research for populations without a diagnosed disorder (Shinn and Toohey, 2001; Heller, 2001; Reiss, 2001). Despite criticisms of the broadened definition, others noted that regardless of where the line between prevention and treatment is drawn, benefits could be gained from closer integration of prevention and treatment research, so that methodological advances in one area could be applied to the other (Pearson and Koretz, 2001). Similarly, it was suggested that a more unified approach to improving the public health could be developed with interventions that incorporate elements of targeted screening and treatment in a broader preventive approach (Weisz, Sandler, et al., 2005; Brown and Liao, 1999).

Recently, a related health care concept—personalized medicine—has emerged. The adjectives "predictive," "preventive," and "preemptive" are frequently attached to this concept (Zerhouni, 2006), suggesting that prediction based on early information about an individual can lead to the avoidance of disorder, a form of prevention. Personalized medicine was spawned in large part by new and enabling technologies of genomic analysis and involves the use of information about individual-level risks, including genetic or other biomarkers, to identify and intervene in incipient medical disorders. This concept can and has been applied to prevention and preemption of MEB disorders. While equating it with indicated and selective prevention, Insel (2008) termed this approach "preemptive psychiatry," positing that it offers the greatest potential for the prevention of both physical and mental disorders. The committee views this concept to be a promising dimension of indicated prevention, but as only one component of a broader spectrum of needed approaches.

As discussed in Chapter 5, there have been substantial developments in identifying genetic and epigenetic information that may contribute to MEB disorders, as well as increased recognition that environmental exposures, particularly during early development, can interact with genetic characteristics to affect gene expression. Similarly, as discussed in Chapter 4, a variety of adverse childhood events, such as early trauma (Anda, Brown, et al., 2007) and other family and community adversities, have been associated with later adverse mental, emotional, and behavioral outcomes. This information is beginning to be used in predictive models for physical as well as MEB disorders; for example, as discussed later in this report, its application to potential indicated prevention of schizophrenia is very promising.

However, this approach is in its early stages and likely to evolve over the next decade or two. Before preemptive psychiatry based primarily on genetic information can be considered ready for widespread implementation, a number of substantial hurdles and risks to implementation must be recognized and addressed, such as the issues of creating a "genetic underclass" and differential access to health care and psychopharmacologies (Evans, 2007). More fundamentally, understanding of the causal role of genetic contributors to MEB disorders must be substantially improved. The committee's call for collaborations between prevention scientists and clinical developmental neuroscientists is aimed at better understanding causality and the moderating genetic or environmental factors associated with mental, emotional, and behavioral outcomes.

The public health perspective endorsed by the committee also mandates that prevention not be limited only to those at imminent risk. Indeed, the mandate of agencies such as the National Institute of Mental Health (NIMH) and the Substance Abuse and Mental Health Services Administration (SAMHSA) calls for a broader approach. For example, the ADAMHA Reorganization Act, which created both, states that the research program at NIMH "shall be designed to further the treatment and prevention of mental illness, the promotion of mental health, and the study of the psychological, social, and legal factors that influence behavior." Similarly, the Center for Mental Health Services at SAMHSA is directed to establish national priorities for the prevention of mental illness and the promotion of mental health.

These mandates suggest a broad-based prevention approach that includes a balance between approaches aimed at those at imminent risk, those at elevated risk, and those who currently appear risk free but for whom specific interventions have been demonstrated to reduce future risk. As Chapter 2 emphasized, the prevalence of MEB disorders among young people suggests that few are entirely risk free. Furthermore, as outlined in this report, a substantial body of research established over the past several decades supports the efficacy or effectiveness of universal and selective interventions, particularly for behavioral disorders. A balance of universal, selective, and indicated prevention research and implementation is needed to address the mental, emotional, and behavioral needs of young people. Consistent with the agencies' legislative mandates, targeted attention is also needed to approaches that can promote mental health, regardless of whether a specific disorder is being prevented.

THE CURRENT APPROACH

The classification system used to define the boundaries of prevention and prevention research is critical for assessing the degree to which prevention research and services are being used along with treatment strategies as part of a public health approach to reduce the burden of MEB disorders in the population. And indeed, a variety of approaches have been proposed. The committee recognizes that it may be difficult in some cases to distinguish different prevention approaches from each other or even to identify clear boundaries between prevention and treatment. We also appreciate the importance of treatment, including its preventive aspects in terms of reducing the likelihood and severity of future problems. Interventions to prevent disability, comorbidity, or relapse are clearly important.

However, the committee thinks that these are aspects of quality treatment and are distinct from, though complementary to, prevention, concurring with the perspective in the 1994 IOM report. We also conclude that the progress made since 1994, as outlined in this report, supports continued focus of prevention resources prior to the onset of disorders. We share the concerns, raised by the 1994 IOM committee and commentators on the NAMHC approach, that an overly inclusive definition of prevention research could dilute resources for interventions designed to prevent the onset of disorder and "often underlies a neglect of interventions to reduce risks" (Institute of Medicine, 1994, p. 28).

Therefore, in this report, the committee has adopted the definitions of prevention developed in the 1994 IOM report, along with the distinctions between prevention and treatment. This report focuses on preventive interventions that target multiple populations whose levels of risk vary, but that are not identified on the basis of having a disorder. As discussed below, however, the committee broadened the conceptualization of mental health to include both the prevention of disorders and the promotion of mental health (see Box 3-1).

RECONSIDERING MENTAL HEALTH PROMOTION

Mental health promotion is characterized by a focus on well-being rather than prevention of illness and disorder, although it may also decrease the likelihood of disorder. The 1994 IOM report included a general call for assessment of outcomes of mental health promotion activities. It also acknowledged that health is more than just the absence of disease and that the goals and methods of prevention and promotion overlap, but it concluded that the evidence of effectiveness of mental health promotion was sparse, particularly in comparison to that for prevention.

At this point in time, this committee views the situation differently. There is agreement that mental health promotion can be distinguished from prevention of mental disorders by its focus on healthy outcomes, such as competence and well-being, and that many of these outcomes are intrinsically valued in their own right (e.g., prosocial involvement, spirituality: Catalano, Berglund, et al., 2004; social justice: Sandler, 2007). As stated in the Report of the Surgeon General's Conference on Children's Mental Health (U.S. Public Health Service, 2000), "Mental health is a critical component of children's learning and general health. Fostering social and emotional health in children as part of healthy child development must therefore be a national priority" (p. 3). There is also increasing evidence that promotion of positive aspects of mental health is an important approach to reducing MEB disorders and related problems as well (National Research Council and Institute of Medicine, 2002; Catalano, Berglund, et al., 2002, 2004; Commission on Positive Youth Development, 2005). These developments have led the committee to conclude that mental health promotion should

BOX 3-1
Definitions of Promotion and Prevention Interventions

Mental health promotion interventions: Usually targeted to the general public or a whole population. Interventions aim to enhance individuals' ability to achieve developmentally appropriate tasks (competence) and a positive sense of self-esteem, mastery, well-being, and social inclusion, and strengthen their ability to cope with adversity.

> **Example:** Programs based in schools, community centers, or other community-based settings that promote emotional and social competence through activities emphasizing self-control and problem solving.

Universal preventive interventions: Targeted to the general public or a whole population that has not been identified on the basis of individual risk. The intervention is desirable for everyone in that group. Universal interventions have advantages when their costs per individual are low, the intervention is effective and acceptable to the population, and there is a low risk from the intervention.

> **Example:** School-based programs offered to all children to teach social and emotional skills or to avoid substance abuse. Programs offered to all parents of sixth graders to provide them with skills to communicate to their children about resisting substance use.

Selective preventive interventions: Targeted to individuals or a population subgroup whose risk of developing mental disorders is significantly higher than average. The risk may be imminent or it may be a lifetime risk. Risk groups may be identified on the basis of biological, psychological, or social risk factors that are known to be associated with the onset of a mental, emotional, or behavioral disorder. Selective interventions are most appropriate if their cost is moderate and if the risk of negative effects is minimal or nonexistent.

> **Example:** Programs offered to children exposed to risk factors, such as parental divorce, parental mental illness, death of a close relative, or abuse, to reduce risk for adverse mental, emotional, and behavioral outcomes.

Indicated preventive interventions: Targeted to high-risk individuals who are identified as having minimal but detectable signs or symptoms foreshadowing mental, emotional, or behavioral disorder, or biological markers indicating predisposition for such a disorder, but who do not meet diagnostic levels at the current time. Indicated interventions might be reasonable even if intervention costs are high and even if the intervention entails some risk.

> **Example:** Interventions for children with early problems of aggression or elevated symptoms of depression or anxiety.

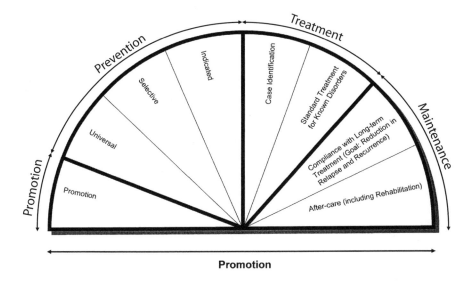

Promotion

FIGURE 3-1 Mental health intervention spectrum.
SOURCE: Adapted from Institute of Medicine (1994, p. 23).

be recognized as an important component of the mental health intervention spectrum, which can serve as a foundation for both prevention and treatment of disorders (see Figure 3-1).

For purposes of this report, the committee has adopted a definition of mental health promotion that is consistent with concepts described in prior reports in the United States (e.g., Substance Abuse and Mental Health Services Administration, 2007a) and used in international contexts (e.g., World Health Organization, 2004; Jané-Llopis and Anderson, 2005):

> Mental health promotion includes efforts to enhance individuals' ability to achieve developmentally appropriate tasks (developmental competence) and a positive sense of self-esteem, mastery, well-being, and social inclusion and to strengthen their ability to cope with adversity.

Inclusion of promotion activities is an important conceptual shift for the field. For the past decade, various prevention researchers have argued for a synthesis of prevention and promotion approaches (Greenberg, Weissberg, et al., 2003; Catalano, Hawkins, et al., 2002; Cowen, 2000; Weissberg and Greenberg, 1998; Durlak and Wells, 1997). Greenberg and colleagues (2003) have maintained that "problem prevention programs are most beneficial when they are coordinated with explicit attempts to enhance [young people's] competence, connections to others and contributions to their community" (p. 427). In the context of youth development, Pittman argued for an increased focus on promotion nearly two decades ago, saying the field needs to move "from thinking that youth problems are merely the principal barriers to youth development to thinking that youth development serves as the most effective strategy for the prevention of youth problems" (Pittman and Fleming, 1991).

In practice there is already considerable overlap between prevention and promotion. Meta-analytic and qualitative reviews of preventive intervention studies demonstrate that many psychosocial prevention programs involve the promotion of child competencies or the healthy functioning of families, schools, or communities (Durlak and Wells, 1997, 1998; Greenberg, Domitrovich, and Bumbarger, 2001). For example, a review of programs that aim to prevent chronic delinquency through early interventions for education and family support found that effective programs have common features of promoting children's cognitive competence and achievement and promoting secure parent-child attachment, positive parenting, and improved educational status for parents (Yoshikawa, 1994). Similarly, reviews of mental health promotion programs for children and young people cite many programs that have been demonstrated both to reduce problems and to increase positive aspects of development (e.g., National Research Council and Institute of Medicine, 2002; Catalano, Berglund, et al., 2002, 2004). Catalano, Berglund, and colleagues (2002, 2004), for example, concluded that several youth development programs that were effective in building positive development in such areas as social, emotional, and cognitive competence as well as self-determination and efficacy were also effective in reducing a range of problem behaviors, such as alcohol and drug use, violence, and aggression. Such findings are compatible with theoretical models in which competence and problem outcomes influence each other over time (see Chapter 4).

Furthermore, the committee's inclusion of mental health promotion in the purview of the mental health field is also consistent with the recognition that health promotion is an important component of public health that goes beyond prevention of disease (Breslow, 1999). Indeed, health has been defined not simply as the absence of disease, but in a positive way as "a resource for everyday life . . . a positive concept emphasizing social and personal resources as well as physical capabilities" (World Health Organization, 1986). Building on this perspective, a 2004 report of the National Research Council (NRC) and the IOM proposed a new definition specifically for children's health: "the extent to which individual children or groups of children are able or enabled to (a) develop and realize their potential, (b) satisfy their needs, and (c) develop the capacities that allow them to interact successfully with their biological, physical, and social environments" (National Research Council and Institute of Medicine, 2004a, p. 33). This approach clearly emphasizes the importance for children of both promotion of mental, emotional, and behavioral health and the prevention of disorders. Adopting a more inclusive approach may also be less stigmatizing for young people and their families and increase participation in relevant programs, as the focus shifts from avoiding the possibility of disorder toward helping young people realize their potential.

CONCLUSION AND RECOMMENDATION

Definitions of prevention are important for identifying the potential contribution of prevention approaches to the overall public health goal of reducing the burden of MEB disorders on children and youth, as well as for distinguishing the complementary contributions of mental health promotion, prevention of disorders, and treatment of disorders. At this time, theory, research, and practice have evolved to support an approach to prevention that aims not only to prevent disorder, but also to promote positive mental, emotional, and behavioral health in young people.

Conclusion: The theoretical grounding and empirical testing of approaches to promote mental health have advanced considerably, making it a valuable component of the intervention spectrum warranting additional rigorous research.

Prevention and treatment are necessary and complementary components of a comprehensive approach to the mental, emotional, and behavioral health of young people. However, to enable distinctions between the two and to monitor the effectiveness of each, delineations must be made. The committee has decided that the definitions of universal, selective, and indicated prevention, as laid out in the 1994 IOM report, with the addition of mental health promotion, offer the most useful framework for the field.

Recommendation 3-1: Research and interventions on the prevention of MEB disorders should focus on interventions that occur before the onset of disorder but should be broadened to include promotion of mental health.

4

Using a Developmental Framework to Guide Prevention and Promotion

Mental, emotional, and behavioral (MEB) disorders among young people, as well as the development of positive health, should be considered in the framework of the individual and contextual characteristics that shape their lives, as well as the risk and protective factors that are expressed in those contexts. This chapter begins by outlining a developmental framework for discussion of risk and protective factors that are central to interventions to promote healthy development and prevent MEB disorders.

The conceptualization and assessment of positive aspects of development, referred to as developmental competencies, are examined as the scientific underpinnings for research on promotion of mental health. The chapter goes on to discuss research on risk factors and protective factors for MEB disorders, with attention given both to factors associated with multiple disorders and to the multiple factors associated with specific disorders. The emphasis is on identifying the implications of findings from this research for the design and evaluation of developmentally appropriate preventive interventions. Specific interventions targeting particular developmental stages are discussed in more detail in Chapter 6, and interventions targeting specific disorders as well as those designed to promote mental health are discussed in Chapter 7.

A DEVELOPMENTAL FRAMEWORK

Prevention and promotion for young people involve interventions to alter developmental processes. That makes it important for the field to be

71

grounded in a conceptual framework that reflects a developmental perspective. Four key features of a developmental framework are important as a basis for prevention and promotion: (1) age-related patterns of competence and disorder, (2) multiple contexts, (3) developmental tasks, and (4) interactions among biological, psychological, and social factors (Masten, Faden, et al., 2008; Cicchetti and Toth, 1992; Kellam and Rebok, 1992; Sameroff and Feise, 1990).

Age-Related Patterns of Competence and Disorder

Understanding the age-related patterns of disorder and competence is essential for developing interventions for prevention and promotion. Healthy human development is characterized by age-related changes in cognitive, emotional, and behavioral abilities, which are sometimes described in terms of developmental milestones or accomplishment of developmental tasks (discussed in further detail below). The period from conception to about age 5 represents a particularly significant stage of development during which changes occur at a pace greater than other stages of a young person's life and the opportunity to establish a foundation for future development is greatest (National Research Council and Institute of Medicine, 2000; see also Chapter 5). Developmental competencies established in one stage of a young person's life course establish the foundation for future competencies as young people face new challenges and opportunities. Adolescence introduces significant new biological and social factors that affect developmental competencies, particularly related to behavioral decision making. A solid foundation of developmental competencies is essential as a young person assumes adult roles and the potential to influence the next generation of young people.

The age at which disorders appear also varies. For example, a national survey on the lifetime prevalence of mental disorders in the United States indicates that the median age of onset is earlier for anxiety disorders (age 11) and impulse control disorders[1] (age 11) than for substance use disorders (age 20) and mood disorders (age 30) (Kessler, Berglund, et al., 2005). The majority of adults report the onset of their disorder by age 24 (Kessler, Berglund, et al., 2005), and evidence suggests that initial symptoms appear 2-4 years prior to onset of a full-blown disorder (see Chapter 2). Other studies also indicate that early onset of symptoms is associated with greater risk of adult disorders, including substance abuse and conduct disorder (Kellam, Ling, et al., 1998; Gregory, Caspi, et al., 2007).

---

[1]Includes intermittent explosive disorder, oppositional defiant disorder, conduct disorder, and attention deficit hyperactivity disorder.

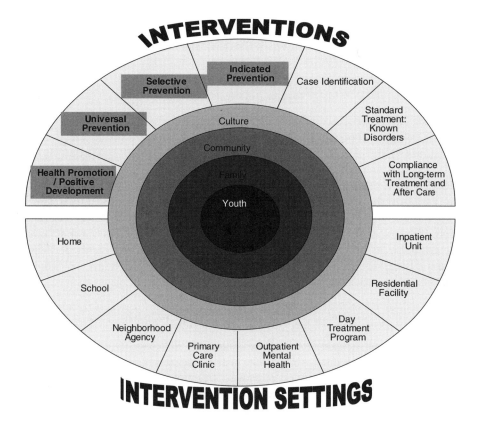

FIGURE 4-1 An ecodevelopmental model of prevention.
SOURCE: Adapted from Weisz, Sandler, et al. (2005).

Multiple Contexts

Development occurs in nested contexts of family, school, neighborhood, and the larger culture (Bronfenbrenner, 1979). Therefore, interventions can occur in a range of settings and in multiple contexts. As illustrated in Figure 4-1, the range of intervention approaches includes promotion of healthy development, prevention of MEB disorders, and treatment of individuals who are experiencing disorders (the outer semicircle). These interventions occur in an ecological framework of human development in which the individual is nested within micro-systems that are in turn nested within a larger community and cultural (including linguistic) context (the central concentric circles). The ecological perspective is widely accepted in the study of mental health, developmental psychopathology (Masten, Faden, et al., 2008), and prevention science (Kellam and Rebok, 1992; Weisz, Sandler, et al., 2005).

Developmental Tasks

Individuals encounter specific expectations for behavior in a given social context. These expectations have been referred to as social task demands or developmental tasks (Kellam and Rebok, 1992; Masten, Burt, and Coatsworth, 2006). Developmental tasks change across phases of development and may also differ by culture, gender, and historical period. Success or failure in meeting these developmental tasks is judged by natural raters (e.g., parents, teachers) as well as by young people themselves. Success with one developmental task can have serious consequences for success or difficulty in others and for the development of later problems and disorders. Developmental competence, discussed below, is strongly influenced by the concept of developmental tasks.

Interactions Among Biological, Psychological, and Social Factors

How young people develop—whether they develop mental, emotional, or behavioral problems or experience healthy development—is a function of complex interactions among genetic and other biological processes (discussed in more detail in Chapter 5), individual psychological processes, and multiple levels of social contexts. Although the precise biopsychosocial processes leading to most disorders are not fully understood, considerable progress has been made in identifying the risk factors and protective factors that predict increased or decreased likelihood of developing disorders. Understanding the pathways of development enables prevention researchers to identify opportunities to change pathological developmental trajectories.

A DEVELOPMENTAL PERSPECTIVE ON THE STUDY OF MENTAL HEALTH PROMOTION

Mental health promotion includes efforts to enhance individuals' ability to achieve developmentally appropriate tasks (developmental competence) and a positive sense of self-esteem, mastery, well-being, and social inclusion and to strengthen their ability to cope with adversity. Understanding the reciprocal pathways by which failures of competence contribute to psychopathology and by which psychopathology undermines healthy development (Masten, Burt, and Coatsworth, 2005) is needed to design promotion activities aimed at strengthening developmental competencies.

Research on mental health promotion is not as fully developed as that on prevention, but progress has been made in defining key concepts and describing biopsychosocial pathways that influence positive development. Important opportunities exist for research to make rapid advances, particularly to improve understanding of how genetic and environmental factors influence developmental pathways (National Research Council and Institute of Medicine, 2000, p. 13).

The discussion that follows focuses on competence or the achievement of developmentally appropriate tasks, which the committee contends should form the basis for mental health promotion research and intervention, and characteristics of healthy development as young people progress from infancy through young adulthood that can be used to operationalize competence.

Defining Competence

Masten and colleagues define competence as "a family of constructs related to the capacity or motivation for, process of, or outcomes of effective adaptation in the environment, often inferred from a track record of effectiveness in age-salient developmental tasks and always embedded in developmental, cultural and historical context" (Masten, Burt, and Coatsworth, 2006, p. 704). Similarly, Kellam, Branch, and colleagues (1975) conceptualize competence from a life-course social field perspective, in which the individual must adapt to new tasks in different social fields (e.g., family, school, peers) at each phase of development. Positive youth development can be viewed as the facilitation of competence during adolescence. Based on a comprehensive review of youth development programs and meetings of experts, Catalano, Berglund, and colleagues (2004) identified multiple goals of programs designed to promote positive youth development: promote bonding; foster resilience; promote social, emotional, cognitive, behavioral, and moral competence; foster self-determination, spirituality, self-efficacy, clear and positive identity, belief in the future and prosocial norms; and provide recognition for positive behavior and prosocial involvement.

The committee uses the term "developmental competencies" to refer to young people's ability to accomplish a broad range of social, emotional, cognitive, moral, and behavioral tasks at various developmental stages. Acquisition of competence in these areas requires young people to adapt to the demands of salient social contexts and to attain a positive sense of identity, efficacy, and well-being. We note, however, that while there is increasing interest in understanding and promoting these positive aspects of development (e.g., Commission on Positive Youth Development, 2005), research in this area is at a relatively early stage. At the same time, research is beginning to identify factors that affect success or failure in accomplishing specific developmental tasks and the relationship to later development of problems or health. For example, various causal models of the links between conduct and academic competence have been developed (e.g., see Hinshaw, 1992).

One longitudinal study of a community cohort of 205 children assessed three dimensions of competence in childhood (academic, social, and conduct) and five dimensions of competence in late adolescence (academic, social, conduct, job, and romantic) (Project Competence; Masten, Burt, and Coatsworth, 2006). Conduct competence (following rules in salient social contexts) in childhood proved to be more likely to lead to academic competence in adolescence than the reverse pathway (see Hinshaw, 1992, for a discussion of alternative causal models of the links between conduct and academic competence). Masten and colleagues proposed the concept of developmental cascades to refer to the process by which competence and problems become linked across time. Illustratively, their study found externalizing, or primarily behavioral, problems (e.g., conduct disorder, oppositional defiant disorder) in childhood leads to lower academic competence in adolescence, which in turn leads to increased internalizing, or primarily emotional, problems (e.g., anxiety, depression) in young adulthood (Masten, Roisman, et al., 2005).

In another study of 1,438 adolescents in two urban, high-poverty public schools in Baltimore and New York (Seidman and Pedersen, 2003), competence was conceptualized as the interaction of the individual with several social contexts: peer, athletic, academic, religious, employment, and cultural. Nine different profiles of engagement with these contexts emerged and showed differing associations with indicators of positive mental health (self-esteem) and mental health problems (depression and delinquency). Youth who were positively engaged in two or more settings had higher self-esteem and lower depression. However, high engagement in athletic contexts along with low engagement in cultural or academic contexts was associated with high rates of delinquency. These authors propose that studying homogeneous at-risk populations can identify diverse profiles of competence (positive or negative) that might be obscured by studying more heterogeneous populations or by studying each aspect of competence separately (Seidman and Pedersen, 2003). Werner and Smith (1982, 1992), in a series of classic studies of youth at high risk on the island of Hawaii, also argue that the resources a child needs to successfully develop vary by developmental stage. Early in life, a close relationship with the primary caregiver is crucially important, whereas in adolescence, the presence of mentors and opportunities in school and the neighborhood are crucial.

Characteristics of Healthy Development

Although there are no universally accepted taxonomy or agreed-on measures of positive mental health, several groups have attempted to integrate research and theory on healthy development at different developmental stages. Table 4-1 summarizes findings related to individual, family, and school and community characteristics that facilitate healthy development from reviews that the committee considers to be particularly informative. These factors differ across developmental periods and across individual, family, and school and community contexts.

For a guide to factors relevant during infancy and early childhood, the committee looked to the influential report *From Neurons to Neighborhoods: The Science of Early Childhood Development* (National Research Council and Institute of Medicine, 2000). Healthy accomplishment of the developmental tasks at these ages—such as secure attachment, emotional regulation, executive functioning, and appropriate conduct—is associated with both positive development and prevention of mental, emotional, and behavioral problems over the long term. The report highlighted the influence of families' socioeconomic resources on healthy development, suggesting that promotion (and prevention) research should include consideration of the influence of poverty on children's caregivers and their physical environment.

The committee drew from several sources on positive development during middle childhood. Masten and Coatsworth (1995) assessed competent functioning in middle childhood in terms of successfully accomplishing developmental tasks, such as academic achievement, following rules for appropriate behavior, and developing positive peer relations. Resilience, or the ability to adapt to life stressors, is a widely accepted aspect of positive development (Catalano, Berglund, et al., 2002; Commission on Positive Youth Development, 2005; Masten, Burt, and Coatsworth, 2005). The Rochester Child Resilience Project identified characteristics of the child and of the family that are associated with resilience for urban children experiencing chronic family stress (Wyman, 2003).

The school is also a social context that can promote the accomplishment of the developmental tasks of academic achievement, rule compliance, and the development of peer relations, as described by Masten and Coatsworth (1995). Aspects of the school context identified by Smith, Swisher, and colleagues (2004) as promoting children's developmental competencies include teacher behavior, pedagogy, organizational characteristics of the school, and family-school relations.

A major review of community programs to promote positive outcomes for adolescent development identified four domains of individual-level assets: physical health, intellectual development, psychological and emotional development, and social development (National Research Council and Institute of Medicine, 2002). The review also identified features of positive developmental settings, which the committee sees as relevant both for the family and for school and the community. Some of these include

TABLE 4-1 Factors That Affect Healthy Development

	Individual	Family	School and Community
Infancy and Early Childhood	**NRC and IOM (2000)** Self-regulation -Attention regulation -Appropriate emotional inhibitions and expression -Early mastery and intrinsic motivation -Executive functioning, planning, and problem solving -Secure attachment Communication and learning -Functional language -School attendance and appropriate conduct Making friends and getting along with peers -Initiating interactions and appropriate conduct -Understanding of self and others' emotions Adequate birth weight	**NRC and IOM (2000)** Healthy physical environment -Adequate prenatal and postnatal health care -Adequate prenatal and postnatal nutrition Nurturing relationships with caregiver including: -Reliable support and discipline from caregiver -Responsiveness -Protection from harms and fears -Affection -Opportunities to resolve conflict -Support for development of new skills -Reciprocal interactions -Experience of being respected -Stability and consistency in caregiver relationship Socioeconomic resources for the family -Adequate income -Ability to provide adequate nutrition, child care, safe housing, health care -Higher parental education -Cognitive stimulation in the home -Parental low economic stress	**NRC and IOM (2000)** Availability of high-quality child care -Nurturance -Support for early learning -Access to supplemental services, such as feeding, screening for vision and hearing, support for working parents -Stable secure attachment to child care provider -Low ratio of caregivers to children -Regulatory systems that support high quality of care

Middle Childhood	Masten and Coatsworth (1995)	Wyman (2003)	Smith, Boutte, et al. (2004)
	-Learning to read and write a language -Learning basic mathematics -Attending and behaving appropriately at school -Following rules for behavior at home, school, public places -Getting along with peers in school -Making friends with peers **Wyman (2003)** -Empathy and acceptance of other children's emotional expressiveness -Preference for prosocial solutions to interpersonal problems -Realistic control attributions -Self-efficacy	-Time in emotionally responsive interactions with children -Consistent discipline -Language-based rather than physically based discipline -Extended family support -Parental resources, including positive personal efficacy, adaptive coping, self-views high on potency and life satisfaction	Features of school environment that are associated with positive development -Positive teacher expectancies -Perceived teacher support -Effective classroom management -Positive partnering between school and family -Culturally relevant pedagogy -School policies and practices to reduce bullying -High academic standards, strong leadership, concrete strategies to promote achievement, assessment of goal achievement, and positive involvement of families

continued

TABLE 4-1 Continued

	Individual	Family	School and Community
Adolescence	**NRC and IOM (2002)** Positive development in adolescence -Physical development (good health habits, good health risk management skills) -Intellectual development (life, school, vocational skills; critical and rational thinking; cultural knowledge and competence) -Psychological and emotional (self-esteem and self-regulation; coping; responsibility; problem solving; motivation and achievement; morality and values) -Social development (connectedness to peers, family, community; attachment to institutions)	**NRC and IOM (2002)** Features of positive developmental settings -Physical and psychological safety -Appropriate structure (limits, rules, monitoring, predictability) -Supportive relationships -Opportunities to belong (sociocultural identity formation, inclusion, etc.) -Positive social norms (expectations, values) -Support for efficacy and mattering -Opportunities for skill building -Integration of family, school, and community efforts	**NRC and IOM (2002)** Features of positive developmental settings -Physical and psychological safety -Appropriate structure (limits, rules, monitoring, predictability) -Supportive relationships -Opportunities to belong (sociocultural identity formation, inclusion, etc.) -Positive social norms (expectations, values) -Support for efficacy and mattering -Opportunities for skill building -Integration of family, school, and community efforts
Young Adulthood	**Arnett (2000)** Identity exploration in love, work, and world view Subjective sense of adult status in self-sufficiency, making independent decisions, becoming financially independent **Masten, Obradovic, and Burt (2006)** Future orientation/achievement motivation	**Arnett (2000)** Balance of autonomy and relatedness to family **Masten, Obradovic, and Burt (2006)** Autonomy (behavioral and emotional)	**Arnett (2000)** Opportunity for exploration in work and school **Masten, Obradovic, and Burt (2006)** Connectedness to adults outside the family

physical and psychological safety, supportive relationships, and positive social norms (National Research Council and Institute of Medicine, 2002). However, the committee notes the review's caveat that additional research is needed to more firmly establish whether these features of positive developmental settings "are the most important features of community programs for youth" (National Research Council and Institute of Medicine, 2002, p. 13).

Arnett (2000) describes the period of the late teens and early 20s as a distinct developmental period in industrialized societies, which he refers to as "emerging adulthood."[2] In these societies, a major demographic shift toward later marriage and parenthood is leaving young adulthood as an age of great variability and exploration in all aspects of life, including where people live, go to school, and work. The developmental tasks of this period are to explore identity in love, work, and world view (e.g., values); to obtain a broad range of life experiences; and to move toward making commitments around which to structure adult life (Arnett, 2000). This work on early adult development continues the tradition of others (e.g., Erikson, 1968; Levinson, 1978) and illustrates the important influence on developmental tasks of modern economic and social conditions in industrialized societies.

A DEVELOPMENTAL PERSPECTIVE ON RISK AND PROTECTIVE FACTORS

Preventive interventions for young people are intended to avert mental, emotional, and behavioral problems throughout the life span. These interventions must be shaped by developmental and contextual considerations, many of which change as children progress from infancy into young adulthood. To develop effective interventions, it is essential to understand both how developmental and contextual factors at younger ages influence outcomes at older ages and how to influence those factors. The concept of risk and protective factors is central to framing and interpreting the research needed to develop and evaluate interventions.

Defining Risk and Protective Factors

Kraemer, Kazdin, and colleagues (1997) define a risk factor as a measurable characteristic of a subject that precedes and is associated with an outcome. Risk factors can occur at multiple levels, including biological, psychological, family, community, and cultural levels. They differentiate

---

[2]The committee uses the term "young adulthood" to be more descriptive and to cut across different theoretical approaches.

risk factors for which there is within-subject change over time (variable risk factors) from those that do not change (e.g., gender, ethnicity, genotype—fixed markers) (Kraemer, Kazdin, et al., 1997). Causal risk factors are those that are modifiable by an intervention and for which modification is associated with change in outcomes. A risk factor that cannot be changed by an intervention or for which change in the factor has not been demonstrated to lead to a change in an outcome is considered a variable marker.

Protective factors are defined as characteristics at the individual, family, or community level that are associated with a lower likelihood of problem outcomes. The distinctions between risk factors discussed above can also be applied to protective factors. The term "protective factors" has also been used to refer to interactive factors that reduce the negative impact of a risk factor on a problem outcome, or resilience (Luthar, 2003). It is often difficult to distinguish the effect of protective factors from that of risk factors, because the same variable may be labeled as either depending on the direction in which it is scored (e.g., good parenting versus poor parenting, high self-esteem versus low self-esteem—Masten, 2001; Luthar, 2003). For example, in a meta-analytic review of studies of risk and protective factors, Crews et al. (2007) reported that low academic achievement was a risk factor for externalizing problems, whereas adequate academic performance was a protective factor.

One approach to distinguishing the effect of protective factors from risk factors is to consider them as the extreme ends of a continuous variable (Luthar, 2003; Rutter, 2003; Stouthamer-Loeber, Loeber, et al., 1993). For example Stouthamer-Loeber, Loeber, and colleagues (1993), in a study of schoolchildren in grades 1, 4, and 7, trichotomized 35 predictors of delinquency at the 25th and 75th percentile to refer to risk and protection, respectively. They found that for 43 percent of the variables both the risk and protective effects were significant predictors, whereas for 11 percent of the variables only the protective effect was significant. Similarly, Luthar and Lantendresse (2005), in a study of wealthy and poor preadolescents, assessed the relations of mental health problems with high or low scores on each of seven aspects of the parent–child relationship. They found that some dimensions (e.g., perceived closeness to parents) had both risk and protective effects (both high scores and low scores were related to symptoms), whereas for other parenting variables (e.g., criticism) there was only a risk effect. Thus, for many commonly studied predictor variables, it is likely that both the risk and protective effects may contribute to children's mental, emotional, and behavioral problems, although studies that carefully differentiate whether the effects of these variables are at the risk or protective pole are not common.

Considering Risk and Protective Factors in the
Design and Evaluation of Preventive Interventions

Over the past several decades a voluminous literature has emerged on risk and protective factors associated with specific disorders (e.g., Garber, 2006; Biglan, Brennan, et al., 2004) and on the multiple disorders and problems that are associated with exposure to specific risk and protective factors (e.g., Luthar, 2003; Cicchetti, Rappaport, et al., 2000). This literature provides the research base for the design of preventive interventions. When potentially modifiable risk and protective factors have been identified through epidemiological and developmental research, preventive approaches can be developed to change those factors to prevent the development of mental, emotional, and behavioral problems. Other risk factors can help define populations that are potential candidates for prevention, such as children exposed to divorce, poverty, bereavement, a mentally ill or substance-abusing parent, abuse, or neglect. Although interventions aimed at these children typically do not target the risk factor itself (e.g., a divorce has already occurred), they can be designed to reduce the likelihood of problem outcomes given elevated risk.

A preventive intervention trial tests whether the intervention is effective in changing the targeted risk and protective factors and whether change in these factors mediates, or accounts for, changes in the problem outcome. Because prevention is aimed at averting problems that may occur across developmental stages, a critical feature of a prevention trial is longitudinal follow-up of participants to assess the intervention's impact on trajectories of development. A randomized preventive trial that provides evidence that an intervention has successfully changed a risk or protective factor and that the change is associated with a later change in a problem outcome is a uniquely powerful scientific tool in moving from passive correlational studies to identification of causal risk or protective factors (Rutter, Pickles, et al., 2001; Howe, Reiss, and Yuh, 2002; see also Chapter 10). Preintervention research that tests models of the pathways between risk and protective factors and the development of mental, emotional, and behavioral problems provides evidence for the theoretical models on which preventive interventions are based. Evidence from randomized prevention trials provides experimental evidence to support or counter those models (Coie, Watt, et al., 1993).

The committee examined four specific aspects of risk and protective factors, their relations to each other and to mental, emotional, and behavioral outcomes, and implications for the design and evaluation of preventive interventions (see Table 4-2).

TABLE 4-2 Summary of Findings from Studies of Risk and Protective Factors and Their Implications for Design and Evaluation of Prevention and Promotion Programs

Findings from Studies of Risk and Protective Factors	Implications for the Design and Evaluation of Prevention Programs
Risk and protective factors operate at multiple levels of analysis	• High-risk groups for prevention programs can be identified at multiple levels, including individuals, families, and communities • Preventive interventions can be directed to change malleable risk and protective factors at multiple levels of analysis
The effects of risk and protective factors are correlated and cumulative • Risk factors tend to be positively correlated with each other and negatively correlated with protective factors • Risk factors tend to have a cumulative effect on the development of mental, emotional, and behavioral problems • Protective factors have a cumulative effect to reduce the development of mental, emotional, and behavioral problems	• Children in high-risk groups are likely to have multiple risk factors • Prevention programs may be most effective when they impact multiple risk and protective factors • Evaluation of prevention trials may indicate which risk or protective factors account for program effects, leading to more efficient prevention strategies over time
Risk and protective factors have effects on both specific mental, emotional, and behavioral problems and on multiple problems • Some risk and protective factors have general effects to impact multiple mental, emotional, and behavioral outcomes • Some risk and protective factors have specific effects on single MEB disorders • Specific effects of risk and protective factors may be found in subgroups of gender or age	• Preventive interventions with high-risk groups may impact multiple outcomes • Preventive interventions with general risk factors should be designed to identify multiple outcomes across developmental stages • Preventive interventions can target risk factors specific to particular MEB disorders

TABLE 4-2 Continued

Findings from Studies of Risk and Protective Factors	Implications for the Design and Evaluation of Prevention Programs
Risk and protective factors influence each other over time • Risk and protective factors are dynamically related to each other over time. They may influence the occurrence of later risk and protective factors • Protective factors may have additive effects, moderation effects, or mediation effects • Risk and protective factors at one level of analysis affect those at another level of analysis	• Evaluation of preventive trials can inform theory concerning the effects of risk and protective factors • Prevention programs can have effects across levels of analysis. For example, risk at the biological, individual, or family level can be modified by interventions at different levels, including social policy interventions • Evaluation of prevention programs should test for mediating and moderating effects • Prevention programs can have promotion effects to strengthen positive outcomes, and promotion programs can have preventive effects to decrease problem outcomes • Prevention programs can impact chains of effects of risk and protective factors, leading to long-term effects across developmental periods

Risk and Protective Factors Can Be Found in Multiple Contexts

One of the earliest and most replicated findings from the empirical literature is that risk and protective factors are found at multiple levels of the social ecology, or the relationship between humans and their environments, from biological and psychological characteristics of the individual to the family and the community (Rutter, 1987; Werner and Smith, 1982, 1992; Luthar, 2003; Crews, Bender, et al., 2007). For example, a synthesis of 18 meta-analytic reviews of risk and protective factors for children found that the strongest risk factors for internalizing and externalizing problems include comorbid internalizing or externalizing problems, family environment stress (e.g., divorce, single parenting), corporal punishment, lack of bonding to school, delinquent peers, and poor peer relations (Crews, Bender, et al., 2007).

One implication of the multilevel nature of risk and protection is that high-risk groups can be identified on the basis of their individual, family, or community indices of risk. Similarly, preventive interventions can be developed to change risk and protective factors across levels of the social ecology (Maton, Schellenbach, et al., 2004; Sandler, Ayers, et al., 2004). Possible interventions might include psychosocial programs to directly strengthen family and child protective factors or reduce risk factors; programs in social settings that affect child development, such as preschools, schools, and social welfare agencies; or policy-level changes, such as funding prevention services or directly increasing a family's access to resources.

Risk and Protective Factors Tend to Be Correlated and to Have Cumulative Effects

Risk factors tend to be positively correlated with each other and negatively correlated with protective factors. Thus, some young people have multiple risk factors, and those with multiple risk factors are less likely to have protective factors. For example, in a five-state sample of 6th through 12th graders, those who were in the highest quintile on a cumulative measure of risk factors were likely to be in the lowest quintile on the measure of protective factors (Pollard, Hawkins, and Arthur, 1999).

Furthermore, the presence of multiple risk or protective factors tends to strengthen the prediction of disorder or positive development (Rutter, 1979; Sameroff, Gutman, and Peck, 2003; Goodyer and Altham, 1991; Fergussson and Horwood, 2003). The effect of cumulative risk and protective factors is also found in studies of populations exposed to a common risk factor, such as poverty, parental substance abuse, parental mental illness, or parental divorce (Wyman, 2003; Roosa, Sandler, et al., 1988; Sandler, Wolchik, et al., 1986). In one analysis, for example, although no single risk factor had a strong relation to disorder or positive development, the accumulation of risk factors across family, parent, peers, and community had a substantial effect in predicting multiple problem outcomes (Sameroff, Gutman, and Peck, 2003). When compared with those with eight or more risk factors, youth with three or fewer risk factors had significantly better odds of showing psychological adjustment and self-competence and not showing problem behavior.

One implication of cumulative risk and protection is that preventive interventions may be more effective when they target multiple risk and protective factors rather than just one. In some cases, mediational analysis from an experimental trial can identify which risk and protective factors are responsible for program effects (e.g., Tein, Sandler, et al., 2006). In other cases, when multiple risk and protective factors are targeted, the trial can be designed specifically to test whether components intended to change specific risk and protective factors have additive effects to improve preventive impact (West and Aiken, 1997).

Some Risk and Protective Factors Have Specific Effects, But Others Are Associated with Multiple MEB Disorders and Problem Behaviors

A common finding in the study of major risk factors is that each is associated with an increased likelihood for multiple problem outcomes (e.g., Shanahan, Copeland, et al., 2008; Kessler, Davis, and Kindler, 1997). A rigorous test of the specific versus the general effects of risk factors would require a prospective longitudinal study in order to ensure that the risk factors arise before the onset of disorders and to understand what earlier factors may have contributed to the appearance of a risk factor at a given time (e.g., unemployment leading to parental depression). It would also be necessary to assess a comprehensive set of risk factors and use a meaningful approach to classify them into distinct categories or dimensions. Looking at these effects across meaningful subgroups, such as gender or developmental period, would also be important.

A major analytic issue is whether the associations between the risk factors and multiple disorders are due to the direct effects of these risk factors or to confounding variables that are associated with both the risk factors and with the disorders. One possibility is that the associations between risk factors and multiple disorders could be accounted for by the covariance between risk factors. To test for confounding with other risk factors, studies would need to examine the effects of a given risk factor while controlling for the effects of all associated risk factors. The other possibility is that a risk factor is related to a particular disorder independently of its relations to other disorders. Because childhood disorders are highly comorbid (see Chapter 2), it would be necessary to test the effects of risk factors on disorders while controlling for the effects of other comorbid disorders.

Many studies have attempted to tease apart specific versus general effects of childhood risk factors on mental, emotional, and behavioral problems. One review of more than 200 empirical studies published between 1987 and 2001 found few consistent relations between adverse outcomes and five risk factors: exposure to violence, abuse, divorce/marital conflict, poverty, and illness (McMahon, Grant, et al., 2003). The reviewers also note that serious methodological limitations across the studies precluded drawing strong conclusions from the existing literature.

Several epidemiological studies have found some evidence for associations between specific risk factors and disorders when controlling for the effects of other risk factors (Kessler, Davis, and Kindler, 1997; Shanahan, Copeland, et al., 2008, Cohen, Brook, et al., 1990). Although cross-sectional studies (e.g., Shanahan, Copeland, et al., 2008) have found specific associations with one disorder or disorder domain, they are not able to address the direction of effects between risk factors and disorder or the mechanisms that link risk factors and disorder. An eight-year prospective longitudinal study found that three risk factors—parental mental illness, a mother–stepfather home, and maternal inattention—were significant predictors of more than one problem outcome when controlling for all other risk factors (Cohen, Brook, et al., 1990). Other risk factors had specific effects. For example, somatic risk, social isolation, and lax rules had a specific relation with internalizing problems; parental sociopathy and power-assertive punishment had specific effects on externalizing problems; and neighborhood crime and residential instability had significant relations with substance abuse.

An implication of the findings on specific versus general effects of risk and protective factors is that evaluations of interventions with groups at risk for multiple mental, emotional, and behavioral problems should be designed to detect effects on multiple problem outcomes. For example, parental divorce is associated with other risk factors, such as interparental conflict, parental mental health problems, and harsh and inconsistent parenting. It is also associated with multiple problem outcomes, including substance abuse problems, internalizing and externalizing problems, and academic problems. The potential for multiple benefits from preventive interventions increases the likelihood that they will reduce the burden of disorder on the affected individuals and be a cost-effective investment for society.

Another implication is that preventive interventions should be based on as clear an understanding as possible of the relations between the targeted risk factors and the outcomes of concern. Identification of a risk factor that is specifically associated with some disorders, after the effects of other risk factors and comorbid disorders have been accounted for, increases confidence that it is potentially a causal factor and that modifying that risk will lead to a reduction in the rate of onset of that specific disorder. Prevention strategies that are targeted to high-risk groups would require an understanding of the pathways of risk and protective processes that lead to specific disorders in the risk group and identifying the potentially modifiable processes.

Risk and Protective Factors Influence Each Other and Mental, Emotional, and Behavioral Disorders Over Time

Research in developmental psychopathology (Cichetti and Toth, 1992; Masten, 2006) and resilience (Luthar, 2003) has described multiple models—main effect, moderational, and mediational models—by which risk and protective factors influence each other and the development of emotional and behavior problems over time. Design of prevention interventions should be based on a solid theory grounded in one of these models. In main effect models, risk factors are related to higher levels of disorder, and protective factors have a counterbalancing relation to lower levels of disorder; these effects are often cumulative across multiple risk and protective factors (Rutter, 1979; Sameroff, Guttman, and Peck, 2003; Sandler, Ayers, and Romer, 2001).

In moderational models, a protective factor may reduce the relation between a risk factor and disorder, or a vulnerability factor may exacerbate the relations between a risk factor and disorder. In looking at the relations between stress and psychopathology, for example, such variables as intelligence or academic achievement and positive family environment moderated the adverse effects of stress (Grant, Compas, et al., 2006). Significant interactions have also been found between cumulative indices of risk and protective factors related to community, school, family, and individual variables (e.g., opportunities for school involvement, family attachment, and social problem-solving skills) in predicting substance use, delinquency, and school problems (Pollard, Hawkins, and Arthur, 1999). The aggregated protection measure reduced the odds for a problem outcome when the score on the aggregated risk measure was high, but not when the score was low. However, Grant, Compas, and colleagues (2006) point out that it is difficult to draw general conclusions concerning moderators of stressors because available studies test effects across different stressful situations and different outcomes and use different measures to operationalize the constructs. A clear conceptual framework is needed to integrate findings across putative protective factors. For example, the moderating role of cognitive variables in the effects of stress on depression is established because of well-established theoretical models of depression.

In mediational models, a chain of events is hypothesized in which the effects of risk or protective factors operate through their effects on another risk or protective factor, which in turn affects the development of mental, emotional, and behavioral problems. Particularly when there is a temporal relation among the factors, mediational models provide a powerful approach to looking at the pathways for the development of disorder over time (Cole and Maxwell, 2003; MacKinnon, 2008). Parenting has been found to be a mediator of the effects of multiple risk factors, including poverty, parental divorce, parental bereavement, and parental mental health problems (Sampson and Laub, 1993; Simons, Johnson, et al., 1996; Kwok, Haine, et al., 2005; Grant, Compas, et al., 2003; Wolchik, Wilcox, et al., 2000; Wyman, Sandler, et al., 2000), and multiple interventions have been designed to strengthen parenting (see Chapter 6).

Both moderational and mediational models also show that risk and protective factors in one context (e.g., the family) may influence or be influenced by factors in other contexts. A meta-analysis found that the effects of poverty on children's internalizing and externalizing problems was partially mediated through its effects to impair effective parenting (Grant, Compas, et al., 2003), whereas other studies found that the effects of poverty are mediated through neighborhood or school variables (Gershoff and Aber, 2006).

Similarly, biological factors may mediate the effects of psychosocial risk and protective factors, and conversely psychosocial risk and protective factors may moderate the effects of biological risk factors. For example, Davies, Sturge-Apple, and colleagues (2007) found that diminished cortisol reactivity mediated the relationship between children's exposure to interparental conflict and the development of externalizing problems over a two-year time period. Research has also identified interactions between genetic and environmental factors to predict disorder (see Chapter 5). However, intervention trials that include genetic or other biological information in the design or analysis of the trial are just beginning to emerge. For example, Brody, Kogan, and colleagues (2008) tested whether a psychosocial intervention to improve parent–child communication of parents in rural poor African American families would moderate the effect of genetic risk due to the presence of a specific variant of the serotonin transporter gene on their children's initiation of alcohol use, binge drinking, marijuana use, and sexual intercourse in early adolescence. As predicted, they found that program participation moderated the relationship between genetic risk and high-risk behavior; youth at genetic risk who did not receive the intervention had significantly greater increases in risk behavior initiation (1.91 versus .90 on the risk index) from pretest than youth at genetic risk who were assigned to the program.

In addition to identifying direct or indirect associations between risk and protective factors and outcomes of interest, it is also important for the development of interventions to understand the processes by which these effects occur (Luthar and Cicchetti, 2000). Conceptually, several different mechanisms have been proposed. Rutter (1987), for example, discussed five processes by which the effects of risk factors could be reduced: (1) by altering the experience of the risk factor (e.g., by coping); (2) by altering exposure to the risk factor (e.g., by parental monitoring of child involvement with antisocial peers); (3) by averting negative chain reactions (e.g., when harsh parenting leads to child oppositional behavior, which leads to increased conflict); (4) by strengthening protective factors (e.g., self-esteem, adaptive control beliefs); and (5) by turning points, which change the total context and provide new opportunities for development (e.g., moving from institutional care to a positive school environment). Each of these processes may be targeted by preventive interventions.

Evaluations of mediators and moderators of preventive interventions also enable the development of more efficient prevention programs (Brown and Liao, 1999). For example, a meta-analysis of school-based programs for the prevention of problem behavior, such as substance use and delinquency, found that program effects on two theoretical mediators (bonding to school and school achievement) were related to effects on problem behaviors (Najaka, Gottfredson, and Wilson, 2001). These findings provide guidance that future school-based prevention programs could usefully include components to promote these mediating factors.

TARGETING INTERVENTIONS FOR PREVENTION AND PROMOTION

The developmental and contextual patterns of risk and protective factors and the ways in which those factors relate to each other and to MEB disorders point to two complementary approaches to developing effective interventions for young people: approaches that target a specific disorder and approaches that target prominent risk and protective factors that are associated with multiple problem outcomes.

Targeting Specific Disorders

Disorder-specific risk factors are often identified on the basis of assessment of elevated but subclinical levels of the disorder or prodromal indicators of the disorder, particularly at a developmental stage at which risk for the onset of the disorder is elevated. When high-risk young people can be identified, indicated prevention programs for them can be a very efficient approach. For example, several interventions have demonstrated efficacy in preventing depression in adolescence by targeting adolescents with elevated but subclinical levels of depressive symptoms and providing brief skill-building interventions (see Chapter 7 and review by Horowitz and Garber, 2006).

Four specific MEB disorders—depression, anxiety, substance abuse, and schizophrenia—are used to illustrate disorder-specific risk factors (see Appendix E for tables that list risk factors for each of these disorders across developmental stages and across the various contexts of the social ecology[3]). As mentioned above, individual, family, and community characteristics can convey either a risk or an element of protection (e.g., positive versus punitive parenting). However, the current literature tends to focus on risk factors. Although not exhaustive of the disorders common among young people, these examples demonstrate that there are patterns of factors unique to specific disorders; they are also examples of disorders for which effective or promising preventive interventions are available. Some of the risk factors (e.g., poverty, family dysfunction) also appear across disorders or problem behaviors and are revisited in the next section.

---

[3]This appendix is available only online. Go to http://www.nap.edu and search for *Preventing Mental, Emotional, and Behavioral Disorders Among Young People.*

Depression

The incidence of depression is rare in children through age 6 and low prior to puberty; it increases as young people reach adolescence, with 5 percent of adolescents in a given year experiencing clinical depression and as many as 20 percent having had a clinical episode sometime during their adolescence, rates similar to those found in young adults (Angold and Costello, 2001). Around age 13, depression becomes about twice as common among girls than boys (Angold and Costello, 2001). This changing picture means that prevention programs need to be appropriate for specific developmental periods, taking into account age and gender differences in the mechanisms leading to depression.

Interventions to prevent depression in young people have primarily focused on three risk factors: parents with mood disorders, a depressogenic cognitive style, and elevated levels of depressive symptoms or a history of depression. Across studies, the rates of depression in adolescents with a depressed parent are three to four times higher than rates in those with non-depressed parents (Beardslee, Versage, and Gladstone, 1998). The mechanism is not understood but is likely to involve a combination of genetic and psychosocial influences, including poor parenting, high family stress, and conflict (Garber, 2006; Riley, Valdez, et al., 2008).

For children of depressed parents, preventive interventions have been developed to promote multiple family-level protective processes and to help children cope effectively (Beardslee, Gladstone, et al., 2003). Beardslee and Podorefsky (1988) specifically examined resilience in this population and identified three characteristics in the children: the capacity to accomplish age-appropriate developmental tasks, the capacity to be deeply engaged in relationships, and the capacity for self-reflection and self-understanding. Specifically, the youngsters understood that their parents had an illness, that they were not to blame and were not responsible for it, and that they were free to go on with their own lives. Correspondingly, the researchers found that a commitment to parenting despite depression characterized the parents of resilient children. These resilience characteristics were built into their preventive intervention strategy, illustrating the connection between understanding risk and resilience and developing preventive interventions.

A depressogenic cognitive style is marked by a tendency to ruminate and to see the world without optimism and as not in one's control (Abramson, Alloy, et al., 2002; Kaslow, Abramson, and Collins, 2000). The results of intervention trials to modify depressogenic cognitive styles have been promising in terms of reducing depressive symptoms and disorder. In some cases, improvement in depressive cognitive mediators accounted for program effects to reduce depression (Clarke, Hornbrook, et al., 2001; Gilham,

Reivich, et al., 1995). Clarke's program included both the risk factor of depressogenic cognitive style and the presence of parental depression.

A high level of depressive symptoms is an important risk factor for the onset of the disorder. In addition, depression is a recurrent disorder, with more than half of those who experience an initial episode experiencing a recurrence. Indicated prevention programs for those with symptoms or a history of depression have focused on changing processes thought to be related to the development of depression, such as depressogenic cognitive styles, explanatory style, interpersonal problem solving, and optimistic thinking (see Garber, 2006, for a review).

Anxiety Disorders

Anxiety tends to begin at an early age and to be chronic (McClure and Pine, 2006; Silverman and Pina, 2008). In the Great Smoky Mountains Study, for example, the mean age of onset was about 7 years old for specific phobias, separation anxiety, and social phobia and about 10 years old for agoraphobia, panic, and obsessive-compulsive disorder (Costello, Egger, and Angold, 2004). Research to identify specific protective, risk, or maintaining factors has been limited (e.g., Craske and Zucker, 2001; Donovan and Spence, 2000; Hudson, Flannery-Schroeder, and Kendall, 2004; Shanahan, Copeland, et al., 2008). The factors identified are generally related to the individual, the family, or school and peers.

Although most of the factors associated with anxiety are implicated in other MEB disorders as well, some are more specific. A child's temperament, specifically behavioral inhibition (characterized by irritability in infancy, fearfulness in toddlerhood, and shyness in childhood), has been found to be associated with an increased vulnerability to anxiety disorders (e.g., Biederman, Rosenbaum, et al., 1993). Similarly, anxiety sensitivity (a predisposition to fear anxiety-related sensations arising from the belief that these sensations are signs of physical, psychological, or social harm; Reiss, 1991; Reiss and McNally, 1985) also appears to be a specific risk factor for anxious symptoms (e.g., Reiss, Silverman, and Weems, 2001).

In the family, parents with anxiety disorders are more likely to have children who are at increased risk for anxiety disorders than their nonanxious counterparts (e.g., Rosenbaum, Biederman, et al., 1993). It also appears that anxious children are more likely than their nonanxious counterparts to have anxious parents (e.g., Last, Hersen, et al., 1987; Turner, Beidel, and Costello, 1987). Some of this association is likely to be due to shared genes or inheritable temperamental styles (e.g., behavioral inhibition). Children also learn anxious reactions via parental modeling and reinforcement of anxious behaviors (e.g., Barrett, Dadds, and Rapee, 1996; Rapee, 2002). Parents of anxious children are typically more controlling and intrusive than parents of children without clinical anxiety (Hudson and Rapee, 2001; Muris and Merckelbach, 1998), and parental overcontrol and intrusiveness seem to reinforce child inhibition (Rapee, 2001). Attachment style may influence anxiety in children as well (e.g., Erikson, Sroufe, and Egeland, 1985; Sroufe, Egeland, and Kreutzer, 1990). One study identified an anxious-resistant attachment style in infancy as a predictor of anxiety disorders in young adulthood (Warren, Huston, et al., 1997).

Prevention programs have typically targeted children who are at high risk for anxiety due to parental anxiety disorders (Bienvenu and Ginsburgh, 2007), behavioral risk factors for anxiety disorders (e.g., behavioral inhibition; Rapee, Kennedy, et al., 2005), or environmental risk factors (e.g., witnessing community violence; Cooley, Boyd, and Grados, 2004). Prevention programs also have targeted prodromal youth (Dadds, Spence, et al., 1997) and asymptomatic youth (Barrett, Farrell, et al., 2006). Studies are still needed to clarify both the mechanisms by which a prevention program achieves its effects and models of anxiety disorder development (Kellam, Koretz, and Moscicki, 1999).

Schizophrenia

The diagnostic criteria for schizophrenia and other psychotic disorders in the schizophrenia spectrum are undergoing reexamination and revision (Tsuang and Faraone, 2002), but the current diagnostic measurements have sufficient reliability to permit a clear study of risk factors and the developmental course. The incidence of schizophrenia and other psychotic disorders accelerates dramatically during adolescence and young adulthood. Because risk factors have been identified from the prenatal period through young adulthood, opportunities for prevention span these life stages.

Family history can be an important predictor of schizophrenia, and there is strong evidence that genetic factors increase the risk for schizophrenia, with multiple genes operating and interacting in complex ways (Erlenmeyer-Kimling, Rock, et al., 2000; Gottesman, 1991; Owen, O'Donovan, and Harrison, 2005; Tsuang and Faraone, 1994). Having one affected parent conveys a lifetime risk 5 to 15 times that of the general population; having two parents with schizophrenia conveys a nearly 50 percent risk (Bromet and Fennig, 1999). Thus, youth who have an affected first-degree relative are an important potential target group for selective intervention. However, this strategy would not be sufficient, as 90 percent of cases of schizophrenia do not have a family history (Brown and Faraone, 2004; Faraone, Brown, et al., 2002).

An important identified risk factor for schizophrenia is obstetric complications, which convey twice the risk of that in the general population. These complications are sufficiently common that reducing them would have the potential for reducing the overall population rate of schizophrenia (Geddes and Lawrie, 1995). Malnutrition (Susser, Neugebauer, et al., 1996), hypoxia, or infection (Pearce, 2001) are thought to have an adverse effect on the neurodevelopment of the fetus. Thus, ensuring good prenatal care (and reducing maternal rubella infections in developing countries) for all expectant mothers is a universal prevention strategy for schizophrenia to be investigated. Another selective strategy might be aiming supportive interventions to those born with obstetric complications.

Screening for developmental difficulties through multiple stages of life may be appropriate among children born with obstetric complications or whose family history suggests high risk (Brown and Faraone, 2004). Data from studies of high-risk groups suggest that nearly all those with affected family members who later have a diagnosis of schizophrenia had attention problems in childhood as well as diagnoses and difficulties in meeting the important task demands at successive stages of life (Mirsky, Yardley, et al., 1995; Weiser, Reichenberg, et al., 2001).

Identification of the prodromal stage of schizophrenia may present an opportunity to intervene (McFarlane, 2007). Indeed, there are a number of trials currently under way that use low-dose atypical antipsychotics, often in combination with family-focused psychosocial interventions, to prevent the onset of a first episode of psychosis in adolescents and young adults with prodromal symptoms (see Chapter 7). Another promising line of research involves identification and potential intervention among youth and young adults who have underlying signs and symptoms suggesting a genetic liability for schizophrenia without full manifestation of symptoms. The term "schizotaxia" represents a nonpsychotic construct with signs of brain abnormalities and some degree of cognitive, neuropsychological, and social impairment. Such a constellation of negative symptoms and neuropsychological deficits is common among unaffected first-degree relatives of those with schizophrenia (Faraone, Biederman, et al., 1995; Faraone, Kremen, et al., 1995). Particularly relevant for prevention is some evidence that schizotaxia symptoms among adults are ameliorated with low-dose resperidone (Tsuang and Faraone, 2002). Despite major challenges in nosology and ethical considerations regarding labeling and intervention among young people, this line of research holds promise as a strategy for preventing schizophrenia.

Substance Abuse

Substance abuse and dependence tend to emerge in mid-to-late adolescence and to be more common among boys. Substance abuse is greater among young people who experience early puberty, particularly among girls. It is widely accepted that children of drug and alcohol abusers are more likely to develop substance abuse problems (Mayes and Suchman, 2006; Hawkins, Catalano, and Miller, 1992). Considerable evidence supports that a genetic vulnerability to abuse may be conferred at birth, and that this vulnerability may be most significant in relation to the transition from drug use to dependence later in life (Mayes and Suchman, 2006).

During childhood, risk for substance abuse is higher for those who have a difficult temperament, poor self-regulatory skills, are sensation seeking, are impulsive, and do not tend to avoid harm. Children who have early persistent behavior problems are also more likely to develop a substance use problem (Hawkins, Catalano, and Miller, 1992). Furthermore, substance abuse is also often comorbid with anxiety, depression, and attention deficit hyperactivity disorder (Mayes and Suchman, 2006; Hawkins, Catalano, and Miller, 1992; Sher, Grekin, and Williams, 2005). Evidence suggests that parents who form warm, nonconflictual relationships with their children, provide adequate monitoring and supervision, and do not provide models of drug use help protect their children from developing substance use disorders.

During middle childhood and into adolescence, peers play an increasingly important role in children's psychological functioning. Children who associate with deviant or drug-using peers or who are rejected by peers are more likely to develop substance use problems (Mayes and Suchman, 2006; Hawkins, Catalano, and Miller, 1992; Sher, Grekin, and Williams, 2005). Peers create norms and opportunities for substance use (Mayes and Suchman, 2006; Hawkins, Catalano, and Miller, 1992; Sher, Grekin, and Williams, 2005) and influence attitudes toward substance use. Children and adolescents who have a low commitment to school (Hawkins, Catalano, and Miller, 1992) or experience school failure are more likely to abuse substances. And healthy peer groups and school engagement appear to be protective.

Children and adolescents with more access and availability to alcohol and drugs are more likely to use them (Mayes and Suchman, 2006; Hawkins, Catalano, and Miller, 1992). There is also evidence that child and adolescent substance use is affected by societal norms about use. Norms can be conveyed by laws, perception (or misperception) of peer use, enforcement, taxation, and/or advertising (e.g., alcohol).

Adolescent use of coping strategies involving behavioral disengagement, tendency toward negative emotionality, conduct disorder, and antisocial behavior increase the risk for substance abuse. For both children and adolescents, early drug use predicts later drug use.

In young adulthood, different risk factors appear to represent different pathways to substance abuse. There is consistent evidence of elevated substance abuse, particularly of alcohol, among those attending college, the same group that had lower use in adolescence (Brown, Wang, and

Sandler, 2008). This suggests that dormitory life and the fraternity/sorority system, with their lack of parental oversight and consistent exposure to peer models, may create powerful norms encouraging use (Brown, Wang, and Sandler, 2008). For those who do not attend college, antisocial behavior and lack of commitment to conventional adult roles appear to be pathways to abuse.

Underage Drinking

Although not all those who drink in their youth develop substance abuse or substance dependence, underage drinking has received significant public health attention, given the prevalence of drinking among those under the legal drinking age, problematic drinking patterns, and their deleterious effects. A brief discussion of factors related to underage drinking provides an illustration of the developmental aspects of a problem behavior of significant public health concern and similarities with the trajectory of some MEB disorders. The likelihood of serious alcohol dependence as an adult is greatly increased the earlier that young people start drinking (Grant and Dawson, 1997; Gruber, DiClemente, et al., 1996).

Almost one-third of young people between the ages of 12 and 20 report recent drinking, with the majority engaging in binge drinking (five or more drinks), when they drink. Although at lower rates than those in older age groups, drinking is reported by youth as young as age 12, with patterns of heavy drinking increasing with age (National Research Council and Institute of Medicine, 2004b). After age 25, rates of overall drinking, as well as rates of frequent and heavy drinking, steadily decline.

Alcohol use by children and adolescents is influenced over the developmental course by genetics, family, peers, neighborhood, and broader social contexts through norm development, alcohol expectancies, and availability (see the review by Zucker, Donovan, et al., 2008). Risks are apparent as early as ages 3 to 5 years, when children develop the understanding that adults drink alcoholic beverages and learn norms about its use (e.g., men drink more than women).

Children whose parents are drinkers are more likely to be drinkers, and their own drinking correlates well with their perception of their parents' drinking. This may occur because parents model drinking and help children develop positive expectancies about the effects of alcohol. Children are also exposed to positive images of alcohol use from television and movies. Among adolescents, positive alcohol expectancies are related to initiation of alcohol use.

As children grow older, peer influences become stronger. Peers provide opportunities for modeling of and encouragement for alcohol use. Media and peer culture depicts drinking as a positive part of social life. Adolescents who associate with alcohol-using peers encourage continual use and can be resistant to change. In addition, adolescents tend to overestimate their peer's drinking, which leads to heavier drinking to conform to the perceived norm.

Public policy in the form of drinking-age laws and their enforcement also influences alcohol use. Lowering the drinking age is associated with increases in teen drunk driving and teen traffic fatalities, while raising it is associated with less teen drunk driving (Wagenaar and Toomey, 2002; National Research Council and Institute of Medicine, 2004b). A higher drinking age (and its enforcement) may decrease underage drinking because it limits access to alcohol, but also by communicating social norms against drinking generally and underage drinking specifically (Hawkins, Catalano, and Miller, 1992). In addition, alcohol consumption decreases with price increases from taxation, particularly among young people with less disposable income (Coate and Grossman, 1988; National Research Council and Institute of Medicine, 2004b).

The risk factors for underage drinking suggest that prevention efforts can be formulated to influence the availability of alcohol, norms about alcohol, and alcohol use expectancies. Limiting media exposure of even young children may decrease normative perceptions of drinking and decrease the development of positive alcohol expectancies (National Research Council and Institute of Medicine, 2004b). Within the family, interventions may be designed particularly around limiting exposure to models of excessive drinking in the home, at family events, and through media sources. Family-based efforts may also target adolescents by monitoring exposure to alcohol-using peers and involvement in alcohol-related activities.

Targeting Risk and Protective Factors for Multiple Disorders

Some risk and protective factors are associated with a broad spectrum of MEB disorders and related problem behaviors for young people, either directly or indirectly through their influence on other risk or protective factors. As a result, preventive strategies may be aimed at these especially important risk and protective factors rather than at specific disorders. Biglan, Brennan, and colleagues (2004) spell out the implications of common and linked risk factors for prevention. First, with common risk factors for multiple problems, intervening in any single risk factor should contribute to preventing multiple outcomes, including externalizing problems, sexual activity, substance use, and academic failure. Second, with multiple risk factors across the developmental course, there should be multiple plausible routes to prevention. Third, with developmentally early risk factors influencing later ones, preventive interventions should be timed to protect against developmentally salient risk factors. Poverty, family dysfunction and disruption, and factors associated with school and the community are particularly illustrative.

Risk Factors Associated with Multiple Disorders

Negative life events at the family, school or peer, and community levels have been associated with multiple psychopathological conditions, such as anxiety, depression, and disruptive disorders (see Craske and Zucker, 2001; La Greca and Silverman, 2002). Similarly, social support and problem-solving coping appear to have broad protective effects (e.g., Pina, Villalta, et al., 2008).

Studies using nationally representative samples and studies of diverse ethnic, gender, and age groups have found that behavior problems involving serious antisocial behavior, substance use (cigarettes, alcohol, drugs), and risky sexual behavior have common risk and protective factors across developmental stages and across multiple levels of the social ecology, including individual genetic factors, dysfunctional parent-child interactions, and poverty. They also often occur together in adolescence (Biglan, Brennan, et al., 2004).

There appears to be an interrelated set of developmental factors in which earlier risk (or protective) factors increase the likelihood of later ones and in which earlier manifestations of problem behaviors increase the likelihood of later risk factors and problem behaviors (Biglan, Brennan, et al., 2004). Furthermore, early developmental tasks result in developmental competencies during childhood (e.g., verbal fluency) or deficits (e.g., insecure attachment) that can be risk or protective factors at later developmental stages. For example, difficult temperament, which is biologically determined, affects the parenting an infant receives, which in turn affects development of early attachment.

Under one model of the development of a set of problem behaviors— antisocial behavior, high-risk sex, academic failure, and substance use—early family conflict was found to lead to poor family involvement, which later leads to poor parental monitoring and associating with deviant peers (Ary, Duncan, et al., 1999). Both poor monitoring and association with deviant peers lead to higher levels of problem behaviors.

A multiyear retrospective study of the effects of adverse childhood experiences or childhood trauma (psychological, physical, or sexual abuse, witnessing violence against the mother, living with household members who were substance abusers, mentally ill or suicidal, or incarcerated) identified strong graded relationships between these experiences and a range of negative outcomes in adulthood. Adult outcomes associated with these childhood experiences included alcoholism and alcohol abuse, depression, drug abuse, and suicide attempts. The likelihood of multiple health risk factors in adulthood were greater when multiple types of negative childhood exposures were experienced (Felitti, Anda, et al., 1998). An analysis specific to mental health outcomes identified a significant relationship between an emotionally abusive family environment and the level of adverse experience with negative mental health outcomes (Edwards, Holden, et al., 2003).

Poverty. By whatever index used, poverty is a highly prevalent risk factor for children in the United States. In 2007, 18 percent of all U.S. children lived in families with incomes below 100 percent of the federal poverty line; the percentage was higher among ethnic minorities (10 percent of white children, 28 percent of Latino children, and 35 percent of African American children) (U.S. census). However, this measure does not fully capture the proportion of families who do not have sufficient resources to meet their basic needs for housing, child care, food, transportation, health care, miscellaneous expenses, and taxes. The Economic Policy Institute estimated that more than 2.5 times the number of families with incomes at or below the federal poverty line do not have sufficient budgets to meet their basic needs independent of outside subsidies (Boushey, Brocht, et al., 2001). Families who live in poverty or near poverty continually need to make trade-offs between necessities. For example, 65 percent of families with household incomes between 100 and 200 percent of the federal poverty line experienced at least one serious hardship during the prior year, including food insecurity, lack of health insurance, or lack of adequate child care (Boushey, Brocht, et al., 2001).

Poverty is a risk factor for several MEB disorders and is associated with other developmental challenges. Poor children show difficulties with aspects of social competence, including self-regulation and impulsivity (Takeuchi, Williams, and Adair, 1991), and abilities associated with social-emotional competence (Eisenberg, Fabes, et al., 1996). Furthermore, poverty has been found to be associated with a wide range of problems in physical health, including low birth weight, asthma, lead poisoning, and accidents, as well as cognitive development. Poor children are also more likely to experience developmental delays, lower IQ, and school failure (Gershoff, 2003; Brooks-Gunn and Duncan, 1997).

Gershoff, Aber, and Raver (2003) describe three pathways by which poverty affects child development. With the parent investment pathway, the relations between poverty and children's cognitive development is mediated by the quality of the home environment, which is represented by the amount of cognitively stimulating material in the home (e.g., books, CDs) and how often parents take their children to stimulating places, such as museums and libraries. With the parent behavior and stress pathway, the parents are considered to be under high levels of stress because of their economic difficulties and the occurrence of stressful life events for which they have insufficient resources to cope effectively. Parental stress leads to increased levels of parental depression and interparental conflict, which in turn lead to problems in parenting, including withdrawal from the children, hostility, more frequent use of corporal punishment, and at extreme levels maltreatment. Each of these factors has been found to relate to higher levels of internalizing and externalizing problems in children.

The third pathway involves the neighborhood and community in which poor families are more likely to live. Poor neighborhoods and schools are less likely to have the resources that promote healthy child development and are more likely to be settings that expose children to additional risk factors, such as violence and the availability of drugs and alcohol. Disentangling the effects of the neighborhood and the family is difficult, but there is evidence that many of the factors associated with poor neighborhoods and schools are associated with multiple mental, emotional, and behavioral problems for children (Gershoff and Aber, 2006). More research is needed to tease out these effects and, most importantly, to identify factors that may protect children from the negative effects of living in high-poverty neighborhoods (Roosa, Jones, et al., 2003).

Gershoff, Aber, and Raver (2003) also describe policy- and program-level interventions that may be effective in reducing the negative effects of poverty on children. Their model illustrates interventions to change each of the pathways that lead to adverse outcomes. Parent-directed human capital enhancement policies at the federal and state levels are designed to aid families through programs for job training and education to increase parents' skills and earning capacity and programs to encourage young women to postpone childbearing so that they can stay in school and obtain better jobs. Income support programs, such as the Earned Income Tax Credit and the Child Support Enforcement Program, are designed to increase the economic self-sufficiency of families. Programs also offer in-kind support, including supplemental child nutrition (e.g., Special Supplement Food Program for Women, Infants, and Children), health insurance for children, and high-quality child care. Parent-directed programs are designed to aid children by enhancing parents' own well-being and their ability to provide a healthy childrearing environment. Two-generation programs are designed with multiple components to assist both parents and children. For example, Early Head Start focuses on improving child development, family development, and staff and community development. Finally, child-directed programs include providing additional funds for high-poverty schools and for after-school programs in poor neighborhoods.

A natural experiment found that increases in family income and income-related resources were followed by a reduction in both psychiatric and behavioral symptoms in children (Costello, Compton, et al., 2003; see also Chapter 6).

Family Dysfunction and Disruption. With the family as the primary setting for child development from birth through childhood and adolescence, it is not surprising that dysfunction in family relations, particularly parent–child relations, is associated with multiple mental, emotional, and behavioral problems, including those described above. Many risk factors (e.g., poverty, parental mental illness) influence mental, emotional, and behavioral problems and disorders through their effects on parent–child relations (Grant, Compas, et al., 2003; Riley, Valdez, et al., 2008). The discussion here focuses on two broad categories of risk factors that are related to dysfunctional family relations and that provide opportunities for preventive intervention: child maltreatment, which represents the extreme manifestation of family dysfunction, and disruptions in family structure, which create serious challenges to healthy family functioning.

Child Maltreatment. Maltreatment of children by primary caregivers is one of the most potent risk factors for mental, emotional, and behavioral problems, and it has been found to be associated with other serious risk factors, such as poverty and parental mental illness. Protective factors include children's positive relationship with an alternative caregiver, positive and reciprocal friendships, and higher internal control beliefs (Bolger and Patterson, 2003).

The prevalence of child maltreatment in the United States is unclear. One estimate places it at 1.2 percent of children in 2004 (National Child Abuse Data System). Hussey, Chang, and Kotch (2006) report that 11.8 percent of adolescents report physical neglect, 28.4 percent report physical assault by a parent or caregiver, and 4.5 percent report sexual abuse by a parent or caregiver sometime before they reached the sixth grade. In the National Longitudinal Study of Adolescent Health (Add Health), which includes a nationally representative sample of adolescents, each form of maltreatment was associated with multiple health problems, including depression, substance use, violence, obesity, and poor physical health (Hussey, Chang, and Kotch, 2006). The majority of these associations remained significant after controlling for such demographic variables as family income, age, gender, ethnicity, parent education, region, and immigrant generation (Hussey, Chang, and Kotch, 2006).

In a recent empirical examination in the National Comorbidity Study (Molnar, Buka, and Kessler, 2001), one of the largest and most methodologically sound studies, childhood sexual abuse was reported by 13.5 percent of the women and 2.5 percent of the men. Significant associations were found with 14 mood, anxiety, and substance abuse disorders among women and 5 disorders among men. The analysis controlled for other adversities, including divorced parents, parental psychopathology, parental verbal and physical abuse, parental substance use problems, and having dependents for women.

The lifetime rate of depression was 19.2 percent for those with no childhood sexual abuse and 39.3 percent for those who had experienced abuse (odds ratio = 1.8; Molnar, Buka, and Kessler, 2001). Rates of dysthymia, mania, and posttraumatic stress disorder were also significantly higher for sexually abused women but not for men. The impact of childhood sexual abuse was especially strong for those who had no other adversities; their odds for depression were 3.8 (95 percent confidence interval). For those who reported 5 or more adversities, the odds of depression were 1.7 (95 percent confidence level). There was some evidence that chronic sexual abuse led to higher rates of some disorders (Molnar, Buka, and Kessler, 2001).

Parental psychopathology, especially among mothers, was the most significant family adversity associated with abuse (Molnar, Buka, and Kessler, 2001) and warrants further investigation. However, finding high rates of disorder with abuse but no other risk factors emphasizes the importance of the negative effects of abuse. The persistence of negative effects of child maltreatment is seen in studies that assess functioning across periods of development. For example, the Virginia Longitudinal Study of Child Maltreatment found that of 107 maltreated children who were followed from middle childhood through early adolescence, fewer that 5 percent were functioning well consistently over time (Bolger and Patterson, 2003).

Understanding the factors that influence the linkage between child maltreatment and problem outcomes starts by distinguishing different levels of abuse. In particular, abuse that starts early and is chronic is linked with pervasive and persistent problems across domains of functioning. Children abused in infancy show difficulties in areas that include affect regulation (e.g., high negative affect, blunted affect), hypervigilance, emotional lability, disruptions in their attachment relations, and self-system deficits (e.g., more negative self-representations) (Ialongo, Rogosch, et al., 2006).

The most effective approach to reducing the effects of maltreatment is to prevent its occurrence. Because of the pervasive mental, emotional, and behavioral problems for which maltreated children are at risk, programs that prevent abuse have the potential to avert multiple disorders and promote healthy development across multiple domains of functioning. There is evidence, for example, that a home visiting program for economically poor, single parents has been effective in reducing the occurrence of child abuse (Olds, 2006; see Box 6-1) and that a population-level approach to strengthening parenting reduces rates of abuse in the community (Prinz, Sanders, et al., 2009). Interventions are also aimed at mitigating the impact of abuse after it has occurred. Several randomized trials with maltreated children demonstrated that infant and preschool psychotherapy and a home visiting program were successful in markedly reducing rates of insecure attachment

(Ialongo, Rogosch, et al., 2006). Other program models have demonstrated success to improve maltreated children's relationships with foster parents (Fisher, Gunnar, et al., 2000) and with well-functioning peers (Fantuzzo, Sutton-Smith, et al., 1996).

Family Disruption. Family disruption can occur for many reasons, including separation or divorce, the death of a parent, and incarceration of a parent. The committee focused on parental divorce and bereavement because they have been the subject both of considerable research and of preventive trials.

The rate of divorce in the United States increased from the 1950s through the 1970s and then stabilized or decreased somewhat over the following decades (Bramlett and Mosher, 2002; U.S. Census Bureau, 2005). However, the official divorce rate underestimates the rate of marital disruption, which may occur as separations that do not become divorces or as disruptions of households with unmarried parents (Bramlett and Mosher, 2002). It is estimated that 34 percent of children in the United States will experience parental divorce before reaching age 16 (Bumpass and Lu, 2000). Children can experience a wide range of other stressors following divorce, such as loss of time with one or more parents, continuing interparental conflict, and parental depression (Amato, 2000). Evidence suggests that effective child coping or interpretation of these stressors, quality of parenting received from both parents, and level of interparental conflict is related to postdivorce adjustment (e.g., Kelly and Emery, 2003; Sandler, Tein, et al., 2000).

Death of a parent (i.e., parental bereavement) occurs to 3.5 percent of U.S. children before age 18 (U.S. Social Security Administration, 2000). The effect of parental death on surviving children rises to national concern particularly when rates increase due to such national disasters as the terrorist attacks of September 11, 2001, war, and such epidemics as HIV.

Following parental divorce, children are at increased risk for multiple mental, emotional, and behavioral problems, including physical health problems, elevated levels of alcohol and drug use, premarital childbearing, receiving mental health services, and dropping out of school (Troxel and Matthews, 2004; Furstenberg and Teitler, 1994; Hoffmann and Johnson, 1998; Goldscheider and Goldscheider, 1993; Hetherington, 1999). Meta-analyses of studies conducted through the 1990s have shown that problems have not decreased (Amato and Keith, 1991a; Amato, 2001). McLanahan's (1999) analysis of 10 national probability samples revealed school dropout rates of 31 percent and teen birth rates of 33 percent for adolescents in divorced families versus 13 and 11 percent, respectively, for adolescents in nondivorced families. Adults who were exposed to parental divorce as children have been found to be more likely to divorce and to have an increased risk for mental, emotional, and behavioral problems, including clinical levels of mental health problems, substance abuse, and mental health service use (Chase-Lansdale, Cherlin, and Kiernan, 1995; Kessler, Davis, and Kindler, 1997; Maekikyroe, Sauvola, et al., 1998; Rodgers, Power, and Hope, 1997; Zill, Morrison, and Coiro, 1993; Amato, 1996).

Children who experience parental bereavement appear more likely to experience mental, emotional, and behavioral problems, such as depression, posttraumatic stress disorder, and elevated mental health problems for up to two years following the death (Worden and Silverman, 1996; Geresten, Beals, and Kallgren, 1991). These risks appear to remain after controlling for other risk factors, such as mental disorder of the deceased parent (Melhem, Walker, et al., 2008). Research has shown mixed findings concerning the mental, emotional, and behavioral problems of bereaved children when they reach adulthood (Kessler, Davis, and Kindler, 1997). However, two prospective longitudinal studies supported increased risk of depression in adult women who experienced parental bereavement as children (Reinherz, Giaconia, et al., 1999; Maier and Lachman, 2000).

Although family disruption is associated with multiple MEB disorders and problems, the majority of children who experience these major stressors adapt well. The most consistent predictive factors are interparental conflict and the quality of parenting by both the mother and the father (Kelly and Emery, 2003; Amato and Keith, 1991b). Parent–child relations that are characterized by warmth, positive communication and supportiveness, and high levels of consistent and appropriate discipline have consistently been related to better outcomes following divorce (Kelly and Emery, 2003; Amato and Keith, 1991b). High-quality parenting from both the custodial parent (usually the mother) and the noncustodial parent (usually the father) is related to lower levels of child internalizing and externalizing problems (King and Sobolewski, 2006). But interparental conflict is one of the most damaging stressors for children from divorced families. Conflict often precedes the divorce and is associated with lasting child problems following the divorce (Block, Block, and Gjerde, 1988). In some families, conflict continues long after divorce, which is particularly destructive when children are caught in the middle (Buchanan, Maccoby, and Dornbusch, 1991). Recent research has found that high-quality parenting from both parents related to lower child mental health problems even in the presence of high interparental conflict (Sandler, Miles, et al., 2008).

Several factors have been found to influence outcomes for children who experience parental bereavement. Among parentally bereaved children who had signed up for an intervention program, four factors distinguished bereaved children who had clinical levels of mental health problems from those who did not: positive parenting by the surviving caregiver, lower mental health problems of the surviving parent, the coping efficacy of the child, and children's appraisals of how much recent stressful events threatened their well-being (Lin, Sandler, et al., 2004). Other factors, such as coping efficacy, control beliefs, postbereavement stressful events, and children's fears that they will be abandoned by the surviving caregiver, have been associated with mental health outcomes for bereaved children (Wolchik, Tein, et al., 2006).

An interesting focus of research has investigated the pathways that lead from family disruption due to divorce or bereavement, along with other commonly co-occurring biological and social risk factors, to adult depression. One analysis of longitudinal data on female twins, siblings, and unrelated women found support for three pathways to the development of depression (Kendler, Gardner, and Prescott, 2002). In an internalizing pathway, genetic risk leads to neuroticism, which in turn leads to early-onset anxiety disorder, and these three influences each lead to episodes of major depression. In an externalizing pathway, conduct disorder and substance misuse lead to depressive disorder. In an adversity pathway, early childhood exposure to a disturbed family environment, childhood sexual abuse, and parental loss lead to low educational attainment, lifetime trauma, and low social support, which in turn lead to four adult risk factors (marital problems, difficulties in the past year, dependent stressful events, and independent stressful events), which in turn lead to an episode of major depression. All three pathways include contributions from genetic factors and interconnections among family adversity, externalizing problems, and later adult adversities.

A prospective longitudinal study, the National Collaborative Perinatal project, also considered timing in an examination of the association between family disruption (divorce or separation before age 7), low socioeconomic status, and residential instability and the onset of adult depression (Gilman, Kawachi, et al., 2003). The effect of low socioeconomic status in childhood on depression risk persisted into adulthood, but the effects of family disruption and residential instability were specific to early-onset depression. Early-onset depression is of special concern because it carries with it a poorer prognosis of increased recurrence and, in some studies, more severe depressions.

Community and School Risk Factors

Most prevention research has focused on risk and protective factors at the level of the individual and the family, but there is increasing recognition that child development is powerfully affected by the broader social contexts of schools and communities (Boyce, Frank, et al., 1998). Risk factors, such as victimization, bullying, academic failure, association with deviant peers, norms and laws favoring antisocial behavior, violence, and substance use, are linked primarily with neighborhoods and schools. For example, poor and ethnic minority children in particular are frequently exposed to violence in their neighborhoods and schools. Among 900 low-income, primarily minority adolescents in New York City in 2002-2003, rates of exposure to violence of various kinds were high: someone offering or using drugs (70 percent), someone beaten or mugged (51 percent), someone being stabbed (17 percent), someone being shot at (14 percent), and someone being killed (12 percent) (Gershoff, Pedersen, et al., 2004). Many also reported being the victim of violent acts, such as being asked to sell or use drugs (35 percent), having their home broken into (18 percent), being beaten up (13 percent), and being threatened with death (9 percent). Much of the exposure to violence occurs either at school or on the way to school (DeVoe, Peter, et al., 2003; Bell and Jenkins, 1991; Richters and Martinez, 1993; Gershoff, Aber, and Raver, 2003).

Exposure to violence is associated with children's development of various mental health problems, particularly posttraumatic stress disorder, anxiety, depression, antisocial behavior, and substance use (Jenkins and Bell, 1994; Gorman-Smith and Tolan, 1998). A reciprocal relation exists between academic achievement and mental health outcomes, in which mental health problems adversely affect academic achievement (Adelman and Taylor, 2000), and poor academic achievement is related to the development of multiple problem behaviors (e.g., substance abuse, antisocial behavior) as well as teenage pregnancy and low occupational attainment (Dryfoos, 1990).

The growing empirical research on characteristics of neighborhoods and schools that are linked with problem development as well as positive youth development has implications for the development and evaluation of prevention and promotion interventions. Gershoff, Aber, and Raver (2003) propose that another dimension of schools and neighborhoods that may affect the development of child mental, emotional, and behavioral problems is the degree to which they provide settings that support healthy development. They characterize neighborhood disadvantage as the absence of settings that provide opportunities for healthy child development—settings for learning (e.g., libraries), social and recreational activities (e.g., parks), child care, quality schools, health care services, and employment opportunities. For schools, disadvantage can be assessed as lower per student spending, a high percentage of children from families in poverty, a higher number of inexperienced and academically unprepared teachers, a high student-to-teacher ratio, and school size being either too large or too small. Each of these characteristics of neighborhoods and schools has been linked with mental, emotional, and behavioral problems of children. Although it is difficult to disentangle the causal effects of neighborhood and school disadvantage from the effects of factors in families and children who live in disadvantaged neighborhoods, research has found that neighborhood disadvantage was associated with higher internalizing and externalizing problems over and above the genetic contribution (Caspi, Taylor, et al., 2000) and that an experimental study found that children whose families were moved from a disadvantaged neighborhood had a lower rate of arrest for a violent crime than those who remained in a high-poverty neighborhood (Leventhal and Brooks-Gunn, 2003).

Similarly, the strongest environmental association related to schizophrenia is urbanicity (Krabbendam and van Os, 2005), although the relation with social class is also strong. It appears that living in urban environments during childhood affects later development of schizophrenia, even if there is a move to less urban environments later in life (Pederson and Mortensen, 2001). This relationship is therefore not fully explained by the "drift" hypothesis, in which those who are developing schizophrenia move to urban settings. There are a few hypotheses that are being pursued to explain this relationship, including increased stress and discrimination against minorities, lack of social capital and other resources in impoverished communities, and gene–environment interactions.

Another way in which the community influences child development is through the norms, values, and beliefs of the residents. For example, collective efficacy, a concept developed by Sampson, Raudenbush, and Earls (1997), refers to "shared beliefs in a neighborhood's conjoint capability for action to achieve an intended effect, and hence an active sense of engagement on the part of residents." It provides the informal social controls that counteract antisocial behavior and has been found to be related to levels of community violence (Sampson, 2001). Peer norms favoring the use of drugs, antisocial behavior, or belonging to gangs are also powerful neighborhood factors that contribute to problem behaviors.

Hawkins and Catalano (1992) proposed the construct of bonding to school, community, and family as key in explaining the development of substance use and antisocial behavior. Positive bonds consist of a positive relationship, commitment, and belief about what is healthy and ethical behavior. Positive bonds to a group develop from having the opportunity to be an active contributor, having the skills to be successful, and receiving recognition and reinforcement for their behavior.

In school, students' relationships with their peers and teachers and the social climate in the classroom have a powerful effect on their development of mental, emotional, and behavioral problems as well as their development of age-appropriate competencies. For example, aggregate-level student-perceived norms favoring substance use, violence, or academic achievement are related to antisocial behavior. For boys with elevated levels of externalizing problems, being in a first grade classroom with high aggregate levels of behavior problems has been found to be associated with a marked increase in the odds of having serious externalizing problems when they reached the sixth grade (Kellam, Ling, et al., 1998). But some teacher characteristics are related to lower levels of mental, emotional, and behavioral problems for students. These include using classroom management strategies with a low level of aggressive behavior, having high expectations for students, and having supportive relations with students.

Programs promoting classroom and school procedures that encourage prosocial behavior, academic achievement, or increased positive bonding to school have important implications for children's healthy development. For example, use of a group contingency to promote prosocial behavior in first grade students has been found to reduce aggressive behavior in first grade (Dolan, Kellam, et al., 1993) and through middle school (Muthén, Brown, et al., 2002). The effects persisted with a reduction 13 years later in the rate of diagnosis of alcohol and illicit drug abuse or dependence (Kellam, Brown, et al., 2008). Also, for the subgroup of boys who started first grade with high levels of aggressive behavior, this intervention reduced the rate of antisocial personality disorder (Petras, Kellam, et al., 2008) and mental health service use (Poduska, Kellam, et al., 2008).

Structural and policy changes can reduce risk associated with the transition to senior high school (Seidman, Aber, and French, 2004). This transition is associated with a decline in academic performance as well as an increase in delinquency, depression, suicidal thoughts, and substance use. However, policy changes, such as reduced school size, that create smaller working units with more supportive relations with teachers and peers have been shown to reduce this risk (Felner, Brand, et al., 1993).

CONCLUSIONS AND RECOMMENDATIONS

A voluminous literature has emerged since the 1994 IOM report on the factors associated with MEB disorders in young people, with a consensus that these factors operate at multiple interrelated levels. Factors both specific to a given disorder and that provide a more generalized risk for multiple disorders provide important opportunities for the development of interventions that modify these factors and explore possible mediating mechanisms.

Conclusion: Research has identified well-established risk and protective factors for MEB disorders at the individual, family, school, and community levels that are targets for preventive interventions. However, the pathways by which these factors influence each other to lead to the development of disorders are not well understood.

Conclusion: Specific risk and protective factors have been identified for many of the major disorders, such as specific thinking and behavioral patterns for depression or cognitive deficits for schizophrenia. In addition, nonspecific factors, such as poverty and aversive experiences in families (e.g., marital conflict, poor parenting), schools (e.g., school failure, poor peer relations), and communities (e.g., violence), have been shown to increase the risk for developing most MEB disorders and problems.

A more recent science base has solidified around the concept of developmental competencies that could inform the development of future interventions focused on the promotion of mental, emotional, and behavioral health.

Conclusion: Interventions designed to prevent MEB disorders and problems and those designed to promote mental, emotional, and behavioral health both frequently involve directly strengthening children's competencies and positive mental health or strengthening families, schools, or communities. However, improved knowledge pertaining to the conceptualization and assessment of developmental competencies is needed to better inform interventions.

The ways in which developmental competencies operate in a health-promoting capacity is less well understood, and additional research is needed to develop common measures that can be used in intervention research.

Recommendation 4-1: Research funders led by the National Institutes of Health, should increase funding for research on the etiology and development of competencies and healthy functioning of young people, as well as how healthy functioning protects against the development of MEB disorders.

Recommendation 4-2: The National Institutes of Health should develop measures of developmental competencies and positive mental health across developmental stages that are comparable to measures used for MEB disorders. These measures should be developed in consultation with leading research and other key stakeholders and routinely used in mental health promotion intervention studies.

Current knowledge on the development of MEB disorders among young people and characteristics of healthy development suggest the need for multiple lines of inquiry for future preventive intervention research.

Recommendation 4-3: Research funders should fund preventive intervention research on (1) risk and protective factors for specific disorders; (2) risk and protective factors that lead to multiple mental, emotional, and behavioral problems and disorders; and (3) promotion of individual, family, school, and community competencies.

5

Perspectives from Developmental Neuroscience

C hapter 4 described the multiple risk and protective factors that can play a role in mental, emotional, and behavioral (MEB) disorders and that can inform the design of prevention interventions, placing these contributing factors in the framework of developmental processes. This chapter illustrates research advances in the framework of developmental neuroscience, including the anatomical and functional development of the brain, molecular and behavioral genetics, molecular and cellular neurobiology, and systems-level neuroscience, that relate to the prevention of MEB disorders. Perspectives from developmental neuroscience provide a foundation for understanding the development of cognitive abilities, emotions, and behaviors during childhood and adolescence, and they thereby reveal valuable opportunities for novel advances in future prevention research.

Reducing Risks for Mental Disorders: Frontiers for Preventive Intervention Research, the 1994 Institute of Medicine (IOM) report, emphasized the importance of the relationship between prevention research and a knowledge base that includes both basic and applied research in neurobiology and genetics. This knowledge base contributes to the understanding of the causes, course, and outcomes of MEB disorders, and it continues to be increasingly important for informing how prevention efforts may intervene in causal pathways that lead to disorders.

In the years since the 1994 IOM report, understanding of the biological processes that underlie brain development has grown at an unprecedented rate, and the past several decades have witnessed much greater interest in the neurobiological underpinnings of MEB disorders. These disorders are increasingly being understood as dynamic disruptions in key developmental processes that exert their effects throughout the life span. Unraveling the causes and consequences of complex MEB disorders remains an enormous challenge. However, major advances have been made not only in identifying genetic and environmental factors that play causal roles in the genesis of disorders, but also in understanding more fully the interaction between genetic and environmental influences in causing or protecting against specific diseases. In addition, advances in the emerging field of epigenetics have begun to provide information about the complex ways in which genetic traits are expressed as disease and the possible mechanisms through which environment and experience can influence gene expression.

This chapter begins with the role of genetics and the interplay of genetic and environmental factors in MEB disorders. This is followed by a discussion of brain development and its relationship to MEB disorders. Next is an examination of neural systems and their role in complex processes that underlie the cognitive and social competence that is essential to healthy emotional and behavioral development. The third section addresses the relationship between developmental neuroscience and prevention science. The final section presents conclusions and recommendations.

GENETICS

The importance of understanding genetic influences in brain development goes well beyond simply explaining the hereditary components of disorders. Genes are the basic component from which the brain's structure and function are determined and regulated. Genes encode proteins, and proteins are the building blocks of cells, interacting with the molecular and physical features of their surroundings to determine cellular structure and function. Individual cells interact functionally with other cells within the neural circuits that make up the structure of the brain, which in turn interact with other neural circuits to determine behaviors. Behaving organisms interact with their environments, which can cause adaptive changes in neural systems, circuits, and cells and ultimately in the expression of genes—which in turn modifies brain structure and function. The complexity of the pathways connecting the genes and the environments of organisms to their behaviors has frustrated most attempts to correlate genes directly with behaviors and with specific diagnostic syndromes in the field of psychiatric genetics (Inoue and Lupski, 2003; Joober, Sengupta, and Boksa, 2005; Sanders, Duan, and Gejman, 2004; van den Bree and Owen, 2003).

Inherited or sporadic genetic mutations can profoundly affect the production, structure, or function of the protein that a gene encodes. This can have a dramatic and highly consistent effect in producing disease. However, more subtle variations in the genetic sequence can also affect protein structure and function, producing much more subtle effects. For example, many of the genetic variants that have been associated with MEB disorders are single nucleotide polymorphisms, that is, substitutions of single nucleotides, the structural components of the genetic sequence (van Belzen and Heutnik, 2006; Sanders, Duan, and Gejman, 2004). Variability in the number of copies of a specific gene sequence (known as copy number variants), which can be caused by rearrangements, microdeletions, or microduplications of the sequence, has also emerged as an important contributor to MEB disorders (Lee and Lupski, 2006), such as schizophrenia (Walsh, McClellan, et al., 2008; Xu, Roos, et al., 2008; International Schizophrenia Consortium, 2008; Stefansson, Rujescu, et al., 2008) and autism (Sebat, Lakshmi, et al., 2007; Marshall, Noor, et al., 2008). These kinds of gene variations can have a more graded influence on molecular and cellular functions than do large deletions or rearrangements of genes. The influences of these gene variants on the structural and functional features of cells, neural circuits, and the behaviors they subserve are correspondingly graded as well.

Variations in the genetic sequences that encode proteins are only one level of influence on the expression of those genes in the production of cellular proteins. Variations in the sequence of the nonencoding, regulatory portions of a gene also have important influences on its expression, as can variations in other genes that encode regulatory proteins. In addition, microRNAs (small sequences of RNA, an intermediate genetic component in the process of making proteins from DNA) can influence the expression of genes and their protein products by altering how the proteins are generated from a gene sequence (Boyd, 2008; Stefani and Slack, 2008). These additional levels of regulation can determine when in the course of development, where in the brain, and to what degree a gene is expressed—all without changing the DNA sequence of the gene.

Many studies, including family studies and gene association studies, have demonstrated a genetic component to MEB disorders (Thapar and Stergiakouli, 2008; van Belzen and Heutnik, 2006). However, genetic studies have not yet found an association of single genes with most MEB disorders. Instead, sequence variants in multiple genes have been shown to be associated with an elevated risk or susceptibility for developing many diseases, such as autism (Muhle, Trentacoste, and Rapin, 2004), depression (Levinson, 2006; Lopez-Leon, Janssens, et al., 2008), schizophrenia (Owen, O'Donovan, and Harrison, 2005), addiction (Goldman, Oroszi, and Ducci, 2005), and bipolar disorder (Serretti and Mandelli, 2008). A review of these many reported associations of specific genes with individual disorders is beyond the scope of this report.

In nearly all instances of these reported associations, the influence of individual genes on the risk for developing a disorder is small (Kendler, 2005; Thapar and Stergiakouli, 2008), usually less than the influence of family history and less than that of other nongenetic risk factors. The association is also often nonspecific (Kendler, 2005), with single gene variants being associated with multiple disorders. Moreover, genetic profiles vary greatly among affected individuals. Not everyone with the susceptibility variant in any one of the associated genes will develop the disorder, and not everyone with a particular disorder will have the susceptibility variant of any associated gene. Therefore, a single genetic variant will rarely be necessary or sufficient to produce a disorder, a point similar to findings on the association of environmental risk factors with MEB disorders (described later in this chapter and in Chapter 4). One strategy that has emerged to address the complexity of linking genes to disorders is to identify more narrowly defined behaviors, characteristics, or biological markers, termed "endophenotypes," that correlate with specific disorders or that are common to more than one disorder. These endophenotypes can serve as a simpler, more readily identifiable focus of genetic studies (Caspi and Moffitt, 2006; Gottesman and Gould, 2003; van Belzen and Heutink, 2006).

Beyond finding associations between genetic variants and MEB disorders or endophenotypes, identifying the effects that specific genes have on molecular pathways, cellular organization, functioning of neural networks, and behavior is crucially important to developing effective intervention approaches based on the modifiable components of the pathways from genes to behavior. This level of genetic research requires experimental manipulations in animal models. Most commonly this involves modification of the genome of mice by inserting, deleting, or mutating specific genes and, in some cases, controlling where in the brain, in what cell types, and when during the course of development a gene is turned off or on. This extraordinary degree of spatial and temporal control over gene expression makes animal models invaluable in identifying the molecular processes of normal and pathological brain development. The disadvantage of animal models, however, is the difficulty of representing the complex cognitive, behavioral, and emotional symptoms experienced by humans. Although the effects of experimental manipulation on certain aspects of cognition and memory can be assessed through the ability of animals to learn and repeat standardized tasks, analogues of emotional experience and thought can be inferred only through behavior that must be correlated with subjective human experience (Cryan and Holmes, 2005; Joel, 2006; McKinney, 2001; Murcia, Gulden, and Herrup, 2005; Powell and Miyakawa, 2006; Sousa, Almeida, and Wotjak, 2006).

Animal models are proving to be of central importance in identifying the likely disturbances in molecular and cellular pathways caused by single gene mutations in some neurodevelopmental disorders, including the fragile X, Prader-Willi, Angelman, and Rett syndromes. Knowledge of those molecular pathways already has led to promising treatment approaches in animal models (Chang, Bray, et al., 2008; Bear, Dolen, et al., 2008; Chahrour and Zoghbi, 2007; Dolen, Osterweil, et al., 2007; Giacometti, Luikenhuis, et al., 2007; Guy, Gan, et al., 2007). Animal models have also successfully linked risk genes with disturbances in particular molecular pathways that may predispose to the development of more complex, polygenic disorders, such as depression (Cryan and Holmes, 2005; Urani, Chourbaji, and Gass, 2005), anxiety disorders (Cryan and Holmes, 2005), obsessive compulsive disorder (Joel, 2006), autism (Moy and Nadler, 2008), schizophrenia (O'Tuathaigh, Babovic, et al., 2007), and substance abuse (Kalivas, Peters, and Knackstedt, 2006).

Despite the challenge of studying the role of genes in the etiology of MEB disorders, advances in technology continue to make large-scale genotyping more feasible and affordable, and the combination of human genetics studies and approaches using animal models has proven to be informative in identifying genes of risk in multifactorial, complex non-psychiatric disorders, such as asthma (Moffatt, 2008) and diabetes (Florez, 2008); they will undoubtedly make important contributions in psychiatric genetics in coming years.

Gene–Environment Interactions and Correlations

Most complex behaviors and the most common forms of MEB disorders are likely to arise from a combination of multiple interacting genetic and environmental influences (Caspi and Moffitt, 2006; Rutter, Moffitt, and Caspi, 2006). The effect of a common genetic variant in altering the risk for a disorder, for example, is likely to be conditioned heavily by the experiences of a developing child, just as the effects of experience in producing a disorder are likely to be conditioned by the genetic background that the child inherits from his or her parents (Rutter, Moffitt, and Caspi, 2006; Thapar, Harold, et al., 2007). These so-called gene–environment (GxE) interactions can confer both risk and protective effects on the child relative to the effects of either the genetic or environmental influences in isolation.

A number of interactions between specific identified genes and specific environmental risk factors have been demonstrated in MEB disorders (Rutter, Moffitt, and Caspi, 2006). For example, a landmark prospective epidemiological study found that the number of copies an individual carries of the short variant of a region of the serotonin transporter gene (5-HTTLPR) significantly increases, in a dose-dependent fashion, the risk for developing depressive symptoms, major depressive disorder, and suicidality—but only in the context of adverse or stressful early life experiences (Caspi, Sugden, et al., 2003) (see Figure 5-1). Similarly, a polymorphism in the gene that encodes monoamine oxidase A (MAOA), an enzyme that metabolizes neurotransmitters, moderates the effect of maltreatment on developing antisocial

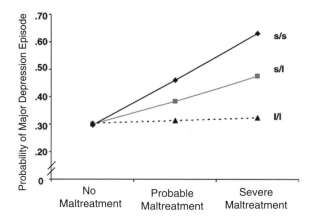

FIGURE 5-1 Gene–environment interaction between effects of prior maltreatment and genotype for the 5-HTTLPR allele on developing depression later in life. Maltreatment has the biggest effect for two copies of the short (s/s) allele and the smallest effect for two copies of the long (l/l) allele. There is an intermediate effect for one copy of each allele (s/l).
SOURCE: Caspi, Sugden, et al. (2003).

problems later in life (Kim-Cohen, Caspi, et al., 2006; Caspi, McClay, et al., 2002): Maltreated children who have the genotype that confers high levels of MAOA expression are less likely to develop conduct disorder, antisocial personality, or adult violent crime. In another domain, a common polymorphism of the dopamine transporter gene has been reported to interact with the risk conferred by prenatal exposure to tobacco smoke, leading to increased hyperactive-impulsive and oppositional behaviors in later childhood (Kahn, Khoury, et al., 2003).

In contrast to GxE interactions, gene–environment correlations are genetic influences on variations in the likelihood that an individual will experience specific environmental circumstances (Jaffee and Price, 2007; Rutter and Silberg, 2002; Rutter, Moffitt, and Caspi, 2006). Gene–environment correlations can confound cause and effect and hinder measurement of GxE interactions because a genetically determined behavioral trait can produce a systematic variation in environmental exposure, and that environmental variation can be deemed erroneously to be a cause of a behavioral trait under study (Jaffee and Price, 2007; Lau and Eley, 2008). Children with autism, for example, are chronically and consistently withdrawn from their caregivers. This chronic withdrawal might induce in the caregiver a sense of hopelessness about ever making a deep interpersonal connection with the child, prompting a secondary withdrawal on the part of the caregiver. An unsuspecting researcher might inadvertently and erroneously attribute the child's impoverished social relatedness to the caregiver's withdrawal, when in fact it was caused by a particular genetic variant.

Epigenetic Effects

Epigenetic effects are potentially heritable alterations of gene expression that do not involve actual modification of the DNA sequence. Instead, alterations in the level of gene expression are induced by changes in the three-dimensional packaging of DNA that in turn make a gene either more or less amenable to production of a protein product. All known mechanisms that produce epigenetic changes in gene expression involve enzymatic processes that add or remove substrates either from the DNA or from histone proteins that are physically associated with DNA and that determine its three-dimensional packing structure (Tsankova, Renthal, et al., 2007). Epigenetic modifications of gene expression are in continual flux, as competing factors modify and unmodify DNA and its associated proteins, as well as their related behavioral phenotypes.

Epigenetic determinants are increasingly invoked as possible explanations for a multitude of "complex genetic" phenotypes, in which multiple genes are each thought to account for a small amount of variance in the clinical phenotype. Moreover, recent research has shown that epigenetic mechanisms can produce short-term adaptation of the phenotype to a changing environment. For example, abundant naturalistic and experimental evidence in humans and animal models has shown that early experience influences reactivity to stress later in life, even into adulthood, and that epigenetic modification of genes that encode components of the stress response can contribute to these enduring effects (Kaffman and Meaney, 2007; Weaver, 2007).

Perhaps most remarkably, a changing environment has been shown to trigger epigenetic effects that can be transmitted across generations, in species as diverse as yeast and humans (Rakyan and Beck, 2006; Richards, 2006; Whitelaw and Whitelaw, 2006). The quality of maternal care given to rat pups, for example, produces epigenetic modifications of gene expression in the brains of the pups that influence the quality of maternal care they provide as adults to their own offspring. This cross-generation transmission has been shown to account for variability in maternal behavior toward offspring that is either nurturing or neglectful (Champagne, 2008).

Several examples suggest that epigenetic mechanisms are important in understanding the causes and in improving the prevention and treatment of MEB disorders (Tsankova, Renthal, et al., 2007). One well-known example is the Prader-Willi and the Angelman syndromes, disorders with highly distinct phenotypes that are nevertheless both caused by a mutation in the same chromosomal region. Although the locus of the mutation is the same, its effects on the behavioral phenotype of the child differ depending on which parent is the origin of the mutation (Goldstone, 2004; Lalande and Calciano, 2007; Nicholls and Knepper, 2001).

Another example of the importance of epigenetic influences in the cause of a disorder is Rett syndrome, a progressive neurodevelopmental disorder characterized by motor, speech, and social behavioral abnormalities (Chahrour and Zoghbi, 2007). Mutations in the MeCP2 gene cause Rett syndrome and, less commonly, other neurodevelopmental disorders, including classic autism, mental retardation, early-onset bipolar disorder, and early-onset schizophrenia. This gene encodes a protein that epigenetically alters the expression of other genes (Chahrour and Zoghbi, 2007; Zlatanova, 2005). In other words, this specific genetic mutation causes disease through epigenetic mechanisms, underscoring how complex, intimate, and interactive genetic and epigenetic factors are in influencing the development of disorders.

Epigenetic modifications of the genome are also necessary for various learning and memory processes in the brain (Levenson and Sweatt, 2005, 2006; Levenson, Roth, et al., 2006; Reul and Chandramohan, 2007; Fischer, Sananbenesi, et al., 2007), suggesting that these processes may be important in the etiology of various mental retardation syndromes. Epigenetic influences play a prominent role as well in changes in the brain and in behavior related to establishing preferences for drugs of abuse in animal models of addiction (Kumar, Choi, et al., 2005). Finally, epigenetic modifications of the genome have been shown to be necessary to produce the behavioral response to antidepressant medications in a mouse model of depression (Newton and Duman, 2006; Tsankova, Berton, et al., 2006).

BRAIN DEVELOPMENT

MEB disorders in children involve disturbances in the most complex, highly integrated functions of the human brain. Understanding from a biological perspective how these functional capacities develop and how they are disrupted is an immense challenge. This section offers a brief overview of current knowledge about the complex processes that contribute to the normal development of the human brain, along with examples of their relationship to the causes of MEB disorders.

Sources of Knowledge of Human Brain Development

Knowledge of normal human brain development and of the abnormalities that produce disorders is limited by the difficulty of studying the human brain at the level of molecules and cells. The human data on brain development thus far come from a small number of postmortem studies and a larger number of in vivo, or live, brain imaging studies. The scientific value of postmortem studies is limited by the quality and number of tissue samples that are usually available and by the capability to study only a small number of brain regions (Lewis, 2002). In contrast, in vivo imaging has proved to be an important tool for studying postnatal brain development in humans across the life span (Marsh, Gerber, and Peterson, 2008), although thus far it has provided information about brain structure and function mainly at a macroscopic level of brain organization, revealing little molecular or cellular information (Peterson, 2003b).

Understanding of the molecular and cellular development of the human brain is therefore gleaned largely from studies of animal models, extrapolated to the maturational timeline of humans. Although a great deal has been learned from those animal models across a wide range of species, how well those findings relate to the development and function of the human brain is not fully known. Moreover, as noted earlier, the molecular bases of the highest-order functions of the human brain cannot be studied easily in animals.

Despite limited data from human and nonhuman primates, the consistency in findings across species suggests that the general features of brain development in animal models are likely to apply to humans as well. Those findings indicate that the wiring of neural architecture is neither fixed nor static. Instead, it is a dynamic entity that is shaped and reshaped continually throughout development by processes that have their own maturational timetables within and across brain regions. These processes are described briefly here and summarized in Figure 5-2.

Overview: Complexities of Brain Development

At the visible anatomical level, the human brain develops during gestation into a complex structure having distinct anatomical regions and a highly convoluted surface. Similarly, at the level of cellular architecture, the human brain is a highly complex, layered structure made up of many distinct kinds of cells that have highly specific interconnections. During fetal brain development, undifferentiated precursor cells need to divide and multiply. The resulting cells must then differentiate into the correct cell types, migrate to the correct place in the brain, and connect properly with other cells. These links among cells must then be organized into functional circuits that support sensation, perception, cognition, emotion, learning, and behavior. In a healthy intrauterine environment, this series of complex and interrelated neurodevelopmental events is initially under the predetermined control of regulatory genes (Rhinn, Picker, and Brand, 2006). In contrast, much of the fine detail of brain organization—how the brain is "wired"—develops

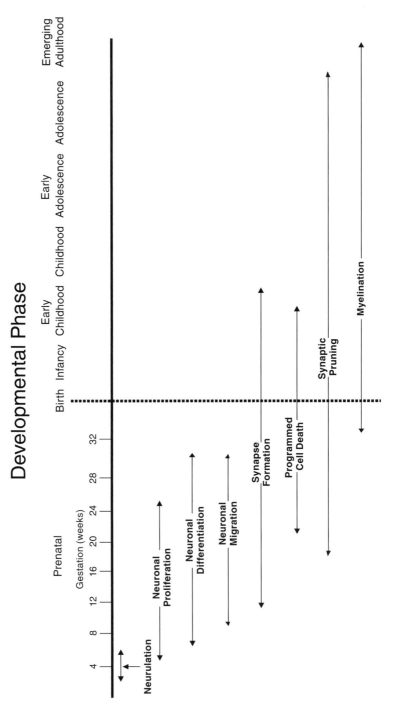

FIGURE 5-2 Timeline of major events in brain development.

through a combination of genetic influences, experience and other external influences, and the interaction of genes and experience.

Setting Up the Nervous System

The nervous system begins to develop in the human fetus 2 to 3 weeks after conception in a process called neurulation, starting as a layer of undifferentiated precursor cells called the neural plate. These cells eventually give rise to all components of the nervous system. As the initial cells divide to create more cells, the neural plate expands, folds, and fuses to form the neural tube (Detrait, George, et al., 2005; Kibar, Capra, and Gros, 2007). The neural tube continues to enlarge while cells in different parts of the tube become specialized, following a spatial pattern established by predetermined molecular mechanisms. From front to back, the neural tube becomes the forebrain (the cerebral cortices), the midbrain (containing neural pathways to and from the forebrain), the hindbrain (the brainstem and cerebellum), and the spinal cord and peripheral nervous system (Rhinn, Picker, and Brand, 2006).

Various physiological and environmental factors can affect prenatal brain development in ways that are either lethal or seriously debilitating (Detrait, George, et al., 2005; Kibar, Capra, and Gros, 2007). Low levels of the vitamin folic acid, for example, produce anencephaly and spina bifida, disorders of formation of the neural tube. Other prenatal environmental exposures can predispose a developing fetus to the development of MEB disorders later in life. For example, common prenatal infections, such as influenza, and less common ones, such as rubella, toxoplasmosis, and cytomegalovirus, can increase the risk of developing mental retardation, schizophrenia, and autism (Fruntes and Limosin, 2008; Jones, Lopez, and Wilson, 2003; Meyer, Yee, and Feldon, 2007; Pearce, 2001; Penner and Brown, 2007). Prenatal exposure to various environmental toxins, including certain insecticides used in homes and for agricultural purposes (Rauh, Garfinkel, et al., 2006), tobacco smoke (Herrmann, King, and Weitzman, 2008), and alcohol (Alcohol Research and Health, 2000), can impair behavior and cognition later in childhood (Williams and Ross, 2007). Premature birth and low birth weight can also predispose to a wide variety of disorders (Peterson, 2003a), including schizophrenia (Kunugi, Nanko, and Murray, 2001), autism (Kolevzon, Gross, and Reichenberg, 2007), and learning disabilities and educational difficulties (Peterson, 2003a).

The Right Cells in the Right Place

Between weeks 5 and 25 of human fetal gestation, undifferentiated precursor cells divide repeatedly, rapidly giving rise to large numbers of cells that will become neurons. Glial cells, the supporting cells of the nervous system, are also generated, but somewhat later than neurons, between weeks 20 and 40 (de Graaf-Peters and Hadders-Algra, 2006). Once cells are generated, two different processes overlap in time. First, the identity or "fate" of these cells becomes progressively more restricted, until the cells are fully differentiated into a specific type of neuron or glial cell. Second, neurons must travel from the site of their origin to their appropriate final location in the brain to provide the function they will ultimately serve, a process called neuronal migration (de Graaf-Peters and Hadders-Algra, 2006; Levitt, 2003; Rakic, 2003). The precise path of neuronal migration is determined by the timing and position of a cell when it is generated, together with a molecular "map" composed of a variety of molecular signals from neighboring cells that guide the migrating cell to its proper final position in a precise and reproducible manner (de Graaf-Peters and Hadders-Algra, 2006; Levitt, 2003; Rakic, 2003). The number of migrating neurons in the human fetus peaks by about week 20 of gestation, and migration stops by about week 30 (de Graaf-Peters and Hadders-Algra, 2006).

Disturbances in neuronal migration have emerged as a key area of interest in understanding the developmental basis of MEB disorders. Failures in neuronal migration produce an accumulation of neurons in the wrong areas of the brain and, consequently, can lead to disorganized brain structure and function. This can be seen in major malformations of the brain, such as lissencephaly (a brain that lacks the usual, complex folded surface) (Guerrini and Filippi, 2005). More subtle disturbances of neuronal migration can create isolated islands of neurons or disruptions of normal circuit function, leading to seizures (Guerrini and Filippi, 2005). Genetic and environmental influences on neuronal migration can produce even more subtle disturbances in the locations of cells that may not be visible at the gross anatomical level but may nevertheless affect functional circuits. In cortical areas involved in higher-level cognitive functions, these effects potentially can produce subtle changes in the brain's behavioral, emotional, and cognitive capacities that may not manifest until later in life (Rakic, 2002, 2003).

Establishing Connections

Once cells are properly differentiated and as they are migrating to their final locations in the brain, they grow extensions, called axons and dendrites, that allow them to connect to and communicate with other neurons. Axons are primarily responsible for sending signals to other cells, and dendrites are processes that primarily receive signals from other cells. Axons use the guidance of external molecular signals to find their way to the right target cells with which they will connect and communicate. A combination of growth-promoting and growth-inhibiting signals provides the growing tip of the axon with a map of connectivity to get to the right location and connect with the right target cell (Chilton, 2006; Tessier-Lavigne and Goodman, 1996).

Dendritic growth and branching begins early in development, initially proceeding slowly but then accelerating rapidly starting in the third trimester (de Graaf-Peters and Hadders-Algra, 2006), producing a thickening of the cortex (the complex, multilayered collection of cells composing the entire outer surface of the brain) (Huisman, Martin, et al., 2002). The timing of dendritic growth differs by brain region and by layer of the cortex. For example, dendritic elaboration is slower in frontal than in visual cortex, and it begins in the deeper layers earlier than in more superficial ones (Becker, Armstrong, et al., 1984; de Graaf-Peters and Hadders-Algra, 2006; Huttenlocher, 1990; Michel and Garey, 1984; Mrzljak, Uylings, et al., 1992). Overall, dendritic development is highly active from the third trimester of gestation through the first postnatal year, continuing at lower rates through age 5 years (de Graaf-Peters and Hadders-Algra, 2006).

Differing neuronal cell types have diverse shapes and sizes. Some have relatively simple shapes. Others have many axonal branches, allowing them to innervate and influence more target cells. Some have complex dendritic trees that provide a greater range of input from other cells. This diversity of form and structure provides for a range of computational functions across different kinds of neurons, from a limited signal input and response to a complex integration of multiple signals. Connections are established with cells that are nearby and cells that are much more distant, eventually linking and integrating information from different regions of the brain.

The basis of this communication between neurons is their physical connection, called a synapse. The formation of synapses requires the development of specialized cellular machinery on both the presynaptic side of the synapse (where neurotransmitters are prepared and released from the terminals of axons) and at the postsynaptic target (where receptors for those neurotransmitters receive and process the signal) (Waites, Craig, and Garner, 2005). The rate of synapse formation increases rapidly after about weeks 24-28 and peaks, at the rate of almost 40,000 new synapses per second, between 3 and 15 months after birth (in the primary sensory and prefrontal cortices, respectively) (de Graaf-Peters and Hadders-Algra, 2006; Levitt, 2003).

The synapse is the primary site of information transfer in the nervous system, and it is also likely to be the primary site of learning and memory. Several disorders that begin early in life and are associated with profound intellectual and emotional disability can be considered disturbances of learning and memory. These include fragile X and other causes of mental retardation, Rett syndrome, and autistic spectrum disorders. Genes that have been identified as either causing or increasing the risk for developing these disorders can be conceived as having in common the disruption of normal development and function of synapses (Chao, Zoghbi, and Rosenmund, 2007; Dierssen and Ramakers, 2006; Willemsen, Oostra, et al., 2004; Zoghbi, 2003).

Refining the Nervous System: Use It or Lose It

Neurons and the connections between them are produced in an overabundance during fetal life relative to their levels at birth and in adulthood. The number of neurons in the human brain, for example, peaks around midgestation. Thereafter, overproduction is reduced through a process of molecularly programmed cell death, called apoptosis (de Graaf-Peters and Hadders-Algra, 2006; Levitt, 2003). For continued survival, neurons require a successful interaction with a target cell, and neurons that do not achieve this interaction will die. Neuronal survival is mediated in part by the limited availability of neurotrophic factors, a class of molecules that are derived from the target cells (Monk, Webb, and Nelson, 2001).

The process of brain development also produces an initial surplus of connections between neurons. Early in postnatal life, the density of synapses in the brain increases dramatically, reaching its peak during infancy (de Graaf-Peters and Hadders-Algra, 2006; Huttenlocher, 1984; Huttenlocher and Dabholkar, 1997; Levitt, 2003). The process of forming synapses, or synaptogenesis, is paired with the complementary process of synaptic pruning, in which some synaptic connections are eliminated. Primates are widely believed to have evolved synaptic pruning as a means for removing synaptic connections that are unused and therefore not needed in the environmental context in which the animal finds itself, while conserving and increasing the efficiency of connections that are useful in that context. Thus, survival of most of the synaptic connections that subserve human behavior is influenced by patterns of neural activity, which in turn are the product of environmental influences and experience (Kandel, Schwartz, and Jessell, 2000).

Studies in humans during childhood are limited but, in combination with data from studies in monkeys, indicate that after the peak of synaptogenesis in infancy, synapse formation and synaptic pruning plateau during childhood and then reach a regressive phase between puberty and adulthood. At that point, a massive, activity-dependent pruning eliminates more than 40 percent of synapses (de Graaf-Peters and Hadders-Algra, 2006; Huttenlocher and Dabholkar, 1997; Levitt, 2003; Rakic, 2002; Rakic, Bourgeois, and Goldman-Rakic, 1994).

Another important process in developing and refining appropriate connectivity in the brain is the wrapping of neuronal axons in an insulating sheath of myelin, which promotes the rapid and efficient conduction of electrical impulses. In humans, myelination progresses rapidly from 1 to 2 months prior to birth through the first 1 to 2 years of life, but it also continues through adolescence and into adulthood (Levitt, 2003; Paus, Collins, et al., 2001; Yakovlev and Lecours, 1967). This timing is similar to the developmental timing of dendritic elaboration and synapse formation.

The survival of cells and synapses requires their ongoing neural activity, suggesting that external stimuli and environmental conditions, including relative deprivation, can have important long-term influences on brain development. These influences have been demonstrated in animal models, from rodents to nonhuman primates (Sanchez, Ladd, and Plotsky, 2001). Their demonstration in humans has been more indirect. It includes evidence that differences in cognitive and psychosocial stimulation are associated with modest differences in cognitive development (Gottlieb and Blair, 2004; Santos, Assis, et al., 2008; Walker, Wachs, et al., 2007), and that the more severe environmental deprivation that occurs with institutionalized infants reduces head size and overall physical growth and impairs emotional and social responsiveness, attentional abilities, and cognitive development (Smyke, Koga, et al., 2007).

Pathological synaptic pruning in particular may contribute to the genesis of at least some MEB disorders, although in the absence of direct longitudinal data, this hypothesis has not yet been confirmed (Levitt, 2003; Rakic, 2002). Disturbances in synaptic pruning that occur during adolescence are hypothesized to underlie many of the anatomical and functional disturbances seen in brain imaging of persons with schizophrenia (Lewis and Levitt, 2002; McGlashan and Hoffman, 2000). Longitudinal studies have reported exaggerated rates of cortical thinning in the dorsal prefrontal, parietal, and temporal cortices compared with healthy developing controls (Mathalon, Sullivan, et al., 2001; Thompson, Vidal, et al., 2001). Nevertheless, the cellular bases for this cortical thinning, as well as the mechanism whereby exaggerated cortical thinning would produce psychotic symptoms, are unknown.

Continuing Development and Mechanisms of Change

As noted, many developmental processes in the brain continue into childhood, adolescence, and young adulthood. This appears to be true of the frontal lobe in particular. In fact, several large human imaging studies have reported a progressive reduction in the thickness or volume of gray matter (regions containing neuronal cell bodies) in the cerebral cortex that begins in childhood and continues through young adulthood, particularly in areas of the frontal and parietal cortices (Giedd, Blumenthal, et al.,

1999; Sowell, Peterson, et al., 2003). These are higher cortical areas that contribute to attentional processes and the regulation of thought and behavior. The decline in cortical gray matter may represent a synaptic pruning in adolescence and young adulthood that could produce more efficient processing in the neural pathways that support improvements in these cognitive processes, which constitute a vitally important feature of adolescent development.

The brain is subject to continual change even after its fundamental architecture and functional circuitry have been established, as evidenced by the capacity to learn new skills and establish new memories throughout life. Changes in brain structure in response to experience, learning, various physiological processes, and pharmacological or environmental agents are known as neural plasticity. Although the molecular mechanisms underlying neural plasticity are not fully understood, experience is known to induce anatomical changes across all levels of the nervous system, from molecular and cellular processes to entire neural pathways.

Such changes in brain structure begin with changes in the architecture of the synapse. Experience in the short term produces transient changes in the strength of communication across synaptic connections primarily by changing the availability of neurotransmitters and other signaling molecules. Experience in the longer term produces changes in synaptic activity, which can influence signaling pathways to regulate the function of receptors and other proteins or to change the number of receptors at the synapse. In addition, ongoing synaptic activity induces changes in gene expression that alter the production of proteins either to build up new synapses or to break down existing ones (Purves, Augustine, et al., 2000). The molecular pathways that alter gene expression and modify synaptic architecture have been studied most extensively in brain regions that subserve learning and memory, especially the hippocampus and the cerebellum. Whether and how these molecular pathways produce changes in the strength of synapses that encode other complex behaviors are not yet known.

In addition to these neuroplastic changes at the level of individual synapses, the brain is plastic at the level of cortical organization. Studies in monkeys have demonstrated that when a digit is amputated, the amount of tissue in the brain that controls movement and sensation changes over a period of weeks, so that the areas representing the remaining digits, which continue to receive sensory input, expand to take over the regions previously occupied by the missing digit (Merzenich, Nelson, et al., 1984; Purves, Augustine, et al., 2000). Similarly, if a monkey is trained to use a digit disproportionately to accomplish a task, the representation of that digit in the motor cortex expands to take over areas previously mapped to neighboring digits (Jenkins, Merzenich, et al., 1990; Purves, Augustine, et al., 2000). In addition, new connections in the cortex are generated when monkeys learn a new skill, such as using a tool, or after localized brain damage (Dancause, Barbay, et al., 2005; Hihara, Notoya, et al., 2006; Johansen-Berg, 2007). Similarly, the learning of new skills in humans leads to changes in the cortical regions that subserve that task (Doyon and Benali, 2005; Ungerleider, Doyon, and Karni, 2002).

One emerging question in the study of neural plasticity is the role that newly generated neurons may have in the postnatal brain. Mature, differentiated neurons have generally lost the capacity to divide to produce new cells, and a central dogma in neuroscience for most of the past century has been that all proliferation of new neurons ends during fetal life. However, many studies have recently provided indisputable evidence that postnatal production of new neurons, or neurogenesis, does in fact occur, even in adult life, in a small number of brain regions and in a large range of species (Gould, 2007). These neurons are generated from a population of neural stem cells that are retained in the brain. Although the full range of triggers for neurogenesis has yet to be identified, it appears to include a broad array of stimuli from experience and the environment, including physical activity and even antidepressant medications (Lledo, Alonso, and Grubb, 2006). The birth of new neurons in postnatal life is one of many means through which experience can modify anatomical circuitry and functional activity in the brain. The number of new neurons generated is small, however, and whether and to what extent these neurons are able to integrate into synaptic circuits and exert a significant functional influence in the brain are at present unclear (Ghashghaei, Lai, and Anton, 2007; Gould, 2007; Lledo, Alonso, and Grubb, 2006).

The ongoing capacity for change in the brain underlies potential mechanisms through which brain function can compensate for, or even recover from, a disorder, whether that disorder derives primarily from adverse genetic or environmental influences or a combination of both. In a broad sense, then, virtually all responses in the brain that help compensate for the presence of a disorder can be considered neuroplastic responses, and they are likely to have their structural basis in the remodeling of synaptic connections and neural systems in the brain. Moreover, the causes of certain MEB disorders are thought to involve the exaggeration or "hijacking" of certain learning and memory processes. This is thought to be a prominent feature of the pathogenesis of addictive disorders, for example, in which substances of abuse pharmacologically induce plasticity in brain circuits that are involved in reward and associative learning. This exaggerated plasticity helps establish new, abnormal stimulus–response associations among the substance, the cues that accompany it, and the behavioral responses to those cues that define disorders of addiction (Kalivas and O'Brien, 2008; Kauer and Malenka, 2007).

Sensitive Periods in Brain Development

Environmental influences that affect specific developmental processes have maximal effects during the developmental stages when those processes are under way. These developmental time periods, referred to as either "critical" or "sensitive" periods, thus constitute a window of influence for experience that is crucially important for proper brain development or for vulnerability of the developing brain to pathogenic influences from the environment. Perhaps the paradigmatic example of this point is the effect of monocular occlusion, in which one eye is sutured closed and prevented from receiving any sensory input. In adult animals, monocular occlusion produces no effect on vision or on brain structure and function. When imposed early in development, however, it permanently alters both: It impairs vision in that eye, it reduces cortical representation of the sutured eye, and it expands cortical representation of the open eye. Binocular occlusion produces perhaps even more extraordinary reorganization of the brain during an early critical period, as neurons in the would-be visual area respond not to light or visual stimuli, but to auditory and somatosensory stimuli instead (Purves, Augustine, et al., 2000; Wiesel, 1982).

Sensitive periods in humans are most clearly identified for disturbances in development of gross sensory and motor functions. For example, problems that create an imbalance in the activity of the two eyes early in life can have a permanent effect on the function of the cortical visual system. Failure to correct congenital cataracts by about age 4 months in human infants produces irreversible impairments in the visual system (Purves, Augustine, et al., 2000). Similarly, correction of strabismus, a misalignment of eye orientation, by age 7 produces optimal prevention of permanent visual impairment (Flynn, Schiffman, et al., 1998), possibly because synaptic elimination in the visual cortex is complete by that time.

Evidence in humans for the existence of sensitive periods when exposure to specific environmental and experiential influences confers enhanced vulnerability to the development of MEB disorders is thus far modest and largely circumstantial. The effects on cognitive development of environmental deprivation and separation from human caregivers may be more severe during early development (Nelson, Zeanah, et al., 2007), an observation consistent with the effects of early separation that have been documented in nonhuman primates (O'Connor and Cameron, 2006; Sabatini, Ebert, et al., 2007). Furthermore, traumatic experiences in childhood and adolescence appear to predispose to the development of severe character pathologies in adulthood; these effects are distinct from the effects of trauma experienced later in life (Bierer, Yehuda, et al., 2003; Golier, Yehuda, et al., 2003; Goodman, New, and Siever, 2004). These effects of childhood maltreatment in humans are consistent with animal models of child abuse and neglect that suggest that early maltreatment alters emotional responses and behaviors in adulthood while supporting learned preferences that are necessary for attachment to abusive caregivers (Moriceau and Sullivan, 2006; Roth and Sullivan, 2005; Sevelinges, Moriceau, et al., 2007). Additional evidence for sensitive periods in humans comes from studies reporting that prenatal but not postnatal exposure to tobacco smoke increases the risk of attention disorders in school-age children (Braun, Kahn, et al., 2006). The neural bases for the effects of early experience on higher-order neurodevelopmental outcomes in humans and in animal models are thus far largely unknown.

NEURAL SYSTEMS

Developmental processes early in brain development establish fundamental brain structure and circuitry. To achieve the complex functions of the brain, signaling circuits that serve similar functions are grouped and integrated in networks both within the cortex and between the cortex and other regions of the brain. These neural systems subserve complex processes, such as learning and memory, attachment, social relatedness, and self-regulatory control. These behaviors underlie the cognitive and social competence that is an essential part of healthy emotional and behavioral development, and deficits in these systems play a role in many MEB disorders.

Learning and Memory

Multiple systems for learning and memory exist in the brain. Working memory, for example, is the "scratch pad" where information is retained for conscious manipulation (D'Esposito, 2007). Declarative memory, in contrast, is the conscious recall of facts, prior experiences, and semantic knowledge that is rapidly acquired and then consolidated for storage as long-term memory (Kandel, 2001; Purves, Augustine, et al., 2000). The hippocampus, working within networks with cortical regions, is important for remembering spatial and temporal relationships and for associative learning processes. It is centrally important for conscious learning and memory, contributing significantly to overall intellectual capacity (Amat, Bansal, et al., 2008; Atallah, Frank, and O'Reilly, 2004; Eichenbaum, 2000; Moser and Moser, 1998). A form of memory that often stands in starkest contrast to declarative memory is the incremental learning and memory of motor skills, procedures, and habits, which collectively is termed "procedural," "habit," or "stimulus-response" (S-R) learning. S-R learning relies on a neural system that is distinct anatomically and functionally from the hippocampus-based declarative memory system and includes the striatum, a portion of the basal ganglia deep within the brain (Packard and Knowlton, 2002). Changes in activity of dopaminergic neurons within the striatum also support learning in response to reward. Reward is an essential component of many learning processes, and it is thought to be involved in both declarative and S-R learning (Adcock, Thangavel, et al., 2006; Shohamy, Myers, et al., 2008).

Emotional experiences have powerful influences on memory, particularly on the accuracy and emotional tone of recalled memories in the declarative memory system. Emotional learning depends heavily on the interactions of the amygdala with the physically adjacent hippocampus, as well as with more remote structures that include the striatum and the frontal cortex. The interaction of the amygdala with memory systems imbues memories with the emotional tone experienced during and following the recalled event (McGaugh, 2004). Experimental emulation and manipulation of various emotions in animal models have shown that the interactions between the amygdala and the hippocampus are influenced heavily by the actions of various neurotransmitters and hormones that mediate the effects of emotional experience on the recall of arousing, rewarding, and stressful life events (McGaugh, 2004; Roozendaal, Okuda, et al., 2006).

In addition to declarative, S-R, and working memory systems, the brain supports associative or conditioned learning, as originally described by Pavlov. This form of learning involves the pairing of a stimulus that does not produce an innate behavioral response (the to-be "conditioned stimulus" or "CS," such as a tone) with a stimulus that does produce an innate behavioral response (the "unconditioned stimulus" or "US," such as a food odor that produces salivation). After repeated pairings of the CS and the US, the CS alone will elicit the unconditioned response (salivation). Conditioned learning involves numerous brain regions, including the hippocampus and the cerebellum (Thompson, 2005; Daum, Schugens, et al., 1993; Logan and Grafton, 1995).

The obverse of conditioned learning is extinction, in which the unconditioned response to the CS is modulated downward over time. Extinction involves exposing an animal repeatedly to a stimulus that has been previously conditioned to elicit fear, but now in the absence of any aversive event. This will extinguish the fearful, conditioned response. Extinction is therefore an active process and not simply a passive, dissipating process of forgetting (Myers and Davis, 2007; Quirk and Mueller, 2008). Extinction is cue-specific, in that extinction to one CS does not induce or accompany extinction to another CS (Myers and Davis, 2007). When extinction fails, as it can during times of stress, the conditioned behavior can reappear (Akirav and Maroun, 2007). The neural basis of fear extinction is thought to include the amygdala, the hippocampus, and the medial prefrontal cortex (Myers and Davis, 2007; Quirk and Mueller, 2008).

Disturbances in one or more of these various learning and memory systems have been implicated in the pathogenesis of a wide range of disorders.

This may not be surprising if the brain is viewed as having been constructed quintessentially for the processes of learning and remembering in order to enhance adaptation and survival efficacy. The diverse and spatially distributed neural systems subserving a great variety of learning and memory systems can give rise to equally numerous and diverse illnesses.

For example, attention deficit hyperactivity disorder (ADHD) has been conceptualized as a disturbance in emotional and reward-based learning, given the difficulty that children with ADHD have learning from prior mistakes, as well as their poor performance on delay aversion tasks, their preferences for smaller immediate rewards over larger delayed ones, and their more frequent risk-taking behaviors (Farmer and Peterson, 1995; Oosterlaan and Sergeant, 1998; Sonuga-Barke, Taylor, et al., 1992). Localized reductions in volumes of the amygdala have been reported in ADHD, primarily over the basolateral nuclear complex (Plessen et al., 2006). Structural disturbances in the basolateral complex may disrupt emotional learning and the affective drive to sustain attention to otherwise mundane sensory stimuli (Cardinal, Parkinson, et al., 2002; Holland and Gallagher, 1999). The basolateral complex is densely connected with the inferior prefrontal cortex (Baxter and Murray, 2002), another region in which reduced volumes have been reported in youth with ADHD (Sowell, Thompson, et al., 2003). Limbic-prefrontal circuits support the ability to tolerate delayed rewards and to suppress unwanted behaviors (Elliott, Dolan, and Frith, 2000), areas of difficulty that are defining hallmarks of ADHD (Barkley, Cook, et al., 2002; Rowland, Lesesne, and Abramowitz, 2002).

Disturbances in the extinction of conditioned fear responses have been postulated in the pathogenesis of a wide range of anxiety disorders. For example, fear is a normative response following exposure to trauma, and in most individuals it soon extinguishes completely. In a minority of individuals, however, fear will fail to extinguish, and they subsequently manifest symptoms of posttraumatic stress disorder (PTSD) (Yehuda, Flory, et al., 2006). Consequently, PTSD has been conceptualized as a disturbance of insufficient inhibitory control over conditioned fear responses (Liberzon and Sripada, 2008; Yehuda et al., 2006). Human imaging studies of PTSD patients have reported (1) exaggerated amygdala responses to a variety of emotional stimuli, presumably representing exaggerated fear responses; (2) deficient activation of frontal cortices, which is thought to mediate disordered fear extinction and impaired suppression of attention to trauma-related stimuli; and (3) reduced volumes and deficient activation of the hippocampus, which may mediate deficits in recognizing safe contexts (Bremner, Elzinga, et al., 2008; Rauch, Shin, and Phelps, 2006). Similar circuit-based disturbances have been postulated in other pediatric anxiety disorders, and they are thought to account for the minority of children whose anxiety disorders do not remit by adulthood (Pine, 2007). Preclinical and clinical studies have suggested that cognition-enhancing medications and repetitive exposure-based interventions, either alone or in combination, may offer a paradigm shift in anxiety disorders. Instead of treating the symptoms of anxiety pharmacologically, this strategy attempts to improve the extinction learning that occurs during cognitive-behavioral therapy (Myers and Davis, 2007; Quirk and Mueller, 2008).

Attachment

Early bonding to a primary caregiver is an innate predisposition for children. It is an important feature of infant development that contributes to social and emotional learning, as well as to resilience and risk for psychopathology (Bakermans-Kranenburg and van Ijzendoorn, 2007; Corbin, 2007; Swain, Lorberbaum, et al., 2007). The classic model for early attachment is visual imprinting in newly hatched chicks. During a specific sensitive period, they develop an enduring selectivity for following either their mother or a replacement object. This imprinting consists of three independent behavioral processes: approaching the mother, learning and remembering her identity, and avoiding others while maintaining an affiliation with her. Specific cortical brain regions and synaptic changes are involved in the memory of and response to the imprinted object in chicks (Insel and Young, 2001).

Mammalian animal models of the attachment of an infant to a caregiver, as well as the behavioral and neuroendocrine responses to separation from that caregiver, have revealed physiological mediators of attachment and separation responses that have specific and long-term regulatory effects on the hormonal, physiological, and behavioral reactivity of the infant (Hofer, 1994). The interactions of the parent and child that are involved in attachment and separation responses include tactile sensation, motor activity, the warmth and temperature of the mother's body, and nutritional factors (Hofer, 1994, 1996). The cry of the infant upon separation, for example, is released by loss of the warmth, specific odors, and passive tactile cues of the mother (Shair, Brunelli, et al., 2003). Nutritional and tactile factors also regulate hormone release and thereby cause abnormal levels of stress-response hormones during separation. Loss of the maternal nutrient supply affects hormone production by the adrenal gland, whereas loss of the tactile interaction between mother and infant affects hormone release by the pituitary gland (Hofer, 1996). These physiological regulators constitute the building blocks from which attachment develops.

Infants attach regardless of the quality of care provided by the object of attachment. During the imprinting-sensitive period, for example, chicks will follow their mother even while being shocked. Similarly, rat pups attach strongly even to a handler providing a shock or rough treatment, and infant monkeys will attach to abusive mothers (Moriceau and Sullivan, 2005). Indeed, human children develop strong attachment to a primary caregiver even when that individual subjects them to extreme abuse and neglect. Attachment studies of infant development have revealed that pathological caregiving manifests not as an absence of attachment, but instead as a disordered pattern of attachment that can be either of an anxious, insecure, or disorganized type, standing in contrast to the secure type of attachment that is the product of sensitive and protective caregiving and provides a necessary foundation for healthy emotional development (Bakermans-Kranenburg and van Ijzendoorn, 2007; Swain, Lorberbaum, et al., 2007).

Nonhuman primate models have demonstrated the importance of early attachment experiences in the development of subsequent attachment behaviors, social relatedness, and emotional regulation (O'Connor and Cameron, 2006; Pryce, Dettling, et al., 2004; Sabatini, Ebert, et al., 2007). Early, but not late, separation from a maternal caregiver, for example, has been shown to impair behaviors that promote effective socialization and to increase anxiety-related behaviors in social situations in adulthood (O'Connor and Cameron, 2006). Human evidence likewise suggests that the disruption of caregiving and social bonding early in life can exert dramatic, lifelong disruptive effects on the social competence and mental health of children. Dramatic reductions in the interactions of infants with caregivers, as can occur in extreme examples of institutionalized and socially deprived infants, can produce long-term impairments in emotional and social responsiveness and in attentional and intellectual capacities (Gunnar, 2001; Gunnar, Morison, et al., 2001; O'Connor, Marvin, et al., 2003; Rutter, Kreppner, and O'Connor, 2001; Smyke, Koga, et al., 2007). That the levels of disturbance in social behavioral and emotional regulation are dramatically greater following an earlier disruption of social bonds suggests that attachment to caregivers may be subject to a sensitive period early in postnatal development and that early deprivation may lead to subsequent social and emotional disturbances in a dose-dependent manner (Nelson, Zeanah, et al., 2007; O'Connor, Marvin, et al., 2003; Smyke, Dumitrescu, and Zeanah, 2002). In this context, it may be noted that the pairing of a separated infant with a very attentive adult can reverse the behavioral effects of early disruption in social bonds, but only when instituted early in life (O'Connor and Cameron, 2006; Cameron, 2007). This finding suggests that, for human infants, appropriate surrogate parents and foster care may have the potential to attenuate significantly the long-term effects of seriously deficient early parenting.

Although most MEB disorders involve the ability to develop and maintain healthy relationships, several disorders appear to arise from a primary disturbance of attachment. An example is borderline personality disorder, whose pathogenesis is thought to be closely linked to disturbances in early relationships, often involving either abuse and neglect or an inconsistency in parental nurturance (Fruzzetti, Shenk, and Hoffman, 2005; Johnson, Cohen, et al., 2006; Lieb, Zanarini, et al., 2004).

Perhaps the human condition that most obviously represents a disturbance in the formation of interpersonal attachments is reactive attachment disorder, which typically is manifested as an excessively inhibited or hypervigilant response to social interaction or, at the other extreme, as an excessively diffuse and indiscriminate sociability. Although its neurobiological underpinnings are not well understood, it is thought to be caused by a persistent disregard of the child's basic emotional or physical needs or by repeated changes in the primary caregiver, which prevent formation of stable attachments during early development (Corbin, 2007).

Social Relatedness

Social relatedness is a complex construct that includes, among other components, the processing of sensory aspects of social stimuli, imitation and perspective taking, emotions induced by social interactions, and awareness of self and others. Distinct neural systems are likely to subserve each of these components.

Extensive evidence from human imaging studies suggests that the neural systems responsible for processing social stimuli are based primarily in the superior temporal cortex (Zilbovicius, Meresse, et al., 2006; Zahn, Moll, et al., 2007). A large body of recent work suggests that a "mirror neuron" system subserves knowledge of imitation, thought to be a precursor skill for the acquisition of knowledge of the intentional states that underlie the actions of others, although this evidence is not conclusive (Agnew, Bhakoo, and Puri, 2007; Iacoboni and Dapretto, 2006; Iriki, 2006; Lyons, Santos, and Keil, 2006; Rizzolatti and Craighero, 2004). Processing the sensory and conceptual aspects of social stimuli in the superior temporal cortex and understanding the actions of others through activity in the mirror neuron system are likely to work in concert with the medial prefrontal cortex to gain an understanding of one's own and others' intentional states. This understanding is referred to as having a "theory of mind" or the ability to "mentalize"—the knowledge that others have perspectives, beliefs, desires, and motivations that are different from one's own.

Social relationships are an essential component of human mental health. Almost all forms of psychopathology involve difficulties in developing and maintaining healthy relationships. A primary example is autism, which is defined by the presence of qualitative deficits in social interaction and affiliation. Each of the systems that subserve the various aspects of social relatedness has been implicated in the pathogenesis of the socialization deficits in autistic children. For example, reductions in gray matter volume, reduced activation during the presentation of social stimuli, and reduced resting blood flow have all been reported in the superior temporal sulcus in individuals with autism (Gendry Meresse, Zilbovicius, et al., 2005; Gervais, Belin, et al., 2004; Zilbovicius, Boddaert, et al., 2000; Zilbovicius, Meresse, et al., 2006). In addition, several functional magnetic resonance imaging studies have implicated dysfunction of the mirror neuron system in persons with autism (Dapretto et al., 2006; Williams, Waiter, et al., 2006).

Self-Regulatory Control

Self-regulatory control is the capacity to weigh prospects for short-term gain from an action against its potential, more remote adverse consequences and to monitor and update the action plan as it unfolds. Broad expanses of the cortex and subcortex subserve the functions of self-regulatory control (Leung, Skudlarski, et al., 2000; Peterson, Skudlarski, et al., 1999; Peterson, Staib, et al., 2001). Both children and adults engage frontostriatal circuits to perform tasks that require self-regulatory control, but they do so progressively more with increasing age. Thus increasing activity of these systems during development is likely to be responsible for the superior performance of adolescents and adults compared with children on tasks that require self-regulatory control (Marsh, Zhu, et al., 2006).

Regulatory control involves control not only of actions, but also of emotions. Reassigning emotional labels to emotion-provoking stimuli, such as emotional faces and scenes, can alter the perceived pleasantness and arousal that the stimuli produce. Known as cognitive reappraisal, this reassignment produces activation of the lateral prefrontal, dorsomedial prefrontal, anterior cingulate, and occipital cortices. Activation of the ventral prefrontal cortex correlates inversely with activity in the amygdala, suggesting that cognitive reappraisal activates the frontal cortex and that the frontal cortex in turn modulates emotion-processing activity in the amygdala (Ochsner, Bunge, et al., 2002). Successful voluntary suppression of the unpleasant emotions activates similar circuits in direct proportion to the intensity of those emotions (Phan, Fitzgerald, et al., 2005). The circuits that cognitive reappraisal and emotional regulation engage are remarkably similar to the circuits activated by other, more purely cognitive, tasks that require self-regulatory control (Ochsner and Gross, 2005).

Maturation of self-regulatory functions largely defines human development, and the self-regulatory circuits that have been identified in normal individuals have been implicated in the pathogenesis of a wide range of neuropsychiatric illnesses. In fact, the capacity for self-regulatory control is one of the strongest predictors of outcome in longitudinal studies of psychopathology in children (Masten, 2004, 2007). Disturbances in these circuits are unlikely to cause disorders in and of themselves. Instead, they are likely to act in concert with underlying disturbances in other neural circuits that subserve important neuropsychiatric functions, such as motor planning and execution, mood and affect, or attention. The combination of disturbances in these latter circuits with dysfunction in self-regulatory systems may then transform a vulnerability or predisposition for developing an illness into the manifestation of symptoms and functional impairments that constitute an overt disorder. Age-specific vulnerabilities in the maturation of varying components of the neural circuits that mediate these self-regulatory functions are likely to contribute to the differences in age-specific prevalence and characteristic ages of onset of the various disorders described in Chapter 4.

ADHD is a prototypical example of a disorder of self-regulatory control. The largest anatomical studies have suggested that overall brain size is approximately 3 percent smaller in children with ADHD than in healthy children (Castellanos et al., 2002), an abnormality that probably derives from a disproportionate reduction in volume of the inferior prefrontal and anterior temporal cortices bilaterally (Sowell, Thompson, et al., 2003). These anatomical disturbances are consistent with the self-regulatory deficits that manifest as the hyperactivity, distractibility, and impulsivity of children with ADHD. Additional anatomical and functional disturbances involve the basal ganglia, the subcortical portions of the frontostriatal circuits that subserve self-regulatory control (Plessen and Peterson, 2008; Shafritz, Marchione, et al., 2004; Vaidya et al., 1998). Anatomical and functional disturbances in these regulatory control systems, though in different portions and subsystems than in ADHD, have also been reported in bipolar disorder (Blumberg, Leung, et al., 2003; Blumberg, Martin, et al., 2003), Tourette syndrome (Marsh, Zhu, et al., 2007; Peterson et al., 2001), obsessive compulsive disorder (Rosenberg and Keshavan, 1998), and eating disorders (Marsh, Gerber, et al., 2009).

Cognitive reappraisal already is a prominent component of the cognitive-behavioral therapies commonly used in the treatment of depression and anxiety disorders. Self-regulatory control tasks are being developed to treat various forms of psychopathology, including tic disorders and ADHD (Posner, 2005; Rueda, Rothbart, et al., 2005; Tang, Ma, et al., 2007; Woods, Himle, et al., 2008). Whether these interventions hold promise as prevention strategies is unknown.

Compensatory and Neuromodulatory Systems

Compensatory responses are attempts to correct for disturbances elsewhere in a biological system and to reestablish a biological balance, known as homeostasis. The quintessential purpose of the brain is to strive to achieve and to maintain homeostasis, both in its internal operations and in the external environment. The brain is likely to attempt to achieve homeostasis in the presence of a mental, emotional, or behavioral disorder by engaging neural systems that help compensate for the functional impairment due to the disorder.

Indeed, findings from human brain imaging studies have increasingly suggested that many differences previously documented in disorders may not represent a primary dysfunction but compensatory responses to the presence of neural dysfunction elsewhere. For example, although longitudinal studies suggest that most cortical abnormalities in children with ADHD represent a maturational delay, some of the differences compared with healthy control children appear to represent a compensatory response. In one study, the right parietal cortex was initially thinner in children with ADHD, similar to most other cortical regions, but then normalized over time only in those with favorable clinical outcomes. These findings suggest that the relative thickening of the right parietal cortex represents a compensatory response (Shaw, Lerch, et al., 2006). In addition, in a different sample of youth with ADHD, the head of the hippocampus was found to be enlarged, with the degree of enlargement being inversely proportional to the severity of the ADHD symptoms, suggesting that the relative hypertrophy of this structure also represents a compensatory response (Plessen, Bansal, et al., 2006). This interpretation has added plausibility in light of the connections of the hippocampus with frontal and parietal cortices and the fact that neurons and synapses in the head of the hippocampus increase in number and size in response to experiential demand (Bruel-Jungerman, Davis, et al., 2006; Cameron and McKay, 2001; Christie and Cameron, 2006; Eriksson, Perfilieva, et al., 1998; Kempermann, Kuhn, and Gage, 1997; van Praag, Shubert, et al., 2005).

Evidence for brain-based compensatory responses is perhaps strongest in children with Tourette syndrome (TS) (Spessot, Plessen, and Peterson, 2004). The dorsal prefrontal and parietal cortices of children with TS have larger volume in inverse proportion to the severity of their tic symptoms, suggesting that the hypertrophy is a compensatory response to the presence of tics (Peterson, Staib, et al., 2001). This hypertrophy is likely to be a consequence of the need to suppress tic symptoms frequently in social settings, which has been shown to produce massive activation of the prefrontal, anterior temporal, and parietal cortices (Peterson, Skudlarski, et al., 1998). The hypertrophy increases inhibitory reserve for the self-regulatory functions that these regions subserve, so that children with TS perform normally and activate frontal tissues similarly to healthy controls. Adults with TS appear to fail to generate this compensatory frontal hypertrophy; as a result, they have more severe symptoms and require greater activation of frontal cortices to maintain adequate performance on tasks that require self-regulatory control (Marsh, Zhu, et al., 2007).

Hormonal Influences on Brain Development and Behavior

Differences between the sexes have been observed across multiple domains of cognitive, emotional, and behavioral development. Boys, for example, appear on average to be predisposed to more physical activity; less tolerance for frustration; and more aggression, impulsivity, and dys-regulated emotions (Eaton and Enns, 1986; Else-Quest, Hyde, et al., 2006; Zahn-Waxler, Shirtcliff, and Marceau, 2008). Girls on average exhibit more rapid language acquisition, greater empathy and social skills, and more fearfulness and anxiety (Else-Quest, Hyde, et al., 2006; Zahn-Waxler, Shirtcliff, and Marceau, 2008).

Several processes, ranging from differences in environmental exposures to innate differences in the biological processes that underlie either emotion and behavior or responses to the environment, could produce these gender differences (Zahn-Waxler, Shirtcliff, and Marceau, 2008). The differences are thought to have their basis at least in part in differences in brain structure and function, which are determined largely by the effects on brain development of both sex hormones and genes encoded on sex chromosomes (Arnold, 2004; Davies and Wilkinson, 2006; Hines, 2003). Hormone-dependent sexual differentiation of the brain is thought to be driven primarily by differences in androgen levels in fetal and early post-natal life. Production of testicular androgen in the human male fetus begins during the sixth week of gestation, producing higher testosterone levels in males than in females between weeks 8 and 24 of gestation (Knickmeyer and Baron-Cohen, 2006; Warne and Zajac, 1998). Studies in animal models demonstrate that differences between the sexes in the levels of various steroid hormones in the brain during fetal life produce sex-specific differences in neuronal proliferation, cell migration, apoptosis, dendritic branching, and the density of dendritic spines (Cooke, Hegstrom, et al., 1998). These differences between the sexes in fetal brain development in turn produce gender differences in brain form and structure that endure throughout postnatal life (Knickmeyer and Baron-Cohen, 2006; Hines, 2003). Changes in levels of steroidal hormones during puberty are then thought to lead to further modification of brain structure and function across both sexes (Romeo, 2003).

Differences between the sexes in brain structure and function are thought to underlie the well-documented gender differences in the diagnostic and age specificity of MEB disorders. For example, females overall are more likely than males to develop major depression and anxiety disorders (Pigott, 1999; Rutter, Caspi, and Moffitt, 2003; Zahn-Waxler, Shirtcliff, and Marceau, 2008), while males are more likely to develop ADHD, conduct disorder, substance abuse, tic disorders, and learning disorders (Rutter, Caspi, and Moffitt, 2003; Zahn-Waxler, Shirtcliff, and

Marceau, 2008; Apter, Pauls, et al., 1993; Tallal, 1991). The age of onset of MEB disorders is generally earlier in boys than in girls, producing a male predominance of these disorders in prepubertal children. This sex-specific difference in rates of illness reverses following puberty, when the prevalence of disorders is higher in girls.

RELEVANCE OF DEVELOPMENTAL NEUROSCIENCE TO PREVENTION

Relationship to Prevention Interventions

Developmental neuroscience provides a great deal of knowledge that will increasingly support preventive intervention approaches for MEB disorders. Knowledge is growing about the determinants of mental health in the prenatal and early postnatal periods of brain development; the importance of consistent and nurturing parental care on development of the brain; and the neural systems that support healthy attachment, socialization, adaptive learning, and self-regulation throughout infancy, childhood, and adolescence. All of this knowledge has important implications for interventions that can not only prevent MEB disorders but also actively promote positive, adaptive, prosocial behaviors and well-being. Specific opportunities to support healthy brain and behavioral development and to protect against environmental factors present themselves at distinct developmental stages, when they are most likely to have a beneficial effect.

During the prenatal period and the early years of a child's life, neurobiological processes establish the potential for healthy development or, in the presence of various risk factors, the potential for the development of significant cognitive, emotional, and behavioral difficulties. Knowledge of these processes informs preventive approaches in a number of ways.

First, as discussed throughout this report, mental and physical health are inseparable, as are brain and physical development. Programs and interventions that support healthy pregnancy are therefore crucial. These can include efforts to ensure adequate and proper nutrition, such as requiring the fortification of foods with folic acid, a universal preventive intervention that has reduced the rates of neural tube defects in the United States by 25-30 percent (Pitkin, 2007). Similarly, reducing exposure to environmental toxins and infections during pregnancy and minimizing obstetrical complications during childbirth can have powerful effects on preventing MEB disorders (see Chapter 6).

Second, this chapter has emphasized the importance of nurturing care for healthy brain development and the lifelong adverse effects that disruptions in this care and exposure to harmful experiences early in life can have on both the development and functioning of the brain. Considerable evidence now suggests that these effects can be prevented or reduced by appropriately designed interventions if they are delivered at the proper time. Thus, for example, interventions focused on fostering the bonding and attachment of caregiver and child should begin at birth and be supported for the first several years of a child's life. This is the aim of such approaches as home visitation and high-quality preschool, which are discussed in the following chapters. On the other hand, the brain continues to develop and retains a large capacity for plasticity throughout infancy, childhood, adolescence, and early adulthood as the neural systems that support such behaviors as attachment, socialization, learning, and self-regulation are refined to achieve healthy cognitive, emotional, and behavioral functioning. Evidence from both traditional models of learned behavior and more novel fields of investigation, such as epigenetics, suggests that environmental improvements can produce long-term changes in brain structure and function, and thus interventions applied even after the optimal sensitive periods of development can attenuate the effects of early adverse experiences.

Later developmental stages also bring developmentally specific opportunities to promote protective factors related to more mature behaviors—for example, building social relationships. Difficulties in developing and maintaining healthy relationships are an important aspect of many MEB disorders. Therefore, influencing social relationships positively and building networks of support in families, schools, and communities are among the primary aims of a wide array of prevention programs, as described in Chapters 6 and 7.

The development of the neural systems that support self-regulatory functions is important for acquiring developmentally appropriate neuro-cognitive skills that affect mental health and risk for MEB disorders (Blair, 2002; Fishbein, 2000; Greenberg, 2006; Pennington and Ozonoff, 1996; Rothbart and Posner, 2006; Riggs and Greenberg, 2004). Numerous studies have shown that appropriately designed and implemented interventions can improve self-regulatory control of thoughts, emotions, and behavior in people of all ages, even young children (Dowsett and Livesey, 2000; Rueda, Posner, and Rothbart, 2005), and several curricula and training programs have been designed to promote self-regulation in prevention frameworks. For example, the Promoting Alternative Thinking Strategies (PATHS) program (described in Box 6-7 in Chapter 6) has been shown to increase inhibitory control and working memory (Greenberg, 2006). Likewise, the preschool curriculum Tools of the Mind, designed to build inhibitory control, working memory, and cognitive flexibility, has been shown to improve these functions in an at-risk population (Diamond, Barnett, et al., 2007).

Another area in which research in developmental neuroscience has implications for prevention of MEB disorders is targeting the appropriate individuals for the delivery of interventions. The identification of children who are at either increased or diminished risk for developing an MEB disorder based on phenotypic characteristics, genotype, or other biological markers (such as physiological or brain imaging measures), or who have a history of environmental exposure offers the prospect for applying indicated prevention strategies. The possibility of targeting interventions based on evidence from developmental neuroscience is genuine and valid if the following criteria are met: (1) the evidence for the association between a marker or exposure and a disorder is sufficient to identify children at risk reliably, (2) a sufficiently powerful strategy for preventive intervention is identified that is relevant for the disorder and the risk factors in question, and (3) the magnitude of the risk or protection that the marker or exposure confers is sufficiently large to justify screening for the marker or exposure.

The potential use of individually identified biological information to determine risk raises important ethical concerns (Institute of Medicine, 2006a; Evans, 2007). These concerns frequently arise in the context of acquiring genetic information, and the rapid increase in genetic research related to MEB disorders has coincided with an increase in public interest and also in private-sector endeavors to provide commercially available access to individual genetic information (Couzin, 2008; Hill and Sahhar, 2006). One concern is appropriate interpretation of the available evidence to determine whether the above criteria have been met before a marker is implemented as a basis for determining individual risk. Genetic and other biological markers are often perceived to be more deterministic than other risk factors in their potential to predict future disease (Austin and Honer, 2005; Hill and Sahhar, 2006; Kendler, 2005; Institute of Medicine, 2006a). However, given the complex, multifactorial etiology of MEB disorders, single genetic variants have very limited predictive power. This is also likely to be true for physiological or brain imaging measures that are being studied in relationship to MEB disorders. Clearly and accurately communicating research findings, including both their promise and limitations, to the public, policy makers, practitioners, and researchers in related disciplines is of paramount importance.

If the evidence does support gathering individual genetic and other biological information for research studies, and especially if testing for MEB disorders becomes available outside the research environment as it has for other health conditions, important decisions must be made. These include who determines whether to test an individual, who can gain access to the test results, who counsels the individual about those results, and who can act on the information (Institute of Medicine, 2006a). On the one hand, limiting access to information about individual risk raises concerns about withholding health information. On the other hand, the availability of individualized information leads to concerns about privacy, stigmatization, and bias and could potentially have negative effects on employment and the ability to obtain adequate health, life, and disability insurance (Institute of Medicine, 2006a). To address these concerns, a broad array of social, ethical, and legal factors should ultimately contribute to decisions about how research findings are applied and how tests to gather information about individual risk are implemented. Such decisions need to incorporate a research-informed, evidence-based understanding of how practitioners, policy makers, and the public will interpret the information and how systems and individuals will make use of the information. These concerns are also important in considering how to use individually identified psychological, social, and other environmental risk factors to screen for the risk of developing MEB disorders (see also Chapter 8).

Relationship to Prevention Research

Defining the neural substrates of healthy cognitive, behavioral, and emotional development and, in particular, understanding the plasticity of such substrates in the face of environmental interventions can provide an important basis for prevention research and for identifying many promising avenues for future study.

Rich theories of the pathogenesis of MEB disorders in young people can be developed using animal models and other methods of basic science research, as well as neurobiological studies in humans. Accordingly, theories derived from developmental neuroscience should have a prominent role in informing the design of such interventions. Research that further identifies how environmental factors affect basic neurodevelopmental processes, such as neuronal migration, synaptogenesis, synaptic pruning, and myelination, may reveal potential new targets for preventive interventions. These targets might range from more specific reduction of exposures to potential pharmacological approaches that can enhance neurobiological processes or attenuate some of the deleterious effects of adverse environmental exposures. Similarly, a greater understanding of the functional activity in neural systems that subserve emotion and behavior might aid in developing improved cognitive training strategies that can protect against the development of disorder by enhancing regulatory or compensatory systems capable of reducing the risk for psychopathology.

Strategies to alter the genome are not a near-term prospect. However, identifying genetic variants that are associated with disorders and understanding the underlying molecular mechanisms may lead to prevention strategies based on correcting molecular disturbances in the pathways that lead from genes to behavior, including the molecular pathways that underlie the effects of known risk factors for disorders. Identifying gene–environment interactions can also suggest ways of correcting pathogenic mechanisms that can be used in new prevention strategies designed to target molecular mechanisms and bolster resilience to the effects of adverse environmental exposures.

In addition to uncovering causal mechanisms, an improved understanding of the genetic determinants of MEB disorders can provide a powerful tool for the study of environmental influences on the development of disorders. Accounting experimentally or statistically for genetic determinants allows for a much more powerful and experimentally controllable assessment of environmental determinants. Thus, genetic approaches should ultimately help to clarify which are the most potent environmental influences in the development of disorders and to prioritize possible biological targets for prevention interventions.

Epigenetics research not only provides support for preventive intervention approaches, as described in this chapter, but also can lead to novel ways of thinking about the design of new and more effective prevention strategies. For example, although the epigenetic causes of disorders are difficult to disentangle from the more traditional effects of learned behavior, growing knowledge of the epigenetically based, transgenerational transmission of maternal care and other behavioral adaptations to the environment raises the possibility that future prevention approaches targeting epigenetic mechanisms may be able to help break cross-generational cycles of such behaviors as violence and substance abuse.

In designing these new interventions, however, it is important to remember that epigenetically transmitted behavioral and emotional dispositions, including stress responsivity, are adaptive for different environmental circumstances (Fish, Shahrokh, et al., 2004). One must therefore take care to ensure that the interventions do not unwittingly produce a mismatch between the newly modified environment and the epigenetically transmitted behavior that was optimized for enhanced survival in the previous, unmodified environment. Such a mismatch could conceivably serve as a risk for pathology, adding a level of complexity to the optimal design of preventive interventions despite the best of intentions in the design and implementation of an intervention.

While theories from developmental neuroscience can inform prevention approaches, findings from prevention trials that suggest causal mechanisms should generate hypotheses that can be tested and further elaborated by basic and clinical neuroscientists using animal models and other neuroscience-based approaches. Therapeutic interventions for already-established human disorders generally offer little insight into the causes of disorders. The fact that penicillin treats pneumonia, for example, does not indicate that the pneumonia is caused by a deficiency of penicillin. As discussed in Chapters 4 and 10, prevention trials permit rigorous testing of causal mechanisms, as well as mediating and moderating effects. If designed in partnership with developmental neuroscientists, such trials therefore offer an unprecedented opportunity to evaluate the neurobiological correlates of preventive interventions by identifying and measuring the anatomical, functional, and neural systems–level effects of those interventions. Because longitudinal studies can identify environmental influences on intervention outcomes and phenotypes over the course of disorders, preventive trials also offer a context for evaluating the hypothesized mechanisms and effects of genetic factors by examining how genetic predispositions may inhibit or enhance the effects of an intervention (an example is the study described in Chapter 4 on serotonin transporter genotype in a prevention intervention trial by Brody, Kogan, et al., 2008). Because the effect sizes of interventions are often small, this kind of information should help in tailoring an intervention to specific individuals, thereby enhancing the magnitude of its beneficial effects.

CONCLUSIONS AND RECOMMENDATIONS

Advances in neuroscience since 1994 have contributed to the growing knowledge of the determinants of mental health, the pathogenesis of disorders, and the ways in which the determinants of those disorders can be influenced through intervention strategies. Much evidence points to the central importance of brain development during the prenatal and early postnatal periods and of nurturing care for the development of the neural systems that support healthy attachment, socialization, adaptive learning, and self-regulation throughout infancy, childhood, and adolescence. The growing knowledge base in these areas has important implications in support of strategies to promote healthy cognitive, emotional, and behavioral development and to prevent MEB disorders.

Conclusion: Environment and experience have powerful effects on modifying brain structure and function at all stages of development in young people. Intervention strategies that modify environment and experience have great potential to promote healthy development of the brain and to prevent MEB disorders.

The growth of knowledge in developmental neuroscience has been particularly rapid in the defining of the roles of genetic, epigenetics, and gene–environment interactions on brain development. First, in the field of genetics, a great deal has been learned about the specific genes and molecular pathways that cause specific but fairly rare neurodevelopmental disorders. These advances have made realistic the previously remote hope that these devastating conditions might one day be treated or prevented. These advances have helped to point the way toward similar progress in understanding more common MEB disorders in children. Technological advances in large-scale, rapid-throughput genotyping have made feasible the study of the genetic vulnerabilities and underpinnings of more common disorders.

Second, advances in understanding and identifying gene–environment interactions have illuminated the ways in which specific genetic variants and life experiences both confer risk for and protect against developing MEB disorders. Third, much has been learned about the mechanisms of epigenetic modification of the genome that can confer enduring changes in gene expression and behavior. These epigenetic modifications have provided a much greater appreciation of the importance of biological adaptation of the developing organism to its environment. Bringing together knowledge in these three areas has important implications for the prospects of influencing causal biological pathways through modifications of the environment in new prevention intervention strategies (see Figure 5-3).

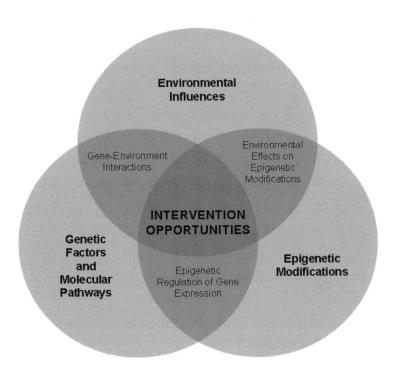

FIGURE 5-3 Intervention opportunities.

Conclusion: Genetic and other neurobiological factors contribute to the development of MEB disorders in young people, but their relative contribution is influenced by environmental factors. Similarly, the effects of environmental manipulations are constrained by genetic and other neurobiological factors.

Thus, efforts to understand the neurological basis of cognitive, emotional, and behavioral development, and especially to understand how these neural substrates can be modified through environmental intervention, are clearly an important basis for prevention research. Although research efforts are justified for intervention strategies at all stages of development in young people, developmental neuroscience has provided overwhelming evidence for the particular importance of fetal and early postnatal development for establishing the fundamental anatomical and functional architecture of the human brain that will endure throughout life, as well as evidence for the existence of sensitive periods for environmental influences in infancy. Therefore, the prenatal period and early infancy warrant a relatively high level of focus in research efforts.

Recommendation 5-1: Research funders, led by the National Institutes of Health, should dedicate more resources to formulating and testing hypotheses of the effects of genetic, environmental, and epigenetic influences on brain development across the developmental span of childhood, with a special focus on pregnancy, infancy, and early childhood.

Greater collaboration between prevention researchers and developmental neuroscientists could provide a powerful scientific synergy. Theories of pathogenesis derived from developmental neuroscience should inform the design of preventive interventions, and prevention trials should be used to inform and evaluate hypotheses of causal mechanisms derived from developmental neuroscience. Likewise, prevention trials should be designed to identify, measure, and evaluate neurobiological effects as possible mediators in preventive interventions. Hypotheses about causal mechanisms generated from prevention research should be tested and expanded using basic and clinical neuroscience approaches.

Conclusion: Collaborations among prevention scientists and basic and clinical developmental neuroscientists could strengthen understanding of disease mechanisms and improve preventive interventions by mutually informing and testing hypotheses of causal mechanisms and theories of pathogenesis.

In order to take greatest advantage of the potential for progress through collaboration, more detailed strategies to link prevention science with clinical and basic neuroscience are needed. This link needs to be supported both at the level of funding for individual investigators and also at the level of institutional infrastructure and support through funding for multidisciplinary research consortia.

Recommendation 5-2: Research funders, led by the National Institutes of Health, should dedicate resources to support collaborations between prevention scientists and basic and clinical developmental neuroscientists. Such collaborations should include both basic science approaches and evaluations of the effects of prevention trials on neurobiological outcomes, as well as the use of animal models to identify and test causal mechanisms and theories of pathogenesis.

Recommendation 5-3: Research funders, led by the National Institutes of Health, should fund research consortia to develop multidisciplinary teams with expertise in developmental neuroscience, developmental psychopathology, and preventive intervention science to foster translational research studies leading to more effective prevention efforts.

A well-supported collaborative research approach of this kind would provide an opportunity to investigate the potential use of genotyping and other biological markers as a basis for indicated prevention strategies. This opportunity needs to be approached with appropriate attention to social, ethical, and legal issues related to the use of individually identified biological information.

Conclusion: The prospect of using genetic and other neurobiological markers to identify young people at risk of MEB disorders raises important concerns, such as potential stigma, bias, and denial of insurance coverage. However, knowingly withholding scientific knowledge from populations who can benefit from them also raises ethical issues.

Recommendation 5-4: The National Institutes of Health should lead efforts to study the feasibility and ethics of using individually identified genetic and other neurobiological risk factors to target preventive interventions for MEB disorders.

Part II:

Preventive Intervention Research

There have been many areas of progress in preventive intervention research since the 1994 Institute of Medicine (IOM) report *Reducing Risks for Mental Disorders: Frontiers for Preventive Intervention Research*. The volume, reliability, and richness of experimental research have significantly improved in part because of significant advances in the methodological approaches applied to intervention research. Randomized trials, which were strongly recommended in the 1994 IOM report, have expanded (see Figure 1-1). Research has identified beneficial preventive interventions throughout young people's development and for a range of outcomes. As the body of intervention research has increased, the number of studies that include economic analyses to explore the costs and benefits of these interventions has also increased, further supporting the value of these approaches. This makes a case for supplementing traditional universal health care approaches, such as prenatal care, immunizations, and policies that support families, to support the healthy development of young people.

This report cannot cover the hundreds of randomized controlled trials that have been conducted since the 1994 IOM report. Instead, the analysis cites and draws on the findings of the several dozen relevant meta-analyses and systematic reviews, which themselves are testimony to the substantial increase in relevant research. The analysis also highlights specific interventions that have been tested and refined in several well-designed randomized controlled trials; some include analyses of cost-effectiveness or long-term outcomes. Although this does not include the many interventions for which some evidence is available, or even all that have been labeled by other groups as effective, it does focus on interventions that have been most rigorously evaluated and illustrates the potential to prevent numerous mental, emotional, and behavioral (MEB) disorders and the problem behaviors related to them. Box II-1 highlights some of the major outcomes of these interventions. In some areas in which evidence is more limited but there is clear conceptual potential, we mention interventions that appear promising but have not been tested in multiple experimental evaluations.

BOX II-1
Outcome Highlights of Preventive Interventions

Prevention of Child Maltreatment
- Meta-analyses have found that interventions that promote family wellness and provide family support are successful in preventing child maltreatment.
- Home visiting programs have demonstrated reduced physical abuse, aggression, and harsh parenting.
- Comprehensive early education programs have demonstrated reduced child maltreatment.

Academic Achievement
- School-based social and emotional learning programs that include academic achievement as an outcome had effects equivalent to a 10 percentage point gain in academic test performance (Durlak, Weissberg, et al., 2007).

Violence Prevention
- School-based violence prevention programs have effects that would lead to a 25-33 percent reduction in the base rate of aggressive problems in an average school (Wilson and Lipsey, 2007).

Conduct Problems
- The Good Behavior Game reduced disruptive and aggressive behavior and reduced the likelihood that initially aggressive students would receive a diagnosis of conduct disorder by sixth grade (Wilcox, Kellam, et al., 2008), or that persistently highly aggressive boys would receive a diagnosis of antisocial personality disorder as a young adult (Petras, Kellam, et al., 2008).
- Linking Interests of Families and Teachers reduced levels of aggressive behavior (Eddy, Reid, and Fetrow, 2000).
- Fast Track reduced self-reported antisocial behavior and, for children at highest risk, reduced incidence of conduct disorder and attention deficit hyperactivity disorder (Conduct Problems Prevention Research Group, 2007).

Depression
- Meta-analyses have found that interventions to prevent depression can both reduce the number of new cases of depression in adolescents and reduce

The prevention science field draws a valuable distinction between efficacy trials, which demonstrate results in a research environment, and effectiveness trials, which demonstrate results in a real-world environment. Although efficacy trials can be helpful in validating the conceptual basis for an intervention, the findings of effectiveness trials are viewed as being more relevant to community settings and the interventions as they will be imple-

depressive symptomatology among children and youth (Cuijpers, van Straten, et al., 2008; Horowitz and Garber, 2006).
- For children at heightened risk, one particularly promising intervention uses a cognitive-behavioral approach and significantly reduced major depressive episodes (Clarke, Hornbrook, et al., 2001).

Substance Abuse
- The Good Behavior Game significantly reduced the risk of illicit drug abuse or dependence disorder at age 19-21 (Kellam, Brown, et al., 2008).
- Life Skills Training significantly reduced drug and polydrug (tobacco, alcohol, and marijuana) use three years after the program (Botvin, Griffin, et al., 2000).
- Linking Interests of Families and Teachers reduced use of alcohol and marijuana.
- EcoFIT (Ecological Approach to Family Intervention and Treatment, a graduated version of the Adolescent Transition Program) reduced rates of growth in tobacco, alcohol, and marijuana use between the ages of 11 and 17 and reduced the likelihood of being diagnosed with a substance use disorder (Connell, Dishion, et al., 2007).

Multiple Disorders
- The Seattle Social Development project, a quasi-experimental combined parent and teacher training intervention, significantly reduced multiple diagnosable mental health disorders (major depression, generalized anxiety disorder, posttraumatic stress disorder, social phobia) at age 24 (Hawkins, Kosterman, et al., 2008).

Anxiety
- As suggestive evidence of prevention potential, a selective intervention for people with high anxiety symptoms led to significantly fewer participants developing anxiety disorders one to two years after the intervention (Schmidt, Eggleston, et al., 2007). An indicated intervention for 7- to 14-year-olds with elevated anxiety symptoms resulted in significantly fewer anxiety disorders at six-month and two-year follow-up (Dadds, Spence, et al., 1997).

mented in everyday practice. The tide has begun to turn, with effectiveness trials beginning to emerge.

As discussed in Part I, young people develop in the context of their families, schools, and communities. Interventions designed to support healthy emotional and behavioral development and prevent disorder take place largely in the contexts of these support systems. Such interventions as prenatal care, home visiting, parenting skills training, programs designed to mitigate specific family-based strain (e.g., bereavement, dealing with a mentally ill parent), and some public policies share a goal of improving family functioning and creating nurturing environments. Many other interventions aimed at a range of problem behaviors have been developed to reach young people through schools, and community-wide approaches have begun to emerge. Some interventions combine aspects of family-based interventions with school-based approaches. These family, school, and community-wide approaches are discussed in Chapter 6.

Chapter 7 includes a discussion of preventive interventions that are targeted at specific disorders rather than at specific settings. Delivered in mental health, health, and school settings, these interventions deal directly with children, with parents, and with the whole family. Chapter 7 also includes interventions targeted at mental health promotion, including intervention strategies related to modifiable lifestyle factors.

The range of developmental phases in a young person's life offers variable opportunities for intervention. Interventions are designed to address differential risk and protective factors prominent in a particular developmental stage or the emergence of symptoms that tend to occur at different ages. Most of the interventions discussed in Chapters 6 and 7, regardless of their mechanism, target young people during one or more developmental phases (see Figure II-1).

Preventive interventions are characterized by the level of risk of the population targeted for intervention. Screening, typically thought of in the context of indicated preventive interventions, in which individuals demonstrate elevated symptom levels that precede a diagnosis of disorder, may have applications for universal and selective interventions as well. The nation should proceed with caution, however. These issues are discussed in Chapter 8.

Family-, school-, and community-based interventions can help reduce the significant personal, family, and social costs of MEB disorders and related problem behaviors. These costs and available economic analyses of some of the interventions discussed in Chapters 6 and 7 are outlined in Chapter 9.

Finally, significant methodological advances since 1994 have increased the reliability of causal inferences possible from preventive intervention research and provided the field with solid guidelines on the design and

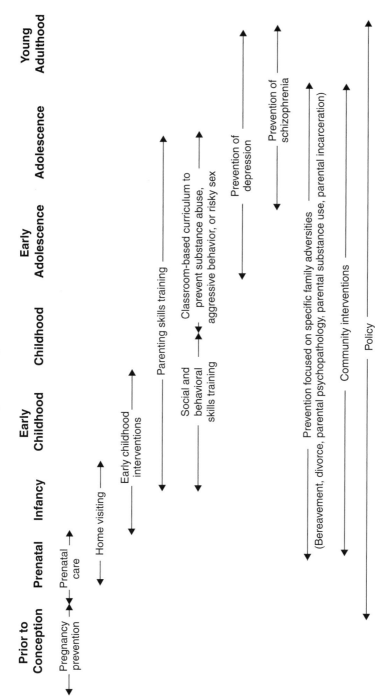

FIGURE II-1 Interventions and their targeted developmental stages.

conduct of quality research. These developments are discussed in Chapter 9, which also provides a bridge to Part III, New Frontiers, by outlining some of the methodological challenges and opportunities for the next generation of prevention research.

The evidence presented here has important practical implications for the practices of the schools, family service agencies, and health care providers that are involved at each stage of the development of young people. Taken together, the evidence shows that the nation could support the healthy development of many more young people.

6

Family, School, and Community Interventions

Young people develop in the contexts of their family, their school, their community, and the larger culture, which offer multiple opportunities to support healthy development and prevent disorder. This chapter first reviews interventions in a variety of settings directed primarily at improving family functioning. These interventions target both expectant parents and families with children of different ages and are discussed in order of developmental stage. The chapter then examines interventions delivered in various school settings that seek to address risks for mental, emotional, and behavioral (MEB) disorders and problems or to foster positive development by focusing on change in developmental processes; this discussion is organized according to school level (e.g., early childhood education) and the developmental processes or behavior(s) targeted. Box 6-1, based on the studies discussed in the chapter, illustrates key results of family and school interventions. The section on community interventions describes approaches aimed at community-wide change. The final section offers concluding comments based on the information presented in the chapter, but does not include recommendations. Chapter 7 reviews preventive interventions that target specific MEB disorders, as well as those aimed at mental health promotion. The discussion in that chapter includes school and community interventions that specifically target substance abuse. Chapter 7 concludes with conclusions and recommendations that draw together the evidence from that and the present chapter.

BOX 6-1
Results of Family and School Interventions

Parenting Programs (examples: Incredible Years, Positive Parenting Program [Triple P], Strengthening Families Program: for Parents and Youth [SFP 10-14], Adolescent Transitions Program [ATP])

- Reduced aggressive, disruptive, or antisocial behavior
- Improved parent–child interaction
- Reduced substance abuse
- Improved academic success

Home Visiting Programs (examples: Nurse Family Partnership and Healthy Families New York)
Home visiting programs that start during pregnancy have demonstrated:

- Improved pregnancy outcomes, maternal caregiving, and maternal life course
- Prevention of the development of antisocial behavior
- Reduced physical abuse, aggression, and harsh parenting

Comprehensive Early Education Programs (examples: Perry Preschool Program, Carolina Abecedarian Project, Child-Parent Centers)

- Less child maltreatment
- Less use of special education services, less grade retention, higher grade completion
- Higher rates of high school graduation and college attendance
- Fewer arrests by age 19, higher rates of employment, and higher monthly earnings

Family Disruption Interventions
New Beginnings Program, an intervention for families undergoing divorce:

- Reduced odds of the child reaching diagnostic criteria for any mental disorder
- Increased grade point average for adolescents
- Reduced number of sexual partners reported by adolescents

School-Based Programs
Good Behavior Game, a first grade classroom management intervention:

- Reduced disruptive behavior and increased academic engaged time
- Reduced likelihood that initially aggressive students would receive a diagnosis of conduct disorder by sixth grade
- Significantly reduced likelihood that persistently highly aggressive males would receive a diagnosis of antisocial personality disorder as a young adult

- Prevention of suicidal ideation and suicide attempts
- Significantly reduced risk of illicit drug abuse or dependence disorder at ages 19-21

Life Skills Training, a school-based substance use prevention program:

- Significantly reduced drug and polydrug (tobacco, alcohol, and marijuana) use three years after the program
- Strongest effects when delivered with fidelity—44 percent fewer drug users; 66 percent fewer polydrug users
- Significantly reduced methamphetamine use up to 4.5 years later when combined with the Strengthening Families Program

Linking Interests of Families and Teachers, a combined family–school intervention focused on skills and communication:

- Reduced levels of aggressive behavior, less involvement with deviant peers and lower arrest rates, less use of alcohol and marijuana
- For fifth graders, continued preventive effects three years later

Fast Track, a multicomponent intervention in grades K-10:

- Reduced self-reported antisocial behavior and significantly reduced incidence of conduct disorder for children at highest initial risk
- Significantly reduced incidence of a diagnosis of attention deficit hyperactivity disorder for children at highest initial risk

Seattle Social Development Project, a combined elementary grade parent–teacher training intervention:

- Reduced diagnosable mental health disorders by age 24 and heavy alcohol use and violence by age 18
- Effects particularly strong for African Americans

Adolescent Transitions Program, a parenting intervention delivered in schools:

- Reduced rates of growth in tobacco, alcohol, and marijuana use between ages 11 and 17 and lowered likelihood of being diagnosed with a substance use disorder
- Reduced rates of arrest

PREVENTION AIMED AT FAMILY FUNCTIONING

Families are the primary socializing agent of young people. Whether young people develop successfully depends substantially on whether families provide the physical and psychological conditions children need to acquire developmental competencies. This section begins with a review of the available evidence regarding family-focused prevention at each developmental phase. It then moves to discussion of interventions that can affect family functioning and mental, emotional, and behavioral outcomes regardless of developmental phase. The section closes with a discussion of the effects of family economic well-being on diverse internalizing and externalizing disorders.

Pregnancy, Infancy, and Early Development

Preconception: Preventing High-Risk Pregnancies Among Teenagers

Pregnancies among teenagers, particularly those younger than 16 years of age, are a risk factor for preterm birth, intrauterine growth retardation, and perinatal complications. Adolescent pregnancies are associated with single motherhood, low educational attainment, and low wages, all of which jeopardize children's development (Ayoola, Brewer, and Nettleman, 2006). Empirical evidence that unintended pregnancies can be prevented by specific pregnancy prevention programs is limited. Higher-quality studies on average show discouraging outcomes for pregnancy, and most studies are pre-post or quasi-experimental. One meta-analysis of prevention strategies aimed at delaying sexual intercourse, improving use of birth control, and reducing the incidence of unintended pregnancy among adolescents found no evidence of beneficial effects for any targeted outcomes (DiCenso, Guyett, et al., 2002). Another found evidence of an effect on contraception and pregnancy but not on sexual activity (Franklin, Grant, et al., 1997).

Although effective methods of intervening to prevent teenage pregnancies through family-, school-, or clinic-based programs are elusive, further research on the larger normative and cultural context for teenage sexuality may lead to approaches that are more effective. The recent decline in teenage pregnancies in the United States (Ventura, Mosher, et al., 2001), for example, suggests that opportunities to address malleable influences do exist.

Fetal Development and Infancy

Significant risks during fetal development for adverse neurobehavioral outcomes include genetic anomalies, poor maternal nutrition, maternal smoking and alcohol and drug use, exposure to neurotoxic substances, maternal depression or stress, low birth weight, and perinatal insults. Interventions that prevent these conditions have the potential to prevent many subsequent problems for the child. For example, recent evidence suggests that reduced exposure of pregnant mothers to lead results in reduced total arrests and arrests for violent crimes of their children at ages 19-24 (Wright, Dietrich, et al., 2008).

Universal preventive measures that have been adopted throughout the United States include the removal of lead from paint and gasoline. Another universal preventive measure (U.S. Environmental Protection Agency, 2004) has been warning pregnant women or those anticipating conception about the high methyl mercury content of fish at the top of the marine food chain. Prenatal exposure to this heavy metal has been linked to adverse cognitive and behavioral childhood outcomes (Gao, Yan, et al., 2007; Transande, Schechter, et al., 2006). However, some studies have reported increases in postpartum depression (Hibbeln, 2002) and reductions in children's IQ (Hibbeln, Davis, et al., 2007) as a result of reduced seafood intake, suggesting that this area may warrant further study.

Preterm Births and Prenatal Care

The rate of preterm births in the United States has increased from approximately 8 to 12.5 percent over the past two decades, and attempts to prevent or reduce their frequency (such as by providing access to prenatal care) have been unsuccessful (Institute of Medicine, 2007c). Reducing preterm births remains a significant opportunity for prevention of MEB disorders in childhood.

Half of all mothers and infants in the United States are enrolled in the Special Supplemental Nutrition Program for Women, Infants, and Children (WIC), a federal program that serves pregnant and lactating women and children up to age 5 (see http://www.fns.usda.gov/pdWIC_Monthly.htm). Participation in WIC has been associated with improved birth outcomes, such as longer pregnancies, fewer preterm births, decreased prevalence of anemia in childhood, and improved cognitive outcomes (Ryan and Zhou, 2006). Although it is likely that the WIC program contributes to the promotion of mental health of children and youth, the magnitude of this contribution is unknown.

Peripartum Depression

Changes in sleep, appetite, weight, energy level, and physical comfort in women during pregnancy and postpartum can cause significant emotional strain. Screening for peripartum (prenatal and postpartum) depression is routinely recommended for women in primary care (Pignone, Gaynes, et al., 2002; U.S. Preventive Services Task Force, 2002). Specific screening tools exist for peripartum depression, such as the Edinburgh Postnatal Depression Scale (EPDS) (Cox and Holden, 2003), one of several tools recommended by the U.S. Department of Health and Human Services' Agency for Healthcare Research and Quality (Gaynes, Gavin, et al., 2005). Such screening tools as the EPDS have the potential to be modified to identify pregnant women with elevated symptoms of depression who would benefit from indicated interventions.

In addition, some self-care tools can be useful as the first step in alleviating symptoms of depression (Bower, Richards, and Lovell, 2001). Such tools, commonly based on cognitive-behavioral therapy (CBT), have emerged in a variety of formats, including booklets, manuals, CD-ROMs, audiotapes, and videotapes (Blenkiron, 2001; Williams and Whitfield, 2001; Gega, Marks, and Mataix-Cols, 2004). CBT has a significant evidence base (e.g., Williams and Whitfield, 2001; Richards, Barkham, et al., 2003; Scogin, Hanson, and Welsh, 2003; Gega, Marks, and Mataix-Cols, 2004), and self-care tools have been successfully incorporated into stepped-care models of depression treatment in primary care settings (for patients with mild to moderate depression), with psychotherapy provided for those who fail to improve (Scogin, Hanson, and Welsh, 2003).

Maternal Sensitivity and Infant Attachment

Mother–infant attachment has been the focus of research and is a well-established influence on infants' successful development (National Research Council and Institute of Medicine, 2000; see also Chapter 5). A meta-analysis of 51 studies that evaluated interventions to increase maternal sensitivity and infant attachment using randomized controlled designs found that on average, the interventions were moderately effective in enhancing sensitivity (Bakersman-Kranenburg, van Ijzendoorn, and Juffer, 2003). A total of 23 of the studies used a randomized design to assess impact on attachment and demonstrated a slight effect; interventions focused on directly enhancing sensitivity were significantly more effective than other types of interventions.

Home Visiting

Home visiting is an intensive intervention that targets successful pregnancies and infant development. In these highly variable programs, a nurse or paraprofessional begins visiting the mother during the pregnancy or just after birth and continues to do so through the first few years of the child's life. The majority of programs provide parenting education, information about child development, social support to parents, encouragement of positive parent–child interactions, and social and health services. Some also provide case management services and health and developmental screening for children (Sweet and Appelbaum, 2004).

Sweet and Appelbaum (2004) conducted a meta-analysis of experimental and quasi-experimental evaluations of 60 home visiting programs. Only a fourth of these programs included home visiting during pregnancy. The authors conclude that on average, families receiving home visiting did better than those in control conditions. Mothers were more likely to pursue education but did not differ in their employment, self-sufficiency, or welfare dependence. The programs produced better outcomes in three of five areas of children's cognitive and social-emotional functioning. However, the authors also note that the significant variability across programs makes it difficult to evaluate them as a group. Aos, Lieb, and colleagues (2004) found that average benefits of the 25 programs reviewed exceeded costs.

The home visiting program with the best experimental evaluations and strongest results to date is the Nurse-Family Partnership (NFP), which has been evaluated in three randomized controlled trials. NFP is unique in targeting only first-time mothers. The theory of change is that women may be more open to support and guidance during their initial pregnancies (Olds, Hill, et al., 2003), which may contribute to the strength of the program's outcomes. This theory is supported by a randomized controlled trial of another home visiting program, which had a significant impact on first-time mothers' positive caregiving but not on that of women who were already mothers (Stolk, Mesman, et al., 2007). In the first two trials (in New York and Tennessee), the program improved pregnancy outcomes, maternal caregiving, and the maternal life course and prevented the development of antisocial behavior. The third trial (in Colorado) showed benefits as well.

NFP has other distinguishing features that may contribute to the strength of its outcomes. First, the program providers are nurses with both substantial training and credibility regarding pregnancy and infants. The Colorado trial experimentally evaluated the impact of nurses versus paraprofessionals and found that nurse visitation produced more benefits compared with the control condition (Olds, Robinson, et al., 2002, 2004). None of the other home visitation interventions reviewed by Gomby (1999) employed nurses as providers. Second, NFP uses well-established techniques to guide changes in specific behaviors, such as smoking, seeking an education, and getting social support. The focus on smoking in the New York study, in which more than 50 percent of mothers smoked, is especially noteworthy given the well-established relationship between smoking during pregnancy and children's subsequent antisocial behavior and substance use (see Brennan, Grekin, et al., 2002; Wakschlag, Lahey, et al., 1997; Weissman, Warner, et al., 1999).

Since nurses who delivered the NFP trial interventions were also expected to deliver the program in the communities to which it would be disseminated, the trials had elements of effectiveness studies. However, the cost of training and the limited pool of nursing professionals in some communities may impede community-wide implementation.

A randomized controlled study by DuMont, Mitchell-Herzfeld, et al. (2008) of the Healthy Families New York (HFNY) program suggests that the use of paraprofessionals can achieve prevention benefits when targeting women during their first pregnancy. The results of this study are consistent with those for NFP in at least two ways. First, like NFP, HFNY worked with young mothers enrolled during their pregnancy (DuMont, Mitchell-Herzfeld, et al., 2008). Second, HFNY had a greater impact on psychologically vulnerable mothers, results that parallel findings for NFP (Olds, Robinson, et al., 2004).

Important differences were also reported. DuMont, Mitchell-Herzfeld, et al. (2008) found greater benefit from delivery of HFNY by paraprofessionals than was found in the NFP trial in Colorado (Olds, Robinson, et al., 2002, 2004). This result may be attributable to the larger number of cases in the HFNY study and the limited statistical power of the Colorado NFP trial (Olds, Robinson, et al., 2002). However, further research is needed to determine conclusively whether paraprofessional home visitors can achieve results comparable to those of nurse visitors.

Early Childhood and Childhood

Aggressive social behavior, which typically begins to emerge during childhood, is a key risk factor for progression of externalizing disorders (see Brook, Cohen, et al., 1992; Kellam, Ling, et al., 1998; Lipsey and Derzon, 1998; Robins and McEvoy, 1990; Tremblay and Schaal, 1996; Woodward and Fergusson, 1999) and also is a predictor of internalizing disorders (Kaltiala-Heino, Rimpela, et al., 2000; Keenan, Shaw, et al., 1998; Kellam, Brown, et al., 2008). There is now extensive evidence on interventions designed to help families develop practices that prevent the development of aggressive and antisocial behavior and its associated problems. These interventions focus on providing training in parenting skills.

Seminal research on family interactions by Patterson and colleagues over the past 40 years has shown that harsh and inconsistent parenting practices contribute to aggressive and uncooperative behavior and that positive involvement with children and positive reinforcement of desirable behavior contribute to cooperative and prosocial behavior (e.g., Patterson and Cobb, 1971; Patterson, 1976, 1982). Building on the early parenting interventions by Patterson's group (e.g., Patterson and Gullion, 1968;

Patterson, 1969, 1974), a number of programs have emerged that target parents of children at different developmental stages, including childhood (e.g., Forgatch and DeGarmo, 1999; Webster-Stratton, 1990; Sanders, Markie-Dodds, et al., 2000), early adolescence (e.g., Dishion and Andrews, 1995; Spoth, Goldberg, and Redmond, 1999), and adolescence (Chamberlain, 1990; Henggeler, Clingempeel, et al., 2002). All of these programs teach and encourage parents to (1) use praise and rewards to reinforce desirable behavior; (2) replace criticism and physical punishment with mild and consistent negative consequences for undesirable behavior, such as time-out and brief loss of privileges; and (3) increase positive involvement with their children, such as playing with them, reading to them, and listening to them.

The efficacy of interventions focused on parenting skills is well established (see Lochman and van-den-Steenhoven, 2002; Petrie, Bunn, and Byrne, 2007; Prinz and Jones, 2003; Serketich and Dumas, 1996). In addition, several meta-analyses report positive effects of such interventions across a range of child and parent outcomes for parents of young children (Barlow, Coren, and Stewart-Brown, 2002; Lundahl, Nimer, and Parsons, 2006; Serketich and Dumas, 1996; Kaminski, Valle, et al., 2008). Kaminski, Valle, and colleagues (2008) report the greatest effect sizes for programs that include parent training in creating positive parent–child interactions, increasing effective emotional communication skills, and using time-out and that emphasize parenting consistency. Many parenting programs have been shown in two or more experimental trials to produce positive behavioral outcomes.

Two examples of parenting interventions with substantial empirical evidence are highlighted in Boxes 6-2 and 6-3. The Incredible Years (see Box 6-2), a combined parent–school intervention, has been tested as a selective and indicated intervention for children with aggressive behavior and related problems that have not yet reached clinical levels. It also has been tested in effectiveness trials using indigenous family support personnel and is one of few interventions that has been tested by independent investigators rather than the program developer. The Positive Parenting Program (Triple P) (see Box 6-3) is a multilevel intervention with universal, selective, and indicated components. It recently demonstrated positive results when tested on a population-wide basis in Australia (Sanders, Ralph, et al., 2008). Both programs have also been evaluated as treatment interventions, with positive results for those diagnosed with specific disorders, such as attention deficit hyperactivity disorder (ADHD; e.g., Hoath and Sanders, 2002).

Additional parenting interventions are highlighted in the next section. Interventions that combine training in parenting skills with school-based interventions are described later in the chapter.

BOX 6-2
The Incredible Years Program:
A Combined Parent–School Intervention

The Incredible Years Program (Webster-Stratton, 1990) includes parent, teacher, and social skills training components.

The parent-training program shows parents brief videotaped vignettes of parent–child interactions as examples of positive interactions and communication with their children, the value of praise and reward, and the use of time-out and other mild negative consequences. The program has been extensively evaluated in treating children with conduct disorders and in preventing further aggressive behavior and related problems in children whose behavior is not yet at the clinical level. It has been shown to improve parents' use of positive parenting practices; to reduce harsh, critical parenting; and to reduce diverse problem behaviors (Gardner, Burton, and Klimes, 2006; Linares, Montalto, et al., 2006; Patterson, Reid, and Eddy, 2002; Reid, Webster-Stratton, and Beauchaine, 2001). These benefits have been shown for a variety of ethnic groups (Reid, Webster-Stratton, and Beauchaine, 2002; Patterson, Reid, and Eddy, 2002) and when provided by diverse professionals, including teachers, nurses, family support specialists, and social workers (Hutchings, Bywater, et al., 2007; Gardner, Burton, and Klimes, 2006). Barrera, Biglan, and colleagues (2002) evaluated the Incredible Years parenting program as one component of an intervention designed to prevent reading failure and the development of aggressive behavior problems among high-risk elementary schoolchildren. Children who received the intervention displayed less negative social behavior than controls.

The program's teacher training component focuses on effective preschool and elementary classroom management, while the social skills component teaches children these skills using dinosaur puppets (Dinosaur School). Gross, Fogg, et al. (2003) evaluated the individual and combined effects of the parent and teacher training for 2- and 3-year-old children in day care centers serving low-income minority families in Chicago. Parents who received the parent training had higher efficacy scores, were less coercive in their discipline, and behaved more positively toward their children than did mothers in the control condition, although the effect on parent coerciveness was not sustained at one-year follow-up. Toddlers who were classed as at high risk for problem behavior at the outset of the study and who were in the parent or teacher training condition improved significantly more than children in the control condition; this improvement was maintained at one-year follow-up. Toddlers in the teacher plus parenting training condition did significantly worse on this measure than those in either the teacher training– or parent training–alone condition.

Webster-Stratton, Reid, and Stoolmiller (2008) report on an evaluation of the teacher training combined with Dinosaur School. The study involved students in Head Start and first grade classrooms in schools that served children in poverty. Teachers who received the training used more positive classroom management strategies, and their students were rated as more socially competent, better at self-regulation, and having fewer conduct problems.

BOX 6-3
Triple P: A Multilevel Parenting Intervention

The Positive Parenting Program (Triple P) focuses on the general population, not just individual families, and has selected components tailored to at-risk groups (such as young single mothers) or children with behavioral problems. The program includes five levels of parenting guidance based on family needs and preferences. The universal level provides information via mass media about effective parenting and solutions to common childrearing problems. The second level provides brief advice to parents for dealing with specific concerns, such as toileting or bedtime problems; parents are typically reached through contact with primary health care providers, such as pediatricians. The third level provides skills training for parents who are having problems with children's aggressive or uncooperative behavior. The fourth level (standard Triple P) provides up to 12 one-hour sessions on parenting skills for parents whose children have multiple behavioral problems, particularly aggressive behavior. The final level, enhanced Triple P, provides skills and support to deal with parental depression, marital discord, or other family challenges.

Sanders, Markie-Dadds, et al. (2000) evaluated three variants of Triple P (enhanced Triple P, standard Triple P, and self-directed training) and a wait-list condition with families of preschoolers who were at risk of developing conduct problems. The two practitioner-assisted interventions were more effective than the self-directed training or the wait-list condition. At one-year follow-up, all three active intervention conditions had similar levels of change in directly observed disruptive behavior. Another randomized controlled evaluation of standard Triple P and enhanced Triple P likewise showed positive effects (Ireland, Sanders, and Markie-Dadds, 2003). Sanders, Pidgeon, and colleagues (2004) tested an enhanced version of Triple P that had an additional component to help parents deal with anger problems. This trial also demonstrated significant benefits.

A randomized controlled study of the mass media component of Triple P (Sanders, Montgomery, and Brechman-Toussaint, 2000) indicated that children of parents who watched a 12-episode television series had significantly lower levels of disruptive behavior (based on parental reports), and parents expressed higher levels of competence. Prinz, Sanders, and colleagues (2009) recently reported a randomized trial of Triple P in 18 South Carolina counties that was accompanied by a media campaign. This study is noteworthy for being the first to show significant positive effects of a parenting intervention in an entire population.

Early Adolescence

Early adolescence is a developmental period during which the prevalence of substance use, delinquency, and depression begins to rise. There is also evidence of an increase in the rates of teasing and harassment in middle school. Significant physical changes occur with the onset of puberty, along with social changes, including the transition from elementary school to middle school or junior high school, increased concern about peer acceptance (Steinberg, 1999), and increased demand for autonomy (Eccles, Midgley, et al., 1993).

Major environmental risk factors that are especially important in early adolescence include family poverty and family conflict, as well as inadequate parental monitoring and deviant peer group formation. A key behavioral risk factor is aggressive social behavior, which contributes to social rejection and deviant peer group formation (Patterson, DeBaryshe, and Ramsey, 1989). In addition, young people who use cigarettes and alcohol are more likely to use other drugs (Kandel, Johnson, et al., 1999). More generally, psychological and behavioral problems tend to be interrelated (Biglan, Brennan, et al., 2004).

Boxes 6-4 and 6-5 describe two parenting interventions using the parenting skills techniques discussed above that have been developed and evaluated in multiple randomized controlled trials. They are adapted to address the unique issues, such as potential substance use and parental monitoring, that arise as young people enter early adolescence. The Strengthening Families Program (SFP) and adaptations of it (see Box 6-4) is a universal intervention that has demonstrated positive results on a range of outcomes. The Adolescent Transitions Program (see Box 6-5) has evolved over a series of trials to an intervention with universal, selective, and indicated components designed for delivery in schools. It has demonstrated long-term effects on substance use and delinquency among both white and minority youth.

Lessons from HIV/AIDS Prevention

The quality of parents' communication about risky sexual behaviors and positive attitudes about responsible sexual behavior can influence their adolescent children (Yang, Stanton, et al., 2007; Dilorio, Pluha, and Belcher, 2003). Without these conversations, adolescents overestimate the level of parental approval of their sexual behaviors, and mothers underestimate the amount of sexual activity of their adolescents (Jaccard, Dittus, and Gordon, 1998). Such communication appears to depend on warm and supportive parent–child relationships (Donenberg, Bryant, et al., 2003). Conversely, family conflict and negative affect are associated with behavioral problems (Szapocznik and Kurtines, 1993), such as earlier sexual debut (Paikoff, 1995) and generally risky sexual behavior (Biglan, Metzler, et al., 1990). Parental monitoring and an authoritative parenting style are consistently associated with less risky sexual behavior, fewer sexual partners, less pregnancy, and increased condom use among youth in the family (see Biglan, Metzler, et al., 1990; Li, Feigelman, and Stanton, 2000; Bell, Bhana, et al., 2008).

BOX 6-4
Strengthening Families Program and Adaptations:
Adolescent Parenting Interventions

Both the Strengthening Families Program (SFP) and the Strengthening Families Program for Parents and Youth 10-14 (SFP 10-14), a video-based adaptation of the original SFP program, help families develop the skills, values, goals, and interaction patterns needed to avoid substance use and other problem behaviors. Spoth and colleagues evaluated SFP 10-14 in two randomized controlled trials involving white, rural families of sixth grade students. Subsequent analyses indicate significant effects on reducing substance use (Spoth, Redmond, and Lepper, 1999; Trudeau, Spoth, et al., 2007; Spoth, Clair, et al., 2006) and, to some extent, delinquent behavior (Spoth, Redmond, and Shin, 2000) and internalizing disorders (Trudeau, Spoth, 2007). Spoth and colleagues conclude that the program had its impact by changing parent–child interaction patterns. Two analyses have concluded that the benefits of the program exceed its costs (Aos, Lieb, et al., 2004; Spoth, Guyll, and Day, 2002).

Recent analyses of the impact on academic performance found that involvement in the program contributed to increased engagement in academic activities in eighth grade, which was in turn predictive of academic success in 12th grade (Spoth, Randall, and Shin, 2008). Spoth, Shin, and colleagues (2006) found that the significant reduction in initiation of both alcohol use and illicit drug use for SFP 10-14 participants did not differ as a function of the risk status of the family. Other longitudinal studies of SFP 10-14 are under way.

SFP has been tested in diverse ethnic communities (Kumpfer, Alvarado, et al., 2002). Mixed results have been found (Fox, Gottfredson, et al., 2004). However, a randomized controlled trial of an adaptation of SFP 10-14 for rural African American populations, the Strong African American Families Program, demonstrated significant reductions in conduct problems among at-risk groups and improvements in parenting, with indications that parenting improvements had a partial mediating effect (Brody, Kogan, et al., 2008).

Several interventions target HIV risk reduction. Like other parent-oriented interventions, they focus on improving parent–child communication and supportive parental behaviors and increasing parental monitoring and limit setting. Although no meta-analyses have been conducted for these programs, a growing body of evidence is available for such interventions (Krauss, Goldsamt, and Bula, 1997; Wills, Gibbons, et al., 2003), with some emphasis on minority populations at greater risk (Brody, Dorsey, et al., 2002; Murry, Brody, et al., 2005; Wills, Murry, et al., 2007; Jemmott, Jemmott, et al., 2005). Some interventions have targeted and successfully reduced both early sexual intercourse and substance use (McKay, Bannon, et al., 2007; Prado, Pantin, et al., 2007).

BOX 6-5
Adolescent Transitions Program:
A Multilevel School-Based Parenting Intervention

The Adolescent Transitions Program (ATP) is a multilevel, adaptive parenting intervention designed to reach parents through middle schools (Dishion and Kavanagh, 2003; Dishion, Kavanagh, et al., 2003). The first randomized controlled trial of the original ATP compared the impact of four alternative approaches. A version that combined parent and teen elements was shown to improve parent–child relations and reduce family conflict. A parent focus–only version reduced school behavior problems and tobacco use and also had a short-term effect on the incidence of aggressive and delinquent behaviors (Andrews and Dishion, 1995).

A second randomized controlled trial in eight small Oregon communities conducted by Irvine, Biglan, and colleagues (1999) evaluated the effectiveness of ATP when delivered by staff who were not mental health professionals. ATP participants showed a number of significant improvements.

A more recent version of the program, the Ecological Approach to Family Intervention and Treatment (EcoFIT), consists of parenting information provided through a Family Resource Center, along with parent–child homework interactions that encourage effective family management (Dishion and Stormshak, 2007; Dishion, Kavanagh, et al., 2003). Multiethnic students (58.6 percent minority) and their families in each school were randomly assigned to this intervention or a control condition (Dishion, Kavanagh, et al., 2002). Intervention parents maintained their monitoring practices, which had a preventive effect on substance use. In a longer-term follow-up, Connell, Dishion, and colleagues (2007) found that, relative to randomized matched controls, adolescents in the participating families had lower rates of growth in tobacco, alcohol, and marijuana use; lower rates of arrest; and a lower likelihood of being diagnosed with a substance use disorder.

Aos, Lieb, and colleagues (2004) report ATP as a program whose benefits exceed its costs.

Two HIV prevention interventions have been tested in multiple trials. Trials of the Chicago HIV Prevention and Adolescent Mental Health project, a family-based, universal HIV prevention program targeting youth in fourth and fifth grades, showed a number of benefits, such as enhanced family decision making, improved caregiver monitoring, and fewer disruptive difficulties with children (McKay, Chasse, et al., 2004; McBride, Baptiste, et al., 2007; Paikoff, Traube, and McKay, 2007). Familias Unidas, which targets Hispanic immigrant parents and their children, was found to increase parental involvement and improve communication and support, and resulted in fewer adolescent behavior problems (Pantin, Coatsworth, et al., 2003).

Adolescence

Adolescence is a period of more independent decision making and risk taking, when the role of parents remains significant but is matched by the influence of peers. Preventive interventions during this stage of development are typically delivered directly to adolescents through schools, and these are discussed later in this chapter.

Some treatment interventions show positive effects for families with adolescents displaying considerable antisocial behavior or substance use. For example, multisystemic therapy (e.g., Henggeler, Clingempeel, et al., 2002) and multidimensional treatment foster care (e.g., Fisher and Chamberlain, 2000) have both demonstrated the benefits of comprehensive approaches to improving caregivers' monitoring and limit setting, as well as positive reinforcement and support of prosocial behavior. These benefits include reduced escalation of antisocial behavior and substance use. These interventions are based on the same principles of effective parenting as the interventions discussed above and may be adaptable for prevention. Parental monitoring can also reduce adolescent alcohol use (National Research Council and Institute of Medicine, 2003).

Young Adulthood

A growing body of research points to the period between age 21, generally viewed as the end of adolescence, and age 25 as a notable developmental phase in the transition to adulthood (Furstenberg, Kennedy, et al., 2003). These young adults face unique challenges involving the transition to and from college or full-time jobs (including the military), formation of marriage and families, and assumption of increasingly more responsible roles. At the same time, many of these young adults are living at or returning home for long periods of time, increasing the potential role of parents and other family members. Yet little research has been done on family-oriented interventions during this developmental phase.

Some environments in which young people live introduce new factors that may affect their mental, emotional, and behavioral health, such as the presence of binge drinking and pressures to drink on college campuses. Preliminary evidence suggests that parents can decrease tendencies to drink excessively and alter perceptions about drinking by talking about binge drinking prior to their child's departure for college (Turrisi, Jaccard, et al., 2001).

For young adults who enter the military, exposure to combat and serious trauma can have severe mental, emotional, and behavioral consequences. Some of the service branches and other groups are undertaking efforts to deal with such stressors (Saltzman, Babayon, et al., 2008). Many of the preventive interventions described in this report are conceptually relevant to members of the armed forces and their families. However, consideration of how these interventions could be used in the military context, given differences in service systems and many other aspects of military and civilian life, is beyond the scope of this report.

Family Interventions That Span Developmental Periods

Such family situations as mental illness, divorce, death, and abuse can affect family functioning and contribute to MEB disorders. Selective interventions to help families deal with these adversities and prevent negative outcomes among children have been developed and tested. Interventions designed for families dealing with parental depression are discussed in Chapter 7.

Family Disruption Due to Divorce or Parental Death

Compared with adolescents in two-parent homes, those with divorced parents exhibit higher levels of mental, emotional, and behavioral problems and lower levels of success in developmental tasks in childhood and adolescence; this increased risk persists into adulthood (Amato and Soboleski, 2001; Amato and Keith, 1991a, 1991b). Parental death is also associated with multiple problems in childhood and adulthood, including more symptoms of depression and anxiety and higher rates of depression and posttraumatic stress disorder (Cerel, Fristad, et al., 2006; Gersten, Beals, and Kallgren, 1991; Kendler, Gardner, and Prescott, 2002; Melhem, Walker, et al., 2008).

Preventive Interventions for Divorcing Families. A number of prevention programs focus on improving outcomes for children who experience parental divorce (Braver, Griffin, and Cookston, 2005; Emery, Sbarra, and Grover, 2005; Grych and Fincham, 1992; Haine, Sandler, et al., 2003; Lee, Picard, and Bain, 1994; Pedro-Carroll, 2005; Sobolewski and King, 2005; Wolchik, Sandler, et al., 2005). Many of these programs work with parents during and after the divorce or target changing the divorce process. At least two programs with positive results work with the mother during and after the divorce to deal with the stressors involved: the Parenting Through Change (PTC; Forgatch and DeGarmo, 1999) program and the New Beginnings Program (Wolchik, Sandler, et al., 2007). A randomized controlled trial of the PTC program demonstrated reductions in coercive parenting, antisocial behavior, and internalizing behavior at 30-month follow-up and reductions in delinquency at 36-month follow-up (DeGarmo, Patterson, and Forgatch, 2004; Martinez and Forgatch, 2001; Patterson, DeGarmo, and Forgatch,

**BOX 6-6
The New Beginnings Program:
A Parenting Intervention for Families Dealing with Divorce**

The New Beginnings Program (NBP) (Wolchik, Sandler, et al., 2007) is designed to strengthen parenting (warmth and discipline), increase father–child contact and nonparental adult support, and reduce divorce stressors. The first randomized controlled trial of NBP, which involved an 11-session group program designed to work with divorced residential mothers of children ages 8-15, led to significantly lower levels of child-reported aggression and parent-reported behavior problems and improved parental warmth and discipline. Improvements in maternal warmth partially mediated program effects on children's mental health problems. A second trial involved 240 divorced mothers of children ages 9-12. Compared with a literature-only control group, children whose mothers participated in NBP demonstrated significantly fewer internalizing and externalizing behavior problems; participating mothers had more effective disciplinary techniques and more positive relationships with their children (Wolchik, West, et al., 2000). At six-year follow-up (Wolchik, Sandler, et al., 2002), exposure to the program continued to show positive effects. The effects of fewer mental health problems and improved grade point average were mediated by improvements in parental warmth and discipline attributable to the program (Zhou, Sandler, et al., 2008).

2004). Two trials of the New Beginnings Program demonstrated positive results, with some benefits sustained at six-year follow-up (see Box 6-6).

One randomized controlled trial of a program for noncustodial fathers, Dads for Life, has shown positive effects. The program teaches skills to improve father–child relationships and reduce postdivorce interparental conflict. Over a 12-month period, the program reduced children's internalizing problems, increased parental alliance, and reduced conflict between the parents (Braver, Griffin, and Cookston, 2005). Two studies evaluating the effects of programs targeted at changes in the divorce process have shown positive effects in improving the postdivorce relationship between the parents (Emery, Sbarra, and Grover, 2005; Pruett, Insabella, and Gustafson, 2005). Finally, programs directed at children through schools have had benefits in reducing internalizing and externalizing problems (Pedro-Carroll, Sutton, and Wyman, 1999; Stolberg and Mahler, 1994).

Parental Death. A meta-analysis of 13 evaluations of interventions (Currier, Holland, and Neimeyer, 2007) to address the needs of parentally bereaved children failed to find significant effects. The studies had numerous methodological weaknesses, however, including small sample sizes and a lack of follow-up assessments.

Two programs that produced mental health outcomes each were tested in a single randomized controlled trial. The Family Bereavement Program was tested in a randomized controlled trial involving 156 families. Compared with a literature-only control, results for parents in the program included improved positive parenting, mental health, and coping and a reduction in stressful life events; for children, inhibition of expression of feelings was reduced. No effects were found on measures of children's mental health (Sandler, Ayers, et al., 2003). At 11-month follow-up, the program participants continued to show improvement, and children who had greater internalizing problems when they began the program showed significant decreases. In addition, girls in the intervention condition showed a reduction in externalizing and internalizing problems compared with girls in the control condition (Schmiege, Khoo, et al., 2006).

Rotheram-Borus, Lee, and colleagues (2001) report on a randomized controlled trial of an intervention targeting adolescents living with a parent in terminal stages of HIV/AIDS. The program helped parents discuss their disease with their children, prepare them for the transition to a new caretaker, and facilitate their coping. Benefits were also found at two years (Rotheram-Borus, Stein, and Lin, 2001) and four years (Rotheram-Borus, Lee, et al., 2003) postintervention.

Child Maltreatment

Programs that target child maltreatment have the potential to prevent multiple MEB disorders and promote healthy development across several domains of functioning. One meta-analysis reviewed 40 evaluations of selective interventions providing early support (prenatal to age 3) to families at high risk for child maltreatment (Geeraert, Noortgate, et al., 2004). The authors found a significant decrease in abusive and neglectful acts and a significant risk reduction in such factors as child, parent, and family communication and functioning.

A meta-analysis by MacLeod and Nelson (2000) reviewed multiple programs designed to promote family wellness and prevent maltreatment of children up to age 12. Examples included home visiting; community-based, multicomponent interventions (providing services such as family support, preschool education or child care, and community development); media interventions; and intensive family preservation services (in-home support programs for families in which maltreatment had already occurred). The study concluded that most interventions designed to promote family wellness and prevent child maltreatment are successful. Effect sizes were largest for measures of family wellness and smaller for verified or proxy measures of child maltreatment. Differences were also reported between reactive interventions (in response to an incident of maltreatment), which had larger effect sizes at postassessment than at follow-up, and proactive interventions, which had larger effect sizes at follow-up than at postassessment. These differences could be attributable to variations in the risks in the populations served or in the ages of the children at the time of the intervention.

Supported Foster Care

Children and adolescents removed from their parents' homes are at high risk for MEB disorders. Recent research at the Oregon Social Learning Center has shown that significantly improved outcomes can be achieved through substantial training, support, and backup of parents, coupled with direct training of young people placed in foster care.

Early Intervention Foster Care (EIFC) is built on research that defined a set of critical parenting skills and methods for teaching them to parents and other caregivers (e.g., Forgatch and Martinez, 1999). The program involves a team approach to training and supporting foster parents through daily telephone contacts, weekly support group meetings for foster parents, and a 24-hour hotline. Children also participate in weekly therapeutic play group sessions. In a randomized controlled trial, Fisher, Burraston, and Pears (2005) found that children in the EIFC condition who had experienced failed attempts at permanent foster home placement were more likely to have a successful placement than similar children in regular foster care. One reason may be that EIFC children had significantly greater psychological attachment to their foster parents than those in regular foster care. The impact of EIFC was also shown by measures of diurnal variation in cortisol level, which is lowered when young children experience maternal deprivation, including foster care placement (Fisher, Gunnar, et al., 2000). Compared with children in regular foster care, those who received the EIFC intervention had increased diurnal variation in cortisol over the course of the intervention that became similar to the pattern for children who had not been maltreated (Fisher, Stoolmiller, et al., 2007).

Price, Chamberlain, and colleagues (2008) randomized 700 foster families to receive a version of a foster family care program or usual care. The study included a multiethnic and racially diverse sample of children between the ages of 5 and 12. Children who received the foster family care program were significantly more likely to be returned to their biological parents or other relatives and had reduced behavior problems. The intervention reduced the likelihood of a failed placement among those with many prior placements, primarily because of improvements in parenting practices (Chamberlain, Price, et al., 2008).

A quasi-experimental trial of another enhanced foster care program, the Casey Family Program, showed positive effects (Kessler, Heeringa, et al., 2008). Case workers in the program had higher educations and salaries, lower caseloads, and access to a wider range of ancillary services (e.g., mental health counseling, tutoring, summer camps). Casey foster parents were provided with more financial resources and had access to more case manager assistance. Finally, youth in the Casey program were offered post-secondary job training or a college scholarship—a major difference compared with the public programs, which did not provide services after age 18. Adult alumni of the Casey Family Program had significantly lower 12-month prevalence of mental disorders than public program alumni, including major depression, anxiety disorders, and substance use disorders.

Effects of Family Poverty and Material Hardship

Family poverty and the economic strains associated with such events as job loss frequently undermine family functioning. They are associated with multiple negative behavioral outcomes among children in these families, increase parental depression and spousal and parent–child conflict, and undermine effective parenting (Knitzer, 2007). Research on interventions related to these factors has produced three notable findings. First, economic risk factors can be modified by government policies, and some experimental studies have demonstrated that such modifications lead to a reduction in emotional and behavioral problems in children (Huston, Duncan, et al., 2005). Second, several studies have demonstrated that interventions directed toward poor parents of young children as well as children's early cognitive development are associated with long-term improvement in multiple mental, emotional, and behavioral problems and healthy accomplishment of developmental tasks over several decades of follow-up (Olds, Henderson, et al., 1998; Reynolds, Temple, et al., 2001). Third, evaluations of a few programs have found that the mediators that account for these long-term effects include early cognitive development and parental participation in children's education (Reynolds and Ou, 2003), along with strengthening of healthy parenting practices (Epps and Huston, 2007).

Despite considerable evidence of the impact of poverty on child and family well-being, experimental research that explores child outcomes due to reducing poverty remains limited. Morris, Duncan, and Clark-Kauffman (2005) analyzed two approaches with the potential to affect family well-being based on seven randomized controlled trials. Four interventions involved income supplementation that provided incentives for mothers to go to work, increasing family income while also protecting government-provided benefits if the jobs were low-paying. Three other interventions sought to motivate mothers to move from welfare to work through mandates and penalties. The former interventions significantly increased income, while the latter did not. Small but significant benefits of the programs occurred among younger children, but small and significant detriments were reported for children who were transitioning into early adolescence.

Casino Income and Poverty Reduction: Evidence from a Natural Experiment

No existing trial has specifically assessed the impact of poverty reduction programs on MEB disorders among young people. However, a study by Costello, Compton, and colleagues (2003) used a natural experimental situation to provide evidence of the benefit of increasing family income in reducing these disorders. Four years into a longitudinal study of a representative sample of 1,420 children ages 9-13, 350 of whom were American Indian, a casino was opened on the Indian reservation. Income from the casino significantly reduced the percentage of American Indian families in poverty, but did not affect the poverty rate among non-Indian families. Across the eight years of the study, small but significant correlations were seen between family income and the occurrence of psychiatric diagnosis and the number of psychological symptoms in both Indian and non-Indian children.

Costello, Compton, and colleagues (2003) also looked at changes in symptoms of externalizing disorders (conduct disorder and oppositional defiant disorder) and internalizing disorders (anxiety and depression) following the casino's opening. Behavioral symptoms increased significantly among children in families that remained poor as the children moved into adolescence, but declined significantly over the same period for the Indian children who were lifted out of poverty. Similarly, there was a significant decline in the rates of internalizing symptoms for those lifted out of poverty but not in persistently poor Indian children. Although many fewer non-Indian families moved out of poverty, some did. The pattern of changes in total psychological symptoms was the same as in the Indian children.

This study has the key features of a multiple-baseline design (Biglan, Ary, et al., 2000); after baseline observations, some of the participants received an "intervention" and others did not. Although the increases in income were not assigned randomly to both Indian and non-Indian participants, it is difficult to imagine what other variable might have confounded the change in economic fortunes that occurred for the Indian children.

Potential for Future Research on Poverty Reduction

Gershoff, Aber, and Raver (2003) identify multiple programs that could improve families' economic well-being: Medicaid, the earned income tax credit, Temporary Assistance to Needy Families, food stamps, federal housing subsidies, the School Lunch Program, minimum wage policy, and WIC.

The earned income tax credit provides incentives to work because it phases out tax credits gradually as the worker's income rises. In 2002 it lifted 4.9 million people (2.7 million children) out of poverty (Francis, 2009).

The impact of these policies and programs on family economic well-being, family functioning, and mental, emotional, and behavioral outcomes could be evaluated in randomized controlled trials. Such studies would require theory-based hypotheses about the impact of poverty and economic hardship on parental stress, depression, and parenting skills and children's internalizing and externalizing disorders. Developing studies to test these hypotheses empirically should be a public health priority.

PREVENTION THROUGH SCHOOLS

Schools are second only to families in their potential to affect children's mental health. They can contribute to young people's successful development by providing nurturance and the opportunity to develop cooperative social relations and social and psychological skills. Thus, it is natural that a considerable number of preventive interventions have been developed for delivery in schools, including preschool settings.

Most of these interventions have focused on preventing behavioral problems and externalizing disorders or promoting positive child behavior in school, although some positive results have been demonstrated on internalizing disorders, such as depression. Other programs have focused on school structural factors, such as the reward structure for prosocial behavior or school–family relations. Preventive interventions begun early in life may have comparatively stronger effects because of the malleability of several developmentally central risk factors, such as family relationships, peer interactions, cognitive development, and emotional regulation.

Early Childhood Interventions

Early Head Start

Early Head Start, launched in 1995, is a federally funded extension of the Head Start Program (see below) targeting low-income pregnant women and families with infants and toddlers.[1] Early Head Start programs vary in the services provided but are designed to respond to local needs, with a focus on supporting healthy child development through parenting and family support.

A randomized controlled study (Love, Kisker, et al., 2002) involving 3,001 families at 17 sites nationwide indicated that at age 3, children

---

[1] See http://www.ehsnrc.org/AboutUs/ehs.htm.

participating in Early Head Start scored significantly higher than those not participating on the Mental Development Index of the Bayley Scales of Infant Development, and fewer of them were in the "at risk" category on this index. They had significantly larger vocabularies, significantly lower levels of aggressive behavior, higher levels of sustained attention, greater engagement with parents, and less negativity toward parents. Program impact was generally larger among families that enrolled during pregnancy, African American families, and those with a moderate number of risk factors. Families with four or five of the following risk factors did not benefit: no high school education, single parent, teen parent, receiving public assistance, and not employed or in school. Two years after program completion, some of the program benefits had dissipated (positive effects on aggressive behavior or negativity during play were not sustained), and additional benefits emerged (including enrollment in formal education programs and positive interactions in the home).

Preschool

Preschool education has been shown to have positive effects on the language skills, literacy, and general cognitive ability of young children in several evaluations of high-quality programs (Yoshikawa, Schindler, and Caronongen, 2007). Two meta-analyses report overall positive outcomes of preschool programs. In a review of 13 evaluations of state-funded preschool programs for children ages 3-5, Gilliam and Zigler (2001) report improved developmental competence. Although significant impact was limited to kindergarten and first grade, some effects, including increased later school attendance and decreased grade retention, were sustained for several years. Only four of the evaluations assessed behavior problems; one of these showed a significant long-term effect through fourth grade.

A second meta-analysis (Nelson, Westhues, and MacLeod, 2003) of universal and indicated (high-risk) preschool prevention programs—many of which included home visiting, parent training, or preschool education components—found significant program effects on children's cognitive functioning (when assessed during preschool years), children's social-emotional functioning (during elementary school), and family functioning (during elementary school). Effects on social-emotional functioning were sustained even after children had finished high school.

Programs that provided preschool education had significantly greater effects on children's cognitive development than those that did not. Preschool children continued to do better in elementary school, but the differences were not significant. Programs with more child and family contact also had significantly greater impact on both cognitive functioning during preschool years and family functioning when children were in elementary school.

The Centers for Disease Control and Prevention's (CDC's) Community Preventive Services Task Force strongly recommends publicly funded, center-based, comprehensive early childhood development programs for low-income children ages 3-5. This recommendation is based on evidence of the programs' effectiveness in preventing developmental delay, as assessed by improvements in grade retention and placement in special education (Anderson, Shinn, et al., 2003).

Temple and Reynolds (2007) review the benefits of three comprehensive early education programs: the Perry Preschool Program and the Carolina Abecedarian project, both evaluated in randomized controlled trials, and the Child-Parent Centers (CPC), which employed a comparison condition. All three programs sought to improve educational attainment through a focus on cognitive and language skills and use of small class sizes and well-qualified teachers. The Perry Preschool Program and CPC included a parent intervention, but the Carolina Abecedarian project did not.

All three programs conducted follow-up assessments into adulthood, which included at least 87 percent of study participants. Important academic outcomes were found, including less use of special education services, less grade retention (for two of the programs), higher grade completion, a higher rate of high school graduation, and higher rates of college attendance. Other program effects included less child maltreatment (in the only program that assessed that outcome), fewer arrests by age 19 (two programs), higher rates of employment (in the two programs that assessed this outcome), and higher monthly earnings (assessed by one program). A study of adults who participated in the Abecedarian project also demonstrated reduced levels of depressive symptoms (McLaughlin, Campbell, et al., 2007). Temple and Reynolds (2007) conclude that the benefits of these programs exceeded their costs. A meta-analysis by Aos, Lieb, and colleagues (2004) of these and other early childhood education programs draws a similar conclusion (see also Chapter 9).

Although Head Start has been cited by CDC as an example of a feasible program that could diminish harm to young children from disadvantaged environments (Anderson, Shinn, et al., 2003), few experimental evaluations of the program have been conducted. Ludwig and Philips (2007) report only one recent randomized controlled trial of the program (Puma, Bell, et al., 2005) and one regression discontinuity design based on data from the 1970s and 1980s (Flay, Biglan, et al., 2005; Ludwig and Miller, 2007). Both studies showed that Head Start has some benefit in improving children's cognitive functioning. The evidence from these studies, considered in the context of other research on the value of early childhood education, points to the likely value of universal access to Head Start for disadvantaged children. At the same time, given the magnitude of the program, the potential value of conclusive evidence of its effect, and the availability of rigorous experimental methods, it is surprising that more experimental evaluations have not been conducted.

Several preschool classroom curricula are designed to improve teachers' behavior management of classrooms by reducing child behavior problems and strengthening children's social skills or executive functioning (or both). The Promoting Alternative Thinking Strategies (PATHS) curriculum (see Box 6-7) is an example of a curriculum that has been tested in both preschool and elementary school settings.

Elementary, Middle, and Secondary School Interventions

Targeting Child Sexual Abuse

As mentioned earlier, child maltreatment, including sexual abuse, is a potent risk factor for emotional and behavioral problems. Davis and Gidycz (2000) report on a meta-analysis of school-based programs aimed at teaching children to avoid and report sexual abuse. These programs led to significant improvement in child knowledge and skills related to sexual abuse prevention. The most effective programs included four or more sessions, active participant involvement (such as role play), and behavioral skills training. However, none of the studies examined effects on the prevalence of abuse, and it is difficult to draw conclusions about potential downstream effects of these programs on the risk for MEB disorders.

Targeting Problem Behaviors, Aggression, Violence, and Substance Abuse

Many of the target risk factors of preventive interventions are interrelated. In early elementary school, for example, both aggressive and withdrawn behaviors can co-occur, imparting much higher risk than aggressive behavior alone (Kellam, Brown, et al., 1983), and both risk factors are independently linked to concurrent and successive problems in concentration, attention, and poor achievement. Depressive symptoms in this period are also associated with poor achievement (Kellam, Werthamer-Larsson, et al., 1991). Externalizing behavior across different social fields and deviant peer group contact in middle school predict later juvenile arrest and drug use, and much higher levels of risky sexual behavior are seen among those with both internalizing and externalizing problems (Dishion, 2000). The life course of those with multiple problem behaviors is especially negatively affected (Biglan, Brennan, et al., 2004).

A variety of school-based interventions have been designed to address risk and protective factors associated with violence, aggression, antisocial

BOX 6-7
Promoting Alternative Thinking Strategies:
A Preschool and Elementary School Curriculum

Promoting Alternative Thinking Strategies (PATHS) teaches elementary and preschool children about emotion, self-control, and problem solving. A series of evaluations of randomized controlled trials have reported program benefits for children. The PATHS curriculum (Kusche and Greenberg, 1994) has varied across studies as a function of the age of children, their abilities, and curriculum opportunities.

Greenberg, Kusche, and colleagues (1995) report on a randomized controlled trial in which four elementary schools and 14 special education classrooms were randomly assigned to deliver or not deliver the curriculum to students in grades 2 and 3. The school-year curriculum consisted of 60 lessons on emotional and interpersonal understanding, including identifying and appreciating various affective states, and how to control emotions. A Control Signals Poster, modeled after a stop sign with red, yellow, and green lights, taught students emotional control and problem solving in difficult social situations. Students learned to stop and try to calm themselves and think about how to handle the situation, how to implement their plan, and how to evaluate their conduct.

Greenberg, Kusche, and colleagues (1995) found that PATHS increased the students' ability to understand and articulate emotions. Special education students had a greater understanding of other people's ability to hide their feelings and the fact that feelings can change.

In a randomized wait-list controlled trial of a version of PATHS with deaf children in elementary grades, Greenberg and Kusche (1998) found that PATHS students performed significantly better on a number of cognitive, social, and emotional measures. Kam, Greenberg, and Kusche (2004) report on a randomized controlled trial of PATHS in which 18 special education classrooms were assigned to either the intervention or the control. Students received the intervention when they were in first or second grade and completed assessments annually for the following three years. Those who received the program had significantly fewer externalizing and internalizing problems than control students, as well as a greater decrease in depression.

PATHS has also been evaluated as a universal intervention in the Fast Track study of the prevention of antisocial behavior. First grade students in schools (378 classrooms) in high-crime neighborhoods in four regions of the United States were randomized to receive or not receive a 57-lesson version of PATHS. Peer sociometric data indicated that PATHS classrooms had lower levels of aggression and hyperactive behavior and a more positive atmosphere, but they did not differ on any teacher ratings of classroom behavior (Conduct Problems Prevention Research Group, 1999b).

behavior, and substance use, primarily in middle school group settings (see Chapter 7 for discussion of programs that specifically target substance use and abuse). Many of these interventions involve social skills training using cognitive components that alter perception and attributions or a curriculum designed to change behaviors to improve social relationships or promote nonresponse to provocative situations. Universal interventions are often designed to affect school structure; improve classroom management; or improve students' relationships, self-awareness, or decision-making skills. Selective and indicated interventions tend to focus on skill development.

A growing body of research shows that many negative outcomes, such as psychopathology, substance abuse, delinquency, and school failure, have overlapping risk factors and a significant degree of comorbidity (Feinberg, Ridenour, and Greenberg, 2007). Emerging evidence suggests that some programs have positive effects on several of these outcomes (Wilson, Gottfredson, and Najaka, 2001). Numerous meta-analyses of school-based preventive interventions have been conducted, varying in the specific types of programs included, the age range of the interventions, and the target problems. All have reviewed one or more outcomes related to antisocial behavior, violence and aggression, or substance abuse and found significant but small to modest effects on measured outcomes. Although both universal (Centers for Disease Control and Prevention, 2007; Hahn, Fuqua-Whitley, et al., 2007) and selective/indicated interventions show positive effects, effect sizes tend to be greatest for high-risk groups (Wilson and Lipsey, 2006b, 2007; Beelman and Losel, 2006; Mytton, DiGuiseppi, et al., 2006; Wilson, Lipsey, and Derzon, 2003; Wilson, Gottfredson, and Najaka, 2001), and greater for improvements in social competence and antisocial behavior than in substance abuse.

Meta-analyses provide support for the positive effects of behavioral interventions (Wilson and Lipsey, 2007; Mytton, DiGuiseppi, et al., 2006; Wilson, Gottfredson, and Najaka, 2001) as well as cognitively oriented interventions (Wilson and Lipsey, 2006a, 2006b). There is some indication that programs combining behavioral and cognitive aspects can impact multiple outcomes, specifically social competence and antisocial behavior (Beelmann and Losel, 2006). Wilson, Lipsey, and Derzon (2003) found significant effects of school-based programs on aggressive behavior. Wilson and Lipsey (2007) conclude that program effects have practical as well as statistical significance and forecast that such programs would lead to a 25-33 percent reduction in the base rate of aggressive problems in an average school.

Few programs to date have focused on classroom or behavior management. A meta-analysis that included two such programs found them to have a sizable impact on delinquency (Wilson, Gottfredson, and Najaka, 2001). There is strong evidence for the long-term effects of at least

BOX 6-8
The Good Behavior Game:
An Elementary School Universal Intervention
Targeting Classroom Behavior

The Good Behavior Game (GBG) is a simple universal program to reinforce appropriate social and classroom behavior in elementary school. The theory of the program is that reducing early aggressive behavior will change the developmental trajectory leading to multiple problems in later life. Classrooms are divided into teams, and each team can win rewards if the entire team is "on task" (e.g., fewer than a specified number of rule violations during the game period) or otherwise acting in accordance with previously stated teacher expectations. Rewards include extra free time, stars on charts, and special team privileges.

The GBG has been tested in multiple trials, including some that measured long-term results. A review by Embry (2002) emphasizes the strength of the evidence and concludes that the GBG (1) dramatically reduced disruptive behavior and increased academic engaged time, and (2) had effects that have been replicated across elementary school grades, among preschoolers, and in other countries.

Kellam and colleagues (Kellam, Werthamer-Larsson, et al., 1991; Kellam, Rebok, et al., 1994) evaluated the long-term impact of the GBG in a randomized controlled trial with 19 Baltimore schools that compared the program with a test of mastery learning among first graders (Block, 1984) and usual practice. The GBG reduced aggressive and disruptive behavior during first grade (Dolan, Kellam, et al., 1993; Kellam, Rebok, et al., 1994; Rebok, Hawkins, et al., 1996; Kellam, Ling, et al., 1998). By middle school, recipients of the GBG had lower rates of smoking (Kellam and Anthony, 1998), and those who had initially been aggressive had experienced less growth in aggressive behavior (Muthén, Brown, et al., 2002).

Petras, Kellam, et al. (2008) used latent class analysis to assess the long-term (at ages 19-21) impact of the GBG on aggressive male behavior. The program significantly reduced the likelihood that persistently highly aggressive boys would receive a diagnosis of antisocial personality disorder as a young adult. It also prevented suicidal ideation and suicide attempts (Wilcox, Kellam, et al., 2008). Other analyses of outcomes at ages 19-21 showed that the GBG significantly reduced the risk of alcohol or illicit drug abuse or dependence (Kellam, Brown, et al., 2008) and use of mental health and drug services (Poduska, Kellam, et al., 2008); there were no effects on anxiety and depression.

Aos, Lieb, and colleagues (2004) report that the benefits of the GBG exceed its costs.

one classroom intervention, the Good Behavior Game (see Box 6-8), on aggression and mental health and substance abuse–related outcomes, particularly among boys.

Preventive interventions can also have a positive effect on academic outcomes, although few studies have measured this outcome (Hoagwood, Olin, et al., 2007; Durlak, Weissberg, et al., 2007). A meta-analysis of programs that include academic achievement as an outcome concluded that the effects of social and emotional learning programs were equivalent to a 10 percent point gain in test performance (Durlak, Weissberg, et al., 2007). Students participating in the program also demonstrated improvements in school attendance, school discipline, and grades. Hoagwood, Olin, et al. (2007) found similar results in a review of school-based interventions that targeted psychological problems, with 15 of 24 studies showing benefits for both psychological functioning and academic performance. However, the academic effects were modest and often short-lived.

Reviews of violence prevention initiatives support their efficacy in reducing violence and aggressive behavior (Centers for Disease Control and Prevention, 2007; Hahn, Fuqua-Whitley, et al., 2007). Based on a systematic review and meta-analysis of 53 universal prevention interventions, the CDC Task Force on Community Preventive Services recommends the use of universal school-based programs for preventing violence and improving behaviors in school. The effects of the reviewed programs were generally greater among preschool and elementary school-age children (Centers for Disease Control and Prevention, 2007).

A recent report by the surgeon general disputes the myth that nothing works with respect to treating or preventing violent behavior (U.S. Public Health Service, 2001c). The report identifies 7 model and 21 promising programs, primarily school-based, for preventing either violence or risk factors for violence.[2]

The Center for the Study and Prevention of Violence applies a rigorous set of criteria (experimental design, effect size, replication capacity, sustainability) to identify programs effective in reducing adolescent violent crime, aggression, violence, or substance abuse. The center has identified 11 model programs and 17 promising programs,[3] several of which are highlighted in this and the next chapter. Most have demonstrated positive effects on multiple problem outcomes.

Combined School and Family Interventions in Elementary School

A number of interventions that combine multiple types of programs (e.g., parenting and schools) or multiple levels (e.g., universal and selective) are beginning to emerge, primarily in elementary schools. The Incredible Years Program (see Box 6-2) combines parent and school interventions and has been tested in both preschool and elementary settings.

In some cases, integrated efforts have included a family or school-based

---

[2]See http://www.surgeongeneral.gov/library/youthviolence/toc.html.

[3]See http://www.colorado.edu/cspv/blueprints. Other recommended school-based programs not highlighted in these chapters listed on this site include the Olweus Bullying Prevention Program and the I Can Problem Solve Program.

BOX 6-9
Fast Track:
A Comprehensive, Long-Term, Multilevel Intervention
for Students at High Risk of Antisocial Behavior

Fast Track is a multisite randomized controlled trial of a comprehensive and extended intervention to prevent antisocial behavior (Conduct Problems Research Group, 1999a, 1999b). Schools in Washington State, North Carolina, Tennessee, and rural Pennsylvania were chosen to participate because they had high rates of crime and poverty in their neighborhoods. Schools at each site were matched on demographics and randomized to the intervention or a usual care control condition. Three successive cohorts of kindergarten students in these schools were screened for teacher-rated conduct problems. Those who scored among the top 40 percent were further screened using parent ratings of behavior problems. The standardized sum of these scores was used to select a sample of 446 control children and 445 intervention children who scored highest in conduct problems.

The intervention continued through 10th grade. In the younger grades, it included parenting behavior management training, social and cognitive skills training for students, tutoring in reading, and home visiting. In 5th and 6th grades there was increased focus on monitoring and limit setting. In 7th and 8th grades, students received lessons on identity and vocational goal setting.

During 7th and 10th grades, assessments occurred three times a year, and further individualized interventions were implemented with each youth, based on his or her behavior and needs. The children and their families were also exposed to the PATHS program (see Box 6-7).

The Conduct Problems Research Group (2007) reports the effects of the intervention as of 9th grade, primary among which was less antisocial behavior for the intervention students. There were no main effects on the incidence of diagnoses of conduct disorder, oppositional defiant disorder, or attention deficit hyperactivity disorder (ADHD). Among the highest-risk youth who received the intervention, only 5 percent received a conduct disorder diagnosis, while 21 percent received it in the usual care condition (the rate was 4 percent in the normative sample). The rate of ADHD diagnosis was also significantly lower in the high-risk intervention sample than in the high-risk usual care sample. It is likely that providing this intervention only to high-risk children would have a favorable benefit-to-cost ratio.

---

intervention that has already demonstrated positive effects separately. For example, the Linking Interests of Families and Teachers (LIFT) project incorporated behavioral parent skills training and a variant of the Good Behavior Game, with preventive effects sustained at three-year follow-up (Eddy, Reid, and Fetrow, 2000). The Fast Track project (see Box 6-9) incorporates PATHS as one part of a comprehensive, long-term intervention with universal, selective, and indicated components. The long-term effects of Fast Track were most significant for the highest-risk participants.

The Seattle Social Development project, a universal quasi-experimental intervention in the elementary grades, was designed to reduce risk and build protective strengths in schools, families, and children themselves. Long-term follow-up revealed multiple positive effects on mental health, functioning in school and work, and sexual health 15 years after the intervention ended (Hawkins, Kosterman, et al., 2005, 2008).

COMMUNITY INTERVENTIONS

Preventive interventions in communities generally have two features. First, they target the prevention of an outcome in an entire population in the community, such as tobacco use among adolescents. Community intervention research provides a target of manageable size for testing whether such population-wide effects can be achieved. Second, these interventions target multiple influences on the behavior of interest, often through multiple channels. Community interventions are attractive because they can encompass all major influences on a behavior.

Most experimental evaluations of community interventions involve the prevention of adolescent use of tobacco, alcohol, or other drugs. These studies are discussed in the substance use section of Chapter 7, which focuses on disorder-specific prevention approaches.

Flay, Graumlich, and colleagues (2004) evaluated one comprehensive community intervention and a social skills curriculum for preventing multiple problems among early adolescents. A total of 12 poor predominantly African American schools in Chicago were randomly assigned to receive the social skills curriculum, a school/community intervention, or a health education control condition. The social skills curriculum was especially designed for African American young people. The school/community intervention added several elements to the social skills curriculum: (1) in-service training of school staff; (2) a local task force to develop policies, conduct schoolwide fairs, seek funds for the school, and conduct field trips for parents and children; and (3) parent training workshops. Both the social skills curriculum and the school/community intervention significantly reduced the rate of increase in violent behavior, provoking behavior, school delinquency, drug use, and recent sexual intercourse and condom use among boys compared with the control condition. The school/community interventions were significantly more effective than the social skills intervention on a combined behavioral measure. Girls, who generally had lower rates of problem behavior, were not affected by the program. A subsequent analysis showed that the effects were due to changes in the boys who were at highest risk (Segawa, Ngwe, et al., 2005).

Much remains to be learned about how to mount effective interventions in entire communities. The predominance of the single-problem focus on substance use in existing evaluations of community interventions high-lights a significant gap in the field given that community-wide interven-tions, including those that incorporate components targeting families and schools, have the potential to address a wider set of common risk factors comprehensively. Communities That Care, a system to help communities identify and prioritize risk factors and implement tested interventions that address those factors, is being tested in a randomized trial with positive initial results (see Box 11-1).

The media and the Internet are emerging as means to reach local com-munities beyond schools and families, as well as the broader community, more widely. Their extensive use by today's young people makes develop-ment and testing of evidence-based promotion and prevention interventions using these venues particularly attractive. For example, Triple P (see Box 6-3) has had some positive results in communicating information about parenting via the media. If effective media-based interventions were avail-able, they could be especially valuable in cases in which the local health care system has not allocated resources for preventive services, or the com-munity, school, workplace, or family unit has chosen not to participate in preventive programs. There are early indications that interventions pro-vided on CD-ROM can be effective at reducing risk of alcohol use, drug use, and violence (Schinke, Schwinn, et al., 2004; Schinke, Di Noia, and Galssman, 2004).

A series of creative studies has demonstrated the wide reach and effec-tiveness of entertainment media approaches. One of the pioneers in this area is Miguel Sabido (Singhal, Cody, et al., 2003). Using social-cognitive techniques developed by Albert Bandura (2006), Sabido has documented significant impact of these approaches in Mexico on such practices as the utilization of national literacy resources and family planning. The latter was measured by documenting the use of contraceptives, which showed annual increases of 4 percent and 7 percent, respectively, in the two years preceding the airing of a television serial novel (*telenovela*) addressing family planning and 23 percent in the year the program was aired.

Studies of the impact of electronic media (such as television, computer-assisted interventions, and websites) on other health-related behaviors have also found positive effects in such areas as cognitive-behavioral mood management skills (Muñoz, Glish, et al., 1982), mental health interven-tions (Marks, Cavanagh, and Gega, 2007; Barak, Hen, et al., 2008), and smoking cessation (Muñoz, Lenert, et al., 2006). The National Institute for Health and Clinical Excellence in the United Kingdom has approved two computerized cognitive-behavioral therapy interventions for depression and panic/phobia disorders (Christensen and Griffiths, 2002).[4] The Psychosocial

---

[4]See http://www.nice.org.uk/TA97.

Intervention Development Workgroup of the National Institute of Mental Health has recommended the development and testing of Internet-based preventive interventions focused on many disorders and many languages (Hollon, Muñoz, et al., 2002). The potential of media-based interventions for the prevention of MEB disorders warrants additional research.

CONCLUDING COMMENTS

Meta-analyses and numerous randomized controlled trials have demonstrated strong empirical support for interventions aimed at improving parenting and family functioning. Interventions focused on reducing aggressive behavior, avoiding substance use, reducing HIV risk, securing permanent foster care placement, and dealing with difficult family situations such as divorce have all produced beneficial effects. The interventions emphasize improving communication; promoting positive parenting techniques, such as parents' supportive behaviors toward their children; reducing the use of harsh discipline practices; and increasing parental monitoring and limit setting. Many interventions have demonstrated effects on multiple problem behaviors, shown positive effects in both prevention and treatment contexts, and produced lasting effects.

Generic efforts to improve parenting skills in families with children and early adolescents could have benefits in preventing a range of problem behaviors, particularly externalizing behaviors. This possibility deserves more exploration through assessment of the impact of family interventions on the entire range of child and adolescent problems.

Substantial development of empirically validated school-based programs that can reduce risk for MEB disorders in young people has also occurred. Many of these interventions focus on promoting positive child behavior or preventing behavior problems, with some positive results targeting MEB disorders more specifically. Interventions are often designed to address risk and protective factors associated with violence, aggression, and substance use. Many tend to focus on skill development to improve students' relationships, self-awareness, and decision-making skills. Some programs have also focused on school structural factors, teacher classroom management, or school–family relations.

Universal, selected, and indicated interventions have been developed for both school and family settings, with some programs including multilevel interventions. Studies have shown differential results in terms of effectiveness with different risk groups. There are some indications that interventions provided on a CD-ROM can be effective at reducing risk of alcohol use, particularly with parent involvement (Schinke, Schwinn, et al., 2004). Some studies have demonstrated better results for higher-risk groups, while others have shown positive effects overall but reduced benefits for groups with multiple risk factors.

Several interventions highlighted in this chapter have been tested in two or more randomized controlled trials and in evaluations by researchers other than the developers of the interventions. Evidence has been found for long-term results with different populations. Many other promising interventions have not yet been subjected to this level of testing.

Given the convergence of evidence related to the positive effects of interventions aimed at improving family functioning and family support, the committee concludes that this area warrants both concerted dissemination and continued research. Some factors, such as poverty, that have notable effects on multiple disorders but have not been subjected to much empirical research merit rigorous evaluation.

Similarly, the evidence of positive effects from school-based interventions points to the considerable potential—with the support of continued evaluation and implementation research in collaboration with educators—of prevention practices in schools aimed at increasing the resilience of children and reducing the risk for MEB disorders. Also promising are interventions at the level of communities, including local community interventions, as well as mass media and Internet interventions, and approaches targeting policies, which warrant continued and rigorous research.

7

Prevention of Specific Disorders and Promotion of Mental Health

The preceding chapter focused on preventive interventions that target change in the systems that most influence the cognitive, emotional, and behavioral development of young people: the family, schools, and the community. This chapter explores available preventive interventions that are targeted at specific mental, emotional, and behavioral (MEB) disorders. Many of these are designed to address the specific risk and protective factors associated with those disorders, although some also target risk factors that are common to multiple disorders.

The disorders targeted by preventive interventions tend to emerge at different development stages; for example, anxiety begins to emerge at a relatively young age, whereas schizophrenia tends to emerge closer to adolescence and young adulthood. Depression, eating disorders, and substance use and abuse tend to become a significant problem in the middle and high school years. The chapter organizes discussion of disorder-specific interventions in terms of the order in which they tend to appear in the developmental course of young people's lives. Many of the interventions discussed in the previous chapter include among their outcomes improvements in one or more disorders, particularly externalizing disorders (e.g., substance abuse, conduct disorder, attention deficit hyperactivity disorder [ADHD]) (see Box II-1). Those results are not repeated here. Similarly, other low-frequency disorders for which little preventive literature is available, such as bipolar disorder, autism spectrum disorder, and pervasive developmental disorders, are not discussed.

The chapter also includes interventions targeted at mental health promotion, including strategies related to fostering positive development among children and adolescents and to modifying lifestyle factors that have been associated with a range of MEB disorders. The programs described here are delivered across mental health, physical health, and school settings and have involved intervention directly with children, with parents, and with the whole family. The chapter closes with conclusions and recommendations based on the evidence presented in both Chapter 6 and Chapter 7.

PREVENTION OF SPECIFIC DISORDERS

Prevention of Anxiety

Anxiety symptoms and disorders typically emerge in childhood (see Chapter 2); lifetime rates of anxiety disorders by adolescence may be as high as 27 percent (Costello, Egger, and Angold, 2005). Anxiety disorders typically precede depression and may contribute to its development (Wittchen, Beesdo, et al., 2004). Although a number of studies have shown the effectiveness of cognitive-behavioral therapy (CBT) in treating anxiety disorders in children and adolescents (Barrett, 1998; Kendall, 1994; Kendall, Safford, et al., 2004; Manassis, Mendlowitz, et al., 2002; Mendlowitz, Manassis, et al., 1999), and there is some evidence of the benefits of anxiety prevention for college-age individuals with anxiety symptoms (Schmidt, Eggleston, et al., 2007; Seligman, Schulman, et al., 1999), relatively little research has been done on the prevention of these disorders. However, Bienvenu and Ginsburg (2007) recently reviewed evaluations of anxiety preventive interventions, most of which were conducted in Australia. All of the interventions are variants of CBT applied to prevention, and most involve parents in some way.

Rapee (2002) and Rapee, Kennedy, et al. (2005) report a selective intervention for 3- to 5-year-olds whose behavior was inhibited according to parent and child reports and a behavioral assessment. Parents were randomly assigned to a no-intervention control condition or to an intervention involving six 9-minute group sessions that taught them how to practice gradual exposure and techniques for dealing with different situations, such as entering school. At 12-month follow-up, the intervention group children had a significantly lower prevalence of anxiety disorders, although there was no effect on parental or maternal ratings of inhibition or inhibition as assessed through behavioral testing.

Barrett and colleagues conducted several studies of universal interventions to prevent anxiety problems among children and adolescents (Barrett, Lock, and Farrell, 2005; Barrett and Turner, 2001). The interventions consist of 10-12 classroom sessions and 4 parent sessions guided by a framework called FRIENDS: Feeling worried; Relax and feel good; Inner helpful thoughts; Explore plans; Nice work, reward yourself; Don't forget to practice; and Stay calm for life (Barrett, Lowry-Webster, and Turner, 2000). Barrett and Turner (2001) randomized 489 children ages 10-12 to one of three conditions: (1) usual care, (2) the program led by a teacher, or (3) the program led by a psychologist. Those assigned to the active interventions had significantly fewer anxiety symptoms at the end of the intervention. In other studies, the program reduced the proportion of 10- to 13-year-olds who were at risk for anxiety problems (Lowry-Webster, Barrett, and Dadds, 2001) and at 12-month follow-up had significantly lowered anxiety among sixth and ninth grade students (Barrett, Lock, and Farrell, 2005). There was some evidence that the intervention produced greater reductions than the control condition for the high- and moderate-risk groups (Barrett, Lock, and Farrell, 2005).

Dadds, Spence, and colleagues (1997) evaluated an indicated intervention for 7- to 14-year-olds who had anxiety symptoms or who met criteria for an anxiety disorder but did not have severe problems. The intervention followed Kendall's FEAR strategy: Feeling good by learning to relax, Expecting good things to happen, Actions to take in facing up to fear stimuli, and Rewarding oneself for efforts to overcome fear or worry (Kendall, 1994; Bienvenu and Ginsburg, 2007). The intervention was provided to young people in 10 weekly group sessions; three sessions were provided to help parents learn to manage their own anxiety and to model and encourage their children's use of the strategies. Six months after the intervention, young people in the intervention group had significantly fewer anxiety disorders than controls (16 compared with 54 percent). The difference was not significant at one-year follow-up, but it was at two-year follow-up (20 compared with 39 percent).

Schmidt, Eggleston, and colleagues (2007) report on a randomized trial of a selective intervention predicated on evidence that sensitivity to anxiety—the fear people have of having anxiety symptoms—is a predictor of the development of anxiety problems. Participants who were high in anxiety sensitivity were randomized to a brief intervention that taught about the symptoms of anxiety and the fact that they are not harmful. Participants were recruited from a university, the community, and local schools, with an average age of 19.3 years. Compared with the no-intervention group, participants had reduced concerns about the physical and social consequences of anxiety by the end of the program, although the effect was not maintained at follow-up. Intervention participants were also significantly more comfortable than control participants when exposed to a CO_2 challenge that elicits anxiety, and significantly fewer had developed anxiety disorders one to two years after the intervention.

Seligman, Schulman, and colleagues (1999) used a randomized design to test an intervention consisting of 10 two-hour group sessions with 231 university students selected on the basis of their pessimistic views compared with controls. The sessions focused on changing cognitions, for example, replacing automatic negative thoughts with more constructive ones. At three-year follow-up, participants had experienced significantly fewer episodes of generalized anxiety disorder and fewer moderate (but not severe) depressive episodes than controls.

Although the preventive interventions for anxiety disorders evaluated to date are all based on CBT approaches, recent research suggests that these approaches may not be optimal (Biglan, Hayes, and Pistorello, 2008). Growing evidence suggests greater effectiveness for acceptance-based interventions (Hayes, 2004; Hayes, Luoma, et al., 2006), which teach people to accept anxiety as a normal part of living a value-focused life. Support for this approach also comes from evidence that efforts to control unwanted thoughts and feelings may exacerbate them (e.g., Wegner, 1992, 1994). Additional research is needed to develop and evaluate preventive interventions based on acceptance-based approaches and to determine the effectiveness of these approaches relative to traditional CBT.

Prevention of Posttraumatic Stress Disorder (PTSD)

Although it appears plausible that providing some sort of counseling to all trauma victims could prevent PTSD, empirical research has not shown this to be the case. Critical incident stress debriefing (CISD) is a technique widely used to prevent adverse reactions to trauma. As soon as possible after the traumatic event, victims are encouraged to discuss the details of their experience, their emotional reactions, any actions they have taken, and any symptoms they have experienced. They are reassured that their reactions are normal, told of adverse reactions that are typical, and encouraged to resume usual activities. The intervener tries to assess whether any adverse reactions have occurred and, if so, refers the person for further assistance. Typically there is a follow-up contact with the victim. Recent research found that CISD is ineffective and possibly harmful (American Psychiatric Association, 2004). A meta-analysis found no benefit from its use and suggested a detrimental effect compared with no intervention or minimal help (van Emmerik, Kamphuis, et al., 2002).

In contrast, randomized controlled trials of CBT for individuals who are symptomatic in the weeks after a trauma reveal significant efficacy (Boris, Ou, and Singh, 2005). Some evidence suggests that this includes children (Chemtob, Nakashima, and Hamada, 2002).

In a quasi-randomized controlled trial, Berger, Pat-Horenczyk, and Gelkopf (2007) evaluated a school-based intervention consisting of an eight-session structured program designed to prevent and reduce children's stress-related symptoms, including PTSD. Compared with the wait-list controls, the study group reported significant improvement on all measures.

Finally, there is some evidence that adolescents who maintain their routines have less posttraumatic stress (Pat-Horenczyk, Schiff, and Doppelt, 2006), a finding consistent with other findings that catastrophizing puts individuals at risk for developing PTSD (Bryant and Guthrie, 2005).

Prevention of Depression

In 1994, when the Institute of Medicine (IOM) report *Reducing Risks for Mental Disorders: Frontiers for Preventive Intervention Research* was released, available trials of interventions targeting depression were able to demonstrate only a reduction in symptoms (Muñoz and Ying, 1993). Since that time, methods have been developed for consistently identifying individuals at significant risk of experiencing depression within the next year, and some trials have demonstrated a reduction in the incidence of major depressive episodes, particularly among those at high risk (Muñoz, Le, et al., 2008). Of the trials that have shown a significant reduction in new episodes, all have focused either on high-risk adolescents (Clarke, Hawkins, et al., 1995; Clarke, Hornbrook, et al., 2001; Young, Mufson, and Davies, 2006) or pregnant women (Elliott, Leverton, et al., 2000; Zlotnick, Johnson, et al., 2001; Zlotnick, Miller, et al., 2006), and at least one intervention prevented episodes among those who had prior episodes (Clarke, Hornbrook, et al., 2001). On the basis of these advances, Barrera, Torres, and Muñoz (2007) assert that prevention of depression is a feasible goal for the 21st century, with the promise of being able to reduce incidence by as much as half.

Preventive Interventions for Children and Adolescents

Recent meta-analyses have concluded that interventions to prevent depression can reduce both the number of new cases in adolescents (Cuijpers, van Straten, et al., 2008) and depressive symptomatology among children and youth (Horowitz and Garber, 2006). In a review that included seven trials targeting adolescents, Cuijpers and colleagues (2008) report that preventive interventions for adolescents can reduce the incidence of depressive disorders by 23 percent. They caution, however, that since the follow-up period in most studies did not exceed two years, the projects may have delayed onset rather than incidence. Both meta-analyses showed slightly higher effect sizes for selective and indicated interventions, although the number of universal interventions was very small.

Significant benefit has been reported for preventive interventions for reducing depressive symptoms in children and adolescents, with small to modest effect sizes (Horowitz and Garber, 2006; Jané-Llopis, Hosman, et al., 2003). In a systematic review of preventive interventions with children and adolescents, Merry and Spence (2007) highlight several promising approaches. However, they also describe failed attempts to repeat results in real-world school and primary care settings, limited follow-up periods, and methodological flaws, and they conclude that there is not yet sufficient evidence of effectiveness for preventive interventions for depression. In an analysis of the high-quality studies reviewed by Horowitz and Garber (2006), Gladstone and Beardslee (in press) demonstrate that although symptom reduction, a powerful goal in itself, is possible, very few studies of adolescents have examined actual reduction in new episodes of major depression, the work of Clarke and colleagues cited above being the notable exception. They emphasize that future studies should examine prevention of episodes as well as reductions in symptomatology.

In the committee's judgment, the balance of evidence suggests that some interventions can significantly reduce the symptomatology and incidence of depression. The potential to increase the sample sizes and reach of interventions has been highlighted by work done to adapt behavioral interventions to a range of settings and cultural groups, including conducting worldwide randomized controlled trials via the Internet (Muñoz, Lenart, et al., 2006).

The Clarke Cognitive-Behavioral Prevention Intervention (see Box 7-1), an indicated program targeting adolescents at risk for future depression, has successfully prevented episodes of major depression in several randomized trials. A recent replication indicated that it is not as effective for adolescents with a depressed parent (Garber, Clarke, et al., 2007). The Penn Resiliency Program (PRP) (see Box 7-2), a school-based group intervention that teaches cognitive-behavioral and social problem-solving skills to prevent the onset of clinical depression, has also had promising results.

Preventive Interventions for Families with Depressed Parents

Children of parents with depression and related difficulties have a substantially higher rate of depression than their counterparts in homes with no mental illness (Beardslee and Podorefsky, 1988; Hammen and Brennan, 2003; Lewinsohn and Esau, 2002; Beardslee, Versage, and Gladstone, 1998; Weissman, Wickramaratne, et al., 2006). They are also at risk for a variety of other difficulties in such areas as school performance and interpersonal relationships (Goodman and Gotlib, 1999). Beardslee and colleagues developed two public health preventive interventions (see Box 7-3) specifically aimed at providing information and assistance in parenting to children of depressed parents, both of which have shown positive results in multiple randomized trials.

BOX 7-1
Clarke Cognitive-Behavioral Prevention Intervention Program:
A Promising Indicated Intervention to Prevent Depression

The Clarke Cognitive-Behavioral Prevention Intervention, a 15-session group cognitive-behavioral intervention focused on coping with stress, is modeled after an effective cognitive-behavioral treatment for depression. The first randomized trial targeted adolescents with elevated depressive symptoms and was delivered in schools. At one-year follow-up, intervention participants had a much lower incidence of major depressive disorder or dysthymia (14.5 percent) than participants in the usual care control group (25.7 percent) (Clarke, Hawkins, et al., 1995). A second trial broadened the definition of high-risk adolescents to include parental depression and subsyndromal symptoms and recruited 95 adolescents from a health maintenance organization rather than from classrooms (Clarke, Hornbrook, et al., 2001). At 15-month follow-up, participants in the experimental condition showed a much lower rate of major depressive episodes (9.3 percent) than those in the usual care condition (28.8 percent) (p = .003). These results were recently replicated in a four-site randomized trial involving 316 at-risk youths (Garber, Clarke, et al., 2007, in press). Parental depression at the beginning of the intervention significantly moderated the effect, however; thus adolescents who had a parent with current depression did not experience a significant reduction in rates of incident depression versus those receiving usual care. Further follow-up of this sample is under way.

PREVENTION OF SUBSTANCE USE AND ABUSE

School-Based Approaches

Many of the interventions discussed in Chapter 6 have had effects on outcomes related to substance abuse. Additional intervention strategies specifically targeting prevention of substance abuse are discussed here. School-based programs with this focus emerge primarily in the middle school years, when initial risk for use is greatest.

Cuijpers (2002) reviewed three meta-analyses of classroom-based substance abuse prevention programs (Rooney and Murray, 1996; Tobler, Roona, et al., 2000; White and Pitts, 1998) and a set of studies that analyzed mediators of the effects of these programs. Their synthesis led to six conclusions about effective programs. First, programs that involve interactions among participants and encourage them to learn drug refusal skills are more effective than noninteractive programs. Second, interventions that focus on direct and indirect (e.g., media) influences on use of drugs appear to be more effective than those that do not focus on social influences.

BOX 7-2
Penn Resiliency Program:
A Promising Universal Intervention to Prevent Depression

The Penn Resiliency Program (PRP) strives to prevent depression by teaching middle school students to think flexibly and accurately about the challenges and problems they confront. Students learn, for example, about the links among beliefs, feelings, and behaviors and how to challenge negative thinking by evaluating the accuracy of beliefs and generating alternative interpretations. The original evaluation of the program (Gillham, Reivich, et al., 1995) found that it halved the rate of moderate to severe symptoms among youths in a predominantly middle-income white sample. Another study (Jaycox, Reivich, et al., 1994) found that depressive symptoms were significantly reduced and classroom behavior was significantly improved in the treatment group compared with controls at posttest and six-month follow-up. The reduction in symptoms was most pronounced in the students who were most at risk. Positive results of PRP in preventing depressive symptoms have likewise been reported by Cutuli, Chaplin, and colleagues (2006) and Gillham, Hamilton, and colleagues (2006). The program has also been found to reduce anxiety (Roberts, Kane, et al., 2004). Similarly, students in a program patterned after PRP—the Penn Optimism Program—experienced decreased depressive symptoms relative to controls (Yu and Seligman, 2002).

On the other hand, a study of a culturally tailored version of PRP with low-income minority middle school students had mixed results. The program had beneficial immediate and long-term effects on depressive symptoms for Latino children, but no clear effects for African American children (Cardemil, Reivich, and Seligman, 2002). Pattison and Lynd-Stevenson (2001) and Roberts, Reivich, and colleagues (2004) failed to replicate the findings reported by Gillham and colleagues (1995). These authors also found that a similar intervention—the Penn Prevention Program—showed no evidence of reducing depressive symptoms in youths, although Roberts, Kane, and colleagues (2004) noted that the intervention group reported less anxiety.

Third, programs that emphasize norms for and a social commitment to not using drugs are superior to those without this emphasis. Fourth, adding community components to school-based programs appears to add to their effectiveness (see also Biglan, Ary, et al., 2000). Fifth, use of peer leaders may enhance short-term effectiveness (see also Gottfredson and Wilson, 2003). Sixth, adding training in life skills to that in social resistance skills may increase program effectiveness (see also Faggiano, Vigna-Taglianti, et al., 2005).

A meta-analysis to assess potential moderators of program effectiveness by Gottfredson and Wilson (2003) determined that programs that can be delivered primarily by peer leaders have increased effectiveness. An analysis by Faggiano, Vigna-Taglianti, et al. (2005) found that the most effective

BOX 7-3
Preventive Interventions Designed for
Families with Parental Depression

Two preventive interventions are aimed at providing education and support to families facing depression, helping them understand the illness and the value of obtaining treatment, and improving their capacity to reflect and solve problems together. One intervention involves two lectures followed by a group discussion with parents only. The other—the Family Talk Intervention—is clinician-facilitated; it consists of five to seven sessions (clinician-centered) that include discussion of the history of the illness and psychoeducation for the parents, meeting with the children (ages 8-14 at the time of enrollment), a family meeting planned and conducted by parents with the clinician's help, and follow-up over several years. In a randomized efficacy trial of these two interventions, significantly more children in the Family Talk group reported gaining a better understanding of parental affective illness as a result of their participation in the intervention. These results were sustained during the year following the intervention (Beardslee, Salt, et al., 1997; Beardslee, Versage, et al., 1997; Beardslee, Wright, et al., 1997). For long-term follow-up, the researchers followed 105 families. Analysis of the entire sample 2.5 years after enrollment showed sustained gains for both sets of intervention groups, with an increase in the main target of intervention—understanding in the children—as well as sustained changes in attitudes and behaviors in the parents; however, the improvement was significantly greater in the Family Talk group. There was an overall effect in both groups of a reduction in depressive symptomatology (Beardslee, Gladstone, et al., 2003). In the most recent follow-up, 4.5 years after enrollment, the same effects were found (Beardslee, Wright, et al., 2008). Also, both intervention groups showed an overall decline in depressive symptomatology, an increase in family functioning, and better recognition of when youngsters became depressed (Beardslee, Wright, et al., 2008).

In another trial, these interventions were adapted for use with inner-city single-parent minority families (Podorefsky, McDonald-Dowdell, and Beardslee, 2001). The intervention proved safe and feasible, and there was more change in the families receiving the clinician approach than the lecture approach, although both interventions showed gains. The interventions have also been adapted for use with Hispanic families, and an open trial has demonstrated that they are safe and feasible and lead to significant gains for both parents and children, with stronger effects in the parents (D'Angelo, Llerena-Quinn, et al., in press). Additionally, the principles of the Family Talk intervention have been applied in a program to help teachers develop skills to deal with depressed parents in Head Start and Early Head Start (Beardslee, Hosman, et al., 2005; Beardslee, Ayoub, et al., in press). Family Talk is now being used in a number of country-wide efforts to develop programs for children of the mentally ill (see Box 13-1 in Chapter 13).

programs are those focused on life and social skills. Skills-based programs increased drug knowledge, decision-making skills, self-esteem, and peer pressure resistance and were effective in deterring early-stage drug use.

Derzon, Sale, and colleagues (2005) report on an analysis of a 46-site, five-year evaluation of school- and community-based substance abuse prevention programs that included behavioral skills programs, information-focused programs, recreation-focused programs, and affective programs. Using a meta-analytic technique to project potential impact by accounting for methodological and procedural differences, they calculated a mean adjusted effect size of 0.24 for decreasing 30-day substance use (tobacco, alcohol, and marijuana).

Life Skills Training (see Box 7-4) is one of the most prevalent substance use prevention curricula in the nation's public schools and has been endorsed as a model program by both the Blueprints for Violence Prevention and the Surgeon's General's Youth Violence Report. Another successful alcohol, tobacco, and marijuana preventive intervention for middle school students is Project ALERT (see Box 7-5). The Drug Abuse Resistance Education (DARE) Program, based primarily on scare tactics, has been found

---

BOX 7-4
Life Skills Training:
A Universal Substance Use Prevention Program

The current goal of the Life Skills Training (LST) Program (Botvin, 1996, 2000) is providing adolescents with the knowledge and skills needed to resist social influences to use cigarettes, alcohol, and other drugs, as well as reducing potential motivations to use these substances by increasing general personal and social competence (Botvin, 1986). Middle (or junior high) school students attend 15 45-minute class periods during or after school, with 10 booster class periods in the second year, 5 booster class periods in the third year, and optional violence prevention units. Botvin and colleagues evaluated LST in a three-year randomized controlled trial of predominantly white seventh grade students from 56 schools. Significant prevention effects were found for cigarette smoking, marijuana use, and immoderate alcohol use. Prevention effects were also found for normative expectations and knowledge concerning substance use, interpersonal skills, and communication skills. Three years later, approximately 60 percent of the initial seventh grade sample was surveyed again during a long-term follow-up study (Botvin, Baker, et al., 1995; Botvin, Griffin, et al., 2000). Significant reductions were found in both drug and polydrug use. Positive effects have also been found for a version of LST modified for minority studies (Botvin, Griffin, et al., 2001) and for an intervention combining LST and the Strengthening Families Program, which is described in Chapter 6 (Spoth, Redmond, et al., 2002; Spoth, Clair, et al., 2006). The benefits of LST have been reported to exceed its costs (Aos, Lieb, et al., 2004).

BOX 7-5
Project ALERT:
A Middle School Substance Abuse Prevention Curriculum

Project ALERT seeks to motivate middle school students not to use alcohol, tobacco, or marijuana and to impart skills needed to translate that motivation into effective resistance behavior. The curriculum includes lesson plans, handouts, interactive videos, posters, unlimited access to online training and resources, toll-free phone support, an ongoing *ALERT Educator* newsletter, and unlimited ability to download additional copies of lesson plans.

The first evaluation of Project ALERT, conducted in the late 1980s, showed positive results in terms of drug use and associated cognitive risk factors (Ellickson and Bell, 1990). A second large-scale randomized controlled trial found similar results (Ellickson, McCaffrey, et al., 2003; Ghosh-Dastidar, Longshore, et al., 2004). On the other hand, a randomized, two-cohort longitudinal evaluation of the program found no positive effects, although this may have been due to implementation differences (St. Pierre, Osgood, et al., 2005). The program is among the substance abuse prevention programs for which Aos, Lieb, and colleagues report that benefits exceed costs (2004).

Project ALERT has evolved over time into a combined middle school and high school curriculum called ALERT Plus, which extends the basic curriculum to ninth grade with five booster lessons to help sustain the program's positive effects. Longshore, Ellickson, and colleagues (2007) found weak results for Project ALERT in a randomized controlled field trial of the intervention with ninth grade at-risk adolescents.

---

in multiple trials to be ineffective in its original form; a modified version is currently being tested.

College Interventions Targeting Prevention of Alcohol and Drug Use and Abuse

The evidence on alcohol and drug abuse prevention in colleges is limited and inconclusive because, although many colleges have such programs, very few studies have evaluated them (Larimer, Kilmer, and Lee, 2005). More robust evaluation has been done of interventions focused on reducing drinking among college students. Carey, Scott-Sheldon, et al. (2007) report on a meta-analysis of 62 interventions. They found that, although on average the interventions reduced alcohol consumption both immediately and at follow-up, the majority of studies failed to produce a significant effect. Variables associated with positive outcomes include motivational interviewing (MI, a nonconfrontational approach to asking students to describe their drinking behavior and its consequences), feedback about expectancies and motives for drinking, and decision-making procedures that prompt the individual to weigh the benefits and negative aspects of drinking. Skills training approaches were less effective, as were interventions for men and for those who were already drinking heavily.

An intervention reported by Carey, Carey, and colleagues (2006) did produce significant benefit. They evaluated MI as a means of reducing problematic drinking among 509 heavy-drinking undergraduates who were randomly assigned to one of six conditions. The students received one of two versions of MI or no interviews. The standard version of MI stressed the students' autonomy in deciding what they wanted to do, discussed norms about drinking, provided tips for reducing drinking, and reinforced talk about change. The second, "enhanced" version included a worksheet containing a decisional grid to help students clarify the pros and cons of changing their behavior. Students were also assigned to receive or not receive a Timeline Follow Back (TLFB) interview that took the students back through the previous 90 days, starting with the most recent period, and helped them reconstruct their drinking behavior during this time. Assessment of the students' drinking behavior and alcohol-related problems occurred at baseline and 1, 6, and 12 months postintervention. They found that the TLFB by itself reduced alcohol consumption compared with the no-intervention control. The standard MI produced significantly greater reductions in alcohol use and alcohol problems than did the TLFB; those who received the enhanced MI did not improve as much. On the basis of this evidence, motivational interviewing coupled with the TLFB appears to have the greatest potential to reduce drinking significantly among undergraduates.

Other Approaches

In addition to school-based and college interventions, efforts to prevent substance use and abuse among young people often include other community, media, regulatory, or policy approaches. These more broadly based strategies tend to target norms and policies rather than trying to reach individuals with behavior change strategies, although in many cases they are combined with components that target individuals more directly through schools and families. Many of these interventions, particularly those targeting alcohol, also focus on reducing the consequences of substance use as much as use itself.

The Centers for Disease Control and Prevention's Guide to Community Preventive Services (n.d.) recommends restrictions on outlet density and zoning to reduce excessive alcohol consumption and enhanced enforcement of laws prohibiting the sale of alcohol to minors. Nationally oriented recommendations related to reducing and preventing underage drinking call for these and other approaches, such as limiting the marketing of alcohol and specifically youth-oriented alcohol products, use of media campaigns targeted at parents, and creation of community coalitions; two policy reports also call for continued research on developmental considerations and early alcohol use (National Research Council and Institute of Medicine, 2002; U.S. Public Health Service, 2007). The Task Force on College Drinking concluded that evidence was strongest for indicated interventions that included cognitive skills training, norms or values clarification, motivational enhancements, or challenging of expectancies, but it recommended comprehensive integrated community coalitions targeting individuals, the student population as a whole, and the college and surrounding community (National Institute on Alcohol Abuse and Alcoholism, 2001).

A review of interventions in nonschool settings designed to prevent substance abuse among those under age 25 found insufficient evidence to draw conclusions about the effectiveness of these programs (Gates, McCambridge, et al., 2006). The authors were able to identify only 17 randomized controlled trials, which varied greatly in their program components and included four types of interventions: MI or brief interventions, education or skills training, family interventions, and multicomponent community interventions. Some interventions, including three family interventions, MI, and two interventions with both community and school components, showed potential benefit in reducing marijuana use. Compared with the more robust data on school-based substance abuse prevention programs, existing research is insufficient to determine the effectiveness of efforts to prevent substance abuse through interventions in other settings.

A review of the impact of universal prevention programs on alcohol use (Foxcroft, Ireland, et al., 2002) found a lack of clear evidence for effectiveness in the short or medium term. This analysis, which included school-based, family, and community interventions, found the most promising effects for long-term outcomes of a culturally focused school and community skills-based intervention with American Indians, which reduced the likelihood of weekly drinking over 3.5 years, and the Strengthening Families Program (described in Chapter 6), which reduced alcohol initiation behaviors over four years.

Almost none of the community interventions aimed at preventing adolescent tobacco, alcohol, or other drug use have been in the subject of more than one experimental evaluation. However, the emphasis on these more broad-based approaches in national recommendations and the progress that has been made since 1994 in this area warrant some discussion of a few example programs that include a significant community and policy component.

The Midwestern Prevention Program (MPP), a multimodal community-wide drug prevention program, evaluated effects on high-risk and general youth populations (Chou, Bentler, and Pentz, 1998; Johnson, Pentz, et al.,

1990; Pentz, MacKinnon, et al., 1989a, 1989b; Pentz, Trebow, et al., 1990). The intervention included the following: (1) classroom curriculum targeting students in sixth and seventh grades, (2) parent training addressing prevention policy and parent–child communication skills, (3) training of community leaders in development of a drug abuse prevention task force, and (4) media promotion of prevention policies and norms (Pentz, MacKinnon, et al., 1989b). The intervention was evaluated in a quasi-experimental trial and a subsequent experimental trial. In the formal trial, the intervention was equally effective for both high- and low-risk youth (Johnson, Pentz, et al., 1990). In the latter trial, there was significantly less tobacco and marijuana (but not alcohol) use in the MPP schools than in control schools, with effects found primarily in private and parochial schools (Pentz, Trebow, et al., 1990); through 3.5 years postbaseline, the percentage of students with reports of substance abuse during the past month declined from one assessment to the next (Chou, Bentler, and Pentz, 1998). MPP produced significant declines in cigarette, alcohol, and marijuana use across all follow-ups. There were limited effects for baseline marijuana users and diminishing effects for early alcohol and cigarette users over time.

Project Northland was a multimodal intervention aimed at delaying the onset of and reducing underage drinking (Perry, Williams, et al., 1996; Perry, Williams, and Komro, 2000, 2002). It was initially evaluated in a randomized trial of 24 small Minnesota communities and subsequently in a randomized trial in Chicago inner-city schools. The intervention included social-environmental approaches and individual behavior change strategies along with community organizing, youth action teams, print media regarding healthy norms about underage drinking, parent education and involvement, and classroom-based social-behavioral curricula. In the Minnesota trial, alcohol use was prevented among 8th grade students, and those who were not using alcohol at the beginning of the project reported significantly less alcohol, marijuana, and cigarette use at the end of 8th grade. The effects were not maintained by the time students were in 10th grade. The results were not replicated in the Chicago trial (Komro, Perry, and Veblen-Mortenson, 2008).

Other programs have focused primarily on changing community policies and norms. Communities Mobilizing for Change on Alcohol developed a social-environmental intervention to reduce underage alcohol access through changes in policies and practices of major community institutions (Wagenaar, Murray, et al., 2000). Strategy teams comprised community groups and organizations focused on decreasing the number of alcohol outlets selling to youth, reducing access to alcohol from noncommercial sources (e.g., parents, siblings, peers), and changing cultural norms that tolerate underage access to and consumption of alcoholic beverages. Fifteen communities in Minnesota and Wisconsin were randomized into intervention or control groups. The intervention reduced youths' commercial access to alcohol and arrests for driving under the influence of alcohol among 18- to 20-year-olds (Wagenaar, Murray, et al., 2000).

Two quasi-experimental studies have also shown benefits in reducing alcohol-related problems. The Community Trials project reduced alcohol-related injuries and deaths among all age groups through community-wide environmental prevention activities and policy change (Holder, Saltz, et al., 1997). The study matched but did not randomize communities in California and South Carolina. In the intervention communities, the following were targeted: (1) community mobilization, (2) responsible beverage service, (3) increased enforcement of drunk driving laws and perceived risk of drunk driving detection, (4) reduced underage access, and (5) reduced availability of alcohol through the use of local zoning and other municipal controls on outlet quantity and density. The intervention produced significant reductions in nighttime injury crashes, alcohol-related crashes, assault injuries, and hospitalizations. Adults reported lower rates of drinking and driving, and sales of alcohol to minors were reduced. Adolescent alcohol use was not assessed.

Saving Lives (Hingson, McGovern, et al., 1996) aimed to reduce alcohol-impaired driving and related risks. The study compared six Massachusetts intervention communities and five control communities using a quasi-experimental design. The intervention involved a task force that designed specific activities for its community, including business information programs, media campaigns, speeding and drunk driving awareness days, high school peer-led education, speed-watch telephone hotlines, and police training. During the five years of program activity there was a 25 percent decline in fatal crashes and a 25 percent decrease in fatal crashes involving alcohol compared with the prior five years.

In contrast with the positive results of media messages related to smoking, however, evaluations of the National Anti-Drug Media Campaign have yielded mixed results. While there is some evidence consistent with a favorable effect of the campaign on parent outcomes, there is no evidence that the effect on parents translates into improved outcomes for their children (Orwin, Cadell, and Chu, 2006).

Derzon and Lipsey (2002) reviewed 72 studies evaluating the effects of a broad range of media interventions on substance use behavior, attitudes, or knowledge. Using pre-post gain effect size statistics, they found positive effects for those receiving media interventions compared with controls, including smaller increases in substance use, greater improvement in substance use attitudes, and larger gains in substance use knowledge. Intervention characteristics consistently associated with greater gains include communications directed at parents and other adults with influence over young people; messages communicated by video (compared with television, radio, or print); and the use of supplementary components, such as group discussion, role play, or supportive services. The authors acknowledge significant methodological challenges for both the research evaluating media interventions and the meta-analysis, and the effect sizes they found were small. However, they conclude that media interventions can be effective, and that the wide reach of such interventions can potentially translate a small effect into significant cumulative changes for large numbers of young people.

Prevention of Eating Disorders

The lifetime prevalence of eating disorders, including anorexia nervosa, bulimia nervosa, and binge eating disorder, is relatively small, more common among females, and most likely to occur during the teen years (Stice and Peterson, 2007). In a meta-analysis of 53 randomized and quasi-experimental trials focused on prevention of eating disorders, Stice and Shaw (2004) found, on average, significant effects (generally small to modest) for each of the included dependent variables: body mass, thin-ideal internalization, body dissatisfaction, dieting, negative affect, and eating pathology. Some effects were detectable as much as two years after the intervention. The effect sizes were smaller for universal interventions, which included many participants not at risk for eating disorders. Didactic programs were less effective than those that engaged participants in interactions. Single-session programs were less effective than longer ones, and programs were more effective if they targeted those over age 15. Interventions that simply provided education about eating disorders were significantly less effective than other interventions for most outcomes. The effective interventions varied in content and included ones that focused on resistance to cultural pressure for thinness, addressed body dissatisfaction, and taught healthy weight management. A meta-analysis of five studies of Internet-based interventions to prevent eating disorders found no statistical significance for pooled outcome data but recommended additional research given the small number of studies (Newton and Ciliska, 2006). Stice and Shaw (2004) similarly point to the need for improved methodological rigor and theoretical rationale in order to progress from promising to conclusive interventions.

PREVENTION OF SCHIZOPHRENIA DURING A PRODROMAL STAGE

There has been limited work on early prevention of psychotic disorders. Given the severity of such disorders as schizophrenia and bipolar disorder (McFarlane, 2007) and their extraordinarily high associated lifetime risk for suicide (Palmer, Pankratz, and Bostwick, 2005) and early mortality (Fenton,

2000), it is essential to investigate opportunities for prevention before onset or when symptoms are in the prodromal stage (a period of nonpsychotic symptoms that precedes onset). Findings from a number of treatment studies of early detection and intervention indicate that both atypical antipsychotic drugs and psychosocial interventions are good candidates for testing in youth who are at high risk for a psychotic episode (Haas, Garrett, and Sweeney, 1998; Leucht, Pitschel-Walz, et al., 1999; Lieberman, Perkins, et al., 2001; Loebel, Lieberman, et al., 1992; Marshall, Lewis, et al., 2005; McFarlane, 2007; Pilling, Bebbington, et al., 2002a, 2002b).

To be effective, however, these preventive and early intervention strategies need to overcome some important challenges. First, epidemiological and developmental factors make it challenging to conduct universal, selective, or indicated preventive intervention trials aimed at those who have not yet had an episode (Faraone, Brown, et al., 2002; Brown and Faraone, 2004). Second, preventive intervention strategies are limited by incomplete understanding of the genetic, neurological, and environmental factors leading to these disorders. Third, ethical challenges are posed by the testing of interventions that may do harm and the stigma regarding labeling someone as being at high risk for psychosis. None of these challenges appears insurmountable, however. Moreover, the very high costs of these illnesses when they occur and the fact that experiencing the illness itself predisposes to more episodes make effort in this area warranted.

A number of prodromal clinics worldwide identify subjects from the community at high risk for a psychotic episode. These clinics provide training to mental health professionals, school and community professionals, and the public regarding early warning signs and opportunities for referral. Several are testing an active intervention, including early pharmacological intervention, against a control condition. The prodromal phase is characterized by schizoid characteristics or familial risk, brief or attenuated psychotic symptoms, and social deterioration or negative symptoms (McFarlane, 2007). The criteria used by these clinics to distinguish those in the prodromal phase from those who are not at elevated risk or have already had a psychotic episode are not identical across clinics. However, there is compelling evidence that those identified in such prodromal stages have a very elevated risk for experiencing a psychotic episode in the near future (Yung and McGory, 1996a, 1996b; Yung, McGorry, et al., 1996; McGlashan, Addington, et al., 2007).

The published studies of these preventive interventions indicate a substantial reduction in rates of development of frank psychosis and in prodromal and psychotic symptoms, although one study did not show statistical significance. Using a simple meta-analysis, McFarlane (2007) estimated that the mean conversion rate across studies is about 11 percent of treated cases and 36 percent of untreated or treatment-as-usual control cases.

Given the limitations of many of these studies and the risk of serious adverse events, the positive results found are not sufficient to recommend such interventions as a standard for practice. However, the interventions show considerable promise, and several studies are under way. Continued research in this area should be a high priority. The existence of standard criteria across multiple sites, such as in the North American Prodrome Longitudinal Study (a collaborative, multisite investigation into the earliest phase of psychotic illness), would be invaluable in conducting such research.

MENTAL HEALTH PROMOTION

Mental health promotion programs aim to improve positive outcomes among young people. Some programs share elements with universal prevention programs when they attempt to reduce negative emotional and behavioral outcomes as well as to improve positive mental health outcomes. As a natural consequence of shared risk and protective factors, mental health promotion and prevention strategies also have shared outcomes. As mentioned in Chapter 3, meta-analytic and qualitative reviews demonstrate significant overlap between the strategies, although promotion programs are distinguished by their primary emphasis on positive aspects of development, including developmentally appropriate competencies. This section first reviews interventions aimed at fostering positive development. It then examines lifestyle factors that promote mental health.

Interventions Aimed at Fostering Positive Development

A common feature of most validated programs aimed at fostering positive development and preventing the development of problems is the emphasis on supportive environments or "nurturance." From the prenatal period through emerging adulthood, such interventions are supportive of individuals and their caretakers and provide positive reinforcement for prosocial behavior. Home visitors encourage young mothers to develop new skills, including how to comfort and interact warmly with their infant. Preschool teachers attend to, praise, and reward the developing skills of their children. The Good Behavior Game reinforces cooperative behavior among teams of children. Trainers praise parents for trying new skills in nurturing their children.

The creation of supportive environments also involves acceptance. Parents who are aggressive toward their children are not confronted; they are simply prompted to try more positive methods of being with their children (Webster-Stratton, 1990). College students who are drinking too much are gently questioned about their drinking and its consequences and are given tips for changing their behavior if they choose to do so. People who have been exposed to traumatic events are helped to accept that these events have happened and to move forward in their lives. Families struggling with parental depression are helped to understand and accept and to develop a shared approach to coping with it. Adolescents and young adults experiencing psychotic symptoms for the first time receive assistance in dealing with them.

In contrast to many punitive societal reactions to young people's problem behavior, none of these interventions emphasizes punishment. The Good Behavior Game helps teachers reinforce desirable behavior and thereby reduce the behaviors that commonly draw punitive responses. Parenting programs help families replace harsh and inconsistent discipline practices with time-outs and brief removal of privileges, while parents are prompted to greatly increase positive reinforcement for desirable behavior. Several studies with families that have experienced major disruptions, such as marital separation and bereavement, have provided consistent evidence that the ability of such parenting programs to increase nurturance (warmth) and improve effective discipline accounts for their effectiveness in reducing internalizing and externalizing of problems in the short term and up to six years following the intervention (DeGarmo, Patterson, and Forgatch, 2004; Forgatch, Beldavs, et al., 2008; Tein, Sandler, et al., 2004, 2006; Zhou, Sandler, et al., 2008; Martinez and Forgatch, 2001). The principles of richly reinforcing desirable behavior and minimizing punishment are practices that may go a long way toward reducing problem behaviors among young people (see also Chapter 11).

Durlak and Wells (1997) reviewed 177 interventions targeted at reducing behavioral and social problems in children and adolescents, including both prevention and mental health promotion interventions. They found significant mean effects for programs that modified the school environment, helped children negotiate stressful transitions, and provided individually focused mental health promotion. Most of these programs both significantly increased competencies and significantly reduced problems.

Catalano, Berglund, and colleagues (2002, 2004) identified 25 youth development programs that focused on building positive constructs, such as social, emotional, and cognitive competence; self-determination; and self-efficacy. They concluded that the programs showed evidence of improving measures of positive development and reducing a range of problem behaviors, such as risky sexual behavior, alcohol and drug use, violence, and aggression. For example, Raising Healthy Children (Catalano, Mazza, et al., 2003), an extension of the successful Seattle Social Development Program, focuses on promoting positive youth development by improving classroom and family support for prosocial behavior. A trial matched 10 schools and randomized first or second grade students to the Raising Healthy Children intervention or a no-intervention group. At 18-month follow-up, program participants had higher teacher-rated academic performance and commitment to school, lower antisocial behavior, and higher social competency. Participants also showed less increase in the use of alcohol and marijuana in their middle school years (Brown, Catalano, et al., 2005).

Similarly, in a meta-analytic review of 237 school-based mental health promotion programs, Durlak, Weissberg, and colleagues (2007) reported improvements in aspects of positive development (e.g., social-emotional skills, prosocial norms, school bonding, positive social behavior), as well as reductions in problem outcomes (e.g., aggressive behavior, internalizing symptoms, substance use). Kraag, Zeegers, and colleagues (2006) reviewed 19 trials of school-based programs that teach coping skills or stress management through relaxation training, social problem solving, or social adjustment and emotional self-control. Although there was significant heterogeneity in methodological quality, they found large pooled effect sizes for both enhanced coping skills and reduced stress symptoms.

A recent evaluation by the RAND Corporation of a widely implemented after-school program, Spirituality for Kids, demonstrated a causal link between spiritual development and resilience. In a randomized trial involving 19 program sites, the program showed medium to large effects on positive behaviors, such as adaptability and communication, and small to medium effects on behavioral problems, such as attention problems, hyperactivity, and withdrawal (Maestas and Gaillot, 2008).

Embry (2004) has suggested that the dissemination of a set of simple behavior-influence procedures, or "kernels," would be helpful for parents, teachers, health care providers, and youth workers in fostering positive development among children and adolescents. Examples include praise notes (Gupta, Stringer, and Meakin, 1990; Hutton, 1983; Kelley, Carper, et al., 1988; McCain and Kelley, 1993), peer-to-peer tutoring (Greenwood, 1991a, 1991b), the Beat the Timer game (Adams and Drabman, 1995), and some of the skills that are used in parent–child interaction therapy (Eyberg, Funderburk, et al., 2001) and other caregiver training approaches. Others have similarly called for the study of core components of programs to facilitate their implementation in schools and other community settings (e.g., Greenberg, Feinberg, et al., 2007). Discerning generic principles that are common to diverse interventions could foster their broader use.

Illustratively, because they achieve their preventive effects through promotion of family and child competencies, several programs discussed earlier in this report, including the Promoting Alternative Thinking Strategies (PATHS) curriculum (see Box 6-7), Fast Track (see Box 6-9), and Life Skills Training (see Box 7-4), as well as the Big Brothers Big Sisters Program (see Box 7-6) are frequently cited as successful promotion and prevention

---

BOX 7-6
Big Brothers Big Sisters

Big Brothers Big Sisters is a community-based mentoring program that matches an adult volunteer (Big Brother or Sister) to a child ages 6-18 from a single-parent household (Little Brother or Sister), with the expectation that a supportive relationship will solidify. The match is well supported by mentor training and ongoing supervision and monitoring by professional staff. An experimental design using random assignment was used to evaluate the Big Brother Big Sisters Program at eight sites across the country (Grossman and Tierney, 1998; Tierney, Grossman, and Resch, 1995). This study, although limited by the lack of long-term follow-up data after the 18-month intervention period and little information about site-level variability, had several positive findings. Youth in the treatment group (including both those who received a mentor and those who did not) had higher grade point averages, attended school more often, and reported better parental relationships and more parental trust despite lack of improvement in other related areas. They were less likely to initiate drug and alcohol use than those in the control group and also reported hitting others less often. Aos, Lieb, and colleagues (2004) cite Big Brothers Big Sisters as a mentoring program whose benefits exceed its costs.

---

programs; they have also been recommended by Blueprints for Violence Prevention.

Lifestyle Factors That Promote Mental Health and Prevent Mental, Emotional, and Behavioral Disorders

Evidence from a small but growing set of observational and interventional studies indicates that modifications in a number of lifestyle factors, including sleep, diet, activity and physical fitness, sunshine and light, and television viewing, can promote mental health. Of these factors, the opportunity is perhaps strongest for the salutary effects of adequate sleep and certain nutritional elements, such as adequate iron content in the diet. In many cases, intervention studies related to lifestyle factors have documented physical health benefits. Given the strong connections between physical and mental health, improvements in both may be achievable using common approaches.

Attempts to modify lifestyle factors can appropriately be centered on families and the activities of the medical care community, promoted in the context of schools and community organizations, or accomplished through policy decisions. It should be noted that in many families, there are substantial barriers to promotion and prevention related to lack of knowledge, as well as factors that interfere with healthy decisions, such as poverty, neighborhood stresses, family tensions, and a general lack of child supervision.

While there is a commonsense element to interventions aimed at improving modifiable lifestyle factors, future efforts must rigorously document the promotion and prevention outcomes of their adoption. Promotion of mental health early in young people's lives using such universal strategies that are feasible, inexpensive, and scientifically compelling holds great promise.

Sleep

Sleep deprivation and sleep-related breathing disorder (SBD) are linked to emotional and behavioral problems that include hyperactivity, inattention, impulsivity, mood lability, and aggression (Institute of Medicine, 2006c; Rosen, Storfer-Isser, et al., 2004; Wolraich, Drotar, et al., 2008). Hyperactivity and attention disorders are associated with two other sleep disorders—restless leg syndrome and periodic limb movement disorders (Chervin, Hedger Archbold, et al., 2002).

Given that 20 percent or more of children have sleep problems, the contribution of SBD and other sleep problems to behavioral disorders is potentially enormous, though largely underrecognized. Interventions to improve sleep duration and quality must be rigorously assessed to determine their potential for improving emotional and behavioral outcomes. For example, a program to screen all children in primary care based on a history of snoring, interrupted sleep, and insufficient hours of sleep could be followed by a behavioral assessment using validated instruments and behavioral interventions as indicated. Studies are needed to demonstrate that the treatment of obstructive sleep apnea with tonsillectomy and adenoidectomy or other measures reduces the occurrence of behavioral consequences. A more general proposed approach to healthy sleep is the establishment of a multimedia public education campaign targeting specific populations, such as children, their parents, teachers in preschool and elementary school, college students, and young adults (Institute of Medicine, 2006c). The intent of such a campaign would be awareness concerning the consequences of insufficient or disrupted sleep, leading to identification of these problems and reestablishment of healthy sleeping patterns.

Diet and Nutrition

Adverse emotional and behavioral outcomes for children have long been linked to dietary factors. However, many suggested nutritional interventions have little or no evidence base. Prenatal nutrition was addressed in Chapter 6. Postnatal nutrition factors include hunger, undernutrition, and failure to thrive, which have been linked to cognitive and behavioral consequences (Dykman and Casey, 2003). Other factors that may be more modifiable include knowledge about optimal food intake and content, which can be addressed with education.

Breastfeeding has been studied extensively concerning its relevance to emotional and behavioral health. On the one hand, mounting evidence suggests that breastfeeding can contribute to enhanced cognitive capabilities independently of confounding factors (Kramer, Aboud, et al., 2008). While the IQ effect is modest in most studies, intelligence is a protective factor for MEB disorders and related problems. On the other hand, the weight of evidence at this time does not support superior behavioral outcomes for children who have been breastfed (Kramer, 2008). Based on current information, breastfeeding should be promoted for many reasons, but prevention of MEB disorders in childhood or in later life is not one of them.

Avoidance of nutritional deficiencies is important for promotion of mental health. High on the list of critical nutritional elements is iron. Children shown to have severe chronic iron deficiency in infancy score lower on measures of mental and motor functioning and are rated by both parents and teachers after 10 years of follow-up as more problematic in the areas of anxiety, depression, social problems, and attention problems (Lozoff, Jimenez, et al., 2000). This study is one of several that suggests an important relationship between iron deficiency and subsequent behavior. A concern, of course, is that iron repletion does not reverse long-term adverse outcomes and that iron deficiency remains very common in the United States (e.g., Schneider, Fuji, et al., 2005). U.S. Hispanic children and overweight children are particularly vulnerable (Brotanek, Halterman, et al., 2005). Strategies for avoiding iron deficiency include iron supplementation of exclusively breastfed babies (Dallman, Siimes, and Steckel, 1980), avoidance of prolonged bottle feeding (Brotanek, Halterman, et al., 2005), and routine testing of certain populations of infants for iron deficiency in the course of medical care. Given the magnitude of potential adverse outcomes, systematic efforts to inform parents of childbearing age about the importance of adequate iron intake for both mother and child should be adopted and sustained at the national level.

Attention has been focused for the past decade or two on the omega-3 fatty acid content of prenatal maternal diets and diets for children postnatally. Low levels of DHA and EPA—omega-3 fatty acid products—and corresponding high levels of arachadonic acid have been shown in animal studies to be detrimental to brain development (Innis, 2008) and are related to indices of brain inflammation (Orr and Bazinet, 2008). Cognitive and some behavioral consequences of this imbalance have been described in animals and correlated with effects on cell membranes in the central nervous system (Mahieu, Denis, et al., 2008). In human studies, alterations in omega-3 fatty acid levels have been associated with cardiovascular disease;

stroke; cancer; cognition problems; and a number of behavioral problems, including attention deficit disorders, depression, autism, and suicide.

A number of randomized trials of omega-3 supplementation for mothers during gestation or for infants indicate benefits for cognitive and motor skills, including language development. These improvements could serve as protective factors for MEB disorders. Trials of the effects of omega-3 supplementation on aggression have also been conducted. Studies involving children have had mixed results, with three studies demonstrating a reduction in some symptoms of ADHD and related problem behaviors (Richardson and Montgomery, 2005; Richardson and Puri, 2002; Sinn and Bryan; 2007); one showing a reduction in hostility and aggression, primarily among girls (Itomura, Hamazaki, et al., 2005); two showing no effect on aggressive or disruptive behavior (Hirayama, Hamazaki, and Terasawa, 2004; Voigt, Llorente, et al., 2001); and one finding only limited effectiveness (Stevens, Zhang, et al., 2003). While not yet conclusive, however, the available evidence warrants well-designed experimental trials of the impact of omega-3 in preventing depression and behavioral disorders involving aggression.

The majority of randomized controlled trials of omega-3 supplementation have focused on its use to treat adults with mental disorders. Although two recent meta-analyses report evidence for the potential value of omega-3 supplementation, particularly for depression (Freeman, Hibbeln, et al., 2006; Lin and Su, 2007), another suggests that the effects are negligible (Appleton, Hayward, et al., 2006). All concur, however, regarding the troublesome variability of results; the heterogeneity and poor quality of many studies; and the need for large-scale, well-designed and -executed studies to permit conclusive statements.

Other associations between dietary content and MEB disorders are focused on the potential effects of allergenic foods and large boluses of sugar on the occurrence of ADHD (Wolraich, 1998). More study in this area is warranted.

Neurotoxins

Exposure to neurotoxins, such as lead and mercury, is a significant risk during gestation (see Chapter 5). Postnatal exposures are also of concern. Blood levels of neurotoxins in childhood are correlated with cognitive deficits and MEB disorders, including ADHD and conduct disorder (Braun, Kahn, et al., 2006; Braun, Froehlich, et al., 2008). Evidence has accumulated that blood lead levels once thought to be safe (>10 mg/ml) can be detrimental to infants (Canfield, Henderson, et al., 2003). Protection against exposure to lead, as well as other potential neurotoxins whose effects are not as well documented, is deserving of greater national attention, and demands the concerted efforts of medical caregivers, environment health specialists, community organizations, and lawmakers, as well as regulatory officials at all levels of government.

Physical Fitness and Exercise

Physical fitness and exercise are widely recognized as important modulators of stress, and there is some evidence of their effectiveness for the treatment of depression (Craft, Freund, et al., 2008). A meta-analysis of exercise interventions targeting depression and anxiety, primarily in college students, showed significant positive effects related to depression and positive but not significant effects related to anxiety (Larun, Nordheim, et al., 2006). However, the 16 available trials were of low methodological quality. A clear relationship between physical fitness and exercise and the prevention of MEB disorders in children is even less well documented. Given the clear relationship between exercise and stress, however, both general and medical education for children and their families should include discussion of appropriate exercise and advocacy for overall family fitness.

Television Viewing

Extended television viewing has been linked to the occurrence of ADHD (Christakos, Zimmerman, et al., 2004) and limiting television time for children as a preventive measure has received increasing attention. The American Academy of Pediatrics recommends no television viewing for children under two years of age and no more than two hours a day thereafter. Exposure of children to violence through television and other media has been linked to conduct problems in children and adolescents (Bushman and Huesmann, 2006; Huesmann, Moise-Titus, et al., 2003). Attempts to reduce exposure of children to violence have had very little effect on the content of entertainment programming, and management of this risk falls largely to in-home restriction.

Sunlight

Exposure to adequate sunlight and light in general may affect mental health. Vitamin D deficiency can occur because children today are outside for shorter periods of time and are often protected by sunscreen. Vitamin D may have effects not only on bone mineralization, but also on immunity to infectious agents. Vitamin D plays an important role as well in brain development and function. Subtle effects of vitamin D deficiency on behavior have been suggested, but a causal relationship has not been firmly established (McCann and Ames, 2008). Whether prevention of vitamin D deficiency truly contributes to mental health in childhood deserves further study. Furthermore, limited exposure to light is related, in some individuals, to the occurrence of seasonal affective disorder. More brightly lit classrooms are associated with fewer classroom problems for children with ADHD (Kemper and Shannon, 2007).

CONCLUSIONS AND RECOMMENDATIONS: CHAPTERS 6 AND 7

This and the preceding chapter have documented substantial progress since the 1994 IOM report in approaches to prevention in multiple developmental stages. The strength of evidence related to prevention of symptoms and incidence of externalizing disorders and problem behaviors has significantly increased, particularly through school-based interventions. There is emerging evidence that preventive interventions not only can reduce symptomatology, but also can reduce the number of new cases of depression. And there is promising evidence of the potential to intervene in the lives of young people in the early stage of schizophrenia, prior to full-blown disorder.

Many programs that have been tested in multiple randomized controlled trials demonstrate efficacy, and an increasing number have demonstrated effectiveness in real-world environments. Increasing numbers of programs are culturally adapted and, while still relatively limited, some have been tested with multiple racial, ethnic, or cultural groups. It is no longer accurate to argue that emotional and behavioral problems cannot be prevented or that there is no evidence for the prevention of MEB disorders experienced during childhood, adolescence, and early adulthood.

> **Conclusion: Substantial progress has been realized since 1994 in demonstrating that evidence-based interventions that target risk and protective factors at various stages of development can prevent many problem behaviors and cases of MEB disorders.**

Interventions variously target strengthening families by modifying discipline practices or parenting style; strengthening individuals by increasing resilience and modifying cognitive processes and behaviors of young people themselves; or strengthening institutions, such as schools, that work with young people by modifying their structure or management processes. Parenting and family-based interventions have demonstrated positive effects on reducing risk for specific externalizing disorders, for multiple problem outcomes in adolescence, for reducing prevalence of diagnosed MEB disorders, and for reducing parenting and family risk factors.

> **Conclusion: Interventions that strengthen families, individuals, schools, and other community organizations and structures have been shown to**

reduce MEB disorders and related problems. Family and early childhood interventions appear to be associated with the strongest evidence at this time.

Interventions based in schools have demonstrated positive effects on violence, aggressive behavior, and substance use and abuse. Emerging evidence has indicated the potential for a positive impact of some of these interventions on academic outcomes. Communities have a role in supporting preventive interventions and in developing responses that address community needs and build on community needs.

Conclusion: Community-based organizations, particularly schools and health care providers, can help prevent the development of MEB disorders and related problems.

Although an increasing number of interventions have shown positive results related to reductions in the incidence or prevalence of MEB disorders, most measure highly relevant risk and protective factors but do not measure disorders per se.

Conclusion: Preventive interventions can affect risk and protective factors strongly associated with MEB disorders. Future research must determine the full impact of these interventions on MEB disorders.

Preventive interventions have increasingly demonstrated positive effects on multiple outcomes, but the range of outcomes assessed is also limited. The same type of intervention may demonstrate positive effects on different outcomes, given the limited nature of the outcomes assessed. Similarly, although academic outcomes are likely to be important to schools considering adoption of preventive interventions, because there is some indication of positive effects on academic achievement, this has been assessed in only a few studies. Inclusion of a broader range of outcomes could help in the identification of potential iatrogenic effects that can meaningfully inform the development of future interventions.

Recommendation 7-1: Prevention researchers should broaden the range of outcomes included in evaluations of prevention programs and policies to include relevant MEB disorders and related problems, as well as common positive outcomes, such as accomplishment of age-appropriate developmental tasks (e.g., school, social, and work outcomes). They should also adequately explore and report on potential iatrogenic effects.

Although there are now multiple, well-tested interventions, the effect sizes for most interventions are small to modest. Similarly, though several studies have now demonstrated results with strong empirical designs and statistical techniques, meta-analyses consistently highlight the methodological weaknesses of many studies. As discussed in Chapter 10, this is not because of a lack of appropriate methodological techniques. There is a convergence among both meta-analyses and individual studies suggesting that interventions are more effective for participants with elevated risk, including for participants in many universal interventions. However, most interventions have been tested with a single cultural group, and few have been tested in community-wide interventions that reach large numbers of at-risk youth. Continued rigorous research is needed to improve the reach of current interventions and to expand interventions that are culturally relevant and responsive to community priorities (see Chapter 11).

> **Conclusion: Although evidence-based interventions are now available for broad implementation in some communities, there is a need to increase the effectiveness of prevention programs and to develop interventions that reach a larger portion of at-risk populations.**

> **Recommendation 7-2:** Research funders should strongly support research to improve the effectiveness of current interventions and the creation of new, more effective interventions with the goal of wide-scale implementation of these interventions.

Mass media and the Internet present a potential opportunity to reach large numbers of young people with readily disseminable interventions. Although the currently available evidence does not support particular interventions, this is an area that warrants additional research. Mass media also offers the potential to address concerns related to stigma that serve as a barrier to prevention.

> **Recommendation 7-3:** Research funders should support research on the effectiveness of mass media and Internet interventions, including approaches to reduce stigma.

Although the research base of preventive interventions has expanded significantly, there are several groups or settings that have not been represented in this expansion. With the exception of college populations, very little research has been done related to young adulthood. Adolescence is also less well represented than earlier developmental periods. In addition, there has been limited research following young people across developmental stages. Although there is converging evidence that approaches that combine multiple interventions, such as family and school interventions, have greater effects, this is a relatively new area of inquiry.

> **Recommendation 7-4:** Research funders should address significant research gaps, such as preventive interventions with adolescents and young adults, in certain high-risk groups (e.g., children with chronic diseases, children in foster care) and in primary care settings; interventions to address poverty; approaches that combine interventions at multiple developmental phases; and approaches that integrate individual, family, school, and community-level interventions.

In addition, as discussed in the chapters that follow, achieving the widespread benefits of evidence-based preventive interventions will also require further research on how to train those who implement interventions, how to influence organizations to adopt evidence-based interventions and to implement them with fidelity, and establishing an infrastructure with the capacity to implement and evaluate proven approaches. These problems might seem to be political and beyond the purview of public health and the behavioral sciences. However, policy decisions and the public support needed to influence those decisions are matters of human behavior. Just as a behavior like cigarette smoking is seen as something to change because it is a risk factor for cancer and heart disease, the lack of public understanding and support for prevention can be seen as a risk factor for societal failure to prevent problem development in childhood and adolescence. Research on how to generate public support for the implementation of evidence-based practices is a next logical step in the centuries-long struggle of the public health community to improve human well-being.

8

Screening for Prevention

Broadly defined, prevention screening is a two-part process that first identifies risk factors or early phenotypic features (behaviors, biomarkers) whose presence in individuals makes the development of psychological or behavioral problems more likely, and then segments the relevant subset of the population to receive a unique preventive intervention. As outlined in Figure 8-1, screening can be carried out at the community level, focused on population-based risks (for universal prevention efforts, e.g., training of clerks to check for underage alcohol sales); at group or individual levels (for selective prevention efforts, e.g., screening for the risk factor, maternal depression, when children receive care in the emergency room); or at individuals based on their unique behaviors or biomarkers that may be prodromal features of mental, emotional, and behavioral (MEB) disorders (for indicated prevention efforts, e.g., screening for risk factors when a child's grades in school fall unexpectedly). Screening for community-level and group- or individual-level risks is based on identification of risk exposures. Indicated prevention requires screening for individual characteristics.

There is a long list of possible community-level exposures that represent risks. Examples include poverty, violence and other neighborhood stressors, lack of safe schools, and lack of access to health care. High-risk exposures for subsets of the population include maternal depression, separation of parents as a result of divorce or a death of one of the parents, physical or sexual maltreatment, any events that lead to placement of a child in foster care, and catastrophic events, such as suicide of a classmate. Individual characteristics are also numerous and can include behaviors or

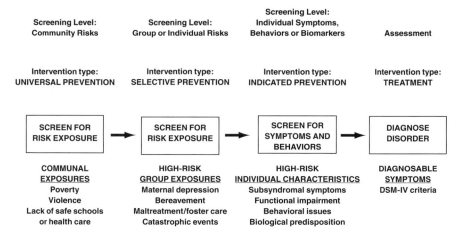

FIGURE 8-1 Schema of opportunities for screening and prevention.

symptoms that do not yet qualify for a *Diagnostic and Statistical Manual of Mental Disorders*, 4th Edition (DSM-IV) diagnosis; chronic disease and other functional impairments, such as neurodevelopmental disabilities; and genetic, environmental exposure, or other biological predisposing factors (see also Chapter 4). Screening at any of these levels will identify youth, individually or collectively, who should be candidates for preventive interventions, assessment, and (if indicated) specific treatment.

Screening should be easily and quickly performed, affordable, and reasonably accurate as a detection tool. There are a number of screening measures and approaches related to MEB disorders that meet these criteria (Stancin and Mizell Palermo, 1997). However, for a number of reasons discussed in this chapter, screening for risks and behaviors or biomarkers associated with a higher likelihood of future MEB disorders has not been widely adopted. The idea of screening for risk factors is considerably different than screening for specific disorders, as is carried out in newborn screening for metabolic disorders that need immediate treatment, such as phenylketonuria. Nevertheless, identification of elevated risks can guide public investments and mobilize communities to pursue needed resources to reduce these risks. While individual risks and behaviors or biomarkers can be identified and receive attention through such settings as primary health care and the school system, there are few specifically identified systems for screening and follow-up at the community or group risk levels. One exception is the Communities That Care approach (see Chapter 11), which has a protocol for helping communities profile their community-level risk and protective factors to aid in selecting an intervention or interventions for implementation.

This chapter outlines criteria for assessing the applicability of screening for selective and indicated preventive interventions, building on criteria published by the World Health Organization (WHO). It also addresses issues related to each of the three levels of screening—community, group, and individual. The chapter closes with conclusions and recommendations on where the field should move to further consider screening in the context of prevention. Although screening approaches have been used in a research context to identify potential participants in indicated preventive interventions, the focus here is on prevention in real-world environments.

CRITERIA FOR SELECTIVE AND INDICATED PREVENTION SCREENING

Fifty years ago, WHO established guidelines to use in determining the public health applicability of screening (Wilson and Jungner, 1968). The 10 basic principles, in various forms, are used today to assess applicability of biomarkers or other diagnostic information for presymptomatic detection of serious disorders. However, the WHO criteria were developed from the perspective of early detection of disease, with the goal of providing treatment before the disorder becomes symptomatic.

For prevention, one of the goals of screening should be to identify communities, groups, or individuals exposed to risks or experiencing early symptoms that increase the potential that they will have negative emotional or behavioral outcomes and take action prior to there being a diagnosable disorder. Successful screening and preventive interventions can reduce diagnosable disorders that require treatment. Thus, considering screening in the context of prevention requires a shift in thinking and adaptation of some of the WHO criteria. For example, mental health screening targets both risk factors and early behaviors or biomarkers that predict MEB disorders. Table 8-1 presents a revised set of criteria that are likely to lead to successful prevention through screening at the individual level. We discuss below the extent to which the amended criteria are met.

1. The MEB disorders to be prevented through identification of this risk factor should be a serious threat to mental health or increase the likelihood of substance abuse or delinquent or violent behavior. MEB disorders among young people result in significant personal and family suffering and substantial societal costs associated with service use and lost productivity (see Chapter 9). Available data on the prevalence of MEB disorders suggest that one in five or six young people is currently experiencing a significant disorder (see Chapter 2), and there are strong links between childhood and

TABLE 8-1 Adaptation of World Health Organization Criteria to Prevention

World Health Organization Criteria	Adaptation for Selective and Indicated Prevention
The condition should be an important health problem.	The MEB disorders to be prevented through identification of this risk factor should be a serious threat to mental health or increase the likelihood of substance abuse or delinquent or violent behavior.
The natural history of the disease should be adequately understood.	The antecedent history of the disorder and its developmental link to target risk factors should be adequately described.
There should be a treatment for the condition.	There should be an effective intervention to address the identified risks or early symptoms and signs of the MEB disorder. Early preventive intervention should lead to better outcomes than a treatment after onset.
Facilities for diagnosis and treatment should be available.	Facilities or settings for screening and intervention should be available.
There should be a latent stage of the disease.	There should be identifiable risk or protective factors or a latent stage of the disorder to be addressed by prevention.
There should be a test or examination for the condition.	There should be validated screening tools or interview techniques to identify risks or early symptoms. Tools should have acceptable accuracy when compared with formal assessments.
The test should be acceptable to the population.	Screening approaches and guidelines should be acceptable to the population and not cause labeling.
There should be an agreed policy on whom to treat.	There should be agreed-on guidelines for whom to refer for assessment, prevention services, or treatment.
The total cost of finding a case should be economically balanced in relation to medical expenditure as a whole.	The cost of finding a case should be affordable, cost-effective, and reimbursable.
Case-finding should be a continuous process, not just a "once and for all" project.	Screening can be population-based or targeted to at-risk groups or individuals. It should be longitudinally implemented, as risks and early signs or markers of MEB disorders may develop over time.

adolescent risk factors and specific MEB disorders. For example, parental depression greatly increases the likelihood of a child's being depressed; similarly, the risk of schizophrenia or other major mental disorders is much higher among those with parents or siblings who have the disorder (see Chapter 4).

2. The antecedent history of the disorder and its developmental link to target risk factors should be adequately described. Although the origins of most MEB disorders and problems are still incompletely understood, the temporal relationship between early behavioral phenotypes and DSM-IV diagnosable conditions has been documented extensively. There are valuable models of how antecedent risk factors relate to the onset of these disorders. The taxonomy of these disorders, although less precise than physical disorders, has also been standardized using DSM criteria. Perhaps most importantly for this discussion, many risk factors for MEB disorders are measurable with scientifically verified assessment tools, facilitating the linkage of their recognition to the onset of later MEB disorder outcomes. While protective factors are less thoroughly documented than are risk factors, they can be recognized in some cases and associated with mental health outcomes.

3. There should be an effective intervention to address the identified risks or early symptoms and signs of the MEB disorder. Early preventive intervention should lead to better outcomes than treatment after onset. We note first that there are treatments available for most MEB disorders. However, the effectiveness of these treatments is highly variable. However, if these disorders can be prevented or delayed, a much larger benefit can be obtained than through early treatment. Parental concern about young children's behavior is a strong risk factor for later emergence of MEB disorders meeting DSM-IV criteria (Perrin and Stancin, 2002). There is some evidence that reduction of risk or presymptomatic intervention prevents, delays, or modifies disorder symptoms. As discussed in Chapter 7, recognition of the risk for depression has led to interventions that reduce the incidence of the full-blown disorder. Interventions for families struggling with divorce have been protective for downstream MEB disorders in the children (see Box 6-9). School or community-wide interventions following a catastrophic event appear to reduce the occurrence of posttraumatic stress disorder (PTSD) in young people (Layne, Saltzman, et al., 2008). Many more such examples could be cited and undoubtedly will surface in the future. The ability to screen for adverse events or conditions has led to effective early interventions in several but not all situations.

Prodromal identification of behaviors or biomarkers for schizophrenia could provide an intervention advantage; studies are suggestive but not yet conclusive that this screening improves clinical outcomes (see Chapter 7). Abused and neglected children are more likely to be abusive and neglectful when they become parents (an intergenerational risk factor) (Noll, Trickett, et al., 2009). It is potentially important to recognize, but there are limited studies that document effectiveness of a specific intervention for children or adolescents known to be abused that reduces their abusive behaviors as they mature. The rationale for screening is strong; however, a robust evidence base must be assembled to demonstrate where investment in broad screening efforts is effective and cost-efficient. In particular, studies should address identification of types of risks that can lead to mobilization of community resources to address risk.

For some disorders, effective prevention strategies are available. Before implementing an individual screening strategy, it would be important to compare its impact with that of a universal strategy. For the prevention of conduct disorder, youth can be identified through screening of teachers and parents for those exhibiting aggressive behavior (Perrin and Stancin, 2002). A number of individual-level interventions are available, ranging from behavioral reinforcement with a mental health professional to long-term intervention, as used in the Fast Track project (see Box 6-9). Alternatively, universal preventive interventions have been shown to have lasting impact on those with the highest levels of aggressive behavior early on (Kellam, Brown, et al., 2008), and they do not encounter the kinds of stigma or labeling that occur from individual-level interventions. Where multiple levels of preventive intervention are available, universal interventions may serve as an informal screening mechanism, with those who do not respond to the intervention being identified for more targeted approaches based on elevated risk.

We note that screening should target not only young people, but also their extended family members and caretakers as well as peers and community environments, including norms and policies, for example, around substance use. Home visitation has been one useful strategy for screening of relevant figures and experiences in a child's life. For example, postpartum depression was detected in more than 40 percent of socioeconomically disadvantaged mothers by home visitation (Stevens, Ammerman, et al., 2002). Situational stresses, such as death of a parent, affect all family members (Melhem, Walker, et al., 2008). Screening for parental mental disorders, such as depression, PTSD, domestic violence, and substance use, is key to designing interventions to reduce children's risk and has been recommended for primary care (Whitaker, Orgol, and Kahn, 2006) as well as emergency room (Grupp-Phelan, Wade, et al., 2007) settings. Preventing behavior problems in young children requires family-oriented strategies that address the needs of both parents and their children.

4. Facilities or settings for screening and intervention should be available. Screening for risks or for precursors of MEB disorders is not limited by the availability of screening settings. Three settings appear to have particular advantages: (1) primary medical care, (2) schools, and (3) preschools or day care. However, none has become a site for the routine screening of children.

Primary Care. A number of screening tools have been proposed for use in the medical office (Perrin and Stancin, 2002). One of the best indicators of risk for emergence of MEB disorders in the future is the presence of parental or caretaker concern about a particular child's behavior. The office visit can screen for risk by routinely inquiring about parental concern. Computerized screening has demonstrated enhanced recognition of behavioral problems in the office setting (Stevens, Kelleher, et al., 2008). There are several barriers to widespread adoption of medical office screening for risks or behavioral indicators of future MEB disorder (Perrin and Stancin, 2002). First, most physicians, including pediatricians and their office staff, have not been trained to include screening in their routine well child or sick child visits (see Chapter 12). Second, good systems frequently are not in place to further assess children who are identified as being at risk. Many pediatric or family medicine offices are neither prepared to take necessary steps, nor are they linked to behavioral care capabilities (psychiatry, psychology, social work expertise) for follow-up of the screening outcomes. Third, in most medical office settings, neither public nor private payers will reimburse for behavioral screening. Early and Periodic Screening, Diagnostic, and Treatment (EPSDT), a Medicaid program, has been used largely to promote developmental screening. For a number of reasons, the intent of the program to include behavioral screening has not been fully realized; the EPSDT screening tools in nearly half the states do not address behavioral health issues at all (Semansky, Koyanagi, and Vandivort-Warren, 2003). States use a variety of tools with variable coverage of mental health and substance abuse issues (Judge David L. Bazelon Center for Mental Health Law, 2009). The state of Massachusetts, as the result of a court decision, has mandated behavioral screening for all children enrolled in Medicaid at each physician visit, starting in January 2008. Physicians' practices are reimbursed $12 for each screening session, so compensation is not a barrier. The effectiveness of the screening and outcomes of children at risk in this program are as yet unmeasured.

Assuring Better Child Health and Development (ABCD) is a program funded by the Commonwealth Fund and administered by the National Academy of State Health Policy. It has created two state health consortia, the second of which (ABCD II) employs standardized, validated screening tools to assess the mental development of young children and to provide follow-up services for those at risk. The successes of this program provide

BOX 8-1
Assuring Better Child Health and Development Initiative

The Assuring Better Child Health and Development (ABCD) Initiative is a program funded by the Commonwealth Fund and administered by the National Academy for State Health Policy. It is designed to strengthen the capacity of states to deliver early child development services to low-income children and their families through their Medicaid programs. Two state consortia were formed under the ABCD initiative. The first, ABCD I, created in 2000, provided grants to four states (North Carolina, Utah, Vermont, and Washington) to develop or expand service delivery and financing strategies aimed at enhancing healthy child development, including efforts to strengthen developmental screening, surveillance, and assessment efforts. The second, ABCD II, formed in 2004, is aimed at strengthening primary health care services and systems that support the healthy mental development of young children from birth to age 3 in five states (California, Illinois, Iowa, Minnesota, and Utah). The initiative was carried out primarily through a small number of pilot programs in clinical practice settings. Many of the states also included an effort to identify and address systematic policy barriers, including clarifying or amending state Medicaid policies.

In an effort to improve the identification of children at risk for or with social or emotional development delays, the ABCD II consortium states each identified standardized, validated screening tools and encouraged pediatric primary care providers to use them as a routine part of their regular delivery of care. Each state sought tools that would accurately identify children who may need behavioral developmental care and follow-up services, be inexpensive and rapid to administer, and provide information that could lead to action. The final selections included the Ages and States Questionnaire® (ASQ), the Ages and Stages Questionnaire®: Social-Emotional (ASQ:SE), the Brief Infant-Toddler Social and Emotional Assessment (BITSEA), the Child Development Review, the Infant Development Inventory, the Parents' Evaluation of Developmental Status (PEDS), and the Temperament and Atypical Behavior Scale (TABS). Most are designed to elicit information from

encouragement that the primary medical care setting can effectively identify children who can benefit from early attention (see Box 8-1). Initial lessons from implementation of this program in Iowa have been made available (Silow-Carroll, 2008), but evaluation of the program is still in progress. Other efforts to screen for MEB disorders in the primary care setting include (1) routinely questioning adolescents about symptoms suggesting depression (ACGME, Adolescent Medicine Training Program Requirements), (2) surveillance (ongoing observation) and screening young children for behaviors suggestive of autism (Johnson, Myers, and the American Academy of Pediatrics Council on Children with Disabilities, 2007), and (3) screening for suicidal ideation (Institute of Medicine, 2002). All of these efforts span parents rather than through clinician observation, requiring minimal staff time to administer. Clinicians felt these tools also helped parents learn about child development, identify concerns, and organize questions prior to an appointment.

ABCD II found that to ensure young children's healthy mental development and to successfully change provider practices, it was necessary not only to improve screening of young children for potential social and emotional development problems but also to help families and clinicians access resources for appropriate follow-up services. Thus, the states also undertook efforts to identify existing resources for assessment and treatment, remove policy barriers to accessing those services, and facilitate referrals. All five ABCD II states were able to increase screening in selected practices, and most states also increased the percentage of children referred for services, including assessment, secondary developmental surveillance, child psychologist evaluation, rehabilitation, early intervention, and school services. There was no consistent measurement of follow-up services received after referral, and child outcomes as a result of screening and referral were not assessed. The states also initiated policy changes that improved program coverage, reimbursement, and system performance; worked with physician practices to test and spread practice innovations; and relied on key partnerships with other state agencies and provider organizations.

Building on this work as well as other advances in the field, the ABCD Screening Academy was established in 2007. It provides technical assistance to help implement practices and policies designed to increase the use of developmental screening tools as part of the standard practice of well-child care delivered by primary care providers.

SOURCES: Pelletier and Abrams (2003); Kaye, May, and Abrams (2006); Kaye and Rosenthal (2008).

the boundary between screening for risk or early indicators and diagnostic efforts. Nevertheless, they offer the potential to intervene early and, in some cases, to prevent fully developed MEB disorders.

Schools. Universal screening to identify students at risk for school failure or psychological or behavioral problems is increasingly recognized as an important professional practice (Burns and Hoagwood, 2002; Glover and Albers, 2007; Levitt, Saka, et al., 2007). For example, both the President's Commission on Excellence in Special Education and the No Child Left Behind Act of 2001 (NCLB) (see U.S. Office of Special Education Programs and NCLB, U.S. Department of Education) have strongly endorsed this approach. In its current 2004 reauthorization, up to 15 percent of the funds available through the Individuals with Disabilities Education Act can be used for early screening, intervention, and prevention to reduce referrals to special education and related services. In a 2002 report on minority and gifted students in special education, the National Research Council recommended that states adopt a universal screening and multitiered intervention strategy in addressing the needs of these school populations, in part to provide services before special education services are needed (see National Research Council, 2002). Finally, the U.S. Public Health Service (2000) recommended that early indicators of mental health problems be identified in existing preschool, child care, education, health, welfare, juvenile justice, and substance abuse treatment systems.

School-based screening also has its opponents. Among the objections raised are (1) teachers' concern that their discretion will be reduced (Elliott, Huai, and Roach, 2007); (2) the extra work involved (Levitt, Saka, et al., 2007); (3) potential stigmatization of students who are identified (Levitt, Saka, et al., 2007); (4) questions about the validity of discrepant rates of disorders related to gender, race/ethnicity, and economic status (Barbarin, 2007); and (5) related parental concerns about labeling and consent.

Thus, universal screening procedures, especially those involving multiple stages, must be brief, technically adequate, valid across racial, ethnic, and socioeconomic groups, and produce valued outcomes in order to be acceptable in educational environments. Moreover, they should be accompanied by appropriate safeguards to address and obviate concerns. For example, parents should be contacted in advance whenever such screening initiatives are being planned and provided with transparent and detailed information about their purpose and methods and how results will be used. The wishes of parents who object to their child's inclusion in such efforts should be respected. The goals and design of these initiatives should be targeted to relatively narrow and specific purposes, for example, (1) improving school success for struggling students, (2) preventing bullying and student harassment, (3) improving teacher and peer relationships, (4) increasing school safety and security, or (5) learning to regulate and control behavior.

The ultimate justification for school-based screening is that it can contribute to preventing the development of psychological and behavioral problems, which interfere with school performance. There is evidence that screening can identify young people who are at risk for the development of these problems.

For example the Systematic Screening for Behavior Disorders (SSBD) program is a validated, universal screening system to identify school-related externalizing or internalizing behavior problems for students of elementary school age (Walker and Severson, 1990). It consists of three integrated screening stages: teacher nominations of students with internalizing and externalizing problems, teacher ratings of the three highest children on each list, and direct observation of students whose scores on the teacher ratings exceed normative cutoffs.

SSBD has a national normative base of over 4,400 cases representing schools in eight states distributed across the United States. The two behavioral observation codes in Stage 3 were normed on 1,300 cases drawn from these same participating schools. Elliott and Busse (2004) reported that SSBD reliably differentiated students having and not having behavioral disorders.

Walker, Seeley, and colleagues (in press) reported a randomized control trial in which SSBD was used to identify the 2 percent of primary grade children who were most aggressive. They identified 200 students (70 percent of whom were Hispanic) in two cohorts and provided an evidence-based intervention involving both parenting skills training and a classroom intervention. The intervention resulted in significant improvements in symptoms, function, and academic domains.

Preschool and Day Care. A large proportion of children in the United States regularly attend day care, nursery school, or an alternative out-of-the-home setting prior to age 5. Identification of risk or early indicators of MEB disorders in these settings provides for early detection and the opportunity for preventive interventions. A significant number of children arrive in kindergarten without the self-regulatory skills to function productively in the classroom (Rimm-Kaufman, Pianta, and Cox, 2000) or are expelled from preschool due to behavioral issues (Gilliam, 2005; Gilliam and Shahar, 2006). Although Head Start has adopted standards mandating mental health assessment and intervention for social-emotional problems of enrolled children (Head Start Quality Research Consortium, 2003), it is unclear if they have been fully implemented. Although numerous screening tools are available, there is no single, widely accepted easy-to-use instrument. Barbarin (2007) recently developed a simple tool aimed at identifying children at risk of early onset social-emotional difficulties designed to address barriers to screening in the preschool context. There are promising indications that mental health consultation in preschool settings can improve behavioral outcomes (Perry, Dunne, et al., 2008). McDermott, Mamum, and colleagues (2008) found that screening children ages 2-4 with a standardized questionnaire for irregular eating patterns identified those more likely to have behavioral problems. Children with a chronic illness in the preschool setting are at risk for depressive symptoms and impairment in several social domains (Curtis and Luby, 2008). However, broad implementation of screening for mental, emotional, and behavioral issues linked with prevention programs has not occurred. Reimbursement, the availability of trained staff, and the ability to provide follow-up services impede screening in this setting as well. Federal agencies and knowledgeable professional organizations should address this opportunity singly but, more importantly, in a partnership mode.

Community. Communities and neighborhoods can respond to the emotional and behavioral needs of their youth, aided by information about community-level risks and the prevalence of specific problems and disorders. Mechanisms are available for community self-assessment, for example, Healthy Cities/Healthy Communities, and Communities That Care Programs. Survey and administrative data will be needed to allow communities to move forward on this front, in particular to identify individuals and groups within the community who are most in need of intervention and support. Successful strategies will include partnerships among schools, primary care settings, the mental health professions, community agencies, and local government.

Community-based programs, such as home visitation, have incorporated behavioral screening into their interventions (Olds, Memphis Study). The Ages and Stages Questionnaire-SE, which can be used for children ages 6 months to 5 years, has been adopted by several home visiting programs. The Child Behavior Check List and the Infant Toddler Social-Emotional Assessment have also been used for home-based screening by visitors.

5. There should be identifiable risk or protective factors or a latent stage of the disorder to be addressed by prevention. Chapter 4 summarized published work on identification and application of knowledge concerning risk and protective factors for MEB disorders. The literature is now replete with results of randomized controlled studies that support the contention that interventions directed to these factors, whether at the community, family, school, or individual level, result in some level of protection against the emergence of MEB disorders. Many disorders display prodromal symptoms well in advance of diagnosable conditions.

6. There should be validated screening tools or interview techniques to identify risks or early symptoms. Clinical judgment in medical care identifies fewer than 50 percent of children who have serious emotional and behavioral disturbances (Glascoe, 2000). This percentage is likely to be smaller for identification of risk factors or early behavioral problems.

Numerous tools and procedures are available that can be used to systematically screen for individual mental, emotional, and behavioral risks or early behavioral symptoms in such settings as primary medical care (see Box 8-1; Perrin and Stancin, 2002; Kemper and Kelleher, 1996), emergency rooms (Grupp-Phelan, Wade, et al., 2007), schools (Barbarin, 2007; Aseltine and DeMartino, 2004; Walker, Severson, and Seeley, 2007), and colleges (McCabe, 2008). Tools are available to screen for a variety of risks, including purging in young adolescent girls (Field, Javaras, et al.,

2008), trauma (Cohen, Kelleher, and Mannarino, 2008), maternal depression (Grupp-Phelan, Wade, et al., 2007), suicide (Aseltine and DeMartino, 2004), and drug abuse (McCabe, 2008), to name a few. The large number of tools available reflects the spectrum of problems and developmental stages to be screened, as well as perhaps the lack of standardization of approaches in this field.

The sensitivity (the ability to accurately identify individuals at risk) and specificity (the ability to accurately identify those not at risk) of available screening tools are important considerations (Meisels and Atkins-Burnett, 2005; Glascoe, 2000). On one hand, a high false-positive rate compounds the problem of stigmatization of potentially healthy children. On the other hand, an excessive false-negative rate will preclude many children in need from being identified and getting the early intervention services needed to keep them healthy. Most of the instruments reviewed have sensitivities and specificities in the 70-90 percent range, which is acceptable for screening. Positive and negative predictive values (the probability of disease among those with a positive test and the probability of no disease among those with a negative test, respectively) are usually not reported in these analyses. The committee did not systematically review the evidence related to all screening tools but was struck by the breadth of available tools.

Adaptation of screening tools for specific ethnic/cultural groups may be required. Psychometric properties are not always demonstrated for these groups (Pignone, Gaynes, et al., 2002). Children from culturally or linguistically distinct backgrounds may respond differently than majority youth not only to the screening instrument, but also to the screening process itself (Snowden and Yamada, 2005). In addition, behaviors and emotions that tools identify as dysfunctional may be adaptive in the sociocultural and physical environments of some ethnic minority children and families (Canino and Spurlock, 1994; Dubrow and Garbarino, 1989). Although race and ethnicity are often confounded with socioeconomic status, and socioeconomic status is the stronger predictor of MEB disorders, efforts to increase the cultural relevance, including the linguistic acceptability, of screening tools warrant attention.

7. Screening guidelines should be acceptable to the population and not cause labeling. Historically, the U.S. public has favored the opportunity to gain knowledge of potentially adverse medical situations or outcomes so that action can be taken to avoid the consequences. For example, all states have newborn screening programs in place, many of which test for 20, 30, or even more serious disorders. However, circumstances related to prevention of MEB disorders may frame this point of view differently. Some people do not want to acknowledge or think about mental illness. When screening results have the potential to adversely label or stigmatize young

people, whether healthy or dysfunctional, even if there is a small chance that this may occur, some families are reluctant to allow their children to participate in screening efforts.

Males with a genotype resulting in low MAOA activity who are mal-treated in childhood have a strong chance (85 percent) of developing antisocial behavior (Caspi, McClay, et al., 2002). Screening early in life with genetic testing would appear to be advantageous in that preven-tive interventions are available that focus on cultivating strong family systems. However, screening could be stigmatizing for black males, who are frequently stereotyped and more likely to be harshly punished com-pared with their counterparts (U.S. Public Health Service, 2001a). There has been public and organized opposition to screening programs, such as Teen Screen,[1] a national mental health and suicide risk screening program (Lenzer, 2004). This dilemma represents a barrier for screening programs for MEB disorders.

Stigma has been recognized as a barrier to screening and mental health services in many settings, including schools. The President's New Freedom Commission called for a national campaign to reduce the stigma of seeking mental health care and the delivery of universal preventive interventions, especially in schools (Mills, Stephan, et al., 2006). Stigma has been charac-terized as public, self, and label avoidance. General approaches to changing stigma include protest, education, and exposure (public) as well as fostering group identity, cognitive rehabilitation, and disclosure for self-stigma and label avoidance (Corrigan and Wassel, 2008). Positive Attitudes Toward Learning in Schools (PALS) is one organized effort to reduce stigma that emphasizes families as partners with schools and the use of community con-sultants (Atkins, Graczyk, et al., 2003; Atkins, Frazier, et al., 2006). Other approaches have embraced the term "mental health" as a positive concept in their communication with the public in an attempt to avoid stigma.

Several states have adopted antistigma programs, including advertise-ments (New Mexico) and a Youth Speakers Bureau (Ohio). The magnitude of the impact of stigma and antistigma efforts on prevention programs for MEB disorders remains to be determined. A survey of adult attitudes of chil-dren's mental health problems found that among adults able to differentiate depression and attention deficit hyperactivity disorder (ADHD) from "daily troubles," a significant percentage rejected the label of mental illness (13 and 19 percent for depression and ADHD, respectively) (Pescosolido, Jensen, et al., 2008). Existing stigma reduction efforts have not been widely supported, probably contributing to the persistence of this barrier. Routine screening for mental, emotional, and behavioral problems may help alleviate concerns about stigma and labeling.

---

[1]See http://www.teenscreen.org.

Other ethical issues enter into screening considerations. Screening in the absence of available preventive or early treatment services is a formula for frustration and serves to heighten the potential for emotionally isolating the identified child. Accordingly, in the committee's view, screening is warranted if follow-up intervention is available and accessible that could protect against risk factors becoming predictive factors. If follow-up intervention is not available, the community will have to weigh other potential benefits, such as community awareness and the potential leveraging of resources against the potential issues raised. The committee also concludes that in cases of individual- or group-level screening, all families should be able to make an informed choice about the participation of their child in screening activities, including being provided information on the goals, methods, and intended use of collected information. Ensuring that families are fully informed, however, is an enormous task.

Screening as a pathway to better mental health will succeed only if all the attendant ethical issues are managed transparently. The most important element of screening programs going forward may be education of the public concerning the benefits of screening, including avoidance of risks and the importance of early interventions.

Public acceptance of screening for risks or early emotional and behavioral problems also becomes a factor in arranging for reimbursement of screening efforts. Costs of newborn screening are borne by the state as the result of legislation. This is not the case for screening related to mental, emotional, and behavioral health. A recent expert forum convened by the Substance Abuse and Mental Health Services Administration (SAMHSA) identified lack of reimbursement incentives for screening and preventive mental health services as one of seven primary mental health barriers (Kautz, Mauch, and Smith, 2008). Economic issues also play a role in decisions about school-based screening because of reimbursement constraints, tight budgets, and reduced staffing in many districts. The future of prevention screening rests in part on public policy decisions.

8. There should be agreed-on guidelines for whom to refer for assessment, prevention services, or treatment. Validated screening tools have cut points or thresholds for concern that would make a child eligible for preventive services or treatment. The first step, following a positive screen, should be the performance of a more detailed psychological assessment to verify the screening results and to determine the nature and the severity of the risk or emotional or behavioral problem. This may take the form of more extensive psychological testing or a psychiatric interview (Perrin and Stancin, 2002). Too often, delay or lack of availability of psychological or psychiatric consultation becomes a barrier for timely assessment and creation of an action plan for the child or adolescent. Lack of training and failure of the health care reimbursement system to compensate primary care providers for behavioral care has been an impediment to expansion of an engaged workforce. Greater capacity for behavioral evaluation and care is an unaddressed need in the United States. Training and support for individuals and programs that provide behavioral care, whether in the health care, social service, or education system, is a high-priority need.

Another barrier is the nature of many of the risk factors, such as poverty, violence, and other neighborhood-related stressors. Modifying these risk factors requires community action, which does not respond in a timely fashion to the needs of individual children. Interventions for population-wide risk factors often fall back on individually focused efforts that identify or build on protective factors, such as parental or other caregiver support in the home. Partnerships with schools can also address risk and protective factors from the individual or group perspective, for example, interventions for exposure to aggressive behaviors (Wilson and Lipsey, 2007).

9. The cost of finding a case should be affordable, cost-effective, and reimbursable. As suggested from the discussion above, screening in the primary health care system can be carried out and reimbursed, as demonstrated by the program for Medicaid children mandated by the courts in the state of Massachusetts. A study of the costs of both developmental and behavioral screening for preschool-age children in a general pediatric practice estimated a per member, per month cost of $4 to $7, depending on the screening objectives and methods (Dobrez, LoSasso, et al., 2001). If effectiveness of screening for, detecting, and preventing cases of MEB disorders can be demonstrated, it is likely that screening in the primary health care setting will be cost-effective. Walker, Severson, and Seeley (2007) report positive outcomes associated with use of a behavioral screening tool paired with family and classroom interventions. No data were found for the cost of screening in school systems. It appears that the biggest economic barrier is not cost, but arriving at societal decisions about who will pay for screening and what the mechanisms for reimbursement of the cost will be.

10. Screening can be population-based or targeted to at-risk groups or individuals. It should be longitudinally implemented, as risks and early signs or markers of evidence-based disorders may develop over time. Contrary to the experience with newborn screening for specific diseases, for which markers are not time-sensitive, risks and early signs or symptoms of MEB disorders may appear or be introduced over time. Therefore, screening for risk factors or the antecedents of these disorders is an ongoing process. The age at which screening should be initiated and the frequency with which it should be repeated have not been subjected to systematic study. These determinations will require judgments based on, among multiple factors, the environment in which youth are raised, the family structure, and direct observation or reports of the child or adolescent behavior. Furthermore, once an intervention to reduce risk is initiated, screening must continue to assess benefits, and the need for repeated screening imposes a burden, both in terms of workforce and economic demands, on present systems of surveillance. This dimension of screening for MEB disorders deserves additional consideration and analysis.

Screening Versus Assessment

Research has demonstrated that some groups of young people are at great risk for emotional or behavioral disorders because they have entered a service system, such as criminal justice or child welfare, or because of their particular life circumstances. Children in foster care, children of depressed or alcohol- or drug-dependent parents, incarcerated children, children with chronic health conditions, children exposed to trauma or violence, or runaway youth all are at heightened risk of emotional or behavioral disorders. In the foster care system, given the known elevated risk, all young people are typically screened or accessed for MEB disorders (Child Welfare League of America, 2007; Stahmer, Leslie, et al., 2005).

CONCLUSIONS AND RECOMMENDATIONS

One of the criteria for assessing the applicability of screening is the availability of facilities to conduct the screening and provide an intervention. The vast majority of young people attend school, see a primary care physician, or both. These settings are likely to be viewed as less stigmatizing than other service environments.

Conclusion: Schools and primary care settings offer an important opportunity for screening to detect risks and early symptoms of mental, emotional, and behavioral problems among young people.

Multiple screening instruments are available for a variety of ages, settings, and behavioral risks. For many reasons, these instruments are not uniformly used. Schools and primary care settings may also be able to readily identify high-risk groups, such as children in divorced families or children in foster care.

Conclusion: A variety of screening instruments and approaches are available, but there is no consensus on the use of these instruments.

Although potential screening settings and tools are available, an overarching principle in determining the applicability of screening should be the availability of an intervention when a risk has been identified. Multiple approaches are available, but few have been tested in conjunction with screening in real-world environments.

> **Recommendation 8-1:** Research funders should support a rigorous research agenda to develop and test community-based partnership models involving systems such as education (including preschool), primary care, and behavioral health to screen for risks and early mental, emotional, and behavioral problems and assess implementation of evidence-based preventive responses to identified needs.

The effectiveness of screening in primary care and emergency departments could be improved if mental health and substance abuse professional organizations were to work with the various professional organizations, such as the American Academy of Pediatrics, the National Association of Pediatric Nurse Practitioners, and the emergency physicians' groups, to develop a consensus on the best instruments for screening for specific behavioral health issues. Policy makers, providers, advocates, and researchers could then provide technical assistance to ensure the use of these tools and evaluate their impact on screening children for behavioral health issues (Semansky et al., 2003). Many of these screening tools are designed to elicit information from parents rather than through clinician observation, requiring minimal staff time to administer. Literacy and language competence must be addressed when using this approach.

Similarly, screening and preventive interventions are more likely to be acceptable and used in a community if members of the community, including parents, are involved in the design of these approaches (see also Chapter 11). Parental involvement in identification of risk, selection of screening tools, and development of follow-up protocols may help address concerns about stigma and labeling. Similarly, involvement by a range of community providers can help ensure that resources are targeted to identified community needs.

There is clear evidence that certain groups of young people face an increased likelihood of negative mental, emotional, and behavioral developmental outcomes. As a result, interventions aimed at assessing and treating these young people have been put in place. Opportunities also exist to provide preventive interventions for groups at known risk.

> **Conclusion: Some groups of young people, such as children in foster care, children in juvenile detention facilities, and children of depressed parents, are known to have a greatly elevated risk for MEB disorders. Targeted screening or in some cases full assessment of individuals in**

**these groups to identify potential preventive services or treatment needs
are warranted.**

Identifying and addressing groups or communities with elevated risk
can serve a preventive function complementary to identification of individuals at risk. This screening level uses public health principles and may
be particularly cost effective.

**Conclusion: Screening for community- and group-level risk factors as
well as individual-level screening for symptoms is an important public
health function.**

Community-level screening in the United States has largely been limited
to communities assessing their own strengths and needs (e.g. Communities
That Care; see Box 11-1) rather than using known risk factors to identify
specific communities with elevated needs. For example, although there is
substantial documentation that factors such as poverty place young people
in communities with these characteristics at greater risk for negative emotional and behavioral outcomes, few programs have targeted resources to
these communities to address community-level risks.

Recommendation 8-2: The U.S. Departments of Health and Human
Services, Education, and Justice should develop strategies to identify
communities with significant community-level risk factors and target
resources to these communities.

Although this would be a novel approach in the United States, there
are models available from the United Kingdom that could guide these
efforts. Since 2000, the United Kingdom has a system for identifying areas
with high need for intervention using the Indices of Multiple Deprivation.
The index is based on the idea that certain areas can be characterized as
deprived on the basis of the proportion of people in the area experiencing
various manifestations of deprivation. The indices include seven domains:
income deprivation; employment deprivation; health deprivation and disability; education, skills, and training deprivation; barriers to housing and
services; living environment deprivation; and crime. These are measured
using 38 indicators based on census and other publicly available data
(Noble, McLennan, and Whitworth, 2009). Areas identified with high
levels of deprivation are targeted for additional local and national-level
resources. In addition to permitting precise focus on areas with high multiple deprivations, this approach provides the ability to track change using
the same criteria. The committee was not aware of any outcomes data on
this approach, however.

9

Benefits and Costs of Prevention[1]

O n an intuitive level, preventing mental, emotional, and behavioral (MEB) disorders among young people is one of the soundest
investments a society could make. The benefits include higher
productivity, lower treatment costs, less suffering and premature mortality,
and more cohesive families—and, of course, happier, better adjusted, more
successful young people. Given the evidence that feasible actions can be
taken to achieve these benefits, the case for action is compelling. Emerging
evidence that some of these interventions are also cost-effective makes the
case even stronger.

In an analysis conducted for the committee, Eisenberg and Neighbors
estimate that the annual costs of MEB disorders among young people
totaled roughly $247 billion in 2007 (see Box 9-1). Demonstrating the
effectiveness of interventions is necessary to establish a scientific basis
for prevention approaches aimed at avoiding these costs. As outlined in
this report, there is reason for optimism about the ability to successfully
intervene in the lives of young people and prevent many negative outcomes. However, decisions about how to invest limited public resources
must consider the cost of delivering the service and demonstrate that the
benefits that can be expected from an intervention—both those that can be
readily valued in dollars (e.g., increased productivity, decreased treatment
costs) and those that cannot (e.g., alleviation of pain and suffering of both

---

[1]This chapter is based in part on a paper written for the committee by Daniel Eisenberg and
Kamilah Neighbors in the Department of Health Management and Policy, School of Public
Health, University of Michigan.

BOX 9-1
Methodology for Cost Estimates

1. Mental Health Service Costs

a. Multiply Ringel and Sturm's 1998 estimate of $11.7 billion by (73.7 + 29.45)/73.7 to expand age group to include ages 18-24 (they only included ages 0-17).
b. Multiply by 2 to account for fact that their estimates do not account for full range of settings, as suggested by Costello, Copeland, and colleagues (2007).
c. Inflate to 2007 dollars (multiply by 1.28), based on the Bureau of Labor Statistics' consumer price index (see http://www.bls.gov/cpi/).
d. Multiply by population growth between 1998 and 2007 for people under age 25 (1.07) = $45 billion.

2. Health, Productivity, and Crime Costs

a. *Mental disorders:* Multiply share of mental health and substance abuse–related DALYs incurred by 0-24 age group (0.355), times National Institute of Mental Health (2002) estimate ($102 billion for 1995—$185 billion less the portion of total costs attributable to health care since counted in part 1), times inflation adjustment from 1995 to 2007 dollars (1.37), times population growth between 1995 and 2007 for people under 25 years old (1.07) = $54 billion.
b. *Drug abuse:* Multiply share of mental health and substance abuse–related DALYs incurred by 0-24 age group (0.355), times Office of National Drug Control Policy (2004) estimate ($165.1 billion for 2002—$180.9 billion less the $15.8 billion in health care costs since counted in part 1), times inflation adjustment from 2002 to 2007 dollars (1.15), times population growth between 2002 and 2007 for people under 25 years old (1.05) = $71 billion.
c. *Alcohol abuse:* Multiply share of mental health and substance abuse–related DALYs incurred by 0-24 age group (0.355), times Harwood (2000) estimate ($158 billion for 1998—$185 billion less the portion of total costs attributable to health care since counted in part 1), times inflation adjustment from 1998 to 2007 dollars (1.27), times population growth between 1998 and 2007 for people under 25 years old (1.07) = $77 billion.

Total = $247 billion, which, divided by 104 million people ages 0-24, equals about $2,380 per young person.

individuals and their families)—outweigh the costs that would be incurred in a real-world environment. As one example of the complexity of measuring costs, a serious mental disorder in a parent or a child has obvious and measurable financial costs associated with treatment and lost productivity. However, the disorder also often profoundly affects the overall functioning of the family in psychosocial ways that are devastatingly costly to the family but not readily susceptible to quantification, much less valuation in dollars and cents.

This chapter opens with a brief tutorial on cost-benefit and cost-effectiveness analysis, as well as an explanation of what the terms "cost-beneficial" and "cost-effective" mean. The chapter then synthesizes existing knowledge on the benefits that could be achieved (namely, avoided costs) if prevention were widely implemented on a national scale. Next the available research on the benefits and costs of individual prevention programs or types of intervention is summarized. The chapter then discusses limitations of the available research and concludes by offering recommendations for future research in these areas.

It is important at the outset to acknowledge the basic purpose and limitations of economic analysis in the context of prevention and prevention research. Economic analysis may be valuable at the beginning of prevention research by quantifying the costs associated with the disorder or problem being targeted for prevention, or at least those costs that lend themselves to quantification. This provides a sense of the potential value of prevention of the problem. Evaluating the cost-effectiveness of an intervention at the end of the prevention research cycle helps determine whether funding the intervention is a wise use of societal resources and hence desirable for dissemination. However, economic analysis has limitations as a decision-making aid. In particular, as mentioned above, even the best analyses are challenged to capture all of the psychological and emotional costs associated with MEB disorders in a manner that would be deemed universally acceptable. As a consequence, estimates of the cost of these disorders may misestimate the true social costs, possibly considerably. Equally importantly, economic analysis addresses efficiency but not equity. In some cases, a society or an organization may prefer investing in a less cost-effective program if it is more likely to reach disadvantaged populations. Also, particularly in the context of prevention, economic analysis may rely on a number of unproven assumptions (see Current Knowledge Regarding Intervention Benefit and Costs, below).

The cost-effectiveness of an intervention also often depends on the perspective of the decision maker. In many cases, an intervention is cost-effective from the perspective of society as a whole, but not from the narrower perspective of a single organization considering whether to fund the intervention. For example, consider the case of an investment in prevention of MEB disorders by a health care provider. That provider incurs the costs of the intervention and derives some of the benefits, in the form of reduced future costs of care. However, major social benefits of the intervention may be realized in other sectors of society, including the education sector (e.g., when students are less disruptive in class) and the criminal justice sector (e.g., when recipients of the intervention are less likely to get into trouble with the law). It is quite plausible that the health care orga-nization may not perceive the intervention as worthwhile from its narrow perspective, whereas from a social perspective the intervention is highly cost-effective (see Chapter 11 for a discussion of implementation issues). Addressing the disjunction between those who bear the costs of an interven-tion and those who experience its benefits may require coordinated plan-ning of interventions and, if possible, aligning of incentives across service systems.

COST-BENEFIT AND COST-EFFECTIVENESS ANALYSIS

Cost-benefit analysis (CBA) and cost-effectiveness analysis (CEA) are two methods of economic analysis used to assess whether an intervention is desirable from an economic perspective; put simply, they evaluate whether the benefits derived from the intervention are worth the cost invested in the intervention. The principal distinction between the two techniques lies in the measurement of desired outcomes. In CBA, all such outcomes are valued in monetary units (dollars), permitting a direct comparison of the benefits produced by the intervention with its costs. When benefits exceed costs, the intervention is said to be cost-beneficial. When benefits fall short of costs—and assuming that one is comfortable that all important posi-tive outcomes have been captured in monetary terms—the conclusion is that the intervention is not worth undertaking. CBA is the ideal form of analysis given that it allows a comparison of desired outcomes (benefits) and undesired outcomes (costs) in the same metric. This permits a precise conclusion about the desirability of the intervention. Is the intervention "worth it"?

CEA, in contrast, is used when one or more major desired outcomes cannot be readily measured in monetary terms but a major outcome, mea-sureable in another metric, is common to the interventions being compared. A notable example in the health care literature pertains to interventions that avoid preventable premature deaths (or preventable illness or disability). Historically, the principal outcome in published studies was measured in terms of life-years saved. Now, most commonly, outcomes are measured as quality-adjusted life years (QALYs). Analysts typically employ CEA when they think that the desired outcome does not lend itself readily to monetization. Thus, breast or prostate cancer screening and treatment avoid premature deaths, but as they do so primarily for people beyond their working years, many analysts are uncomfortable attributing a dollar value to the beneficiaries' extra years. It is possible to do so, using a mea-sure of willingness-to-pay (Gafni, 1997). Since the desired outcomes and the undesired outcomes (costs) are measured in different metrics in CEA (life years and dollars, respectively), the bottom line of a CEA is a ratio, in this case cost per QALY. An intervention is deemed cost-effective if it produces the desired outcome at a reasonable price, typically the lowest cost to realize a QALY among competing interventions. Thus, if an analyst is comparing three different interventions, all other things being equal, the cost-effective intervention is the one for which the cost per QALY is the least. (This simplification ignores additional concerns—the other things *not* being equal—such as *who* benefits from the extra life years.) Often, analysts will label cost-effective an intervention not compared directly with alternative investments. In such instances, typically they are comparing their findings to a standard in the literature. As a rule of thumb, ratios in the range of $50,000 to $100,000 or lower per life year lost are generally considered cost-effective (Ubel, Hirth, et al., 2003).[2]

In theory, a well-designed CBA and CEA of the same intervention should yield the identical conclusion about the desirability of the intervention (Bleichodt and Quiggin, 1999). An intervention will be cost-effective—that is, cost less per unit of benefit than alternative interventions—if its benefits exceed its costs and do so with a net benefit that is greater than that of the alternative interventions. In practice, however, because researchers often focus on somewhat different outcomes depending on the method being used,[3] one cannot assume that CBA and CEA will yield identical conclusions about intervention desirability. Furthermore, all of these analyses rest on assumptions related to the quantification and valuation of important outcomes, assumptions that can drive the conclusions reached. Indeed, standard practice in CBA and CEA should include use of sensitivity analysis, a family of methods to evaluate whether bottom-line conclusions are sensitive to assumptions made in the analysis (Gold, Russell, et al., 1996).

The health care literature is dominated by CEAs; that is, one finds relatively few CBAs (Hammitt, 2002). The principal reason is the inability, or reluctance, of analysts or policy makers to place dollar values on important health outcomes. As we describe below, however, the prevention field seems to be an exception: the majority of studies to date have employed CBA.

ECONOMIC NEED FOR PREVENTION

Prevention, by definition, is undertaken to avoid harmful outcomes; the potential benefits of prevention are therefore equivalent to the net harms, or costs, of those outcomes. MEB disorders among young people account

---

[2]Ubel, Hirth, and colleagues (2003) assert that the cost-effectiveness threshold should be raised to $200,000 or more per QALY.

[3]For example, researchers using CBA may ignore improvements in health-related quality of life, because other benefits, such as reduced crime and increased employment, are easier to quantify in dollar terms.

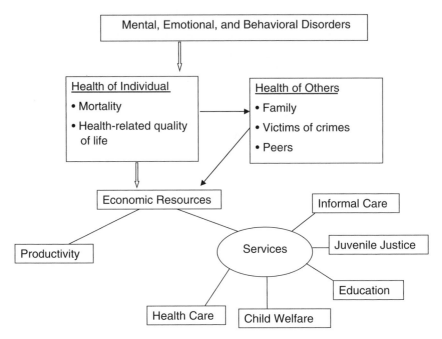

FIGURE 9-1 Costs of mental, emotional, and behavioral disorders among young people.
SOURCE: Adapted from Eisenberg and Neighbors (2007).

for considerable costs to the health care, child welfare, education, juvenile justice, and criminal justice systems, as well as enormous additional costs in terms of the suffering of individuals, families, and others affected (see Figure 9-1). The most direct and probably most significant economic cost is increased morbidity and decreased health-related quality of life of the individual experiencing a MEB disorder.

The individual's health problems, in turn, may lead to adverse consequences for other members of society, such as family members, victims of crime, and peers. Health problems typically also lead to additional costs, in the form of reduced productivity and earnings (Kessler, Heeringa, et al., 2008) and increased use of a range of social services. And, of course, MEB disorders place enormous stress on young people themselves and interfere with healthy development.

Morbidity and Quality of Life

MEB disorders among young people are associated with substantially increased morbidity and reduced health-related quality of life. These health problems are associated with psychological suffering (U.S. Public Health Service, 1999a) as well as increased risks of physical illnesses (Vreeland, 2007). These health consequences represent an enormous burden during childhood (Glied and Cuellar, 2003) and are also correlated with significantly increased risks to health and reduced productivity in adulthood (Kessler, Berglund, et al., 2005; Kessler, Ormel, et al., 2003).

A young person's mental disorder or substance abuse may also lead to negative health consequences for other members of society. For example, mental disorders lead to lost productivity and functioning not only for the children, but also for the parents and caregivers of the children (Tolan and Dodge, 2005). Untreated mental illness may also have intergenerational effects. Having a depressed mother, or having two parents with poor mental health, is associated with mental, behavioral, and emotional problems in children (Kahn, Brandt, and Whitaker, 2004; see also Chapter 7).

Substance abuse, and to a lesser extent other MEB disorders, are also associated with more frequent risky behavior (such as driving under the influence) (Harwood, 2000), which often have substantial health repercussions for others. In addition, an individual's health condition may affect his or her peers; in particular, substance abuse (Gaviria and Raphael, 2001) and suicidal behavior (Gould, Jamieson, and Romer, 2003) are thought to spread among peers via a contagion effect.

To quantify the total health burdens posed by various illnesses and disorders, researchers with the Global Burden of Disease project of the World Health Organization (WHO) and the World Bank calculated disability-adjusted life years (DALYs) lost due to each health condition. This measure accounts for both morbidity (mainly measured by functional impairments) and mortality. For the United States, depression and alcohol use and abuse were among the top five sources of premature death and disability (Michaud, McKenna, et al., 2006). According to the most recent estimates by age group for the United States, in 1996 mental disorders and substance abuse accounted for 30 percent of DALYs lost by people under age 25 (calculation by Eisenberg and Neighbors based on Supplementary Material, Additional File 4 to Michaud, McKenna, et al., 2006).[4] This represents by far the highest burden of any disease category for this broad age range. By more specific age intervals, the proportions were 3 percent for ages 0-4, 18 percent for ages 5-14, and 48 percent for ages 15-24. Given evidence that people with mental disorders are at greater risk for both communicable

---

[4]This percentage was calculated by including all conditions in the Global Burden of Disease project's neuropsychiatric category except epilepsy and multiple sclerosis, which are not typically considered mental disorders. Updated estimates for the United States, for the year 2005, will be available within the next few years, according to Catherine Michaud, the first author of the report used to generate the estimates here.

and noncommunicable diseases and that their disorders contribute to both intentional and unintentional injuries, the percentage may be even higher (Prince, Patel, et al., 2007).

Economic Resource Costs

Health problems associated with MEB disorders decrease productivity and significantly increase the utilization of services, thus reducing economic resources available to society for other purposes.

Productivity[5]

During childhood and adolescence, when most people do not participate in the labor market, the direct impacts of mental disorders and substance use on economic productivity are small but real. Young people with MEB disorders may diminish the productivity of others closely involved in their lives, particularly family members. For example, the stress and unpredictability of having a child with a serious MEB disorder can interfere with parents' work lives (Busch and Barry, 2007), or a disruptive child in a classroom can interfere with other students' learning. There may also be significant costs to the work or educational productivity of siblings (Fletcher and Wolfe, 2008).

The indirect and long-term consequences are also likely to be large. These conditions interfere with young people's ability to invest in their own human capital via education. Many studies show that poor mental health and substance use among young people are negatively related to participation and performance in school (Diego, Field, and Sanders, 2003; Glied and Pine, 2002), as well as high school completion (Vander Stoep, Weiss, et al., 2003), important determinants of productivity in adulthood. These factors can increase risk for such behavioral problems as delinquent and antisocial behavior (Yoshikawa, 1994). Also, to the extent that MEB disorders in childhood carry over into adulthood, there will be further reductions in economic productivity. A large number of studies, many of which focus on depression, document that adults with mental illness and substance abuse disorders are less likely to be employed, and those who are employed work fewer hours and receive lower wages (see Ettner, Frank, and Kessler, 1997; Kessler, Heeringa, et al., 2008). Similarly, as adults, employees with mental

---

[5]When aggregating the costs of mental disorders and substance abuse, it is important to keep in mind that productivity costs may already be reflected, at least to some extent, in measures of health burden, such as DALYs. Thus, one might be double-counting by claiming, for example, that a case of depression accounts for a certain number of DALYs in addition to productivity costs. This caveat, however, does not take away from the fact that in general productivity costs are large and important to consider in their own right.

health or substance abuse disorders can reduce the productivity of other workers, particularly if the job affects the work of others (e.g., assembly line work).

Utilization of Services

As one would expect, mental disorders and substance abuse are strongly associated with increased utilization of mental health and substance abuse services. Ringel and Sturm (2001) estimated the annual national costs of mental health treatment for children under age 18, as of 1998, at $11.68 billion, or $172 per child. They found that expenditures were $293 per child for ages 12-17, $163 per child for ages 6-11, and $35 per child for ages 0-5. Adjusted to current dollars using the consumer price index, the annual national costs in 2007 would be $14.8 billion. We are not aware of analogous estimates for substance abuse treatment of young people, although estimates are available for adults for alcohol abuse (Harwood, 2000) and drug abuse treatment (Office of National Drug Control Policy, 2004). In the past 15 to 20 years, the mix of mental health services for young people has shifted from inpatient to outpatient settings (Ringel and Sturm, 2001), as in the adult population (Wang, Demler, et al., 2006). Also, as in the adult population, the relative treatment mix for children's mental health has shifted from specialty settings to primary care (Wang, Demler, et al., 2006) and from therapy and counseling to medication (Glied and Cuellar, 2003) (although this latter shift was interrupted in 2003 by the Food and Drug Administration's warnings about the use of antidepressant medications for children) (Libby, Brent, et al., 2007). These changes are also not fully reflected in the estimates cited.

Young people with MEB disorders have higher utilization of mental health services across a range of social service systems, not just health care. Costello, Copeland, and colleagues (2007) considered data from a range of settings and demonstrated that mental health service costs in health care settings represent only a modest fraction of the total costs incurred by children with mental disorders for these services. Using a sample of adolescents ages 13-16 in western North Carolina, they estimated that mental health service costs for adolescents with mental disorders equated to $894 per adolescent in the local population, with more than one-quarter (27 percent) of the total costs incurred in the school and juvenile justice systems.[6] The overall estimate is over three times that in the Ringel and Sturm (2001) study,

---

[6]This number is based on converting the total costs per 100,000 population in Table 2 in Costello, Copeland, and colleagues (2007) to total costs per person. The percentage attributable to the school and the juvenile justice systems is based on dividing the sum of these costs ($10.9 million and $13.2 million, respectively) by the total costs ($89.4 million).

which focused mainly on mental health service costs in health care settings. The findings of Costello, Copeland, and colleagues (2007) are consistent with other empirical studies showing that MEB disorders are associated with increased use of services in nonmedical settings, such as foster care (Harman, Childs, and Kelleher, 2000), special education (Bussing, Zima, et al., 1998), and juvenile justice (Teplin, Abram, et al., 2002).

Youth with MEB disorders who become involved with the juvenile justice system also often incur costs related to law enforcement and court expenses, detention, placement and incarceration, and other forms of treatment that are publicly provided (National Center on Addiction and Substance Abuse, 2004). In addition, violent crimes can result in victim costs, such as medical care, treatment through public programs, and property damages to victims. The costs associated with all juvenile (under age 18) arrests in 2004 were estimated at about $14.4 billion (National Center on Addiction and Substance Abuse, 2004), and the costs of medical care, treatment through public programs, and property damages to victims of juvenile violence were estimated at about $95 million (Miller, Sheppard, et al., 2001). Although not all of these crimes were committed by young people with MEB disorders, overall costs of these disorders would be higher if the cost of relevant juvenile crimes were included with service use estimates. In addition, these health problems lead to significantly increased use of informal (unpaid) care by family members and others. For example, family members with a child with mental health care needs are more likely than family members whose children do not have these needs to reduce their working hours or stop working to care for their child (Busch and Barry, 2007).

Using data from the Fast Track project, Foster, Jones, and colleagues (2005) estimated that each youth with conduct disorder incurs public costs of more than $70,000 over a seven-year period, with costs incurred by the juvenile justice, education, and general health care systems in addition to the mental health system. Similarly, a study in the United Kingdom (Scott, Knapp, et al., 2001) documented societal costs from childhood conduct disorder that extended into adulthood. Children who had diagnosed conduct disorder at age 10 incurred public service costs by age 28 that were 10 times higher than those considered to have no problems and 3.5 times higher than those with conduct problems but not diagnosed with conduct disorder. This suggests that preventive interventions aimed at addressing behavioral problems before they reach the threshold for a diagnosis could yield significant savings.

Estimates of Total Costs

Comprehensive "cost of illness" studies quantify and aggregate, in monetary terms, the various costs associated with particular illnesses or disorders. Although there are many recent studies of this type in European countries, the most recent estimates in the United States correspond to 1995 for mental disorders (National Institute of Mental Health, 2000), 2002 for drug abuse (Office of National Drug Control Policy, 2004), and 1998 for alcohol abuse (Harwood, 2000). Aggregating service costs and health and productivity costs[7] for individuals age 18 and older,[8] the annual economic costs of mental disorders were estimated at $185 billion in 1995 (National Institute of Mental Health, 1999), the annual economic costs of drug abuse in 2002 were estimated at $180.9 billion (Office of National Drug Control Policy, 2004), and the annual economic costs of alcohol abused in 1998 were estimated at $185 billion (Harwood, 2000). These reports do not permit an estimate of costs specific to people from birth to age 24. However, in an analysis for the committee, Eisenberg and Neighbors used data in these reports to make a rough approximation, for the year 2007, by making the following two assumptions: (1) the full cost of services for this age group per person is twice as high as the mental health care costs per person estimated by Ringel and Sturm (2001)[9] and (2) the population share of health, productivity, and crime-related costs for people ages 0-24 is 35.5 percent (a calculation based on Supplementary Material, Additional File 4 to Michaud, McKenna, et al., 2006). Under these assumptions, Eisenberg and Neighbors estimated that the total annual economic costs are roughly $247 billion as of 2007 (in 2007 dollars),[10] or about $2,380 per person under age 25. This per-person total includes about $500 in health service costs and $1,900 in health, productivity, and crime-related costs.

Several caveats pertain to this estimate. Perhaps most notably, one would not be able to prevent all of these costs, no matter how much one

---

[7]The authors measured health and productivity costs by estimating the lost or diminished income due to morbidity and mortality. This is typically called a human capital approach to valuing health. Estimates from the human capital approach tend to be lower than estimates from willingness-to-pay approaches and are typically considered lower bound estimates (Hirth, Chernew, et al., 2000). Note that they also accounted for costs to other members of society, such as informal care and crime.

[8]Although the reports are not specific about the age groups included, one can infer that they apply to those age 18 and over based on the data sources used.

[9]This is a conservative assumption in two respects. First, it is lower than the adjustment factor of 3-4 estimated by Costello, Copeland, and colleagues (2007). Second, treatment costs are rising over time; for example, Mark, Coffey, and colleagues (2005) found that mental health and substance abuse treatment costs for the full population increased from $60 billion in 1991 to $104 billion in 2001.

[10]Note also that the estimate of total costs accounted for population growth.

invested in prevention. Not all MEB disorders are preventable, given current knowledge, and some may never be preventable. On one hand, from this perspective, the estimate of $247 billion overstates the potential value of prevention. On the other hand, this estimate includes only costs avoided from preventing disorders that would meet full clinical criteria and does not include costs that would be avoided from reducing problem behaviors and symptoms in the range in which symptoms are not severe enough to meet diagnostic criteria. These costs are generally not included in cost-of-illness studies, but they may be very large. From this perspective, the estimate of $247 billion understates the aggregate costs of MEB disorders among young people. As well, the estimate does not fully capture the quality of life of the children and their families.

Quantifying the costs of MEB disorders among young people is useful as a way to approximate the potential value of prevention and to compare the burden of these disorders[11] among young people with other disease burdens, but very few studies have addressed this topic. In general, as Hu (2006) describes, methodologies in cost-of-illness studies vary and often depend on several assumptions that require further study. In the context of MEB disorders among young people, one important next step for this research literature is to conduct a comprehensive cost-of-illness study for the United States that builds on previous studies, such as Harwood, Ameen, and colleagues (2000) and Ringel and Sturm (2001), and the estimates created for this report by Eisenberg and Neighbors (2007) and accounts for the substantial use of services outside medical settings shown by Costello, Copeland, and colleagues (2007). After the initial work is completed to refine the methodology and identify data sources, periodic updates will be much easier to produce. In addition, further research is needed to improve the ability to project lifetime consequences of mental disorders in childhood. In particular, researchers face the challenge of disentangling confounding factors from true causal relationships in observed relationships between mental disorders in childhood and later outcomes.

Miller (in Biglan, Brennan, et al., 2004) provides a much higher estimate of $435.4 billion in 1998 ($557.3 in 2007 dollars) for the costs of problem behaviors among youth, defined as underage drinking, heroin or cocaine abuse, high-risk sex, youth violence, youth smoking, high school dropout, and youth suicide acts. More than half was attributable to suffering and quality of life, with the balance consisting of work losses, medical spending, and other resource costs. Averaged across all youth, this would be an average cost of $12,300 per youth ages 12-20 ($15,744 in 2007 dollars).

---

[11]The discussion that follows refers specifically to emotional and behavioral disorders rather than problems, as it is referring to costs associated with actual disorders.

COST-EFFECTIVENESS OF PREVENTIVE INTERVENTIONS

Although the potential benefits from preventing MEB disorders are clearly large, and there is a substantial and growing body of evidence documenting the positive outcomes of prevention interventions, relatively few evaluations have been conducted to assess the cost-effectiveness of the interventions. The evaluations that are available tend to be those associated with the interventions with the longest follow-up and include some of the most successful programs. Similarly, cost-effectiveness evaluations tend to be limited to such areas as early childhood development, youth development, and prevention of violence, depression, and substance abuse, in which there has been more research overall. In addition, most of the favorable cost-effectiveness results apply to interventions for higher risk populations, although a small number of universal prevention programs have also been shown to be cost-effective.

Aos, Lieb, and colleagues (2004) reviewed the economic analyses of a large number of relevant interventions. The authors conducted a comprehensive and detailed review and analysis for the Washington State government of prevention and early intervention programs designed to (1) reduce crime; (2) lower substance abuse; (3) improve educational outcomes, such as test scores and graduation rates; (4) decrease teen pregnancy; (5) reduce teen suicide attempts; (6) lower child abuse or neglect; and (7) reduce domestic violence. In addition to the discussion below based in part on their analysis, we refer the reader to this study as a resource for additional empirical results as well as a detailed discussion of methodological issues.

Early Childhood Interventions

Perhaps the most heavily researched preventive programs are early childhood interventions for children from birth to age 5. Some of these programs are primarily home-based, whereas others are primarily center-based. In a meta-analysis of over 25 studies of home visitation programs (by nurses or other trained professionals), Aos, Lieb, and colleagues (2004) concluded that the average benefits per child were about $11,000 and costs were about $5,000.[12] The benefit-cost ratio has been shown to be higher for certain programs; for example, in an economic evaluation of the Nurse-Family Partnership Program, Karoly, Kilburn, and Cannon

---

[12]All dollar values in this section are in 2002 or 2003 dollars. In addition to average effects for this group of programs, Aos, Lieb, and colleagues also estimated the benefits of the Nurse-Family Partnership at $26,298 and the costs at $9,118 and the benefits of the HIPPY (Home Instruction Program for Preschool Youngsters) at $3,313 and the costs at $1,837. They estimated that benefits exceeded costs for the Comprehensive Child Development Program and the Infant Health and Development Program.

(2005) found that the program cost about $7,000 per child and produced total benefits of about $41,000 per child for the higher risk sample and about $9,000 per child for the lower risk sample.[13] In general, some of the main benefits of home visitation programs, converted into dollar estimates of their value, have been reduced child abuse, improved achievement test scores, and decreased likelihood of arrest later in life. The benefits from reduced child abuse are generally estimated on the basis of reductions in medical, child welfare, and other public service costs and crime costs, based on epidemiological evidence showing correlations between child abuse and these costs later in life. Improved achievement test scores are usually valued on the basis of how earnings relate to education. Finally, arrests are valued in terms of both the costs to the criminal justice systems and victims (particularly health costs for crimes involving injuries) and lost productivity while incarcerated (see also the technical appendix to Aos, Lieb, et al., 2004).

Several different center-based early interventions also appear to have benefits that exceed their costs (see Targeting Early Childhood Development in Preschool in Chapter 6 for further discussion of these programs). In a meta-analysis of over 50 studies of early childhood education programs for low-income 3- and 4-year-olds, Aos, Lieb, and colleagues (2004) found that, on average, benefits per child were $17,000 and costs were $7,000. In an economic analysis of the Abecedarian Early Childhood project, an intensive, multiyear intervention for children from birth to age 5, Barnett and Masse (2006) found that per-child benefits were $158,000 and costs were $63,000; the primary benefits were related to cognitive abilities and education, which were valued in terms of estimated impact on future earnings. The intervention was also associated with a reduction in smoking, which was valued in terms of estimated reduction in premature mortality (with a year of life then valued at $150,000, based on willingness-to-pay estimates in the literature). The Perry Preschool project, which included 1-2 years of intensive preschool, home visiting, and group meetings of parents, had estimated per-child benefits of $240,000 and costs of $15,000 (Belfield, Nores, et al., 2006); the primary benefits, some of which were observed well into adulthood, were reduced crime, positive academic outcomes, and reduced smoking. The Chicago Child-Parent Centers, a center-based preschool education for disadvantaged children, had estimated benefits per child of $75,000 and costs of $7,400 (Temple and Reynolds, 2007); the primary benefits were improved academic outcomes and reduced crime.

Temple and Reynolds (2007) compared the benefit-to-cost ratios of

---

[13]Although the estimates provided by Aos, Lieb, and colleagues (2004) and Karoly, Kilburn, and Cannon (2005) differ, the difference between benefits and costs is substantial for both.

the Perry Preschool project, the Carolina Abecedarian project, and the Chicago Child-Parent Centers to other types of interventions designed to benefit children's development. They concluded that preschool education has a more favorable benefit-to-cost ratio than the Special Supplemental Nutrition Program for Women, Infants, and Children, the Nurse-Family Partnership, a class-size reduction initiative for grades K-3, and the Job Corps. There has been debate, however, regarding the benefits and costs of pre-K programs, including Head Start (Cook and Wong, 2007), the most heavily funded and widespread early childhood education program. Ludwig and Phillips (2007) attempt to resolve the debate by pointing out that Head Start costs about $9,000 per child, and would need to produce academic achievement gains only on the order of .1 to .2 standard deviations to confer equivalent benefits. They argue that the evaluation literature on Head Start strongly favors a benefit of this size or more, and that the program should be viewed as cost-beneficial. Heckman (1999, 2007) argues that investments in early childhood development, particularly for disadvantaged children, have greater payoff in terms of the development of skills needed for future success than do investments in any other period of life. A systematic review of economic analyses of programs targeting mental health outcomes or accepted risk factors for mental illness by Zeichmeister, Kilian, and colleagues (2008) concluded that, among the few available studies, the most favorable results were for early childhood education programs.

Youth Development Interventions

Although comprehensive interventions in early childhood have probably received more attention from scholars and policy makers, many comprehensive interventions for older (school-age) children and adolescents also appear to be cost-effective. Aos, Lieb, and colleagues (2004) found that five of the six youth development programs reviewed,[14] whose aims include improving parent–child relationships and reducing problem behaviors, such as substance use and violence, are cost-beneficial, with benefit-cost ratios ranging from 3 to 28. These authors also found that several programs for juvenile offenders, with a range of goals mostly pertaining to improved behavior, are highly cost-effective, yielding net benefits per child well over $10,000 in many cases.

---

[14]The programs determined to have benefits that exceed costs include the Seattle Social Development project, Guiding Good Choices, the Strengthening Families Program for Parents and Youth 10-14, the Child Development project, and the Good Behavior Game. CASASTART was determined to have costs exceeding benefits.

Interventions Targeted at Specific Mental, Emotional, and Behavioral Disorders or Substance Use

There are currently few economic analyses of interventions that target the prevention of specific MEB disorders or substance use among young people, although there are a large number of studies that document efficacy, effectiveness, or both (see Chapters 6 and 7). The interventions in these economic analyses address depression, violence and conduct disorder, and substance use. Lynch, Hornbrook, and colleagues (2005) performed a cost-effectiveness analysis of a highly successful group cognitive-behavioral therapy intervention to prevent depression among adolescent children of depressed parents (see Box 7-4). They found that the intervention is very likely to be cost-effective, with an incremental cost of $610 per child and a cost-effectiveness ratio of $9,275 per QALY[15] (95 percent CI, –$12,148 to $45,641). Foster, Jones, and Conduct Problems Research Group (2006) found that the Fast Track intervention, designed to reduce violence and conduct disorders among at-risk children, was about 70 percent likely to be cost-effective in preventing conduct disorder for the higher risk group, but it had less than a 0.01 probability of being cost-effective for the lower risk group, which represented the majority of the sample. Aos, Lieb, and colleagues (2004) found that 10 of the 12 substance use prevention programs (including two programs that focus on smoking prevention) they analyzed were highly cost-effective, with benefit–cost ratios ranging from 3 to over 100.[16] The estimated benefits per child were generally small (less than $1,000 in most cases), but the costs were even smaller (less than $200 in all but one program).

Current Knowledge Regarding Intervention Benefits and Costs

Overall, knowledge about the benefits and costs of specific interventions aimed at preventing MEB disorders is promising but still limited. Relative to the number of efficacious or effective interventions (see Chapters 6 and 7), few investigators have conducted cost-effectiveness or cost-benefit analyses. There is also considerable uncertainty about many of the estimates in the available literature. For interventions that exhibit dramatically dif-

---

[15] QALYs, like DALYs, are measures of health that account for both morbidity and mortality. As mentioned earlier, ratios under $50,000 per life year lost are generally considered cost-effective; this is regardless of whether life years are adjusted for quality of life (Ubel, Hirth, et al., 2003).

[16] The programs determined to have benefits that exceed costs include the Adolescent Transitions Program, Project Northland, Family Matters, Life Skills Training, Project STAR, the Minnesota Smoking Prevention Program, the Other Social Influence/Skills Building Substance Prevention Program, Project Toward No Tobacco Use, All Stars, and Project Alert. DARE and STARS for Families were ineffective, making the costs exceed the benefits by definition.

ferent levels of benefits compared with costs, this uncertainty may be moot, but in other cases, it is important to consider carefully.

Perhaps the most important source of uncertainty pertains to longer term outcomes. In many economic evaluations, longer term outcomes of participants in an intervention are not observed and instead must be projected on the basis of other data. Many long-term benefits of early prevention programs cannot be measured until middle childhood and adolescence (e.g., juvenile crime). Longitudinal data used to make projections, such as correlations between the incidence of MEB disorders in childhood and in adulthood, do not necessarily represent accurate causal estimates, as Foster, Dodge, and Jones (2003) note. Another important source of uncertainty is a lack of statistical power. As Mrazek and Hall (1997) observe, many studies in this literature have modest sample sizes and are not sufficiently powered to look at key measures of effectiveness; typically, adequately powered estimates of cost-effectiveness require even larger samples than estimates of effectiveness per se (Ramsey, McIntosh, and Sullivan, 2001). A third, related source of uncertainty results from the outcomes measured: that is, whether interventions that appear to be cost-effective in reducing risk factors closely connected to MEB disorders, but do not measure disorders as an outcome, can actually prevent the incidence of these disorders.

Another source of uncertainty includes potential differences between cost-efficacy and cost-effectiveness. Evaluations of interventions conducted in research settings (efficacy studies) may get different results if conducted in real-world settings (effectiveness studies), raising potential questions about whether the cost-effectiveness (or more accurately, cost-efficacy) would be realized if the intervention were implemented in a nonresearch environment (see Foster, Dodge, and Jones, 2003, for a brief discussion of this). Similarly, the costs of interventions implemented in real-world settings may differ from the costs in a research setting.

In addition, as discussed in more detail in Chapter 11, a major challenge in prevention research, particularly when dealing with whole communities, is that preventive interventions are likely to have differential impact on individuals in different contexts because (a) participants have different risk and protective factors that cause different responses to the intervention; (b) the level of participation in interventions varies; and (c) interventions are routinely delivered with varying levels of fidelity and adoption. These factors can reduce overall impact compared to that seen in efficacy trials; thus some analyses of behavioral or economic outcomes in community implementation studies may not find significant effects.

There are challenges in measuring the cost of the time of children and other people involved in interventions. Those challenges can lead to poor estimates of costs, creating either an over- or underestimate. Often, however, analysts omit such time costs, introducing a clear bias toward underestimating total costs. For example, some studies do not consider the opportunity cost incurred by teachers delivering an intervention who might otherwise be engaged in productive teaching activities (Aos, Lieb, et al., 2004). Finally, and importantly, other intangibles, most notably the suffering of children and their families, are likely to be costly but extremely difficult to quantify and assign a monetary value. The difficulty in measuring and valuing these costs restricts the potential of CBA and CEA to accurately evaluate the relative merits of preventive interventions for MEB disorders, which may lead to a substantial underestimation of the benefits of successful interventions. Research needs to be devoted to improving measurement methods that will permit assessment of the economic value associated with suffering related to these disorders.

Another important caveat is that the quality of the underlying evidence used to project costs and benefits varies. Aos, Lieb, and colleagues (2004) account for this in their meta-analysis by assigning different weights to studies based on indicators of quality, but such a solution has unavoidable limitations, as the authors acknowledge. Many evaluations do not meet some of the important guidelines for quality of evidence, as stated by such organizations as the Food and Drug Administration (1998) and the Society for Prevention Research (Flay, Biglan, et al., 2005). For example, evaluators have not always published a specific plan of analysis before collecting data, which leaves open the possibility of selectively reporting positive results among many outcomes and analytical approaches.

A final caveat for this literature is the reminder that, while some studies employ CEA, most of the studies in the prevention field have employed CBA. In practice, CEA and CBA results are not strictly comparable. However, in this literature, because most of the studies yield strong conclusions (positive in most cases), it is unlikely that the basic findings would be sensitive to the choice of method. As this literature evolves and more interventions with borderline cost-effectiveness are evaluated, examining the sensitivity of conclusions to alternative assumptions will be important.

CONCLUSIONS AND RECOMMENDATIONS

The potential value of prevention of MEB disorders among young people is enormous. MEB disorders among young people result in significant costs to multiple service sectors. Such disorders threaten children's future productivity and wellness and disrupt the lives of those around them.

Conclusion: The economic, social, and personal costs of MEB disorders among young people are extraordinarily high.

To date, there is some evidence that the benefits of some specific interventions outweigh the costs. However, the scientific literature on the cost-effectiveness of prevention is still young, and it faces a number of conceptual and practical obstacles.

Conclusion: The current body of research on costs, cost-effectiveness, and cost-benefits of preventive mental, emotional, and behavioral interventions is very limited.

Much of the strongest evidence to date is for interventions that improve protective factors or reduce risk factors demonstrated through research to be closely related to MEB disorders (see Chapter 4). For example, multiple economic evaluations of early childhood development programs have demonstrated benefits that exceed costs.

It is also notable that among the limited number of interventions shown to be cost-effective, many were either targeted to higher risk children (e.g., the early childhood programs such as the Perry Preschool project) or were cost-effective only for a higher risk subgroup within the analysis (e.g., the Fast Track study). Aside from a small number of substance use prevention programs (see review by Aos, Lieb, et al., 2004), few universal interventions have been demonstrated to be cost-effective for preventing MEB disorders. Future research is needed to determine whether selective and indicated prevention programs are inherently more likely to be cost-effective in the context of MEB disorders, or if this finding is an artifact of the programs that happen to have been subjected to economic evaluations thus far.

Conclusion: Of those few intervention evaluations that have included some economic analysis, most have presented cost-benefit findings and demonstrate that intervention benefits exceed costs, often by substantial amounts.

However, few studies measure effects on diagnosable MEB disorders as an outcome, and most do not conduct sufficient longitudinal follow-up to fully capture potential long-term benefits. Also, considerable uncertainty remains about some of these estimates. Economic analyses are important for quantifying the potential value of prevention and assessing the actual value of existing interventions.

Many scholars in the prevention field have called for more regular economic analyses (Flay, Biglan, et al., 2005; Spoth, Greenberg, and Turrisi,

2008; Zeichmeister, Kilian, et al., 2008).[17] Many preventive interventions have been shown to be highly effective but have not yet been evaluated for cost-effectiveness in real-world settings. Guidelines on how to conduct high-quality cost-effectiveness studies are needed to help shape the development of this area of research as it continues to evolve.

> **Recommendation 9-1:** The National Institutes of Health, in consultation with government agencies, private-sector organizations, and key researchers should develop outcome measures and guidelines for economic analyses of prevention and promotion interventions. The guidelines should be widely disseminated to relevant government agencies and foundations and to prevention researchers.

For interventions involving young people, long-term outcomes are often pivotal for determining cost-effectiveness, as significant benefits are likely to accrue into adulthood, yet current knowledge is remarkably weak in most contexts. Long-term follow-up data should be collected whenever possible. As electronic data systems become more integrated and accessible, one promising avenue is through administrative databases, which do not necessarily depend on expensive efforts to track down and interview participants.[18] CEAs should also make clear the various sources of uncertainty. If the cost-effectiveness results are dramatically positive or negative, wide intervals may not raise questions about the overall conclusion that an intervention is cost-effective, but publishing such information will make the assessment more transparent. Special attention should be given to addressing the fact that costs from an intervention in one sector may be evident in other sectors. While this has been done for early childhood, less attention has been focused on this issue in other developmental stages, such as adolescence.

Economic analyses should also be comprehensive in their accounting of relevant costs and benefits. The work by Costello, Copeland, and colleagues (2007), for example, illustrates the importance of measuring costs across a range of service venues. Again, integration of electronic data systems may be a valuable tool for capturing these costs. To capture the benefit of reductions in specific MEB disorders, interventions should measure diagnostic outcomes whenever possible.

---

[17]This is an issue not only for prevention but also for treatment of mental disorders in children. A comprehensive review of economic evaluations of child and adolescent mental health interventions (most of which are treatment, not prevention) found only 14 had been published to date, although the authors speculated that two or three times that many would be in print within five years (Romeo, Byford, and Knapp, 2005).

[18]Of course, researchers would need to overcome hurdles related to informed consent and privacy restrictions.

Evaluations should begin to address the fact that multiple interventions over the span of childhood may have important dynamic complementarities (Heckman, 2007). For example, participation in an early childhood intervention such as Head Start may enhance a child's ability to benefit from a later intervention to prevent substance use. Although it would be difficult to randomize children to different sequences of interventions over a long time span, empirical research to address these complementarities to the extent possible would be very informative.

Similarly, understanding the causal links between aspects of poverty (e.g., food insecurity, disadvantaged neighborhoods, low-quality schools) and mental health should be improved. These links may reveal some of the most important mechanisms by which to prevent MEB disorders in cost-effective ways, but it is very difficult to establish incontrovertible causal relationships due to the many likely confounders in observational data.[19]

While there have been calls for increased economic analyses, the number of projects that include calculation of costs and cost-effectiveness will increase only if guidelines on how to conduct these types of analyses are widely available and the additional costs recognized.

Recommendation 9-2: Funders of intervention research should incorporate guidelines and measures related to economic analysis in their program announcements and provide supplemental funding for projects that include economic analyses. Once available, supplemental funding should also be provided for projects with protocols that incorporate recommended outcome measures.

Although one might argue that grant awards should be increased rather than providing supplemental funding to those that conduct economic analyses, there is a precedent for providing supplemental funding in other areas. For example, the National Institutes of Health (NIH) provides research supplements for projects involving underrepresented minorities and individuals to improve the diversity of the research workforce. Although these supplements are modest, NIH has reported that they are an effective means of encouraging institutions to recruit from currently underrepresented groups.

Evaluations of the costs and cost-effectiveness of prevention interventions will increase only if researchers include them in their protocols. Studies designed to determine the effectiveness of interventions in a real-world setting should be clear not only on what the intervention costs, so that a community can judge the feasibility of funding the project, but also

---

[19]For discussions of links between poverty and mental health among children, see, for example, Ripple and Zigler (2003) and the Center on the Developing Child (2007).

the cost-effectiveness, or expected benefits, so that the community can determine the potential value of their investment.

> **Recommendation 9-3:** Researchers should include analysis of the costs and cost-effectiveness (and whenever possible cost-benefit) of interventions in evaluations of effectiveness studies (in contrast to efficacy trials).

Finally, cost-benefit and cost-effectiveness studies of mental health promotion interventions—scarce in the literature to date—would be very useful in permitting a meaningful comparison of the relative desirability of prevention and promotion approaches.

In concluding this discussion, it is important to note that the significant societal benefits of preventing mental, emotional, and behavioral problems among young people may warrant intervention even when there is no specific cost-effectiveness data available, particularly if there is evidence that an effective intervention is available. Waiting for future cost-effectiveness analyses to become available, which might take years to develop, would put many young people at unnecessary risk.

10

Advances in Prevention Methodology

S ince the 1994 Institute of Medicine (IOM) report *Reducing Risks for Mental Disorders: Frontiers for Preventive Intervention Research*, substantial progress has been made in the development of methodologies for the measurement, design, and analysis of the effects of preventive interventions, as well as in the identification of antecedent risk and protective factors and their effects. These new methodological tools are necessary to assess whether an intervention works as intended, for whom, under what conditions, at what cost, and for how long. Although not unique to prevention, answers to these fundamental research questions are needed to help a policy maker determine whether to recommend an intervention and to help a community know whether it can reasonably expect that a newly implemented program is likely to lead to benefit.

Methodological advances are due in part to technical developments in biostatistical methods, causal inference, epidemiology, and other related quantitative disciplines. However, many of the new approaches have been developed by federally funded methodology centers (see Box 10-1) to respond to specific scientific and practical questions being raised in ongoing evaluations of prevention programs. In particular, evaluations of preventive interventions that have been conducted as randomized field trials (Brown and Liao, 1999; Brown, Wang, et al., 2008) have contributed not only to the development of alternative study designs and statistical models to examine intervention impact, but also to dramatic improvements in statistical computing. This has led to more insightful statistical modeling of intervention effects that takes into account the longitudinal and multilevel nature of prevention data.

BOX 10-1
Centers for Research on Prevention Science and Methodology

The Prevention Science and Methodology Group (PSMG) is an interdisciplinary network that has been supported by the National Institute of Mental Health (NIMH) and the National Institute on Drug Abuse (NIDA) for the past 20 years. It brings together prevention scientists conducting cutting-edge randomized trials and expert methodologists who are committed to addressing the key design and analytic problems in prevention research. PSMG has attempted to anticipate needs for methodological development and to have new methods ready when the trials demand them (Albert and Brown, 1990; Brown, Costigan, and Kendziora, 2008).

As the field of prevention science has matured over the past 15 years, PSMG has worked on such problems as generalized estimating equations as a way to account for uncertainty in longitudinal and multilevel inferences (Zeger, Liang, and Albert, 1988; Brown, 1993b); methods to assess intervention impact with growth models (Muthén, 1997, 2007; Muthén, Jo, and Brown, 2003; Muthén and Curran, 1997; Curran and Muthén, 1999; Muthén and Shedden, 1999; Carlin, Wolfe, et al., 2001; Muthén, Brown, et al., 2002; Wang, Brown, and Banderen-Roche, 2005; Muthén and Asparouhov, 2006; Asparouhov and Muthén, 2007); variation in impact by baseline characteristics (Brown, 1993a, 1993b; Ialongo, Werthamer, et al., 1999; Brown, Costigan, and Kendziora, 2008); mediation analysis (MacKinnon, 2008); multilevel models for behavior observations (Dagne, Howe, et al., 2002; Dagne, Brown, and Howe, 2003, 2007; Howe, Dagne, and Brown, 2005; Snyder, Reid, et al., 2006); modeling of self-selection factors (Jo, 2002; Jo and Muthén 2001; Jo, Asparouhov, et al., in press); and randomized trial designs specifically for prevention studies (Brown and Liao, 1999; Brown, Wyman, et al., 2006; Brown,

Prevention methodology, or the use of statistical methodology and statistical computing, is a core discipline in the field of prevention science (Eddy, Smith, et al., 2005) and is one of the new interdisciplinary fields embodied in the NIH Roadmap.[1] It aims to invent new techniques or apply existing ones to address the fundamental questions that prevention science seeks to answer and to develop ways to present these findings not only to the scientific community but also to policy makers, to advocates and community and institutional leaders, and to families, the ultimate potential beneficiaries of prevention programs and often, their potential consumers.

Methodologists make inferences about program effects by relying on three things: (1) measures of key constructs, such as risk and protective factors or processes, symptoms, disorders, or other outcomes, and program implementation, fidelity, or participation; (2) a study design that

---

[1] See http://nihroadmap.nih.gov/.

Wang, et al., 2008). Besides its close collaboration with ongoing trials (Brown, Costigan, and Kendziora, 2008), PSMG has continued to maintain close ties to the developers of the Mplus statistical package, allowing for a seamless integration of new statistical models, broad application of these models in existing software, and application of these new methods in existing trials.

A similar interdisciplinary methodological group, the Methodology Center, is located at Pennsylvania State University and is funded by NIDA and the National Science Foundation. The Methodology Center works in collaboration with prevention and treatment researchers to advance and disseminate statistical methodology related to research on the prevention and treatment of problem behavior, particularly drug abuse. This group has developed longitudinal models that address the unique aspects of changes in drug use over time including latent transition analyses (Collins, Hyatt, and Graham, 2000; Chung, Park, and Lanza, 2005; Chung, Walls, and Park, 2007; Lanza, Collins, et al., 2005) and two-part growth models (Olsen and Schafer, 2001); missing data routines for large, longitudinal data sets (Schafer, 1997; Schafer and Graham, 2002; Demirtas and Schafer, 2003; Graham, 2003; Graham, Cumsille, and Elek-Fisk, 2003); designs and inferences that take into account varying dosages or levels of exposure to an intervention or adaptive interventions (Bierman, Nix, et al., 2006; Collins, Murphy, and Bierman, 2004; Collins, Murphy, and Strecher, 2007; Murphy, 2005; Murphy, Collins, and Rush, 2007; Murphy, Lynch, et al., 2007), and cost effectiveness (Foster, Porter, et al., 2007; Foster, Johnson-Shelton, and Taylor, 2007; Olchowski, Foster, and Webster-Stratton, 2007).

determines which participants are being examined, how and when they will be assessed, and what interventions they will receive; and (3) statistical analyses that model how those given an intervention differ on outcomes compared with those in a comparison condition. This chapter discusses statistical designs and analyses, as well as offering comments about measures and measurement systems. While there are important technical issues to consider for measurement, design, and analysis, the community and institutional partnerships that are necessary to create and carry out a mutually agreed-on agenda are critical to the development of quality prevention science (Kellam, 2000).

We discuss first the uses of randomized preventive trials, which have led to an extraordinary increase in knowledge about prevention programs (see Chapters 4 and 6). Because well-conducted randomized preventive trials produce high-quality conclusions about intervention effects, they have achieved a prominent place in the field of prevention research. Despite their clear scientific value, randomized experiments of prevention programs are often viewed warily by communities and institutions, and their place in community prevention studies is often questioned. Since trials can be conducted only under the aegis of communities and their organizations, this chapter presents information about these trials so community leaders and policy makers can make informed decisions about whether such trials match their own community values and meet their needs, or if alternative designs are needed.

The chapter also reviews the use of other designs, including natural experimental designs and nonexperimental designs to examine a program's effects, whether a training model works, and whether a program can be implemented with sufficient strength or fidelity in different communities.

Next comes an overview of statistical analysis methods that incorporate longitudinal and multilevel data from prevention studies to model how interventions affect young people's development in different contexts. We discuss the unique strengths of qualitative data in prevention research and ways that qualitative and quantitative data can be used alongside one another. Finally, the chapter identifies challenges that have not yet been met in addressing the fundamental research questions in the prevention field.

EVALUATING A PREVENTIVE INTERVENTION WITH A RANDOMIZED PREVENTIVE TRIAL

Randomized preventive trials are central in evaluating efficacy (impact under ideal conditions) or effectiveness (impact under conditions that are likely to occur in a real-world implementation) of specific intervention programs that are tested in particular contexts (Coie, Watt, et al., 1993; Kellam, Koretz, and Moscicki, 1999; Howe, Reiss, and Yuh, 2002; Kellam and Langevin, 2003). The design for a randomized trial divides participants into equivalent groups that are exposed to different interventions, and analysis that appropriately compares outcomes for those exposed to different interventions leads to inferential statements about each intervention's effects. A well-conducted randomized trial is a high-precision instrument that leads to causal statements about a program's effect so that one can be assured that any observed differences are due to the different interventions and not some other factor.

Randomization strengthens confidence in the conclusions about an intervention's impact by ensuring the equivalence of the intervention and the control groups. Because of random assignment, participants in the two intervention conditions are nearly equivalent prior to the study, both on measured characteristics, such as age, gender, and baseline risk, and on relevant characteristics that may not be measured, such as community readiness. With randomized assignment to these groups, it is possible to test for the effect of an intervention even when a community is undergoing major, uncontrolled societal changes, such as a recession. Other designs, for example those that compare a cohort exposed to intervention with the cohort in a previous year, may be more likely to reach erroneous conclusions because of differences between the two groups (e.g., different economic circumstances) that may be undetected or difficult to account for in the analysis.

In prevention science, evaluation trials are usually conducted only after substantial preliminary data demonstrate that the intervention shows promise. Initially a theoretical model of the development of a disorder, or etiology, is used to specify risk and protective factors that can be selectively targeted in preventive interventions. For example, social learning theory posits that for many children, conduct disorder arises from the learned behavior of children exposed to repeated coercive interactions in the family. This etiological theory is then used to identify potential mediators (risk or protective factors), such as inconsistent and punitive parental responses to the child and association with deviant peers, in a causal model for outcomes of substance abuse disorders or delinquency.

A theory of change is then used to identify an existing intervention or to develop a new preventive intervention aimed at these target risk or protective factors. In a program aimed at preventing substance abuse and delinquency among children who are returning to parental care from a foster placement, a parent training intervention might be designed to reduce punitive statements, to enhance communication with the child, and to improve linkages with the child's own parents and teacher in preparation for the critical transition period of return to the family of origin. The timing of the intervention may be a consideration as well as the content. Key transition periods may occur when a stage of life begins, such as entry into elementary or middle school or during times of stress, such as a parental divorce or separation.

Measures are developed to assess these risk (e.g., punitive and inconsistent parenting) and protective factors (e.g., communication and monitoring of the child over time) to assess the effect of the intervention on parental behavior, and to determine whether changes in these hypothesized mediators actually lead to reductions in deviant behavior among young people.

In a pilot study with a few dozen families, data can be collected to check whether the trainers are delivering the program as designed to the original custodial parents, whether the parents are changing their interactions with their children appropriately, and whether the predicted immediate behavior changes are seen among the children. After successful completion of this initial work, a randomized trial with a larger number of families can then be used to test this preventive intervention on a defined population of foster children (e.g., those in group care) and at a set time preceding their return to their families. Upon the trial's completion, intent-to-treat analyses are typically used to assess overall effects as well as examine the conditions under which the intervention effect varies by child, family, or service provider characteristics. To understand how behavior is modified over the longer term by this intervention, the children are typically followed for a year or more beyond the end of the intervention services. Finally, mediation analyses are used to understand how the effects of an intervention actually take place. Both efficacy and effectiveness trials require appropriate analytical models to produce valid statements about intervention effects (Brown, Wang, et al., 2008).

Substantial investment in both time and money is required to conduct a randomized preventive trial. This process begins with framing the theoretical basis for a preventive intervention; then moves on to partnering with communities around an appropriate design, selection and recruitment of the sample, random assignment to intervention conditions, collection of data while adhering to the protocols specified by the design; and finally analysis of data and reporting of the results. The payoff for this work is described in three sections below.

Evaluating the Effects of Preventive Interventions

Some randomized preventive trials examine questions of program efficacy, or impact under ideal conditions, and can also help determine whether the intervention affects hypothesized mediators and proximal targets in expected ways. These efficacy trials are conducted in settings in which the intervention fidelity is maintained at a high level, usually by having trained researchers deliver the intervention rather than by individuals from the community. The intervention itself can be delivered in research laboratory settings outside the community (Wolchik, Sandler, et al., 2002) or in schools or other settings that serve as the units that are randomized to the intervention or control conditions (Conduct Problems Prevention Research Group, 1992, 1999a, 1999b; Reid, Eddy, et al., 1999; Prado, Schwartz, et al., 2009). Efficacy trials require randomization of youth to either the new intervention or to standard settings so that a comparison of outcomes can be made. Some communities have a concern that youth assigned to the control or standard setting do not receive the intervention and thereby do not receive its potential benefit. These concerns can at times be mitigated, as discussed below.

Other randomized trials address questions of effectiveness, or impact under settings that are likely to occur in a real-world implementation of a preventive intervention (Flay, 1986). An effectiveness trial tests a defined intervention that is delivered by intervention agents in the institutions and communities in a manner that would ultimately be used for large-scale implementation. This typically requires a stronger community partnership and involvement in all aspects of the study design and conduct. Any community concerns about withholding a new intervention from youth who are randomly assigned to the control or standard condition need to be addressed directly, because of ethical and human subject concerns, as well as from the practical side of maintaining the study design in a field setting. Often, communities come to consider randomization as a fair way to assign a novel intervention program to its community, given insufficient resources to deliver to everyone at once. Communities may want to test one intervention that they have already adopted but not fully implemented; it may be acceptable to compare an enhanced version of this intervention to that already being used (Dolan, Kellam, et al., 1993). Also, for some studies, it may be possible to provide the new intervention later to those who were initially assigned to the control setting (Wyman, Brown, et al., 2008); such wait-list designs, however, allow for only short-term, not long-term evaluations of impact.

Using Preventive Trials to Improve an Intervention

An equally important goal of randomized preventive trials is to search for ways to improve in an intervention. A specific intervention that targets a single risk factor, such as early aggressive behavior, can be used in a randomized trial to test a causative link between this risk factor and later behavior or emotional disorders (Kellam, Brown, et al., 2008). Specifically, if one found that the intervention did change the target risk factor, and this led to reduced disorders, it would provide support for the underlying etiological theory. For example, elaborated statistical analyses of intervention impact can show who benefits from or is harmed by an intervention, how long the effects last, and under what environmental circumstances these effects occur. Interventions may deliver different levels of benefit or harm to different kinds of participants or in different environments (Brown, Wang, et al., 2008), and information about these differences can extend the causal theory as well as guide decisions on whether to adopt or expand a prevention program or to attempt to improve outcomes through program modification.

For example, one first-grade intervention was found in a randomized trial to produce improvement in mathematics achievement, but all of this gain occurred among children who began school with better than average mathematics achievement; those who were below average gained nothing compared with children in the control group (Ialongo, Werthamer, et al., 1999). However, a behavioral component of this intervention was found to have a beneficial impact on precursors to adolescent drug use (Ialongo, Werthamer, et al., 1999). In follow-up research studies, the mathematics curriculum has been discontinued but the behavioral program has been continued. For the school district, the benefits of this trial were more immediate.

In another example, a study of young adolescents at risk for delinquency tested three active preventive intervention conditions against a control: a parent intervention alone, a peer-based intervention, and a combined peer and parent intervention. The parent condition alone produced a beneficial outcome; the combined peer–parent intervention produced results similar to the control; and the peer-based intervention produced more delinquency than did the other conditions (Dishion, Spracklen, et al., 1996; Dishion, Burraston, and Poulin, 2001; Dishion, McCord, and Poulin, 1999). Detailed examination revealed that the at-risk adolescents were learning deviant behavior from the more deviant peers in their group before, during, and after the program. This adverse, or iatrogenic, effect when a peer group includes a high proportion of delinquent youth is thought to be a major factor in explaining why boot camps and other similar programs often show a negative impact (Welsh and Farrington, 2001). In this way, analysis of intervention failures can be highly informative in guiding new prevention programs.

Testing Whether a Program's Population Effect Can Be Improved by Increasing the Proportion Who Participate

In randomized trials with individual- or family-level assignment, often a large fraction of those randomly assigned to a particular intervention never participates in that intervention, even after consenting (Braver and Smith, 1996). This minimal exposure from not coming to intervention sessions means that they cannot benefit from the intervention. Would the intervention be more effective if one could increase participation? Or would outreach to a more difficult-to-engage portion of the population be counterproductive, because they already have the skills or resources that the intervention develops, or because the intervention does not meet their needs? Given the generally low level of participation in many effective interventions, it has been increasingly important to identify ways to increase a program's reach into a community to those who could benefit (Glasgow, Vogt, and Boles, 1999).

Some designs help evaluate these self-selection effects. One option is to use "encouragement designs" under which individuals are randomly selected to receive different invitation strategies, reinforcers, or messages to encourage acceptance of an intervention. This approach can be seen in an evaluation of the impact of Head Start programs by the Administration for Children and Families (2005). Because these programs were already available in most counties in the United States, and the program is viewed as a valuable resource, especially for poor families, it was considered unethical to use a design that withheld a child's access to this program. Instead, in selected Head Start sites around the country, 3-year-old children and their families were randomized to one of two conditions: enrolling in a Head Start center at age 3 (early Head Start) or enrolling in the same center at age 4 (later Head Start). Those entering at age 3 were also accepted for enrollment at age 4. About 75 percent of the families enrolled their children in Head Start at the assigned age. Among the remaining 25 percent, some 3-year-olds randomized to early Head Start enrolled at age 4, some randomized to later Head Start enrolled at age 3, and some did not enroll in Head Start at all.

This encouragement trial attempts to modify the time of enrollment in Head Start. If all enrollments matched the assigned condition, standard or intent-to-treat analyses would provide legitimate causal inferences about the effects of the timing of enrollment. Because one-quarter of the parents made enrollment decisions contrary to the assigned condition, the intent-to-treat analysis, which makes no allowance for deviations from the assigned condition, provides a biased estimate of the causal effect of the intervention.

Use of Preventive Interventions to Test and Elaborate Theories of Change and Development

Although using preventive interventions to test and elaborate theories of change and development is the least practical reason for conducting trials, it may be the most important for generating new knowledge. The empirical findings from prevention science experiments can also be used to refine and modify the etiological theories that were used to guide the development of the intervention. Indeed, this bootstrap process—using an incomplete theory to guide the development of an intervention (Sandler, Gersten, et al., 1988) and then using the empirical results to advance the theory and fill in critical gaps—is a hallmark of the current prevention science model. It is also an atypical model in experimental sciences. A traditional epidemiological approach to treatment of an existing disorder, such as schizophrenia, generally uses a randomized trial to test a specific treatment at a certain dosage and length, with the analyses showing whether the treatment had a positive effect. Before conducting a treatment trial using this traditional approach, the hypothesized etiological model is often highly developed, and only when the pharmacokinetics and other factors are well understood is the treatment tested in a rigorous randomized trial.

With modern preventive trials, the experimental trial is, in contrast, often used to inform etiological theory at the same time. An etiological model of drug use, for example, is based on malleable risk and protective factors that can then be targeted by an intervention (Kraemer, Kazdin, et al., 1997; Botvin, Baker, et al., 1990; Botvin, 2004). The preventive intervention tests both the malleability of identified risk factors and the causal chain leading from these risk factors to distal outcomes (Snyder, Reid, et al., 2006). These causal chains can be tested with mediation modeling (MacKinnon, 2008), which decomposes the overall effects into those that follow hypothesized pathways and those whose pathways are not identified. A mediation model that explains most of an intervention's impact through the hypothesized pathways confirms the underlying theoretical model of change, whereas if the hypothesized pathways contribute little explanatory power, a new theory (or better mediating measures) needs to be developed to explain an intervention's effects.

More detailed models of etiology can be developed with analyses that examine the variations across subgroups and environments in the impact of an intervention on both mediators and distal outcomes (Kellam, Koretz, and Moscicki, 1999; Howe, Reiss, and Yuh, 2002; MacKinnon, 2008). For prevention of drug use, for example, a universal intervention that (1) builds social skills to resist the use of drugs, (2) gives feedback to young people about the true rate of peers' drug use, and (3) enhances coping skills could well have very different effects on young people who are current drug users and those who are nonusers. Understanding such differences can lead to an elaboration of knowledge of how peer messages and media images influence initiation and escalation behavior, as well as the roles played by personal and social skills (Botvin and Griffin, 2004). Griffin, Scheier, and colleagues (2001), for example, identified psychological well-being and lower positive expectancy toward drug use as key mediators between competence skills and later substance use.

Preventive trials can also examine the causal role of a particular risk factor when it is targeted by an intervention. For example, continuing aggressive or disruptive behavior early in life is a strong antecedent to a wide range of externalizing behaviors for both boys and girls (Ensminger, Kellam, and Rubin, 1983; Harachi, Fleming, et al., 2006). While these behaviors are much less frequent for girls than for boys, the long-term risk of any problem behavior is high for both sexes (Bierman, Bruschi, et al., 2004). Nevertheless, there are important differences in the specific risks and mediation pathways (Moffitt, Caspi, et al., 2001; Ensminger, Brown, and Kellam, 1984). The long-term link between individual-level aggression in first grade and adult antisocial personality disorder has been found to be both stronger and also more malleable by the Good Behavior Game (see Box 6-8) for boys compared with girls (Kellam, Brown, et al., 2008), which points to differences in the causal role of this risk factor for boys and girls.

Using Randomized Trials to Address Other Questions

Randomization can be used in highly flexible ways in studies of preventive interventions (Brown, Wyman, et al., 2007; Brown, Wang, et al., 2008), often answering different questions from the traditional randomized trial that focuses on efficacy or effectiveness alone (West, Biesanz, and Pitts, 2000). For example:

- **Head-to-Head Impact.** How beneficial is a preventive intervention program compared with another type of intervention? Preventive interventions can be compared not only with one another, but also with a service-based or treatment approach. In elementary school systems in the United States, for example, many incoming first grade children do not do well in the first couple of years of school; nevertheless, most of these failing children are not provided remedial educational services until the third grade. It is feasible to compare the impact of a universal classroom-based preventive intervention aimed at improving children's ability to master the social and educational demands at entry into first grade with a more traditional model that provides similar services at a later stage for children in serious need.
- **Implementability.** What effects come from alternative modes of training or delivery of a defined intervention? After demonstrating that an intervention is effective, one can examine different means of implementing that intervention, holding fixed its content. Webster-Stratton (1984, 2000) has used such trials to demonstrate that self-administered videotapes are effective and a cost-effective way of delivering the Incredible Years Program (see Box 6-2) outside the clinic.
- **Adaptability.** How does a planned variation in the content and delivery of a tested intervention affect its impact? For example, the third-generation Home Visitor Trial, conducted by Olds, Robinson, and colleagues (2004) in Denver, compared the delivery of a home-based intervention by a paraprofessional with the standard intervention delivered by nurse home visitors.
- **Extensibility.** What impact is achieved when an intervention is delivered to persons or in settings different from those in the original trial? One question being addressed is whether Olds's work on nurse home visitors, which originally focused on high-risk new mothers, would work as well for all pregnancies. Encouragement designs (described above) are also extensibility trials, since they can be used to expand the population that would normally participate in these interventions.

- **Sustainability.** Does impact continue as the time since completion of training increases? A sustainability trial compares the outcomes achieved by those who completed training earlier with outcomes for those who have just completed training or have not yet been trained (controls). For example, teachers can be randomized to start training at one of three times. At the end of the second training period, a sustainability trial would compare the outcomes achieved by the teachers who were trained first with those of the newly trained teachers and the teachers in the third training group.

- **Scalability.** What impact is achieved when an intervention is expanded to more settings? Using the same rolling system of teacher training as an example, a scalability trial would assess whether such an intervention maintains its effect as it is expanded system-wide. As it expands, the number of teachers requiring training and supervision increases, and therefore a scalability trial tests the system-level responses to these demands.

Using Randomized Preventive Trials to Meet the Needs of the Community

Field experiments of prevention programs are guided by federal requirements to maintain protection of human subjects. But they also require additional active community support and oversight in the design and conduct of the trial. Through partnerships with researchers, communities and institutions can play a major role in all aspects of the trial, including framing the research around community goals, norms, and values; shaping the questions that are asked during the research, granting access to people, data, and intervention and evaluation sites; and holding researchers accountable for the study and reporting back to the community. These community and institutional partnerships provide an added level of commitment and assurance of ethical conduct of research beyond those regulations required by universities and research institutions for human subjects' protection. Most often these partnerships are facilitated by setting up community and institutional advisory boards that provide direction to researchers and memoranda of understanding between all parties.

As mentioned above, communities often have major concerns about random assignment itself, which can be seen by parents, service providers, and administrators as manipulating, or as providing fewer opportunities for children, or as interference by outside researchers in the ways that children interact with schools, communities, or health systems. Also, service providers are concerned that the assessments made by researchers could be used to evaluate their performance. By active engagement of broadly representative community leaders, institutional leaders, and researchers around the issues of randomization, issues of trust and the social contract with researchers arise and need to be worked through to provide a base for conducting research in the community. For example, randomization can be seen as providing an equal chance for every child to receive a new intervention that cannot immediately be given to everyone. This process of "flipping a fair coin" can be seen as an equitable way of distributing limited resources. From this process can come a study design that is acceptable from the community's and institution's perspectives as well as that of the researchers.

Community-based participatory research, an intensive approach that involves the community in all phases of the research process, including specification of research questions and approaches (see Israel, Schulz, et al., 2003), is another potential approach to ensuring that trials meet the needs of the community. Similarly, partnerships that involve the systematic evaluation of interventions developed by community organizations in response to community priorities and values can increase their value to the community (see also Chapter 11).

Scientific Logic Behind the Use of Randomized Preventive Trials

Some in the scientific community believe that it is not possible to conduct field trials of prevention programs to produce sound causal inferences about these programs. However, good, randomized, preventive trials share many of the qualities that scientists have come to expect from controlled clinical trials, including random assignment to intervention and procedures to limit attrition and selective dropout or bias in measurement (Brown, 2003; Brown, Costigan, and Kendziora, 2008). Preventive trials, however, have some unique aspects.

First, it is virtually impossible to conduct a completely masked (or blind) psychosocial field trial the way double-blind clinical trials are conducted, in which neither the treating physician nor the patient knows whether an active drug or a placebo is used. A double-blind protocol provides a built-in protection against outcomes being influenced by patient or physician preferences, expectations, or beliefs. In psychosocial preventive interventions, this type of blinding does not happen. The intervention agents, often teachers or parents, must receive training in the intervention and participate in its delivery. Furthermore, the participants are generally aware that they are receiving the intervention, if for no other reason than they experience a different environment determined by the intervention.

The fact that randomized field trials cannot blind either the intervention agents or the study participants has important implications for the assessment of outcomes. It is important that these assessments be conducted by staff who do not know the participant's intervention condition. This is much easier to manage when participants are assigned individually to intervention or control conditions. It is more challenging in settings in which the intervention is applied to a whole group, such as a school, a classroom, or a medical or social service setting. Steps to reduce the chance that assessment biases influence conclusions about the intervention's effect include revealing as little of the actual study design to the assessment staff as possible, conducting follow-up assessments in a random order of individuals or groups (e.g., schools), and incorporating direct observations of behaviors whenever possible (Brown and Liao, 1999; Brown, 2003; Snyder, Reid, et al., 2006; Brown, Wang, et al., 2008).

Second, preventive field trials often require long evaluation periods and repeated measures that extend over different stages of life. By contrast, typical clinical trials often have relatively brief follow-up periods. The long follow-up periods for randomized field trials increase the potential for missing observations ("missingness") and loss of study participants, which creates major challenges in both design and analysis. Often, multistage designs or designs with planned missingness can increase the efficiency of follow-up (Brown, Costigan, and Kendziora, 2008) as well as protect against potential sources of attrition bias (Brown, Indurkhya, and Kellam, 2000). Furthermore, effective fieldwork procedures now exist that help maintain low attrition (Murry and Brody, 2004). Advanced analytical techniques are also available for handling missing data, even in the face of high levels of missingness (Schafer, 1997).

Another aspect of psychosocial preventive interventions is that they are often delivered in existing group settings, such as the classroom, school, family, or community. These group settings are "social fields" that are strongly linked to many of the predictive risk or protective factors that affect mental health and drug abuse. They also establish norms, determine the relevant set of task demands for the child, and provide formal or informal evaluations by natural raters that shape and mold children's response to the demands in that particular social field (Kellam, Branch, et al., 1975; Kellam and Rebok, 1992; Kellam, 1990).

Because many preventive interventions are carried out in these existing social fields, they are tested in preventive trials that often randomize whole groups rather than randomize at the level of individuals in the groups (Raudenbush, 1997; Murray, 1998; Brown and Liao, 1999). A major consequence is that the statistical power of such a design depends most heavily on the number of groups in the study rather than the total number of participants. Thus a trial involving 500 students in each of four schools with the schools randomly assigned to two interventions has statistical power similar to a traditional one-level design with four individuals assigned to two interventions. The large number of students in this design contributes relatively little precision to inferences about impact because of the small number of schools in the design.

The requirement for sufficient statistical power in group-based designs has led some researchers to conduct trials in a large number of schools or other group settings. Life Skills Training, for example, was carefully tested in 56 middle schools with approximately 70 children per school (Botvin and Griffin, 2004). Although a modest number of children per school is often sufficient to evaluate the overall strength of a group-based intervention compared with a control setting, additional participants may be required for more complex analyses. An examination of theory-driven hypotheses about how the intervention may vary as a function of baseline risk requires substantially more participants than would be required for examining overall impact (Brown, Costigan, and Kendziora, 2008).

Ways to Reduce Trial Size in Group-Based Randomized Trials

In some circumstances, group-based trials are prohibitively expensive unless special designs and strategies are used to make them cost-effective. One approach is the statistical technique of blocking. Blocks refer to higher level units, such as a school, in which both the intervention and the control conditions are included. For example, assigning classes in the same school to different interventions would be a classroom-based design with the school used as a blocking factor, whereas assigning all classes from the same school to the same intervention would be a school-based trial without blocking.

In deciding whether to randomize at the individual, classroom, or school level, for example, one needs to take into consideration both the most efficient way to deliver the intervention and the possibility of contamination, that is, when controls are inadvertently exposed to the intervention. In general, randomizing units that are at the same level as the unit of intervention (e.g., randomizing classes within a school for a classroom-based intervention) will provide the highest level of statistical power, provided contamination is limited (Brown and Liao, 1999).

Other approaches can also be followed to increase statistical power in group-based randomized trials. Designs that force balance on group-level characteristics and then randomize or that form matched pairs of these groups followed by random assignment of one in each pair to each condition can sometimes lead to increases in statistical power. With small numbers of schools or other units, however, matching can sometime reduce power by decreasing the degrees of freedom that are available for testing intervention effects.

Analytical methods can increase power as well. For example, a group-level covariate, such as the level of positive norms toward drug use in a school at baseline, can be used to adjust for differences by intervention condition that remain after randomization for a school-based drug prevention trial. Indeed, the inclusion of a baseline variable measured at the level at which randomization occurs can often increase statistical power more than the inclusion of individual-level baseline variables.

Even when there are no natural settings (e.g., schools) to use in implementing a prevention program (e.g., for families experiencing divorce), the intervention may still be designed and delivered in a group setting in the community (Wolchik, Sandler, et al., 2002; Sandler, Ayers, et al., 2003).

BUILDING RIGOROUS CAUSAL INFERENCES FROM RANDOMIZED FIELD TRIALS

At the time of the 1994 IOM report, prevention scientists generally had a limited understanding of the underlying framework for drawing causal conclusions about their interventions from randomized and nonrandomized experiments. There is now a greater understanding and appreciation of the design requirements that must be met for a trial to provide an adequate basis for making clear statements about the causal effect of an intervention.

The most commonly used model for making causal inferences about the effects of an intervention is based on the Neyman, Rubin, Holland (NRH) approach of counterfactuals (Neyman, 1990; Rubin, 1974, 1978; Holland, 1986). Although these key publications were available before the 1994 IOM report was written, understanding of the significance of this work and its implications for study designs has matured since then.

This theoretical approach considers that each individual in a two-arm trial could potentially have two outcomes, one when assigned to the first arm of the trial and a second when assigned to the second arm. Using this "potential outcome" model, the true intervention impact for that individual is then defined to be the difference in these two outcomes. However, it is impossible to observe both outcomes for a single participant; the trial makes only one outcome available to measure. The remaining unobserved outcome for each individual is a counterfactual: what would this person have been observed to do if he or she had received the other intervention. Because it is not possible to observe the outcome under both the assigned intervention and the counterfactual, it is not possible to assess this causal impact for a single individual. With a randomized experiment, however, it is possible to compare the average response for those assigned to one intervention with the average response of those assigned to the other condition. The difference in average responses for those assigned to the two conditions (often adjusted for covariates) is generally interpreted as a causal effect of the intervention.

The NRH approach provides conditions under which the difference in the average responses to the treatments is, in fact, an unbiased estimate for the average causal effect in the population. In nontechnical terms, the assumption that the estimate is unbiased depends on the following conditions being met (Rubin, 1974):

- The sample selected for study is representative of the population.
- As a whole, the participants assigned to the two intervention conditions are equivalent to one another.
- The intervention received is the same as the one randomly assigned.
- Any differences in assessment are unrelated to the intervention condition.
- Attrition or loss to follow-up is unrelated to the intervention condition.
- Each individual's response under the assigned intervention is unaffected by the intervention conditions assigned to all others in the sample.

Adhering to a specified study protocol for maintaining equivalence will go a long way toward satisfying many of these criteria. For example, when the assignment to an intervention is in fact random or a stratified random process, the second condition of equivalent intervention groups is satisfied. Likewise, attrition bias and assessment bias can both be minimized if the procedures for recontacting and reassessing participants in the follow-up period are performed blind to intervention condition (Brown and Liao, 1999; Brown, Indurkhya, and Kellam, 2000) or corrections are made for missing data at baseline.

Possible Inferences in Response to Self-Selection

One innovative change in the way prevention trials are now analyzed is to account for self-selection factors that differentiate those who choose to participate in the prevention program from those who do not. Consideration of self-selection factors is critical in examining the effects of prevention programs aimed at individual young people or families. Some decline to participate at all, others may participate in the intervention initially but drop out before the study is completed, and others may continue to participate throughout the intervention period.

It is tempting to compare the outcomes by level of participation and interpret any differences as being due to the effects of the intervention. For example, one might find that, on average, those exposed to the full intervention had poorer outcomes overall compared with those who did not participate. This might suggest the conclusion that the intervention was harmful. However, these observed differences alone are not a sufficient basis for statements about program effect or causality, and indeed such an intervention could well be beneficial for those who participate, despite the finding above. The problem with making conclusions taking into account level of participation is that the participants with greater involvement may have a higher baseline risk than those with more limited or no participation, and therefore those who self-select into the intervention could end up having worse outcomes than those who do not participate, regardless of intervention effect.

The design and analysis of studies can aid in distinguishing the effect of the intervention from the effects of self-selection. Individual participation can be measured only in those randomized to the intervention group, because those in the control group are not offered the opportunity to participate. Nevertheless, a randomized trial design makes it possible to treat the control group as a mixture of would-be participants and would-be nonparticipants. Thus, with appropriate assumptions, it is possible to arrive at causal inferences about the intervention effect on those who would be participants in an intervention. This is an example of the general approach called "principal stratification" (Bloom, 1984; Angrist, Imbens, and Rubin, 1996; Frangakis and Rubin, 1999, 2002; Jo and Muthén, 2001; Jo, 2002; Jo, Asparouhov, et al., in press). Such analyses are extremely valuable in that they characterize not only the effects of an intervention on participants, but also who chooses to participate in an intervention.

Distinct Ethical Issues for Conducting Preventive Trials

In treatment studies, the existing standards for ethical conduct of research dictate that it is improper to withhold an effective, safe treatment from participants. Thus because there are successful treatments for schizophrenia, it would be inappropriate and unethical to evaluate a new antipsychotic drug in a randomized trial that assigned some psychotic individuals to receive a placebo. The ethical considerations are different, however, in testing an antipsychotic drug for its ability to prevent schizophrenia or psychotic episodes in individuals exhibiting prodromal or preclinical signs or symptoms of schizophrenia. Although a few small randomized trials suggest that low-dose resperidone along with family therapy may provide some preventive value for adolescents who are at high risk for developing schizophrenia (McGorry, Yung, et al., 2002), the potential for causing side effects or otherwise harming individuals with these powerful drugs must be considered. In the case of a disorder that has not yet been manifest and an intervention that is known to have significant side effects, "doing no harm" has to be considered in order to decide whether it is ethical to conduct this kind of trial.

One potential way to deal with some of these ethical concerns, when there is a very real possibility of doing harm, is to use a mediational model to predict who is likely to benefit most from this type of antipsychotic drug. This type of mediation design (Pillow, Sandler, et al., 1991) uses the trial's inclusion/exclusion criteria to limit the trial to those whose signs or symptoms most closely match those targeted by the intervention. Limiting participants in the trial to those with prodromal symptoms as well as brain abnormalities associated with schizophrenia identifiable by magnetic resonance imaging, for example, may tip the benefit-cost ratio sufficiently to justify a trial (with appropriate consent) of a potentially risky pharmacological intervention. The burgeoning availability of genetic and other biological information with tenuous links to specific disorders also elevates ethical considerations (see Chapter 5).

Sometimes a design that would clearly be unethical or impractical with individual-level random assignment can be appropriate if conducted with group-level random assignment. This approach was used for practical reasons in a large preventive trial aimed at preventing the spread of HIV among Thai military conscripts through changes in sexual practices. Rather than randomly assign individuals in the same company to two different conditions, companies were matched within battalions and then randomly assigned to an active behavioral intervention or a passive diffusion model (Celentano, Bond, et al., 2000). Part of the rationale in such studies is that a community-wide preventive intervention cannot be implemented across a country at the same time, thus randomly assigning some of the communities to this intervention deviates from what would normally happen simply by using a fair method of assigning which communities receive the intervention first.

Using Wait Lists to Randomly Assign When an Intervention Is Delivered

In many situations, a community or government agency decides that all its young people should receive a new preventive intervention, even though the intervention itself has not yet been well evaluated. Indeed, in suicide prevention, for which few programs have been evaluated rigorously, communities frequently decide to saturate the community with a program. Under certain circumstances it is still possible to evaluate the effectiveness of such an intervention using a randomized design. For example, a standard wait-list design can be used to randomly assign half of the participants or groups to receive the intervention immediately and half to receive it later.

Communities are often accepting of a standard wait-list design because there are benefits to both conditions: a community that initially receives the intervention has an opportunity to benefit immediately; the community with a delayed start has the opportunity to benefit from any enhancements of the intervention made on the basis of the initial experience. A disadvantage with this design is that, because everyone receives this intervention within a short time frame, only short-term effects can be examined. However, if groups are randomized, such as schools, and the wait list is delayed until the following cohort in the delayed schools, evaluation of longer term effects is still possible. This is because the first cohort contains participants who never receive the intervention.

A type of randomized design that has only recently been used in prevention studies is called a dynamic wait-list design (Brown, Wyman, et al., 2006). In contrast to the standard wait-list design, in which an intervention is delivered either immediately or after a specified delay, the dynamic wait-list design randomly assigns participants to one of three or more times to start the intervention. For time-to-event outcomes, the dynamic wait-list design has more statistical power because it increases the number of time periods, with most of the statistical gain occurring in moving from two to four or six time periods (Brown, Wyman, et al., 2006). This design was used in the school-based Georgia Gatekeeper Training Trial (Wyman, Brown, et al., 2008), in which 32 schools were randomly assigned to one of five start times for the training program, and the primary outcome was the rate at which suicidal youth were identified by the school.

Ethical Issues for Prevention When Variation in Intervention Impact Is Found

Researchers are beginning to identify different degrees of benefit or harm from an intervention across different subgroups on the basis of baseline characteristics and contexts. If one finds that one subgroup shows consistent benefits and another shows that the same intervention causes them to do worse, then both the use and the nonuse of this program will cause some harm to a segment of the population. Another situation that may arise is a finding of benefit on some outcomes but compensatory harm on others. There is reason to believe that genetic variations, whose prevalences are due to evolutionary pressures, provide either advantages or disadvantages in adaptive response to specific environments (see Chapter 5). As one begins to look at how a complex preventive intervention affects individuals with specific genetic characteristics, it would not be surprising to find allelomorphic variation in outcomes, or that positive as well as negative outcomes can occur for those with a single allele. Any of these occurrences raises questions about the use of an intervention and should suggest continued work to adapt the intervention to specific individual and environmental situations.

EMERGING OPPORTUNITIES FOR PREVENTION TRIALS

Preventive Trials for Disorders with Low Prevalence

The prevention field still has relatively little information about effective interventions for conditions that occur infrequently. In designing prevention trials for low-base-rate disorders and outcomes, such as schizophrenia (Faraone, Brown, et al., 2002; Brown and Faraone, 2004) and suicide (Brown, Wyman, et al., 2007), the sample sizes necessary to obtain sufficient statistical power often seem prohibitively large. For example, a universal preventive trial aimed at a 50 percent reduction in youth suicide in the general population would require more than 1,000,000 person-years of observation. Although a study this large is often considered impractical, some novel alternatives exist. One approach is to combine data across a cluster of similar trials by using a common outcome, such as death from suicide or unintentional causes, for a long-term follow-up assessment. Data on mortality outcomes can be collected relatively cheaply using the National Death Index. An approach that aggregates data across studies will have to take into account variation in impact across studies with random effects, just as in meta-analysis (Brown, Wang, and Sandler, 2008).

An important strategy that other health fields use to test interventions on low-base-rate outcomes is to assess the impact of the intervention on a more common surrogate endpoint that has been identified as an antecedent risk factor for the outcome of interest. The rate of HIV seroconversion, for example, is sufficiently low in the general U.S. population that most HIV prevention trials use a reduction in HIV risk behavior as their primary outcome. Likewise, suicide attempts can serve as a surrogate for suicide itself, because there are roughly 100 times more suicide attempters than suicide completers, and attempt is a strong predictor of future suicide. The use of suicide attempts as an outcome would allow for sufficient statistical power with a much smaller study population.

Evaluating the Components of Interventions and Adaptive Interventions

Trials to examine the functioning of distinct components of an intervention may be needed, as when a comprehensive prevention program, such as Life Skills Training (see Box 6-1), has multiple components or modules that have been incorporated over the years. Although an intervention is normally tested in its entirety, the contribution of separate components can be examined through such approaches as study designs that deliver selected components (Collins, Murphy, and Bierman, 2004) or by examining the strength of different mediational pathways (West, Aiken, and Todd, 1993; West and Aiken, 1997).

Testing components is also necessary in preventive interventions that are designed to be flexible, so that the program can be tailored to the specific needs of the participants. Fast Track, for example (see Box 6-9), was a randomized trial aimed at preventing the consequences of aggressive behavior from first grade through high school (Conduct Problems Prevention Research Group, 1992, 1999a, 1999b). Over the course of the 10-year study, each participant in the intervention condition received specific program components that were deemed most appropriate based on his or her risks and protective factors at a given point in life. By the end of the study, the set of interventions and their dosages or durations differed substantially from person to person. Analytical techniques are available to disentangle some of the effects of dosage from different levels of need, but the use of designs, especially with multiple levels of randomization, may provide clearer insight into the effects of the intervention components (Murphy, van der Laan, et al., 2001; Murphy, 2003; Collins, Murphy, and Strecher, 2007).

Testing Prevention Components

There is also interest in testing whether small, relatively simple elements of a prevention program can be successfully applied in different contexts. For example, implementation of the Good Behavior Game in first and second grade, which gave teachers an extensive period of training and supervision and included the creation of a support structure in the school and the district, was found to have long-term benefits for high-risk boys (Kellam, Brown, et al., 2008; Petras, Kellam, et al., 2008). In an effort to provide this intervention at reduced cost, others have attempted to implement the Good Behavior Game intervention using much less training and system-level support (Embry, 2004). Because the training received as part of one intervention becomes part of a teacher's toolkit, it would be useful to evaluate the subsequent effects of the differences in teachers' training and support in conjunction with the Good Behavior Game on levels of aggressive behavior in their students. Program components can be tested by themselves by randomizing which teachers, or other such intervention agents, are to receive no training, low training, or high training.

Using the Internet for Randomized Preventive Trials

The Internet presents new opportunities to deliver preventive interventions to a diverse and expanding audience and to test the interventions in large randomized trials. With the delivery of a prevention program through the web, the opportunity exists to test new or refined components using random assignment and to revise the program in response to these results using methods described by Collins, Murphy, and Bierman (2004) and West, Aiken, and Todd (1993).

Internet-based programs are also likely to present methodological challenges. First, a randomized trial would typically depend on data from self-reports obtained through the Internet, and uncertainty as to the validity of these data, as well as the proportion of participants willing to respond to long-term evaluations, could limit the evaluation plan. It may be necessary to use a multistage follow-up design (Brown, Indurkhya, and Kellam, 2000; Brown, Wang, et al., 2008), which would include a phone or face-to-face interview for a stratified sample of study participants.

Sequencing of Preventive Trials and Selective Long-Term Follow-Up

In most health research, trials are staged in a progression from basic to clinical investigations to broad application in target populations, allowing for an ordered and predictable expansion of knowledge in specific areas (e.g., Greenwald and Cullen, 1985). In the prevention field, rigorous evaluations of the efficacy of a preventive intervention can be lengthy, as are studies of replication and implementation. However, opportunities exist for strategic shortcuts. One approach is to combine several trials sequentially. For example, in a school-based trial, consecutive cohorts can serve different purposes. The first cohort of randomly assigned students and their teachers would comprise an effectiveness trial. In the second year, the same teachers, who continue with the same intervention condition as in the first year, along with a second cohort of new students, can be used to test sustainability. Finally, a third student cohort can be used to test scalability to a broader system, with the teachers who originally served as the intervention's controls now also trained to deliver the intervention.

A related issue involving the staging of trials is determining when there is sufficient scientific evidence for moving from a pilot trial of the intervention to a fully funded trial. In the current funding climate, researchers often design a small, pilot trial to demonstrate that an intervention looks sufficiently strong to proceed with a larger trial. Reviewers of these applications for larger trials want to have confidence that the intervention is sufficiently strong before recommending expanded funding. However, as pointed out by Kraemer, Mintz, and colleagues (2006), the effect size estimate from the pilot trial is generally too variable to provide a good decision-making tool to distinguish weak from strong interventions. There is need for alternative sequential design strategies that lead to funding of the promising interventions.

Another methodological challenge involving the review process is deciding when an intervention's early results are sufficiently promising to support additional funding for a long-term follow-up study. A limited number of preventive interventions have now received funding for long-term follow-up, and many of these have demonstrated effects that appear stronger over time (Olds, Henderson, et al., 1998; Wolchik, Sandler, et al., 2002; Hawkins, Kosterman, et al., 2005; Kellam, Brown, et al., 2008; Petras, Kellam, et al., 2008; Wilcox, Kellam, et al., 2008). It is difficult for reviewers to assess whether an intervention's relatively modest early effects are likely to improve over time or diminish, and therefore some of the most promising prevention programs may miss an opportunity for long-term funding.

NONRANDOMIZED EVALUATIONS OF INTERVENTION IMPACT

Conducting high-quality randomized trials is challenging, but the effort and expense are necessary to answer many important questions. However, many critical questions cannot be answered by randomized trials (Greenwald and Cullen, 1985; Institute of Medicine, 1994). For example, Skinner, Matthews, and Burton (2005) examined how existing welfare programs affected the lives of families. Their ethnographic data demonstrated that many families cannot obtain needed services because of enormous logistical constraints in reaching the service locations.

In other situations, there may be no opportunity to conduct a true randomized trial to assess the effects of a defined intervention, because the community is averse to the use of a randomization scheme, because ethical considerations preclude conducting such a trial, or because funds and time are too limited. Even so, many opportunities remain to conduct careful evaluations of prevention programs, and much can be gained from such data if they are carefully collected. Indeed, much has been written about the limits of the knowledge that a standard randomized trial can provide, and natural experiments can sometimes provide complementary information (West and Sagarin, 2000).

When a full randomized trial cannot be used to evaluate an intervention, an alternative study should be designed so that the participants in the intervention conditions differ as little as possible on characteristics other than the intervention itself. For example, it will be difficult to distinguish the effect of an intervention from other factors if a community that has high readiness is compared with a neighboring community that is not at all ready to provide the intervention. It may be necessary to work with both communities to ensure that they receive similar attention before the intervention starts as well as similar efforts for follow-up.

Pre-Post Designs

A pre-post design is another alternative to randomization. Such studies evaluate an intervention on the basis of the changes that occur from a baseline (the "pre" measurement) to after the intervention period (the "post" measurement). This type of design can provide valuable information, particularly when it supports a hypothesized developmental model involving known mediators that lead to expected prevention targets. However, the pre-post design suffers from confounding with developmental changes that are occurring in young people. On one hand, with drug use in adolescents, for example, the sharp increases in drug use with age—as well as seasonal effects—could completely mask the potential benefit of an intervention. On the other hand, lower drug use after the intervention than before would suggest that the intervention has prevention potential. Also, pre-post designs can lead to erroneous conclusions if they involve selecting participants at high risk and assessing whether their risk goes down; improvement might be expected simply because of a regression to the mean effect.

Interrupted Time-Series Designs

An important way to improve pre-post designs is to include multiple measurements of variables of interest. A good example of this is the interrupted time series (or multiple baseline design extended to several groups), in which multiple measurements of the target behavior are made both before and after the intervention. Varying the timing of the intervention across participating individuals or groups, especially if assignment to an intervention time is randomized, can further strengthen the evaluation design. Policy changes, such as wide-scale implementation of a new program, changes in the law or changes in enforcement of existing laws, often provide opportunities to evaluate an intervention in this type of natural experiment. One example is the evaluation of policies that restrict tobacco sales to minors (Stead and Lancaster, 2005). In their examination of the effect of positive reinforcement to tobacco stores and sales clerks to avoid tobacco sales to minors, Biglan, Ary, and colleagues (1996), for example, repeatedly assessed the proportion of stores making underage sales both before and after the intervention, demonstrating that the behavior of clerks is modifiable.

Regression Discontinuity Designs

Another type of natural experiment that provides an opportunity for program evaluation occurs when strict eligibility criteria, such as age or level of risk along a continuum, are imposed for entrance into a program.

In such cases, the difference in regression intercepts, or the expected outcome when other variables are equal, for the outcome measure among those who were eligible and those who were not eligible provides an estimate of the intervention effect (Cook and Campbell, 1979). Gormley, Gayer, and Phillips (2005) used this design in concluding that a universal statewide prekindergarten program had a large impact on achievement.

ADVANCES IN STATISTICAL ANALYSIS OF PREVENTION TRIALS

At the time of the 1994 IOM report, virtually all published analyses were limited to examining an intervention's impact on an outcome variable measured at a single point in time at follow-up. Analyses of impact in randomized field trials and longitudinal analyses were conducted independent of one another. Now, however, it is customary to use growth modeling techniques to examine trajectories of change using more extensive longitudinal data, with corresponding gains in statistical power (Muthén and Curran, 1997) and interpretability (Muthén, Brown, et al., 2002). Growth models can be a valuable tool in understanding the impact of interventions.

Using Growth Models

Most theories of change in prevention research posit an evolving effect on the individual that varies over time as new developmental stages are reached. Although it should be possible to detect intervention effects at a critical transition period using an outcome measured at a single time point, it is also possible to examine the impact of interventions using longitudinal data to show differences in individuals' developmental trajectories or growth patterns (e.g., repeated measures of aggression or symptoms) by intervention condition.

Often the patterns of growth can be summarized with a few parameters. By fitting individual-level data to linear growth curves, for example, an intervention's effect can be summarized based on the difference in mean rates of growth for intervention and control participants. Other approaches might include latent growth modeling of different aspects of growth using quadratics and higher order polynomials, piecewise growth trajectories, and nonlinear growth models (Muthén, 1991).

The effects of interventions may vary not only as a function of time, but also across individuals. For example, a universal intervention may have a stronger effect over time on those who start with higher levels of risk compared with those with lower levels of risk, as is now found in a number of preventive interventions (Brown and Liao, 1999; Brown, Wang, et al., 2008). Growth models that include an interaction between intervention condition and baseline levels of risk (Muthén and Curran, 1997) can capture such variation in impact over time.

Growth mixture modeling is another analytic approach that allows individuals to follow one of several different patterns of change over time (Muthén and Shedden, 1999; Carlin, Wolfe, et al., 2001; Muthén, Brown, et al., 2002; Wang, Brown, and Bardeen-Roche, 2005). Its advantage over the interaction model described in the previous paragraph is its flexibility; for example, if the intervention causes low- and high-risk youth to receive benefit but youth with moderate risk are harmed, growth mixture models should detect these differential effects. Intervention effects can be modeled for each pattern of growth in risk behaviors over time, such as stable low levels of drug use, escalating levels, stable high levels, and decreasing levels. The results of such analyses may show, for example, that although a universal intervention reduces drug usage among those who begin using drugs early, it may have the unintended effect of increasing drug usage in what began as a low-risk group. A result of this type should lead to a redesign of the intervention.

Latent transition analyses (Collins, Graham, et al., 1994) are also used to examine changes in drug usage trajectories over time. These methods can directly model the changes in patterns of drug use over time and changes through exposure to an intervention. To distinguish drug initiation from escalation or similar qualitative versus quantitative differences in delinquency (Nagin and Land, 1993), methods that allow censoring, truncation, and so-called two-part models (Olsen and Schafer, 2001) can now be used in growth mixture modeling and other complex analyses.

For behavioral observation data, which has a prominent place in prevention research (Snyder, Reid, et al., 2006), multilevel random effects can be used to incorporate large tables of contingent responses or associations in complex mediation analyses (Dagne, Brown, and Howe, 2007). Similarly, analysis of trajectories can involve not only continuous data but also binary data (Carlin, Wolfe, et al., 2001), count data (Nagin and Land, 1993), and time-to-event or survival data (Muthén and Masyn, 2005). In addition, many analytical tools are available to examine different types of variables in the same model, so that continuous measures can be used to assess the impact of an intervention on growth trajectories through one stage of life while impact on adult diagnoses is measured as a dichotomous variable (Muthén, Brown, et al., 2002).

All these methods provide opportunities to specify and test precise questions about variation in the impact of an intervention. However, erroneous conclusions are possible if the underlying processes are not carefully modeled (Carlin, Wolfe, et al., 2001; Wang, Brown, and Bandeen-Roche, 2005).

Multilevel Modeling of Intervention Effects

Multilevel modeling of contextual effects, such as the school, has also been well integrated into the evaluation of preventive trials. At the time of the 1994 IOM report, it was rare for published analyses of group-based randomized trials to correct for nonindependence among the participants in a group. As a result, they could erroneously report impact when it was not statistically significant. In a trial with 20 schools, half of which are randomized to a prevention program, the correct statistical test of impact is based on the number of schools, not the number of children, which may be several orders of magnitude larger (Murray, 1998). Now it is expected that published papers of group-based randomized experiments will use multi-level analysis (Raudenbush, 1997) or generalized estimating equations and sandwich-type estimators (Zeger, Liang, and Albert, 1988; Brown, 1993b; Flay, Biglan, et al., 2005) to account for group randomization.

Modeling That Incorporates Growth and Context in the Same Analysis

At the time of the 1994 IOM report, it was customary to report only the overall impact of an intervention in a population. Since then, statistical modeling has advanced so that longitudinal and multilevel modeling can now be handled in the same analysis. It is common to see analyses that include both individual growth and multiple levels of nesting, such as children nested within classrooms and schools (Gibbons, Hedeker, et al., 1988; Brown, Costigan, and Kendziora, 2008). Analyses can examine how change occurs across multiple levels (Raudenbush and Bryk, 2002) and examine impact across both individuals and contextual levels with different types of growth trajectories (Muthén, Brown, et al., 2002; Muthén and Asparouhov, 2006; Asparouhov and Muthén, 2007).

Handling of Missing or Incomplete Data

A major advance has been the treatment of missing data in statistical analysis of longitudinal data. When the previous IOM report was written, most published analyses of intervention impact simply deleted any missing cases. Now most impact analyses make use of full maximum likelihood methods (Dempster, Laird, and Rubin, 1977) or multiple imputations (Rubin, 1987; Schafer, 1997; Schafer and Graham, 2002; Demirtas and Schafer, 2003; Graham, 2003; Graham, Cumsille, and Elek-Fisk, 2003). These techniques are especially important for evaluating impact across long periods of time, because data will be incomplete for many of the participants and differentially across contexts.

Intent-to-Treat and Postintervention Modeling

The traditional standard of intent-to-treat analyses used to analyze clinical trials has been extended to multilevel and growth modeling for randomized field trials. This approach overcomes the challenges in handling dropin and dropout and other types of missing data that regularly occur in prevention trials (Brown, Wang, et al., 2008). So-called intent-to-treat analyses, or analyses based on the assigned rather than the actual intervention or treatment, are generally used as the primary set of models to examine intervention effects overall and for moderating effects involving individual-level and group-level baseline characteristics.

These traditional methods of examining the effects of an intervention can be supplemented with postintervention analyses. The postintervention approach takes into account the intervention actually received by each participant (Wyman, Brown, et al., 2008), the dosage received (Murphy, 2005; Murphy, Collins, and Rush, 2007; Murphy, Lynch, et al., 2007), and the level of adherence (Little and Yau, 1996; Hirano, Imbens, et al., 2000; Barnard, Frangakis, et al., 2003; Jo, Asparouhov, et al., in press), as well as the intervention's effect on different mediators (MacKinnon and Dwyer, 1993; MacKinnon, Weber, and Pentz, 1989; Tein, Sandler, et al., 2004; MacKinnon, Lockwood, et al., 2007; MacKinnon, 2008).

METHODOLOGICAL CHALLENGES AHEAD
FOR PREVENTION RESEARCH

As the field of prevention science matures, important new developments in methodological research will be needed to meet new challenges. Some of these challenges include (1) integrating structural and functional imaging data on the brain; (2) understanding how genetics, particularly gene–environment interactions, can best inform prevention; (3) testing and evaluating implementation strategies for prevention programs; and (4) modeling and expressing effects of prevention for informing public policy.

Incorporating imaging and genetics data into analyses will require the ability to deal with huge numbers of voxels, polymorphisms, and expressed genes. The large literature on data reduction techniques and multiple comparisons may provide a basis for methods for studying mediational pathways, expressed genes, and gene–environment interactions that may influence prevention outcomes and should be considered in intervention designs. Also, as the body of evidence for effective programs continues to grow, demand will increase for evaluations of alternative strategies for implementing such programs. Finally, the ability to model the costs as well as the effectiveness of different preventive interventions for communities will allow for policy decisions made on the basis of the best scientific findings. These issues are discussed in more detail in Part III.

CONCLUSIONS AND RECOMMENDATIONS

Since the 1994 IOM report, new methodological tools have been developed that enable more nuanced analysis of outcomes, more sophisticated designs that enable randomized assignment, and more reliable outcomes. These advances in modern statistical approaches have been particularly useful in the context of field trials of preventive interventions that face particular randomization challenges not usually relevant to clinical trials.

Conclusion: Significant advances in statistical evaluation designs, measures, and analyses used in prevention research have contributed to improved understanding of the etiology of emotional and behavioral disorders and related problem behaviors since 1994.

Prevention methodology has enabled the use of refined statistical and analytical techniques to be used in an iterative manner to refine interventions, for example, by identifying components or groups for which the intervention is most successful and to further develop theories about causal mechanisms that contribute to the development of problems or to an intervention's results.

Conclusion: Improved methodologies have also led to improved interventions, etiological theories, and theories of change.

The highest level of confidence in the results of intervention trials is provided by multiple well-conducted randomized trials. In addition, for some areas of prevention, the types of designs that are typically used have relatively limited ability to produce unambiguous causal inferences about intervention impact because of statistical confounding or inadequate controls, low statistical power, lack of appropriate outcome measures, or attrition. In these situations, it is important to develop additional evaluation designs that provide more rigorous testing of these interventions. Furthermore, few interventions have been tested for long-term outcomes despite the availability of appropriate methodologies. Several interventions have demonstrated effects on reducing multiple disorders and other related outcomes, such as academic performance. The value of preventive interventions would be significantly strengthened if long-term results could be demonstrated on a more consistent basis.

Recommendation 10-1: Research funders should invest in studies that (1) aim to replicate findings from earlier trials, (2) evaluate long-term outcomes of preventive interventions across multiple outcomes (e.g., disorders, academic outcomes), and (3) test the extent to which each prevention program is effective in different race, ethnic, gender, and developmental groups.

Being able to obtain replicable results is one of the hallmarks of science, since lack of replicability raises questions about generalizability. Direct replicability corresponds to a test of the same intervention under very similar conditions. Systematic replicability refers to testing of the intervention under conditions that are deliberately modified (e.g., intervention agent, trainer, length of program, target population) in order to examine whether the results change with these modifications (see Chapter 11 for discussion of adaptation to different populations). Given limited funding, lack of interest by review groups in direct replication, and the current state of knowledge about the effects of preventive interventions, we recommend that systematic replications are more appropriate than direct replications.

Funding is often limited for evaluations that assess outcomes beyond the end of an intervention or a short time after the intervention. Yet demonstrating outcomes that endure increases confidence in an intervention and provides a more comprehensive test of the impact of the intervention on children's lives and its benefit to society. Assessment of long-term outcomes would ideally include consideration of the sustainability of outcomes across developmental periods (Coie, Watt, et al., 1993). Given that most preventive interventions are designed to mitigate developmental processes that can lead to mental, emotional, and behavioral disorders and problems over time, assessment of whether proximal outcomes at one developmental period are sustained in distal outcomes at a later developmental period is needed. Several of the programs discussed in Chapters 6 and 7, including the Nurse-Family Partnership, Life Skills Training, Good Behavior Game, Strengthening Families 10-14, and the Family Check-up, have met this criterion. Although the Society for Prevention Research (Flay, Biglan, et al., 2005) has suggested six months as a minimum follow-up period,[2] the committee considers this to be a necessary but insufficient time frame for the majority of outcomes.

As statistical and methodological approaches have been developed in

---

[2]For "outcomes that may decay over time," the Society for Prevention Research (Flay, Biglan, et al., 2005, p. 2) recommends that evaluations include "at least one long-term follow-up at an interval beyond the end of the intervention (e.g., at least 6 months after the intervention." The Society for Prevention Research standards also acknowledge that the interval may need to differ for different types of interventions.

response to ongoing evaluations over the past 15 years, advances in this area must continue to keep pace with and respond to new knowledge that affects prevention science. The significant rise in interventions with evidence of effectiveness, the importance of implementing interventions with fidelity, and the lack of empirical evidence on how to successfully implement interventions will call for the development of new methodologies to explore various implementation and dissemination strategies (see also Chapter 11). This might include exploration of such questions as implementability, adaptability, extensibility, sustainability, and scalability.

> **Conclusion: Methodologies to evaluate approaches to implementation and dissemination are less well developed than methodologies related to efficacy and effectiveness.**

Other recent research advances, including the results of imaging and other developmental neuroscience studies and findings related to the role of gene–environment interactions (see Chapter 5), provide new challenges and opportunities for intervention research and will require thoughtful consideration of design strategies.

> **Recommendation 10-2:** The National Institutes of Health should be charged with developing methodologies to address major gaps in current prevention science approaches, including the study of dissemination and implementation of successful interventions.

The methodologies developed should include designs to test alternative approaches to implementation and dissemination of evidence-based and community-generated prevention programs (see Chapter 11). Priority areas should also include approaches that link neuroscience methods and clinical research with epidemiology and prevention in understanding the etiology of mental health and of disorders and approaches that link theories developed through neuroscience research with preventive intervention approaches designed to test causal mechanisms (see Chapter 5).

Part III:

New Frontiers

11

Implementation and Dissemination of Prevention Programs

P art II illustrates the substantial progress made in prevention science since 1994. It describes numerous efficacious or effective prevention programs (Chapters 6 and 7), as well as the cost-effectiveness of many of these programs (Chapter 9). It also demonstrates numerous methodological advances that increase confidence in the reliability of evidence that provides a strong basis for believing that the mental, emotional, and behavioral health of the nation's young people could be significantly improved if evidence-based programs and policies were widely used (Chapter 10). Thus far, however, preventive interventions have generally not been widely implemented in schools and communities (Ennet, Ringwalt, et al., 2003; Gottfredson and Gottfredson, 2002; Hallfors and Godette, 2002; Wandersman and Florin, 2003) and have done little to reduce behavioral health problems in American communities (Chinman, Hannah, et al., 2005; Sandler, Ostrom, et al., 2005).

While sustained, high-quality implementation by communities is essential to achieving greater public health impact from the available tested and effective preventive interventions (Elliott and Mihalic, 2004; Glasgow, Klesges, et al., 2004; Spoth and Greenberg, 2005), implementation of existing programs alone is unlikely to be sufficient. Implementation must also include development and evaluation of research-based adaptations of programs to new cultural, linguistic, and socioeconomic groups; evaluation of approaches that have broad community endorsement; and implementation of policies and principles that support healthy development.

This chapter begins with a discussion of alternative implementation approaches. It goes on to review examples of experience with implementation of existing prevention programs, as well as a number of challenges to implementation. The chapter then describes strategies that can complement the implementation of evidence-based interventions. Next is a discussion of research needed to increase understanding of and support successful implementation. The final section presents conclusions and recommendations for moving implementation forward.

IMPLEMENTATION APPROACHES

A major implementation issue is the balance between delivering an evidence-based program as developed and adapting a program to meet the specific needs of the community. This section describes three alternative implementation approaches: (1) direct adoption of a specific evidence-based prevention program, (2) adaptation of an evidence-based intervention to community needs, and (3) community-driven implementation. Table 11-1 summarizes the advantages and disadvantages of each. These three approaches are not mutually exclusive or exhaustive of all potential approaches. Each requires an active partnership among community leaders, organizations and institutions, and researchers and must address issues of trust, power, priority, and action. The appropriate approach in a given community will depend on its characteristics and priorities and the availability of an existing evidence-based program that matches its needs. Ideally, evaluation is a component of all three approaches to shed light on why a specific approach works in a particular community or how to generalize knowledge about successful implementation to other programs, communities, or institutional settings.

Adoption of an Existing Evidence-Based Program

A community's adoption of a specific prevention program involves delivering the program with high fidelity, increasing the likelihood that its impact will be similar to that found in the original studies. Typically, programs have met a specific standard of evidence, often articulated by federal, state, or other external funding sources (Halfors, Pankratz, and Hartman, 2007). Standardized curricula, teaching manuals, or taped media help deliver the program in a manner similar to that used by the original researchers. Generally, there is limited adaptation of the program to the cultural or historical characteristics or the particular interests of the community.

Sites typically need sufficient local capacity and resources and technical assistance from the program developers or other certified trainers to ensure fidelity, monitoring, supervision, and sustainability (Elliott and Mihalic, 2004). Both the Nurse-Family Partnership Program and Life Skills Training, considered strong evidence-based programs backed by research findings

TABLE 11-1 Comparison of Three Implementation Approaches

Model	Advantages	Disadvantages
Implementation of an existing evidence-based program	High program fidelity Relatively high likelihood of achieving intended impact Known resources and requirements for effective implementation Likely continued funding under federal and state supported evidence-based prevention	Program may not fit community needs, strengths, or capacities Real-world implementation may differ dramatically from the way originally tested Lack of ownership in the program Few evidence-based programs have the capacity to provide technical assistance and training An evidence-based program may not target outcomes relevant to community
Adaptation of an existing program to meet community needs	Ownership and high support from community and potentially high adoption Program more relevant to ethnic, racial, or linguistic characteristics of community Reasonably likely to achieve impact	Key program components may be modified, thereby reducing outcomes Essential program components not always evident
Community-driven implementation	Can develop high community acceptance and ownership Potential for broader implementation across different organizations and institutions within the community Opportunity to empirically evaluate the outcomes of programs accepted by the community and use quality improvement methods to enhance outcomes over time	Lengthy period to develop community awareness, common vision, and program Potential for ineffectiveness or iatrogenic effects Challenges in obtaining funding for sustaining a unique program

from multiple randomized trials in different types of communities, are being implemented in specific communities using this approach. There is some evidence that they are flexible enough to provide benefit across communities with diverse ethnic backgrounds (Botvin, Griffin, et al., 2001).

However, it often takes decades of longitudinal follow-up for a program to be designated as evidence-based, and the original program may not address the current needs or priorities of communities. Research-based programs rarely can meet the triple challenges of maintaining an active research program, a successful marketing strategy, and a qualified technical assistance and training program. In addition, it may be difficult to reproduce in the community the level of expertise of staff used to deliver the intervention in the original study. Finally, importing a program may result in a lack of ownership in the community, negatively affecting the ability to sustain the program over time.

Given increasing evidence of the importance of community engagement and technical assistance, several models have been developed to help communities build the infrastructure needed to identify and implement specific evidence-based programs (see Box 11-1). For example, the Communities That Care (CTC) model leads a community through an assessment process to select specific evidence-based programs. The CTC model strongly discourages

---

BOX 11-1
Models for Community Implementation
of Evidence-Based Programs

Communities That Care

Communities That Care (CTC), a prevention system designed to reduce adolescent delinquency and substance use, was built as part of the Center for Substance Abuse Prevention approach to effective implementation (see http://ncadi. samhsa.gov/features/ctc/resources.aspx). It provides a process for communities, through a community prevention board, to identify their prevention priorities and develop a profile of community risk and protective factors. The CTC logic model involves community-level training and technical assistance for three steps: (1) community adoption of a science-based prevention framework, (2) creation of a plan for changing outcomes through a menu of evidence-based programs that target risk and protective factors identified by the community, and (3) implementation and evaluation of these programs using both process and outcome evaluations. Currently, there are 56 available programs that meet CTC's required standard of evidence.

BOX 11-1 Continued

CTC's theory of change hypothesizes that it takes two to five years to observe changes in prioritized risk factors and five or more years to observe effects on delinquency or substance use. CTC's data driven process is being evaluated in multiple steps. The first step, a five-year nonexperimental study with 40 incorporated towns, assessed the degree to which they reported using tested and effective programs. In the next phase, 24 of these communities who had not reported already using such programs agreed to be part of a large randomized community-level trial to test the CTC model (Hawkins, 2006). Early findings from these communities indicate that CTC has positive effects on targeted risk factors and delinquent behavior (Hawkins, Brown, et al., 2008) as well as alcohol use and binge drinking (Hawkins, Oesterle, et al., in press). Longer term follow-up is under way.

PROmoting School-community-university Partnerships to Enhance Resilience Model

The PROmoting School-community-university Partnerships to Enhance Resilience (PROSPER) model (Spoth, Greenberg, et al., 2004; Greenberg, Feinberg, et al., 2007) has devised a system aimed at broad implementation of evidence-based programs designed to support positive youth development and reduce early substance use delivered to rural areas with supports at the local, regional, and state levels. Underlying this system is the building of an infrastructure that supports local ownership and capacity building as well as leadership and institutional support (Spoth, Greenberg, et al., 2004). Three groups are involved in the PROSPER partnership model: (1) faculty from land grant universities and affiliated cooperative extension staff, (2) the elementary and secondary school systems, and (3) community agency providers of services for children and families, along with other community stakeholders.

The partnership benefited from the existing training and technical assistance infrastructure provided by the Extension System and the U.S. Department of Education's Safe and Drug-Free Schools (SDFS) Program. Because the prevention programs in PROSPER are delivered by local practitioners, it focuses on building strong support of the school–local community team, which chooses interventions and is responsible for their implementation. At the state level, researchers work with regional Extension Service prevention coordinators and coordinators from the SDFS Program. These regional coordinators then provide support to local teams of extension agents, elementary and secondary school faculties and staffs, and community interagency coalition members. The long-term goal is to provide infrastructure support as well as direct assistance to sustain effective, empirically based programs in communities.

This implementation model has national implications, as the Extension Service has more than 9,600 local agents working in 3,150 counties across the United States. The Department of Education has multiple technical assistance centers that support efforts to adopt empirically supported programs that can reduce substance abuse, violence, and other conduct problems in the schools. Furthermore, the SDFS Program currently has coordinators in many schools to facilitate the implementation of such research-based programs.

program adaptation, based on evidence that delivery of evidence-based programs as designed is likely to lead to the most successful prevention efforts.

Adaptation of an Existing Program to the Community

Adaptation of programs focuses on concerns about community or cultural relevance. A community identifies an evidence-based program that matches its needs, values, and resources and modifies or adopts elements of the program to maximize community acceptance, implementation, and sustainability. Researchers often work in close collaboration with community leaders to find ways to integrate components of prevention programs in ways that are acceptable and meaningful to the community and to evaluate results.

There is long-standing consensus that health promotion and prevention programs should be culturally sensitive, along with concerns about whether a given prevention intervention is generic enough to be efficacious and effective with diverse cultures (Resnicow, Baranowski, et al., 1999; Seto, 2001; Woods, Montgomery, and Herring, 2004; Weeks, Schensul, et al., 1995; Hutchinson and Cooney, 1998). Prevention programs must also be mindful of developmental processes, reinforcements of risk behavior, relevant contextual factors, and a population's unique risk profile (Brown, DiClemente, and Park, 1992).

A few studies have shown that making adaptations to different cultural groups while maintaining core elements of programs implemented with fidelity can produce strong results across different cultural groups (Botvin, Schinke, et al., 1994; Botvin, Baker, et al., 1995; Botvin, Schinke, et al., 1995; Reid, Webster-Stratton, and Beauchaine, 2001). However, there is currently no consensus and limited scientific evidence on the key elements that determine the necessary balance between program adaptation and program fidelity.

Bell, Bhana, and colleagues (2008) point out that, for an intervention to be culturally sensitive, it must have content that is welcoming to the target culture, contain issues of relevance to the culture, not be offensive, and be familiar to and endorsed by the culture. If a given intervention embodies generic principles of health behavior change, such as aspects that create social fabric, generate connectedness, help develop social skills, build self-esteem, facilitate some social monitoring, and help minimize trauma (Bell, Flay, and Paikoff, 2002), it can usually be adapted to have an appropriate level of cultural sensitivity (Bhana, Petersen, et al., 2004; Peterson, 2004; LaFromboise and Lewis, 2008; LaFromboise, 1995). For example, if going on a spirit quest builds self-esteem in American Indian culture, efforts to build self-esteem in American Indians might best be served by a spirit quest exercise instead of formation of a soccer team (Bell, 2005; see also

BOX 11-2
A Program Adaptation for an American Indian Population

An American Indian tribe in the Southwest worked in collaboration with academic researchers to create the American Indian Life Skills (AILS) intervention for the purpose of reducing the factors associated with suicidal behavior (LaFromboise and Lewis, 2008). AILS was found to have a positive impact on American Indian high school students' feelings of hopelessness, suicidal ideation, and ability to intervene in a peer suicidal crisis situation (LaFromboise and Howard-Pitney, 1993). When used as a comprehensive suicide prevention approach, the intervention demonstrated a substantial drop in suicidal gestures and attempts. Although suicide deaths neither declined significantly nor increased, the total number of self-destructive acts declined by 73 percent (May, Sena, et al., 2005).

Extensive input was solicited from members of the tribe initiating AILS in order to fit its cultural norms. Key aspects of giving instruction, problem solving, and helping others in that culture were examined. Focus groups members were selected by community leaders to give guidance on intervention content, implementation issues, and intervention refinement. It was believed that suicidal behavior could be attributed to direct modeling influences (e.g., peer or extended family member's suicidal behavior) in conjunction with environmental influences (e.g., geographic isolation) and individual characteristics (e.g., hopelessness, drug use) that mediate decisions related to self-destructive behavior.

Life Skills Training was used throughout the intervention to complement traditional ways of shaping behavior. Each skill-building activity was selected from research supporting best practices for social emotional regulation and cognitive skills development, including methods of group cognitive and behavioral treatment.

Needed modifications were made to strategies identified. For example, in lessons on recognizing and overcoming depression, the Pleasant Events Schedule (Lewinsohn, Munoz, et al., 1986) was modified to reflect American Indian adolescent socialization in the reservation context, renamed "Depression Busters," and used as the basis for both an intervention activity and a homework assignment. Items such as "talking on the telephone" or "playing a musical instrument" were retained, while new items, such as "doing heavy outdoor work (e.g., cutting or chopping wood, clearing land)" or "being at weddings and other ceremonies," were added. In lessons addressing stress management, the eight ways of coping advanced by Folkman and Lazarus were shared in the focus groups to better determine cultural coping preferences and coping styles (Folkman, Lazarus, et al., 1986). The coping strategies most highly endorsed by participants in these groups were emphasized throughout the intervention. This "hybrid-like" approach (Castro, Barrera, and Martinez, 2004) encouraged the inclusion of traditional and contemporary tribal world views in the intervention without compromising its core psychological components.

After several formative evaluations with diverse tribal groups, AILS has been refined to address the needs of both traditional and pan-tribal adolescents (LaFromboise, 1995; LaFromboise, Coleman, and Hernandez, 1991). It has been

continued

BOX 11-2 Continued

implemented by interventionists (including teachers) for work with urban and reservation youth during in-school, after-school, and community-based programs for American Indian youth. AILS is thought to be broad enough to address concerns across diverse American Indian tribal groups yet respectful of distinctive and heterogeneous cultural beliefs and practices. The program received support in 2007 from three suicide prevention projects, funded by the Substance Abuse and Mental Health Services Administration, to train American Indian interventionists on a wide-scale basis, to complete an early adolescent version of the intervention, and to create an implementation guide. Efforts to evaluate AILS in an urban Indian education program are currently under way.

Box 11-2). Bernal, Bonilla, and Bellido (1995) provide a framework for developing culturally sensitive interventions that calls for consideration of language, persons, metaphors, content, concepts, goals, methods, and context.

On the other hand, research has indicated that, although cultural or other adaptations made by practitioners that reduce dosage or eliminate critical core content can increase retention by up to 40 percent, they also reduce positive outcomes (Kumpfer, Alvarado, et al., 2002). For example, efforts to create and disseminate best-practice components of the Nurse-Family Partnership Program failed to produce the same results as the controlled trial replications (Alper, 2002; Olds, 2002). While research on dissemination of tested and effective prevention programs appears warranted, more research to identify the active ingredients of those programs is required before adaptation and dissemination of best practices distilled from these programs are warranted.

In general, there has been a dearth of research on cultural, racial, and ethnic issues involved in interventions aimed at preventing mental, emotional, and behavioral (MEB) disorders (U.S. Public Health Service, 2001a) and even less research on the effectiveness of specific prevention strategies when implemented in a population other than that originally targeted by a trial. However, several models are being used to examine the extent to which program adaptation can be used to address the unique cultural needs of communities. Castro, Barrera, and Martinez (2004), for example, describe a hybrid approach to modifying the content and delivery of an existing prevention program. This area needs more research, as few empirical studies have examined alternative strategies.

One method of enhancing cultural sensitivity and cultural relevance is to involve the community in every aspect of a prevention trial (LaFromboise and Lewis, 2008; LaFromboise, 1996; Madison, McKay, et al., 2000; McCormick, McKay, et al., 2000; Baptiste, Blachman, et al., 2007; Bell, Bhana, et al., 2007; McKay, Hibbert, et al., 2007; Pinto, McKay, et al., 2007). However, developing and maintaining community involvement throughout all stages of program implementation present considerable challenges, as discussed below.

Community-Driven Implementation

Community-driven implementation builds heavily on the decision making of community leaders, often in partnership with researchers, with a focus on improving the community relevance and sustainability of a program. Implementation is guided by a community-driven agenda and staged implementation of a prevention program, in some cases including development, implementation, and testing of a locally developed intervention. Evidence-based programs or principles are often introduced by research partners relatively late in the process. Built on the community-based participatory research approach, an agenda for community action is developed through a cooperative process with community members and multiple community constituencies. The involvement of researchers in identifying priorities may be quite limited or very involved (Minkler, 2004), but it always focuses on community leadership and establishment of an organizational structure for building and sustaining one or more interventions (Baptiste, Blachman, et al., 2007). In many minority communities, there is a history of mistrust of outsiders, government agencies, or researchers in particular (Thomas and Quinn, 1991), which influences the degree to which researchers are involved in decision making (McKay, Hibbert, et al., 2007).

The traditions of research, including reliance on planned research designs, multiple assessments, and legal consent documents, are often viewed negatively by communities. Thus, researchers may begin as outside advisers who listen to the goals and needs of communities, with a partnership in the decision-making processes evolving over time. The wealth of practical experience and wisdom in community-based organizations may offer opportunities for communities to establish an empirical basis for interventions with strong community support through community–research partnerships. Collaborations with key community constituents can (1) enhance the relevance of research questions, (2) help develop research procedures that are acceptable to potential community participants from diverse cultures, (3) address challenges to conducting community-based research, (4) maximize the usefulness of research findings, and (5) foster the development of community-based resources to sustain prevention funding beyond grant funding (Israel, Schulz, et al., 1998; Institute of

Medicine, 1998; Schensul, 1999; Jensen, Hoagwood, and Trickett, 1999; Wandersman, 2003). Efforts to move from efficacy and effectiveness to full-scale implementation can and often do begin early by establishing such partnerships (Fixsen, Naoom, et al., 2005).

A number of prevention specialists have called for the scientific study of community–research partnerships (Chinman, Hannah, et al., 2005; Spoth and Greenberg, 2005; Trickett and Espino, 2004; Wandersman, 2003). The principles that guide such partnerships are clear and involve researchers developing win-win relationships with communities in their efforts to foster trust and mutual respect (see Madison, McKay, et al., 2000; Israel, Schulz, et al., 2003; Trickett and Espino, 2004; Bell, Bhana, et al., 2007; McKay, Hibbert, et al., 2007; Pinto, McKay, et al., 2007). Researchers and community collaborators should attempt to develop shared vision and mission,

---

BOX 11-3
CHAMP: Collaborative HIV Adolescent Mental Health Program

The Community Collaborative Board for the CHAMP project builds on the framework for an academic–community collaborative approach to HIV/AIDS risk reduction with urban adolescents (McKay, Hibbert, et al., 2007). The mission was "if the community likes the program, the research staff will help the community find ways to continue the program on its own" (Madison, McKay, et al., 2000).

The CHAMP Community Collaborative Board structure is characterized by moderate- to high-intensity collaboration (Hatch, Moss, et al., 1993). All of the CHAMP Family Programs use community representatives as liaisons between youth and families in need and prevention programs, as suggested by research (Koroloff, Elliott, et al., 1994; McKay and Paikoff, 2007). Community parent facilitators, who had participated in the program themselves, are trained to reach out to their neighbors and invite them to learn more about the program. In addition to providing factual program information, they are also able to share personal, firsthand program experience.

Community members also play a role in delivering the intervention, helping to address issues of cultural sensitivity and addressing research concerns of efficacy and effectiveness while preparing the community for dissemination. All of the intervention sessions are cofacilitated by a mental health intern/parent facilitator team. The team receives weekly joint training in program content; skills related to facilitation of child, parent, and multiple family groups; and issues related to prevention research and protection of human subjects, including confidentiality and mandated safety issues.

Grant funding to enhance leadership development among community board members was secured to help pave the way for the community to take over the

consensus on strategies, and synergy in execution and implementation (Senge, 1994). Resources should be openly discussed with community members, who should benefit from the resources as much as do the researchers. Thus resources, both tangible (e.g., researchers employing community members and partners providing facilities for programs) and intangible (e.g., partners' knowledge of participants and researchers' knowledge of research methods), should be shared (Suarez-Balcazar, Davis, et al., 2003). Collaboration must also involve team training in which researchers learn community issues and community partners learn research issues. Early involvement of communities, power sharing, mutual respect, community benefit, and cultural sensitivity (Sullivan, Kone, et al., 2001) are needed to meet these challenges. Box 11-3 describes a program aimed at HIV/AIDS risk reduction that is built on such a collaborative model.

intervention from the research team (Madison, McKay, and the CHAMP Collaborative Board, 1998). Community support was hypothesized to facilitate wider dissemination of prevention messages and strategies (Galbraith, Ricardo, et al., 1996; Schenshul, 1999; Stevenson and White, 1994). The team believed that given the business skills necessary to run such programs, large community-based agencies might be more able than academic research teams to retain proven programs within their infrastructure, enhancing the likelihood that a specific program would be sustained over time (Galbraith, Ricardo, et al., 1996; Goark and McCall, 1996). Community leaders were also responsible for the day-to-day research operation (with consultation from university researchers) (McKay, Chasse, et al., 2004).

CHAMP-Chicago and New York were also funded to study how to transfer an academic research project (based at the University of Illinois in Chicago and Mt. Sinai School of Medicine in New York), with both efficacy and effectiveness components. For example, in Chicago the program was transferred to a community-based organization (Habilitative Systems Inc., a social service agency in urban Chicago). Key elements of the framework for this 13-year transfer are (1) ensuring a good academic-agency fit, (2) early planning for sustainability, (3) building in continuous quality improvement, and (4) balancing program adaptation with fidelity (Baptiste, Blachman, et al., 2007).

The experience implementing the CHAMP Program in Chicago and New York helped inform the 2001 CHAMP-South Africa research project. Based on its success, in 2007, the South African HIV prevention intervention obtained private foundation funding to serve 500 families, many of whom were in the control condition during the study.

EXAMPLES OF EXPERIENCE WITH IMPLEMENTATION
OF EXISTING PREVENTION PROGRAMS

In all fields of health, including the prevention of MEB disorders, there is a time lag between documentation that an intervention, program, policy, or practice improves health in a defined community and successful adoption of that program in society (Walker, Grimshaw, et al., 2003; Walker, Seeley, et al., 2008). Levels of implementation of preventive interventions are rarely measured; however, more information is available on implementation of substance abuse prevention in schools than on other prevention interventions. In a national study of middle schools, Ringwalt, Ennett, and colleagues (2002) found that, while 81.8 percent of public and private schools offered a substance abuse prevention curriculum, only 26.8 percent were using 1 of 10 tested and effective curricula. Furthermore, even when schools and communities use tested and effective programs, they often fail to implement them with fidelity to the standards delineated by program designers (Ennett, Ringwalt, et al., 2003; Mitchell, Florin, and Stevenson, 2002; Wandersman and Florin, 2003).

The National Study of Delinquency Prevention in Schools (Gottfredson and Gottfredson, 2002) found that only half of drug prevention curricula and one-fourth of mentoring programs met "dosage" requirements (amount of students' exposure to the subject). The rest delivered fewer and less frequent sessions than were specified by program developers. Moreover, only half of the programs were taught in accordance with the recommended methods of instruction.

Hallfors and Godette (2002) report that only 19 percent of all surveyed school districts faithfully implemented tested and effective prevention curricula. Similarly, Ennett, Ringwalt, and colleagues (2003) found that only 14 percent of middle school teachers of drug prevention curricula exposed their students to adequate content and means of delivery. Yet adherence to core program components is important to ensure outcomes. There is evidence that some tested and effective prevention programs work only when implemented with a high degree of fidelity (Abbott, O'Donnell, et al., 1998; Botvin, Mihalic, and Grotpeter, 1998; Henggeler, Brondino, et al., 1997; Kam, Greenberg, and Wells, 2003; Olweus, Limber, and Mihalic, 1999). Methods for widespread dissemination of tested and effective prevention policies and programs with high levels of fidelity are needed (Farrington and Welsh, 2006; Spoth and Greenberg, 2005; Wandersman and Florin, 2003).

Often, federal or state guidelines dictate reimbursement only for using approved or evidence-based programs. For example, the tobacco settlement money from several states allows for funding of specifically named prevention programs. Colorado amended its revised statutes to provide continued funding for the Colorado Nurse-Family Partnership Program. Recent congressional action related to child abuse programs sets aside funds for competitive state grants to implement evidence-based home visitation models.

Numerous guidelines for best practices in program implementation have been published at the federal and state levels, although somewhat different, and sometimes confusing, criteria have been used for the selection of recommended programs across reviews and federal agencies (see Chapter 12). The Blueprints for Violence Prevention project at the University of Colorado, originally stimulated with federal funds from the U.S. Department of Justice, was institutionalized as an effort to facilitate community-level adoption of specific violence prevention interventions. Similarly, the Safe Schools Healthy Students Initiative, a joint program of three federal agencies, encourages the use of evidence-based programs. However, empirical evidence of the implementation experiences or results of this program are lacking.

One of the most promising approaches to prevention involves early education of children to prepare them for the challenges of reading and learning, as well as to help them develop the social skills necessary to develop positive relations with their peers as well as adults. Yet far fewer children in the United States ages 3-5 receive preschool or center-based early education than is the case in many other developed countries (Yosikawah, Schindler, and Caronongen, 2007). Children from poor families and children with less educated mothers are dramatically less likely to receive these services compared with those with higher incomes and mothers with more education (U.S. Department of Education, 2007).

Although there are exceptions, overall implementation of effective interventions has been modest at best. Scientific evidence of health benefits and standard methods of dissemination alone appear to work only under limited circumstances. Successful examples of implementation that do exist across the life span and across different settings are reviewed below.

Implementation of Prevention Programs in Early Childhood

Chapter 6 outlines a number of early childhood programs that have demonstrated positive outcomes for children and their families. The history of one promising program implemented in multiple states provides important lessons on the significance of implementation fidelity and program design. Healthy Families America (HFA) is a program aiming to prevent child abuse and neglect that was modeled after the Hawaii Healthy Start program and implemented state-wide in several states. The core of this program involves identifying parents at high risk of abuse and neglect of their children. Parents are identified through broad-based screening and then offered voluntary home visiting services delivered by paraprofessionals for a period of three to five years (Duggan, McFarlane, et al., 2004). A study conducted in Hawaii yielded disappointing results, with as many negative as positive impacts on key family process outcomes (Duggan, McFarlane, et al., 2004). The evaluators offered several potential explanations for these results: The program may have been poorly implemented, as half (51 percent) of the parents dropped out within the first year and participating families received fewer home visits than intended; the paraprofessional staff may not have had sufficient skills to identify high-risk situations and engage parents in the process of reducing risks associated with abusive parenting; and a shift away from an emphasis on recognizing and addressing risks for abusive parenting toward an early intervention philosophy of parent-driven goal setting, which was caused by funding requirements, may have compromised its effectiveness.

A recent evaluation of an augmented HFA program, with a sharper focus on using cognitive appraisal theory to reduce risks for abuse and neglect, as well as better implementation practices, yielded considerably more favorable results compared with both the unenhanced HFA program and a control group that did not receive any home visiting services (Bugental, Ellerson, et al., 2002). These positive findings were particularly evident for medically vulnerable infants, such as those born prematurely or those with low Apgar scores (assessing physical condition after delivery) at birth. Although the study was small and thus in need of replication, this finding illustrates the current effort among the nation's largest home visiting models to use evaluation findings to promote program improvement. The lessons learned from this study (i.e., the importance of engaging families, providing high-quality training and ongoing supervision of staff, and ensuring consistent and well-implemented service delivery) illustrate the value of program accountability as a strategy for continuous enhancement rather than as a vehicle for terminating potentially effective services that produce initially disappointing results. Similarly, lessons learned from the Healthy Families New York evaluation (see Chapter 6) reinforce the likely value of targeting first-time mothers with limited resources.

The implementation of quality early childhood programs at scale continues to be a vexing problem in the field. Few evaluations have linked implementation quality to the magnitude of impacts on children's social-emotional or mental health outcomes. Research from Early Head Start's 17-site evaluation has shown that sites with earlier and more complete implementation, as measured by the Early Head Start Program Performance Standards, had stronger positive impacts on child social-emotional and cognitive outcomes than those with later or less complete implementation (Love, Kisker, et al., 2002). Other research on quality in at-scale programs has found that Head Start classrooms in general are in the "good" (though not "excellent") range of quality on the Early Childhood Environment Ratings Scale (Administration for Children and Families, 2006). Research on the impacts of thresholds of quality in this and other scales measuring early childhood care and education environments is currently lacking. Nursery and preschool programs represent a clear opportunity to intervene early in the lives of young children.

Implementation of Prevention Programs in Schools

The implementation of universal school-based interventions faces considerable challenges, including access to and approval of schools that are often overburdened with other academic and policy-related priorities. Multiple levels of approval from superintendents, principals, teachers, and school boards and community partners may also be required. In addition, the relatively low dosage that is common to most universal strategies may not offer sufficient exposure to impact children already at very high risk for a specific disorder (e.g., depression or anxiety). Universal interventions are likely to be most effective when they have sufficient duration and intensity, target the development of protective factors and resilience likely to impact risk for multiple disorders, or target problems common to a large segment of the population (e.g., bullying, early alcohol use).

Nevertheless, there are several opportunities for successful implementation in schools, particularly since there has been a substantial change in legislation focused on evidence-based prevention at both the federal and state levels. Two dramatic examples are the Safe and Drug-Free Schools Act of 1999, which states "principles of effectiveness," and the No Child Left Behind Act of 2001 (NCLB), which calls for school districts to implement evidence-based programming (Hallfors and Godette, 2002). Other opportunities have been created by several state legislatures that have mandated the use of character education in schools.

Prevention programs relevant to schools focus on the school and its structure (organizational features, school rules), classroom behavior management, and curricula that teach students new skills, recently termed social-emotional learning (see Chapters 6 and 7). Some form of curricula-oriented prevention programs for substance abuse is in a large number of the nation's middle schools.

Schools have also become a venue for both targeted and indicated interventions. As an example, Title I Part A provides additional funding to schools that have poverty levels above 40 percent, and such programs can be delivered either universally or in a targeted fashion to those at higher risk. Some school-based indicated interventions focus on children who are showing early indications of a potential disorder (e.g., high rates of aggressive behavior, anxiety, depression, or other forms of maladjustment). These interventions are also usually provided in special groups, and most support the development of social and emotional learning skills. For some prevention programs, school is only one of several components that also may include family or community-based interventions. However, given the extra costs associated with multicomponent interventions, they are more often used with either selective or indicated models (e.g., the Incredible Years; Webster-Stratton, 1998), or with universal models that occur in high-risk neighborhood schools (e.g., Seattle Social Development project; Hawkins, Kosterman, et al., 2005).

Implementation of Prevention in Child Welfare and Juvenile Justice Settings

In one study of scale-up of an intervention to help foster parents improve their children's emotional and behavioral functioning (Multidimensional Treatment Foster Care), a "cascading training model" was used and tested for effectiveness. After an initial phase representing an efficacy trial, a second phase of treatment for foster parents was delivered by paraprofessionals, who were intensively overseen by an onsite supervisor and an experienced clinical consultant. During a third phase, the paraprofessionals trained a second cohort of staff. In this phase, the clinical consultants oversaw the supervision but did not have any direct contact with the new staff. The evaluation found that both phases resulted in decreases in children's problem behaviors, with no significant difference between the two phases. This suggests that intensive training and supervision can enable "third-generation" staff to scale up and implement an intervention with fidelity (Price, Chamberlain, et al., 2008).

Implementation of Prevention in Primary Care Settings

Few preventive interventions have been tested in primary care settings, although collaborative treatment models involving primary care and behavioral health staff have begun to emerge (Forrest, Glade, et al., 1999; Guevara, Rothbard, et al., 2007), and physicians should routinely screen for behavioral and developmental concerns (see Chapter 8). Pediatric primary care settings are seeing significant numbers of patients with mental health problems (Horowitz, Leaf, et al., 1992; Briggs-Gown, Horwitz, et al., 2000; Kelleher, McInerney, et al., 2000), with some estimates that the number of office visits for mental health problems has increased by 2.5 (Kelleher, McInerney, et al., 2000; Zito, Safer, et al., 1999). One promising primary care intervention involves a strategy to encourage teens to use a primary care Internet-based intervention to prevent depression (Van Voorhees, Ellis, et al., 2007). As outlined in Chapter 8, primary care settings represent a significant opportunity for development of new approaches to identify and respond to parents' concerns about their children's behavioral and emotional health. Such approaches would facilitate coordination of all the children's health care needs and reinforce the integral nature of physical and mental health care needs.

IMPLEMENTATION CHALLENGES

Fixsen, Naoom, and colleagues (2005) note that "[successful] implementation is synonymous with coordinated change at system, organization, program, and practice levels." This coordination is not easy to achieve, and indeed these authors note that poor implementation of a beneficial program can come from unsupportive policies or regulations or a lack of funding opportunities at the federal, state, or local level; a lack of organizational commitment, capacity, or leadership; poorly chosen or high turnover among intervention agents or practitioners; or a lack of involvement in or ownership in the program by the community. Until recently there has been little support from the federal or state governments for prevention activities and even less for building an infrastructure that facilitates these efforts. It is also often difficult to sustain attention on a specific problem, as evidenced by the current lowering of priorities for HIV prevention and youth tobacco prevention (U.S. Government Accountability Office, 2007; Institute of Medicine, 2006b).

Coordinating all these issues would be difficult enough if policy makers, organizations, practitioners, community leaders, and consumers all spoke the same language and shared a common vision. However, these groups often have vastly different world views and priorities and are often reluctant to learn about each others' perspectives.

The previous sections have described some key challenges to the implementation of preventive interventions, including the need to balance cultural adaptation and fidelity, the difficulty of forming essential community-research partnerships, and the time lag between documentation that an implementation is effective and its successful adoption. This section reviews additional implementation challenges: funding; service system priorities; training, monitoring, and capacity building; data systems; low participation and retention rates; and organizational context.

Funding

Obtaining adequate funding is a challenge for all types of implementation. Program cost, including the cost of labor, materials, and technical assistance, is often just as or even more important to communities and policy makers than effectiveness. Yet not only are evaluations of the benefits and costs of prevention programs relatively uncommon (see Chapter 9), but also collection of cost data is as well. In one analysis of prevention programs targeting children younger than age 5, cost data were available for only a small percentage of the studies (Brown, Berndt, et al., 2000).

There have been limited commitment and funding for prevention training and materials at government and community levels (Hallfors, Pankratz, and Hartman, 2007), with few targeted funding sources and available sources providing limited amounts. For example, SDFS, which represents 70 percent of school funding for drug prevention programs, provides an average of only $6.30 per child (Hallfors, Pankratz, and Hartman, 2007), well below the copying costs let alone the costs of training and sustaining an effective prevention program. Furthermore, two-thirds of the states do not provide any additional funding beyond that provided by SDFS. A report on Nevada's implementation of school-based substance abuse and violence prevention programs concluded that funding was inadequate in most school districts to implement the type of prevention program needed (Nevada State Department of Education, 1998). Half of the states have two or fewer full-time staff available to support schools' selection and implementation of drug prevention programs statewide (Hallfors, Pankratz, and Hartman, 2007). The Safe Schools/Healthy Students Grant Program, funded jointly by three federal agencies, aims to help local communities develop integrated programming that involves prevention, treatment, and school reform efforts in K-12 based on evidence-based interventions. However, although over 150 communities have been funded through this program, there is as yet little published research on this model.

Service System Priorities

Prevention is often tangential or only weakly related to the mission of the institutions and communities in which its programs could be housed, leading to limited infrastructure to support and sustain prevention programs in their natural settings (Greenberg, 2004; Spoth, Greenberg, et al., 2004). For example, integrating mental health and drug prevention into the existing primary health care system would require more accessible reimbursement mechanisms. The mental health system, which is primarily focused on treatment of disorder, would need to be reoriented.

Similarly, the primary mission of schools is to educate students, with an emphasis on core subjects, like science, math, history, and reading; it is unlikely that they will support a program that does not directly relate to this primary mission (Kellam, 2000). American schools face many competing demands, and education leaders must make difficult choices about priorities (Adelman and Taylor, 2000; Berends, Bodilly, and Kirby, 2002; Hall and Hord, 2001). Currently most education leaders focus on the student academic performance requirements of the NCLB. While a potential benefit of the act is the promotion of academic excellence and equity, it has also led to high-stakes testing, a narrowing of the curriculum, and a loss of the "whole child" in education. Critics caution that, without attending to students' social and emotional needs, many of these actions may be ineffective at best and harmful at worst, especially for economically disadvantaged groups (Meier and Woods, 2004). A consequence of NCLB has been a marginalization of most prevention efforts, as they have not been well linked to educational outcomes (especially achievement test scores). Few prevention programs take the time or effort to integrate into the schools' central mission (Smith, Swisher, et al., 2004). In fact, few even assess academic performance as an outcome (Hoagwood, Olin, et al., 2007; Durlak, Weissberg, et al., 2007), although there is some indication that programs focused on social and emotional learning can increase academic achievement (Durlak, Weissberg, et al., 2007).

As a result of federal and state legislation, U.S. schools are rapidly reorganizing and striving to develop broader and more comprehensive models of reform that use clear goals, standards, and benchmarks for outcomes (Education Commission of the States, 2001; Togerni and Anderson, 2003). As empirically validated programs have accumulated and been increasingly adopted (Ringwalt, Ennett, et al., 2002), schools are searching for integrated models with a clear scope and sequence from prekindergarten through grade 12 (Collaborative for Academic, Social, and Emotional Learning, 2003; Elias, Zins, et al., 1997). Current evidence-based programs span relatively small parts of this age span.

As the process of school reform grows, researchers and practitioners will need to work together to develop pre-K-12 guidelines and consider how all the elements of evidence-based programs and policies fit together in the context of an overall schoolwide or school district effort, how they increase students' school success, and how to ensure that coordinated, multiyear programs will be implemented effectively (Adelman and Taylor, 2000; Osher, Dwyer, and Jackson, 2002). Integration of program models across developmental periods, long-term curricular planning involving both researchers and practitioners, adequate local infrastructure to support prevention activities, teacher training and technical assistance, and appropriate evaluation of process and outcome must be part of this process (Greenberg, Weissberg, et al., 2003). Legislation in both Illinois and New York now requires that schools develop plans for social and emotional learning, models for learning standards, and benchmarks across all grade levels.

School–community systems with programming integrated between universal, classroom programs and either selective prevention (e.g., counselor-led programs with students who are experiencing divorce, bereavement, or other trauma), indicated prevention (for children identified as having aggression, peer problems, prodromal signs of depression, etc.), or treatment are rare. The fragmented nature of the models created by curriculum developers and researchers as well as the often fragmented planning between schools, government agencies, and the private sector of human services contribute to this problem.

Social settings that have not been often targeted to house preventive interventions include important microsystems and exosystems (systems that affect the child but do not directly include the child, such as a parent's workplace) of human development (Bronfenbrenner and Morris, 1998). Workforce development organizations, for example, have the potential to influence parental employment, which in turn is related to early childhood development. Community-based organizations (aside from child care and preschool programs) have also been underutilized. They may be settings that families trust (e.g., organizations serving immigrant populations) and that therefore may be productive settings for child- or family-focused programs. The primary health care system has also generally been overlooked as a setting for preventive interventions. Finally, the bulk of child care–based interventions have occurred in center-based settings, with family day care settings rarely targeted for quality improvement or implementation of specific preventive curricula.

Other service systems also have potentially much to gain from prevention. Communities have to invest significant resources to handle delinquent youth through the juvenile justice system, to counter ineffective or unsafe parenting through the foster care system, and to counter difficulties in learning or behavior through special education. The missions of all these programs are clear: to provide services to those who are in serious need. However, these systems usually do not embrace the mission of preventing these problems from arising in the first place. Unless prevention can find ways to integrate its work into the central missions of these and other community institutions (Kellam, 2000), the prevention focus will continue to be lacking.

Two reports of the Institute of Medicine call for an increase in bidirectional communication between researchers and organizations and social service settings in which prevention can be housed (Institute of Medicine, 1994, 1998). It seems sensible that research efforts should be directed toward understanding and facilitating such communications, although little research has been conducted in this area. One study, surveying both researchers and practitioners who attended the same bereavement conference on modes of communication, found relatively modest overlap (Bridging Work Group, 2005).

Training, Monitoring, and Capacity Building

A review by Mihalic and Irwin (2003) concluded that a consistently important factor in the success or failure of implementation of evidence-based interventions is the quality of ongoing technical assistance. With appropriate training and monitoring, programs can be disseminated with fidelity (Fagan and Mihalic, 2003; Spoth, Guyll, et al., 2007; Spoth, Redmond, et al., 2007). However, systems for delivering proactive technical assistance are limited and generally not up to the task required for large-scale dissemination (Mitchell, Florin, and Stevenson, 2002). For example, the Blueprints project attempted to implement a set of 10 empirically supported programs, but only 4 of these programs had sufficient organizational capacity to implement the intervention in 10 different communities per year (Elliott and Mihalic, 2004). The Blueprints project has a rigorous system for identifying violence prevention programs with a very high level of evidence, facilitates tests of replication of promising programs, disseminates knowledge of these programs to communities, and provides technical support for community implementation, with the direct involvement of the program's developers. One of its key findings was that both the program developers and the implementation sites often required substantial multiyear technical assistance. For schools, the major training difficulties were lack of time to work with the model and the need for continual training due to staff turnover (Elliott and Mihalic, 2004). With intensive effort, however, sites were able to implement chosen programs with high fidelity, often approaching or exceeding the level of fidelity achieved by the program developers in the original study.

The Blueprints project examined the degree to which chosen programs were adapted locally, even though most of the intervention trainers discouraged adaptation. Very little local adaptation in these particular programs was needed to achieve acceptance, participation, and quality implementation, even in diverse communities, and fidelity and sustainability were emphasized. However, by design, Blueprints does not evaluate impact on behavioral outcomes in the implementation communities, relying instead on each program's earlier empirical success. It is possible that the programs had different rates of success in the implementation sites compared with those in the original studies.

To address capacity-building and training needs, the Nurse-Family Partnership has established a nonprofit National Service Office to develop community capacity to implement a home visitation program with high fidelity and provide training and technical assistance (Olds, Hill, et al., 2003).

In addition to training and technical assistance provided by program developers, other organizations, including federally funded technical assistance centers (see Box 12-2) and state-level organizations (Pennsylvania Commission on Crime and Delinquency;[1] Neal, Altman and Burritt, 2003; New York State Office of Mental Health[2]) are providing assistance in implementing prevention programs, particularly substance abuse and violence prevention programs. In addition, programs are being encouraged to provide manuals and other materials to assist in the implementation of programs.

Data Systems

Data systems that integrate family, school, and developmental information could be a useful tool for targeting and monitoring prevention programs. NCLB legislation has provided an as yet unattained opportunity to use academic information to inform prevention needs. Integration of service and data systems for early childhood health, learning, and mental health, for example, could reduce duplication of services, track families across systems, identify children and families who are particularly vulnerable, link family need levels to services, and assess delivery and outcomes for diverse families in particular communities (Knitzer and Lefkowitz, 2006; Schorr and Marchand, 2007).

Such integration has recently become a policy focus in the early childhood field. For example, the Maternal and Child Health Bureau's Early Childhood Comprehensive Systems initiative funds states (currently 47) to help coordinate services related to early health care, education, mental health, and family support (Johnson and Theberge, 2007). Studies in other state policy areas (e.g., state-level expenditures on state prekindergarten related to children's cognitive and social-emotional outcomes in the Early Childhood Longitudinal Study-Kindergarten Cohort; Magnuson, Ruhm, and Waldfogel, 2007) could be applied to future studies on state variation in early childhood policies, such as systems coordination. Controlling for other unobserved state policy characteristics, such as concurrent policy change in other areas, is a challenge. In general, evaluation and quality improvement approaches require adequate data collection, storage, and analysis.

Low Participation and Retention Rates

An intervention may be poorly implemented due to a community's being overly optimistic about its capacity to provide the intervention to

---

[1] See http://prevention.psu.edu/project/delinquencyandviolenceprevention.html.

[2] See http://www.omh.state.ny.us/omhweb/sv/schlviol.htm.

sufficient numbers of the target population (Chinman, Hannah, et al., 2005; Miller and Shinn, 2005). Brown and Liao (1999) note that "even well-designed, efficacious interventions may fail when they are not delivered or implemented at full strength." These authors opine that an intervention may not succeed if a high level of participation cannot be sustained throughout the intervention period. They note, as well, that an intervention's benefit vanishes if there is low participation or if the intervention is not delivered to those who are likely to benefit from it. Individual choice to participate is not a major factor in the adoption of universal classroom or school prevention programs by a school because they generally involve all students. The same is not true of programs that require individuals to choose to participate, including most selective or indicated prevention programs. Often, when one of these prevention programs administered individually or by a small group is available in a community, proportionally few families opt to participate in it (Flay, Biglan, et al., 2005).

When there is low individual-level participation, the overall benefit of the program in the community will typically also be low (population-level benefit is the proportion who participate times the effect size for the participants) (Braver and Smith, 1996; Brown and Liao, 1999). The overall effectiveness of family-based prevention programs (Reid, Webster-Stratton, and Hammond, 2003; Spoth and Redmond, 2000; Epstein, 1991; Eccles and Harold, 1996; Sheldon, 2003; Ialongo, Werthamer, et al., 1999) is particularly affected by low participation levels because families often make individual choices to participate, both initially and over time.

For example, a significant number of families enrolled in home visitation programs drop out over the course of two to three years. Ialongo, Werthamer, and colleagues (1999) had reasonably high population-based participation rates (35 percent of all first grade parents attended six of the seven sessions, 13 percent attended none of the sessions), with families on average receiving half the intervention, and positive long-term results. Family-based programs focusing on stressful events, such as divorce (Wolchik, Sandler, et al., 2002; Forgatch and DeGarmo, 1999) or bereavement (Sandler, Ayers, et al., 2003), as well as community-wide parent training (Brody, Murray, 2006b), also require extensive community engagement and recruitment to get acceptable participation levels. A critical concern for family-based programs is to increase participation, particularly for the subset at high risk that could most benefit (Brown and Liao, 1999). In addition, attention is needed for strategies for increasing participation rates in real-world contexts that may not be able to offer the same incentives possible in the research context.

Lack of cultural relevance may contribute to low participation. However, universal family prevention programs designed specifically for specific minority groups (Brody, Murry, 2006b; Prado, Pantin, et al., 2007) have also experienced significant recruitment challenges. The use of focus groups and community partnerships to adapt the intervention and select settings for data collection and intervention, as well as inclusion of program and evaluation staff with similar cultural backgrounds, have allowed these studies to maintain excellent participation rates over time (Murry and Brody, 2004). Other factors may also contribute to low participation rates, including the stigma associated with a program aimed at mental health, substance use, or problem behaviors; competing family demands, including multiple jobs or shift work; and community distrust of researchers.

Organizational Context

Successful implementation, including the ability to sustain a program, requires investments in people, relationships, and time, as well as coordination around such critical issues as staffing and funding (Neumann and Sogolow, 2000). Organizations with little flexibility, fewer connections with professionals, and limited history with innovation may be the most in need of change but least capable of achieving it (Rogers, 1995; Kondrat, Greene, and Winbush, 2002; Hoagwood, Burns, et al., 2001; Schoenwald and Hoagwood, 2001). Many agencies that lack academic or other affiliations often need technical assistance, staff support, and implementation resources to implement preventive interventions (Spoth, Kavanagh, and Dishion, 2002). Community-based agencies often grapple with high staff turnover and lack of adequate space, facilities, and equipment, all of which can interfere with sustainability (Kellam and Langevin, 2003; Swisher, 2000). Technical tasks, such as maintenance of data systems to assess risk factors, fidelity, outcomes, and satisfaction, are especially challenging when implementation is guided by community-based organizations or partnerships (Dzewaltowski, Estabrooks, et al., 2004).

Empirical work demonstrates that the types of changes required to implement and sustain preventive interventions are difficult to achieve. Robertson, Roberts, and Porras (1993) noted in a meta-analysis that organizations that aimed at changing factors, such as organizational climate and culture, along with technological and strategic factors, were more successful than organizations that targeted only one of these areas. Valente's (1996) social network threshold model for innovation, which pairs local champions of a program—who can provide information outside the organization about a program—with those in an organization who can change or shape its agenda is relevant to implementation of prevention programs.

Both organizational climate and culture reflect the norms, expectations, and values of the organization, and they have strong influences on innovation and the adoption of new mental health service programs (Glisson and James, 2002). Glisson and colleagues use a change agent to facilitate stakeholder support in a program, external relationships with the organization, and compatibility between the culture and the innovative program (Glisson, 2002; Glisson, Dukes, and Green, 2006). Because such organizational change approaches have been successful in delivering mental health services, it may be a useful model to promote the adoption of prevention services as well.

STRATEGIES THAT COMPLEMENT THE IMPLEMENTATION OF EVIDENCE-BASED INTERVENTIONS

Despite the potential for preventing MEB disorders through the implementation of evidence-based programs, there are limitations to relying exclusively on this approach. First, as noted above, evidence remains limited about the ability of existing evidence-based programs to be effective for populations other than those that participated in the original evaluations of these programs. Moreover, implementation may be hampered if the original evidence was limited to efficacy trials rather than scientific evaluation based on characteristics as close to real-world conditions as possible. In addition, the widespread adoption, implementation, and maintenance of evidence-based programs will require a significant public investment. This section delineates additional strategies that can complement the implementation of evidence-based programs.

Public Education

Nationwide efforts to reduce cigarette smoking (Biglan and Taylor, 2000; Institute of Medicine, 2007b), one of the most successful public health efforts of the 20th century, illustrate the potential of public education strategies. The prevalence of smoking among adults has decreased by 58.2 percent since 1964, and smoking initiation by adolescent and young adults has also decreased (Institute of Medicine, 2007b). Although multiple factors contributed to this remarkable decline, one contributor is the information that has been communicated to the public about the harm of tobacco use.

At least two levels of government have adopted information and education strategies. At the local level, many school boards have required smoking prevention as a component of health education programs. At the federal level, Congress has mandated the publication of regular surgeon general's reports on smoking and health and, since 1966, has required warning labels on cigarette packs. The first surgeon general's report on smoking (U.S. Department of Health, Education, and Welfare, 1964) had an immediate and profound impact: In the first three months after its issuance, cigarette consumption fell by 15 percent. During a brief period, from 1967 to 1970, the public was exposed to mandated antismoking commercials on television, which produced the first four-year decline in per capita smoking in the history of cigarette smoking. Subsequently, the Public Health Cigarette Smoking Act of 1969 banned cigarette ads on TV and radio effective in 1971 (Warner, 2006).

Experience with antismoking social marketing campaigns in both California and Massachusetts has demonstrated the ability of professionally designed, well-funded, and sustained counteradvertising to decrease smoking. More recently, the highly acclaimed "truth campaign" antismoking ads produced by the American Legacy Foundation have been demonstrated to decrease smoking among youth (Farrelly, Davies, et al., 2006). We conclude that properly produced, financed, and distributed media campaigns can discourage youth smoking and reduce smoking among adults.

Information and education clearly jump-started the antismoking campaign. All told, it seems highly likely that the combination of information and education interventions in the first decade of the antismoking campaign played a critical role in reducing youth smoking.

MEB disorders and related problems are more diverse and complex than the single behavior of smoking. Nonetheless, there is an important potential role for public communication in terms of reducing the stigma associated with MEB disorders, conveying messages about the support structure needed to facilitate healthy development, and generating public support for relevant policies and principles as well as positive attitudes about the potential of the nation's young people.

Dissemination and Adoption of Common Principles

As documented in this report, there are interconnections among MEB disorders, and the factors that contribute to them are interconnected. Similarly, there are common principles across a range of prevention approaches. Widespread communication of these principles to parents, community decision makers, and policy makers could influence individual and collective decisions supportive of common prevention practices. As discussed in Chapter 7, a number of common aspects of effective preventive interventions as well as general lifestyle factors promote physical and mental health. Dissemination and adoption of these principles can contribute to the healthy development of the nation's young people and the prevention of MEB disorders. Specifically:

- Effective preventive interventions reduce young people's exposure to biologically and psychologically toxic events, such as harsh discipline, abuse, and neglect.
- A common feature of most validated prevention programs is an

emphasis on supportive environments or "nurturance" and positive reinforcement for prosocial behavior.

- Acceptance and encouragement in family, school, and community environments are more effective and desirable than confrontation or coercion.
- Such techniques as praise notes, peer-to-peer tutoring, and caregiver training can help facilitate the creation of nurturing environments.
- Adequate sleep, diet, and exercise, and television viewing limits can contribute to positive health outcomes.

Principles such as these can be adopted in home, school, and community environments and need not be attached to specific prevention programs. Communication of the importance of these principles can reinforce desirable behavior, minimize aversiveness, contribute to healthy development, and help promote a societal norm supportive of positive development. As with any interventions, empirical evaluation is also needed on how this information can be communicated to parents, teachers, caregivers, policy makers, and prevention practitioners and whether the communication of such information can have the same benefits that communications about smoking have had in reducing tobacco use.

Public Policy

Public policy changes made a significant contribution to the success of the tobacco control movement (Institute of Medicine, 2007b). Based on growing evidence of the harm of environmental tobacco smoke, tobacco control advocates have been able to push for local and state laws restricting smoking. Smoke-free laws dramatically reduce workplace exposure to noxious chemicals. Such laws also lead to reductions in smoking among workers in the affected establishments. Thus, workers in smoke-free workplaces are 3.8 percent more likely to quit smoking than are workers in workplaces that are not smoke free. Continuing smokers working in smoke-free environments reduce their daily cigarette consumption by an average of 3.1 cigarettes (Fichtenberg and Glantz, 2002).

Public policy has also been a significant contributor to reductions in alcohol use and abuse. Taxation of beer, which increases its price, has been shown to reduce alcohol consumption among young people, especially those who are heavy drinkers (Biglan, Brennan, et al., 2004). Increasing the drinking age from 18 to 21 also has a well-documented impact on alcohol-related auto crash fatalities (Wagenaar and Toomey, 2002). The National Highway Traffic Safety Administration estimated that increasing the drinking age from 18 to 21 saved 17,359 lives between 1975 and 1997. Pentz, Jasuja, and colleagues (2006) similarly argues that policies related to drug use, including national media attention, have contributed to the ebb and flow of drug use among adolescents.

States and the federal government have also enacted numerous laws to protect children from injury (e.g., car seat and bike helmet laws) and disease (e.g., requiring immunizations). Infant seat restraints in cars are now used by the majority of young children nationwide, and bike helmets are now common for children when just years ago they were only seen in bicycle races. Immunization protocols are well established, and proof of relevant immunizations is often required as a condition of school enrollment.

Public policy could play a more significant role in mental health promotion and the prevention of MEB disorders. Given the relationship between poverty and MEB disorders (Conger, Ge, et al., 1994; Gutman, McLoyd, and Tokoyawa, 2005; see also Chapter 6) and the fact that the United States has the highest rate of child poverty among 25 economically developed nations (United Nations Children's Fund, 2001), policies that reduce poverty should have a particularly high priority. Numerous policies can reduce family poverty and its effects, either by increasing available income through such programs as the Earned Income Tax Credit, unemployment insurance, Temporary Assistance to Needy Families, or federal housing subsidies, or by helping address nutritional needs through such programs as food stamps, the School Lunch Program, and the Special Supplemental Nutrition Program for Women, Infants, and Children. Similarly, policies that could contribute to reducing health disparities and differential access to health care services (e.g., Medicaid, expansion of the State Children's Health Insurance Program), as well as public health policies that minimize harmful environmental factors, such as exposure to neurotoxins (e.g., lead), warrant consideration. Policies that promote increased access to early childhood education programs could set children, particularly impoverished children, on a positive life course. Finally, policies that support families, such as parental or family leave policies, access to quality child care, affordable transportation, recreational areas, and safe neighborhoods, facilitate supportive families and communities.

Policies shifting schools and the juvenile justice system away from the use of punishment and toward the use of positive methods of developing desirable social behavior are also needed. For example, the Los Angeles Unified School District recently adopted a policy that requires the implementation of systems of positive reinforcement in schools as an alternative to punishment (Los Angeles Unified School District, 2007). The policy is based in part on empirical evidence that punitive practices increase vandalism and antisocial behavior (Mayer, 1995).

Expanding implementation of relevant public policies should be part of a national implementation strategy to support prevention of MEB disorders and promotion of mental health. At the same time, research on the impact of policies and on strategies for achieving effective public policies should be a portion of the nation's prevention science portfolio.

RESEARCH NEEDS

Implementation and Dissemination Research

An important step prior to implementation should be the availability of effectiveness studies. As more programs have shown efficacy in controlled trials, a next stage in prevention is studies of effectiveness under real-world conditions (Institute of Medicine, 1994). This research focus, often called "type 2 translational" research, occurs after efficacy has been established and focuses on factors associated with the adoption and use of scientifically validated interventions by service systems (Green, 2007). It also includes consideration of maintenance and sustainability issues at the practice level that can be used to guide implementation. In the real world, translation of science-based practices often stumbles, largely unguided, toward uneven, incomplete, and disappointing outcomes.

Translational research explores the factors that influence the quality of implementation; in such studies, implementation quality itself may be the outcome. A developing "science of implementation" (Dane and Schneider, 1998; Durlak, 1998; Domitrovich and Greenberg, 2000) emphasizes the potential to advance the adoption of effective programs and redesign of health systems to ultimately improve health (Madon, Hofman, et al., 2007; Chambers, 2008). There is increasing knowledge regarding a variety of factors that influence implementation quality and recognition that better quality implementation leads to improved outcomes for children (Durlak, Weissberg, et al., 2007).

Translational research related to school-based interventions should focus on a variety of factors: the decision-making process, the curriculum model or policy and the implementation support system, nonprogram factors, such as characteristics of teachers and students, and policies and regulations of school and governmental bodies. For example, a recent community-based study highlighted the interactive influences of high-quality implementation by teachers and level of principal leadership in influencing aggressive behavior in elementary school-age children (Kam, Greenberg, and Wells, 2003). There are at least three conceptual models that may assist in guiding research questions, including those of the National Implementation Research Network (Fixsen, Naoom, et al., 2005), the school ecological model (Greenberg, Domitrovich, et al., 2006), and the REACH model (Glasgow, Klesges, et al., 2004).

In addition, Spoth and Redmond (2002) present a conceptual framework for scaling up preventive interventions and moving from effectiveness to

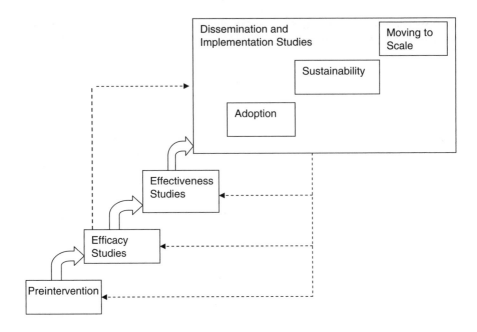

FIGURE 11-1 Stages of research in prevention research cycle.

implementation to achieve greater public health impact. They suggest three interrelated sets of research requirements and findings to accomplish population-based prevention: "(1) rigorously demonstrating intervention effectiveness; (2) attaining sufficient levels of intervention utilization in diverse general populations, requiring study of recruitment/retention strategies, cultural sensitivity, and economic viability; and (3) achieving implementation quality, involving investigation of adherence and dosage effects, along with theory-driven, intervention quality improvement" (p. x). To accomplish this, it may be useful to view implementation as having three phases: adoption, sustainability, and moving to scale (see Figure 11-1). Prevention scientists, government organizations, state and community organizations, and community leaders have major roles throughout this process. Ideally, the results of these phases will feed back to earlier areas of research. Specific research questions related to each of these phases warrant additional attention:

- Research questions related to the adoption of a prevention program into a service system, which routinely involves the formation of partnerships and the development of an infrastructure to support the technical, financial, administrative, monitoring, evaluative, and logistical needs related to the program.

- Research questions pertaining to sustaining the program once it is introduced in a service system. The ability to sustain a program relates to the organizational structures, practices, data monitoring, leadership, and related characteristics in place in the home institution for the program.
- Research questions involving moving to scale, or understanding which steps facilitate the structures and funding necessary to expand the program to other sites.

There are major challenges of introducing and taking effective programs to scale, particularly in poor and underserved communities (Madon, Hofman, et al., 2007; Sanders and Haines, 2006), and clearly the current body of generalizable knowledge is inadequate to provide robust strategies for effective implementation across different populations, systems, and programs. Nevertheless, there is reason for optimism.

First, the dearth of generalizable knowledge is a product of the lack of significant investment in scientific studies of the implementation and dissemination process. Second, while the specific factors regarding successful program implementation may vary from case to case, there are many commonalities in why organizations have difficulties adopting and sustaining prevention programs. For example, poor communities, minority populations, and developing countries often lack professionally trained staff to deliver a program as originally designed, so successful implementation may need to identify unique program delivery agents using existing resources (Sanders and Haines, 2006). Also, there is general agreement in the field about shared dimensions of organizational change that are relevant across widely different interventions; these include system readiness for change, culture, and the role of leaders (Chambers, 2008). Third, the increasing use of more rigorous designs, such as randomized trials that test different implementation strategies (see Chapter 10), social network analysis (Chambers, 2008), and the combined use of qualitative and quantitative data, is likely to lead to more precise implementation inferences around shared research questions. This information can be used as markers to guide the development of successful implementation efforts across diverse fields and settings.

Implementation research turns the traditional efficacy/effectiveness research questions of prevention science into experimental questions about the process of implementation itself. To date the leading model for examining implementation of prevention programs has been to focus on a single region, such as an urban school district or an entire state. With this approach, one can examine how process factors affect the adoption of a program over time, even if there are unique or novel factors operating in that particular system (Biglan, 2004). In addition, some randomized trial designs are beginning to be used to study the process from effectiveness to large-scale implementation. For example, the community epidemiology model of Kellam and colleagues can examine questions related to effectiveness, sustainability, and moving to scale, along with randomization (Kellam, Koretz, and Moscicki, 1999; Kellam, 2000). This approach examines variation in the community through the use of random assignment of the intervention conditions to different contexts and across time. To test effectiveness of a classroom-based intervention, for example, classes in a school can be randomized to intervention, and the impact for intervention and control classrooms can be compared in the first cohort (Brown, Wang, et al., 2008). This can be followed by examination of intervention sustainability by measuring the level of program fidelity that intervention teachers deliver in the second year with new students. Teachers remain in the same intervention condition, but the support structure in the schools for monitoring, supervision, and resource allocation changes from the first year to reflect the way such a program is likely to be delivered over time. Finally, scalability can be examined in a third cohort in which all the teachers implement the full intervention. Again, with resources allocated as one would anticipate in a scaled-up program, this third cohort can be used to compare the level of program fidelity as well as child outcomes with those of previous cohorts subjected to different levels of infrastructure support. This model, however, allows limited testing of the components of a higher level implementation strategy involving the full school district, since there is only one such district studied at a time (Kellam, 2000).

Implementation Trials

A valuable approach that would increase knowledge of successful implementation strategies is to test alternative strategies using a randomized trial design (implementation trials). This would necessarily require multiple location and multilevel analyses to fully examine impact. One such implementation trial is comparing the CTC model (see Box 11-1) to an implementation plan with passive assistance (Hawkins, 2006).

In Project Adapt, Smith, Swisher, and colleagues (2004) tested two types of implementation of Life Skills Training (LST) using group-based random assignment. They compared a standard implementation model in which the LST curriculum stood apart from the day-to-day teaching activities with an infusion model that integrated the curriculum into traditional courses. Three rural school districts were randomly assigned to the traditional LST condition, the infused LST condition, and a control condition. There was some suggestion of beneficial impact of both intervention conditions against control for girls in the first year of the study, although these findings generally disappeared by the second year and did not show at all for boys. There were few differences between the two intervention conditions, although this could have been due to the low statistical power for this school-based design.

An ongoing randomized trial of two different methods of implementing an evidence-based program for foster care in California counties may shed new light on implementation approaches. The trial was driven by a California mandate to use evidence-based practices and interest in identifying ways to facilitate statewide implementation. Although this particular trial involves multidimensional treatment foster care (Chamberlain, Saldana, et al., in press), an evidence-based program that targets high-need children who are in state custody, it can also be enlightening for the implementation of evidence-based prevention. Training had earlier been offered to all California counties, but only about 10 percent of the counties became early adopters, not unlike that of most novel interventions (Rogers, 1995; Valente, 1996). All the remaining 40 eligible counties were randomly assigned to one of two methods for implementation: a standard model and a community development team model, which used cross-county peer-to-peer support to address the administrative, financial, and logistical challenges in implementing the program. The evaluation is assessing whether the rate and length of time for adoption and sustainability is reduced by the team model, taking into account the dependence between team members.

Research on Increasing Rates of Intervention Adoption and Participation

The rate of adoption of a particular program across different communities and the rate of participation in a community are major issues that affect levels of program implementation. A variety of potential approaches to increase these rates could be evaluated in future research.

Encouragement Designs

The general class of randomized "encouragement designs" are ones that randomize individuals to different modalities of recruitment, incentives, or persuasion messages to influence their choice to participate in one or another intervention condition. Such incentives as cash or child care discounts have been used to encourage participation. An important advantage of these designs is that they allow one to take into account self-selection factors in examining impact (Yau and Little, 2001; Frangakis and Rubin, 1999; Barnard, Frangakis, et al., 2002). They also address whether targeted efforts to increase participation reach those most at risk (Brown and Liao, 1999). Randomized encouragement trials have been used to evaluate early versus late enrollment in Early Head Start (Administration for Children and Families, 2005), whether antiviral medications for HIV should adhere to a rigid regimen or be more flexible (HIV SMART AntiRetroviral Trial),

---

BOX 11-4
The Internet as a Potential Tool for Wide-Scale
Dissemination of Preventive Interventions

The enormity of need for mental health services often produces a type of paralysis: since it is not feasible to train enough providers to *treat* all individuals with mental, emotional, and behavioral disorders, how can *preventive* interventions be provided to those at risk? This dilemma is caused in part by the exclusive reliance on consumable interventions, such as face-to-face services, and the use of medications. Once a prevention or therapy session is over, no other individual can benefit from that hour of contact. Once a medication is consumed, no one else can benefit from its therapeutic effect. The development and implementation of interventions delivered via the Internet offers the promise of an approach to make interventions available on a continual basis to a wide range of young people at minimal cost while addressing several dissemination and implementation challenges.

Fidelity: The fidelity of Internet interventions is inherent as the material on the computer screen remains the same, no matter how many times it is used. The content of the intervention can be shared widely exactly as tested in randomized control trials.

Scalability: An Internet intervention can be shared with literally thousands of users beyond the locality in which it was created, while remaining accessible to the original locality. The site of a proven Internet intervention can be immediately opened to use by anyone with web access, which also allows effectiveness evaluation on a wide scale.

Sustainability: The cost of maintaining a website hosting an evidence-based preventive intervention is relatively modest, especially if the site is an automated, self-help intervention.

---

and whether strategic, structural engagement of adolescents increases completion of family therapy more than traditional engagement methods (Szapocznik, Perez-Vidal, and Brickman, 1988). Such designs may have value in exploring ways to increase the reach of prevention programs.

In the years since publication of *Reducing Risks for Mental Disorders: Frontiers for Preventive Intervention Research* (Institute of Medicine, 1994), a modest number of experimental tests have aimed at increasing individual- or family-level participation rates for a preventive intervention. For example, motivational interviewing techniques have been used in trials in an attempt to engage parents around problems or issues that they can relate to their own children (Dishion, Kavanagh, et al., 2002).

Accessibility: Internet interventions can simultaneously serve users across a community, a state, the nation, or the world, at any time of the day or night, including holidays and weekends.

Stigma: The availability of Internet interventions that are used in the privacy of one's own home, educational or work setting, or using a public access computer makes these interventions more likely to be used by people who would not come to a mental health–oriented program.

Reaching multicultural, multilingual communities: Internet interventions can be implemented relatively easily in multiple languages. Similarly, advances in technology now make it possible to create Internet interventions that require a minimum level of reading or writing. The use of video, graphics, and audio allow the creation of Internet interventions that can be used by individuals at any education level.

Internet interventions also have limitations. One of the most troublesome is the lack of access to the web by many low-income, low-education groups. However, Internet access is increasingly available via mobile devices, such as cell phones. Many developing countries have skipped the stage of land-line phones and moved directly to cell phones. As is the case for other venues, Internet interventions will not be effective in preventing all types of MEB disorders. It is useful to think in terms of "market segmentation," in which specific means of reaching populations at risk will need to be developed and evaluated to see which is most effective for which population. Nevertheless, to help make prevention feasible, one must think beyond traditional interventions and harness the power of advanced communication media, such as the Internet.

Use of Current Technologies

The advent of the Internet and modern use of technology presents new opportunities for both dissemination and research. Broadcasting the availability of accessible web-based or CD-ROM programs or making implementation resources (e.g., training, manuals) available could potentially increase the use of prevention programs. Implementation of interventions via the web has the potential to address several implementation barriers (see Box 11-4). Because online interventions can occur anonymously, these technologies also have the potential to be less stigmatizing, a significant potential barrier to participation.

Identification of Early Adopters

Rogers (1995) identified general factors that affect or influence the diffusion of innovations. This early work on program diffusion was based on a synthesis of careful observation from case studies. One major finding is that early adopters share traits that can be readily measured or inferred from behaviors or attitudes. While this earlier work was observational in nature and did not attempt to influence adoption itself, assessments can be used to identify communities, organizations, institutions, families, as well as individuals who are most likely to be early adopters of such programs. Thus identification of those likely to be early adopters and targeting prevention efforts to these groups represent a potential strategy to affect program adoption.

Use of Opinion Leaders

More recently, the same principles underlying research on diffusion of interventions and social influence have been used proactively to increase the adoption of prevention programs and test adoption strategies in group-based randomized trials. One approach used early in HIV prevention is to target opinion leaders in a community who would themselves deliver peer-to-peer messages to promote increased program adoption. Kelly, St. Lawrence, and colleagues (1991), for example, successfully identified and then trained gay opinion leaders in rural communities to encourage safe sexual practices. These leaders were able to modify HIV risk behaviors in their communities. Also, media campaigns for HIV prevention in developing countries are using soap operas in which leading actors talk openly about the use of condoms and getting tested for HIV (Valente, 1996).

A similar approach is now being used in approaches to youth suicide prevention; teenage leaders are trained to deliver messages to both peers and adults in their community aimed at increasing help seeking among suicidal youth. Suicidal youth are often much less likely to talk to adults than are nonsuicidal youth (Wyman, Brown, et al., 2008), yet the vast majority of youth tell a friend before committing suicide. A general strategy for reducing suicide is to increase willingness to talk to a trusted adult by both suicidal youth and their friends. One such program (Sources of Strength) is designed to change peer norms about secrecy and disclosure surrounding distressed youth. A first implementation step is to identify peer leaders from diverse social networks. The program then modifies norms by having each of the peer leaders identify trusted adults in their own lives to whom they would turn at times of stress.

Market Research

Many evidence-based prevention programs are delivered to small portions of the population. A small number of state agencies, schools, communities, or families select programs with the highest levels of evidence, opting instead for programs that have less evidence, or no program at all. One promising approach to improve program reach to individual families is to integrate business models into prevention to address consumer needs from the beginning (Rotheram-Borus and Duan, 2003). By following a prevention service development model that integrates consumer preferences from the beginning (Sandler, Ostrom, et al., 2005), the research team can aim for effectiveness and large-scale implementation from the start of the product development cycle.

Similarly, there is a need for greater consideration of the most effective metrics to report outcomes to the public. Although effect size may be the most appropriate metric for studies of indicated interventions in which all participants begin with a substantial rate of symptoms, it may be a poor metric for universal interventions. In universal interventions, it is usually the case that a large percentage of the population begins with low levels of symptoms, and thus it is unlikely (at least in the short term) that much of this population will benefit from the intervention. In most cases it is only in the higher symptom group of the population that larger effect sizes will be obtained (Wilson and Lipsey, 2007). Thus, for universal interventions, alternative methods are needed to convey the practical and social policy significance (Davis, MacKinnon, et al., 2003; McCartney and Rosenthal, 2000). Cost-effectiveness is one such metric, as universal interventions may achieve more benefit in relation to their cost given their large reach.

Naturalistic Large-Scale Public Health Research

Although their internal validity makes them valuable science, randomized control trials do not always have good external validity. Furthermore, much academic research is rarely applied to the day-to-day world. Science can often benefit from the experience of everyday clinical observations. For example, in 1982 when clinical observations in a community mental health setting found an extraordinary number of children exposed to violence, a plethora of scientific research projects confirmed this observation, culminating in several large-scale strategies to prevent these children from developing mental health sequelae (Jenkins and Bell, 1997; Bell, 2004).

In addition, communities often implement programs because they are based on extensive clinical wisdom and have widespread community support. Research designed to empirically test programs being implemented in naturalistic environments could identify approaches that are readily implementable by other communities. Gibbons, Hur, and colleagues (2007) have developed statistical methodology that provides some evidence in support of such interventions. Conversely, randomized control prevention trials can also inform public health practice. For example, a violence prevention trial, Aban Aya (Flay, Graumlich, et al., 2004) informed a Chicago public school violence prevention initiative with teenage mothers (Bell, Gamm, et al., 2001), which demonstrated significant reductions in pregnant teenage dropout rates. In addition, most teens had only one child despite becoming a mother at very young ages (Lamberg, 2003).

CONCLUSIONS AND RECOMMENDATIONS

There have been clear advances in implementing effective programs since the publication of *Reducing Risks for Mental Disorders: Frontiers for Preventive Intervention Research* (Institute of Medicine, 1994). Indeed, the knowledge base on effective prevention programs at that time was very thin. However, the levels of effective implementation are much lower than the availability of tested interventions suggests.

Conclusion: Implementation of effective preventive interventions is hampered by lack of ongoing resources and competing priorities of the service systems or communities that could implement them.

One of several contributors to the relative lack of implementation is lack of empirical evidence regarding how to effectively approach implementation. A critical next phase of research needs to examine methods for enhancing the implementation of effective programs. The prevention research cycle proposed in the 1994 IOM report assumes a "hierarchical scientist-as-expert perspective and portrays scientists as separate agents conducting research on 'subjects' and 'groups'" (Dumka, Mauricio, and Gonzales, 2007). Although the stages of research in the model require the cooperation of individuals and organizations, the model did not specifically address the relationships and collaborative processes that are critical to accomplishing each stage (Dumka, Mauricio, and Gonzales, 2007).

For implementation to be successful, there needs to be strategic input from science, policy, and practice perspectives that builds on the scientific knowledge base. Evidence is needed on how to make implementation occur in communities, the policy directives that promote or enforce the use of evidence-based programs and data systems, and the effective adoption and sustainability of programs in practice (Greenberg, 2004). Important progress has been made, and there are now new opportunities to make partnerships between scientists, policy makers, and practitioner communities to transport effective prevention programs into community settings. Additional research is needed to identify core components shared across programs. Major implementation challenges suggest new avenues of research.

Conclusion: Knowledge about effective strategies for implementing or adopting evidence-based prevention interventions is limited. New approaches to implementation represent the frontier of prevention research.

Recommendation 11-1: Research funders should support experimental research and evaluation on (1) dissemination strategies designed to identify effective approaches to implementation of evidence-based programs, (2) the effectiveness of programs when implemented by communities, and (3) identification of core elements of evidence-based programs, dissemination, and institutionalization strategies that might facilitate implementation.

Knowledge gained from evaluation of implementation approaches will be more generalizable if it is conducted in multiple settings. A number of evidence-based interventions are viable candidates for implementation. Evaluations that involve partnerships between states or communities ready to implement interventions and researchers could yield valuable results.

Recommendation 11-2: Research funders should fund research on state- or community-wide implementation of interventions to promote mental, emotional, or behavioral health or prevent MEB disorders that meet established scientific standards of effectiveness.

Although there are many evidence-based models, it is not clear how generalizable they are to groups other than the ones with which they were tested. Interest in an intervention is likely to be greater if it is culturally relevant and embraced by the community. Lack of relevance may contribute to interventions being implemented with limited fidelity and resultant limited outcomes. Addressing this may include replication with new populations as well as examining versions that strengthen the cultural competency of interventions.

Conclusion: Despite multiple dissemination venues, evidence-based interventions have not been implemented on a wide-scale basis. Where interventions have been implemented, they are often not implemented with fidelity, with cultural sensitivity, or in settings that have the capacity to sustain the effort.

Conclusion: Little research has addressed the question of how transportable evidence-based interventions developed for one ethnic group are to a range of ethnic and cultural groups.

Recommendation 11-3: Research funders should prioritize the evaluation and implementation of programs to promote mental, emotional, or behavioral health or prevent MEB disorders in ethnic minority communities. Priorities should include the testing of culturally appropriate adaptations of evidence-based interventions developed in one culture to determine if they work in other cultures and encouragement of their adoption when they do.

Finally, multiple opportunities for naturalistic research could enrich the prevention portfolio and convincing evidence that collaborations between researchers and communities can increase the relevance and sustainability of interventions, including through efforts to adapt existing evidence-based interventions.

Recommendation 11-4: Researchers and community organizations should form partnerships to develop evaluations of (1) adaptation of existing interventions in response to community-specific cultural characteristics; (2) preventive interventions designed based on research principles in response to community concerns; and (3) preventive interventions that have been developed in that community, have demonstrated feasibility of implementation and acceptability in the community, but lack experimental evidence of effectiveness.

On a practical level, for tested preventive interventions to become widespread, the available research suggests that successful interventions should include at least the availability of published material, such as handbooks, curriculum, and manuals describing the intervention and prescribing actions to be taken; certification of trainers or an electronic training system; high-quality, data-driven technical assistance; implementation fidelity measures; dissemination efforts that are organized around marketing and delivery; an information management system; and community demand for systems that work.

In addition to development and implementation of effective programs, the nation needs to support implementation of policies and broad prevention principles in order to create a comprehensive, sustained approach to prevention. Policies that support low-income families and promote healthy development are needed as the basic foundation for such an approach.

12

Prevention Infrastructure

The development and ultimate success of efforts to improve mental, emotional, and behavioral outcomes among young people depend heavily on the availability of systems to support efforts in three domains: research and innovation, training, and delivery of successful interventions. This chapter addresses three key interconnected topics: (1) funding for research, training, and service delivery programs; (2) the adequacy of access to prevention delivery systems; and (3) content of training programs directed to enhancing the prevention workforce.

The chapter begins with a discussion of federal funding, highlighting the challenges in determining the level of funding for either prevention research or services, indications that the federal commitment to prevention research may have waned since the publication of *Reducing Risks for Mental Disorders: Frontiers for Preventive Intervention Research* (Institute of Medicine, 1994), and the lack of systematic coordination of either research or service delivery efforts. It then moves to issues related to the development of prevention delivery systems, including discussion of multiple federal efforts related to prevention and promotion, the need for consistent, rigorous standards to identify effective interventions, and illustration of some existing state and local efforts to develop delivery systems. The chapter closes with discussion of gaps in prevention-specific training in a range of disciplines, pointing out that prevention efforts are likely to continue to languish without targeted attention to preparing the future prevention workforce.

FUNDING

It is difficult to quantify current funding for either prevention research or prevention services, due to the many agencies involved, varied definitions and tracking systems used by agencies, and the multiple levels of service funding and delivery. In some cases, prevention is a piece of a larger program or an eligible activity under a block grant, but there is no specific accounting of the proportion targeted to prevention. Similarly, programs that fund services aimed at addressing factors that contribute to prevention of mental, emotional, and behavioral (MEB) disorders clearly have an important role to play in prevention, but they cannot fairly be claimed as prevention programs in their entirety—for example, child abuse prevention programs. In addition, there is no national network or organization that coordinates all preventive efforts, either for research or services, from which funding estimates can be generated. While more states and counties have been investing in prevention activities, the scope of that investment has not been monitored systematically.

Research Funding

Multiple components of the U.S. Department of Health and Human Services (HHS), including the National Institutes of Health (NIH), the Agency for Healthcare Research and Quality (AHRQ), the Maternal and Child Health Bureau (MCHB), the Centers for Disease Control and Prevention (CDC), and the Administration for Children and Families (ACF) fund prevention research involving young people. The research arms of the U.S. Department of Education (ED) and the U.S. Department of Justice and private foundations also fund relevant research. Published randomized controlled trials (see Figure 1-1) tend to be funded primarily by HHS. Of those with an identified funding source,[1] almost three-quarters (74 percent) received some funding from HHS; more than half (57 percent) received all of their funding from HHS. Given that NIH is the largest source of research funding in HHS, particularly for randomized controlled trials, it is reasonable to assume that they are the primary source of this funding. Only one in four published randomized controlled trials received all of its funding from a non-U.S. government source, such as foundations or foreign governments.

---

[1]Funding information was available for 261 of the 424 (62 percent) published randomized controlled trials identified. The Public Health Service, which includes NIH and all of the health agencies within HHS, was the primary source.

National Institutes of Health

NIH publishes online their estimates of funding for various diseases, conditions, and research areas. Although the amount spent on "prevention" declined overall from $7.185 billion in fiscal year (FY) 2004 to $6.739 billion in FY 2009, this includes all NIH institutes, so it is impossible to say to what extent this applies to prevention of MEB disorders among young people (see http://www.nih.gov/news/fundingresearchareas.htm). Determining federal research funding for prevention in this area is also complicated by the current system for categorizing and reporting grants, which lacks a common definition of prevention. This situation exists despite a definition of prevention accepted by the NIH Prevention Research Coordinating Committee,[2] updated in 2007.

NIH is nearing the end of a project to establish an NIH-wide system for coding funded projects, the Research, Condition, and Disease Categorization (RCDC) system.[3] This system has been developed in response to a requirement that was added to the NIH Reauthorization Act in 2006. It will be able to produce a complete annual list of all NIH-funded projects related to each of 360 categories, including prevention, using standard definitions that will be used across all NIH centers and institutes. Projects will be coded for all applicable categories to allow for funding information to be searched and cross-referenced by multiple categories. The first funding report is expected to be available on a public website in spring 2009 for project funding in FY 2008, and it will not be applied retroactively to previous years. Once in place, this new system should improve the availability of consistent, accurate information on NIH funding for the prevention of MEB disorders. It is unclear, however, how prevention will be defined for the RCDC system.

Furthermore, there are no plans for the RCDC system to provide linkage to financial data, limiting opportunities to quantify the federal investment in prevention research.

NIMH, NIDA, and NIAAA Funding

The National Institute of Mental Health (NIMH), the National Institute on Drug Abuse (NIDA), and the National Institute on Alcohol Abuse and Alcoholism (NIAAA) are the NIH institutes with direct responsibility for research related to prevention of MEB disorders, and they are a significant source of funding for intervention research. The National Institute of Child Health and Human Development (NICHD) also plays a critical role

---

[2]See http://odp.od.nih.gov/research.aspx.
[3]See http://rcdc.nih.gov/.

in exploring developmental pathways and healthy development of young people. The committee requested historical data on prevention and treatment research and narrative information on FY 2006 funding from NIMH, NIDA, and NIAAA. However, these institutes were not able to provide uniform data and, with the exception of NIMH, were not able to provide longitudinal data. None routinely tracks its prevention research projects as universal, selective, or indicated.

NIMH was able to provide the most comprehensive financial data. Although both prevention and treatment intervention research funding increased between 1999 and 2006, prevention intervention research funding represented a smaller proportion of the overall NIMH budget than treatment intervention research (6.62 percent versus 8.75 percent, respectively, in FY 2006). If research aimed at "prevention of negative sequelae of clinical episodes, such as comorbidity, disability, and relapse or recurrence" were classified as treatment intervention research, consistent with the committee's definitions of prevention and treatment (see Chapter 3), the discrepancy between funding for prevention (6.72 percent in 2006) and treatment intervention research (14 percent in 2006) would be considerably greater (see Figure 12-1). In addition, both the percentage increase between 1999 and 2006 (80 and 102 percent for prevention and treatment intervention research, respectively) and the total funding ($94.4 and $122.8 million, respectively, in FY 2006) were much less for prevention than for treatment intervention research.

Consistent with the 1994 Institute of Medicine (IOM) report *Reducing Risks for Mental Disorders: Frontiers for Preventive Intervention Research* funding for prevention research[4] on drug abuse was proportionately greater than the funding for prevention research on mental disorders. Between 1999 and 2006, the proportion of NIDA's total appropriation expended for prevention ranged from 13.4 to 14.5 percent, while that of NIMH ranged from 5.7 to 7.6 percent during the same time period. The vast majority of NIAAA prevention research in FY 2007, the only year for which estimates were provided, focused on underage drinking.

Organizational Structure. When the 1994 IOM report was published, NIMH, NIDA, and NIAAA each had a prevention research branch; only NIDA has one today. The NIDA prevention research branch remains in the Division of Epidemiology, Services, and Prevention Research (previously called the Division of Epidemiology and Prevention Research). NIAAA now has a Division of Epidemiology and Prevention Research, which works collaboratively with other divisions. NIMH has established an associate director position in the Office of the Director with coordinating respon-

---

[4]NIDA was not able to provide an accounting of treatment research.

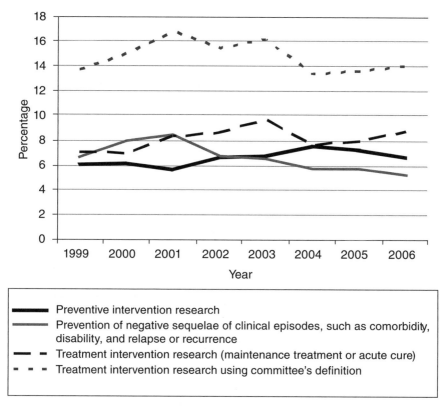

FIGURE 12-1 Proportion of NIMH budget for prevention and treatment in intervention research.
SOURCE: Committee analysis of data provided by NIMH.

sibilities related to prevention. The position, however, has no funding authority. NIMH does have a Child and Adolescent Treatment and Preventive Intervention Research Branch, which funds many of its prevention research projects; HIV prevention programs are funded out of its Primary Prevention Branch.

Research Centers. NIMH, NIDA, and NIAAA also fund university-based prevention research centers[5] (see Table 12-1). The centers conduct training and research related to a range of prevention-related issues, largely focused on young people. The number of NIMH-funded centers decreased from five

---

[5]NIMH and NIDA each also fund a center that addresses prevention methodology (see Chapter 9).

TABLE 12-1 Prevention Research Centers

NIMH	NIDA Transdisciplinary Prevention Research Centers (TPRCs)	NIAAA
Prevention Research Center for Families in Stress, Arizona State University: Focused on interventions with children at risk for developing mental health problems because of exposure to high-stress situations, such as parental divorce or death. **Center for Prevention and Early Intervention, Johns Hopkins University Collaboration:** A collaborative focused on interventions to reduce aggressive/disruptive behavior in children through elementary school-based interventions. **Prevention Programs for Rural African American Families, University of Georgia:** Focused on the implementation of interventions with rural African American families.	**Duke University TPRC:** Focused on the role of peer networks in prevention research. **Drug Abuse Prevention During Developmental Transitions, Rutgers University:** Focused on how individuals transitioning developmental phases acquire and integrate information about substance use into their behavior and how that knowledge can be applied to the design of preventive interventions. **Pathways Home: Reducing Risk in the Child Welfare System, Oregon Social Learning Center:** Focused on developing effective and feasible parenting interventions for children and their families in the child welfare system. **USC Transdisciplinary Drug Abuse PRC, University of Southern California:** Focused on the application of research on memory, implicit cognition, and network analysis theory to the design of prevention interventions. **Drug Abuse Prevention: A Life Course Perspective, University of Kentucky:** Focused on the role of novelty/sensation-seeking behavior in the onset and trajectory of drug abuse and applying this information in the tailoring of prevention efforts.	**Prevention Research Center, Pacific Institute for Research and Evaluation:** Focused on basic and applied research leading to the development of effective prevention programs to reduce alcohol abuse and related problems, with an emphasis on environmental approaches. **Youth Alcohol Prevention Center, Boston University School of Public Health:** Focused on alcohol-related problems among young people.

NOTES: NIAAA = National Institute on Alcohol Abuse and Alcoholism, NIDA = National Institute on Drug Abuse, NIMH = National Institute of Mental Health.

to three between FY 1993 (the last year included in the 1994 IOM report) and FY 2006.

NIDA currently funds five Transdisciplinary Prevention Research Centers (TPRCs) designed to bring together the expertise of basic and applied disciplines to accelerate the development and implementation of preventive interventions. Neuroscientists, behavioral and cognitive scientists, and drug abuse prevention researchers collaborate on discovery and translational research areas that have the potential for producing new approaches to drug abuse prevention. Similar mechanisms do not currently exist in NIMH or NIAAA or across the three institutes. NIAAA funds two prevention centers: the long-standing Prevention Research Center based at the University of California, Berkeley, and a new center focused on youth alcohol prevention.

Intervention Research Portfolio Snapshot. The FY 2006 abstracts for projects focused on young people (ages 0-25)[6] provide a one-year snapshot of NIMH, NIDA, and NIAAA prevention intervention research funding. Abstracts were coded by two reviewers on a variety of categories, including intervention type (universal, selective, indicated), trial type (efficacy, effectiveness, implementation), targeted risk factors, outcomes, and mediators; targeted population; and the location and provider of the intervention.[7] The coding results were analyzed for 35 NIMH abstracts, 77 NIDA abstracts, and 53 NIAAA abstracts.

We conclude from this analysis (see Box 12-1) that there is an emergence of effectiveness trials, but a lack of research that experimentally evaluates factors influencing implementation and dissemination of interventions. Appendix F provides a detailed summary of the analysis results.[8] The analysis argues for greater attention to economic analyses as well as evaluations that assess multiple outcomes. The current research portfolio does not address gaps identified by the committee, including the need to expand research to cover more settings that provide opportunities to prevent MEB

---

[6]At the time the information was submitted by NIMH and NIDA, FY 2006 was the most recent year for which complete data were available. NIAAA, which submitted information later, provided data for FY 2007. NIMH grants provided to the committee included those that are coded in their database as targeting ages 0-25. It did not provide grants coded as "age unspecified," which may include some grants funded by NIMH that target this population.

[7]Abstracts classified by NIMH as prevention of negative sequelae were included, but only projects considered by the committee to be prevention were included in this analysis. The coding was refined through a pilot phase involving multiple reviewers, with final coding conducted by two independent reviewers. Where the two reviewers did not agree on a code, a consensus was reached in consultation with a third coder. This was needed most often for the intervention type (24 percent of the abstracts) and trial type (38 percent of the abstracts).

[8]This appendix is available online only. Go to http://www.nap.edu and search for *Preventing Mental, Emotional, and Behavioral Disorders Among Young People.*

BOX 12-1
Prevention Intervention Research at NIMH, NIDA, and NIAAA,
Fiscal Year 2006

Intervention Type and Trial Type

- NIDA and NIAAA funded a greater proportion of universal intervention trials than NIMH.
- NIMH funded the largest proportion of efficacy trials (51 percent); NIDA grants were more evenly divided between efficacy and effectiveness; and NIAAA funded the largest proportion of effectiveness trials (53 percent).
- Overall, there were relatively few implementation or dissemination projects (4-18 percent), although these were most common for NIDA. Most included an experimental comparison of different strategies.
- A very small number of grants (6-11 percent) included any mention of economic analysis of the intervention.
- Close to half of the projects across institutes mentioned long-term follow-up (more than one year) as part of their protocol.

Outcomes, Risk Factors, and Mediators

- HIV/AIDS (27 percent) and risky sexual behavior (29 percent) were the most common target outcomes for NIMH grants. These were followed closely by depression (25 percent), conduct problems (20 percent), academic performance (18 percent), and anxiety (16 percent).
- HIV/AIDS and risky sexual behavior were also frequently targeted by NIDA and NIAAA. About one-quarter of NIDA projects also targeted academic performance, conduct problems, and other mental health issues.
- The majority of NIMH grants focused on measuring single outcomes, with only a third of the grants targeting multiple outcomes. Grants funded by NIDA and NIAAA were more likely to address multiple outcomes.
- Projects targeted primarily individual-level risk factors, and over three-quarters of grants for all three agencies target the child as the mediator; that is, the project aimed to change the skills or beliefs of the targeted group of young people.

disorders, greater attention to cultural appropriateness and adaptation, and interventions for young adults.

Centers for Disease Control and Prevention

CDC has an active public health research portfolio that includes a focus on child development. In its 2006 publication *Advancing the Nation's Health: Guide to Public Health Research, 2006-2015*, health promotion is

- The family was more likely to be a targeted mediator in NIDA-funded projects.
- NIAAA was the only agency in which policy was identified as a mediator (9 percent).

Population, Location, and Provider

- The majority of grants in all three agencies targeted school-age children, adolescents, or young adults, with fewer than 10 percent focusing on early childhood.
- Around one-quarter of both NIDA and NIMH abstracts focused on children of elementary school age, with the remainder focused primarily on middle school and high school.
- Young adults were an infrequent target of intervention by both NIMH and NIDA projects. NIAAA had both substantially more projects targeting young adults (68 percent) and a large proportion of projects in colleges (47 percent), due to their specific research portfolio focusing on interventions targeted at 21- to 25-year-olds.
- Although a significant number of NIMH and NIDA grants take place in school settings, relatively few have school personnel (rather than research staff) as the provider of the intervention.
- Very few trials take place in the health care system or in other government agencies that serve children and families, and very few projects indicated that they were evaluating cultural adaptations of existing interventions.

NOTES: NIAAA = National Institute on Alcohol Abuse and Alcoholism, NIDA = National Institute on Drug Abuse, NIMH = National Institute of Mental Health.
SOURCE: Based on analysis of 35 NIMH, 77 NIDA, and 53 NIAAA project abstracts.

one of six specified areas, although the role of mental health promotion is unclear. In the area of health promotion, creating healthy schools is one of the target areas. In addition, CDC provides funding for Community-Based Participatory Prevention Research, although prevention of MEB disorders among young people has been a relatively small component of funded projects.

Private Foundations

Currently, apart from religious congregations, total annual charitable expenditures in the United States are about $1 trillion. Depending on funding priorities, the amount of this investment should grow substantially, possibly more than double, as an unprecedented intergenerational transfer of wealth is predicted to occur between 1998 and 2052 (Fleishman, 2007). This will provide an opportunity to increase research for prevention of MEB disorders, especially if foundation boards are educated about the social and economic costs of mental disorders at a time when the United States needs a strong and productive workforce. Some private foundations already support preventive services and research related to mental, emotional, and behavioral problems among young people. Information on the amount of this investment is unavailable, but it is likely to be modest.[9]

Preventive Services Funding

There are no current estimates of overall national spending on preventive services. The most recent estimate concluded that in 1995 federal agencies contributed $1.8 billion, state Medicaid contributed $1.3 billion, and employee assistance/wellness programs contributed $1.2 billion toward the prevention of mental illness (Harwood, Ameen, et al., 2000). This would translate to $5.9 billion in 2007 dollars.

Federal Investments

Similar to the situation at the time of the 1994 IOM report, multiple federal agencies fund programs and services related to the prevention of MEB disorders. Although few are directly targeted to this task, there are many more federal efforts to encourage prevention and promotion activities than was the case in 1994, particularly activities targeted to mental health activities in schools.

The lead federal agency and largest funder of prevention of mental health disorders and substance abuse is the Substance Abuse and Mental Health Services Administration (SAMHSA). Within SAMHSA, this falls to the Center for Substance Abuse Prevention (CSAP) and the Center for Mental Health Services (CMHS), primarily through its Division of Prevention, Traumatic Stress and Special Programs. Unlike CSAP, which has the

---

[9]The Child Mental Health Foundations and Agencies Network, a group of public and private agencies and foundations interested in issues of child development and public policy, aims to improve connections between research, practice, and policy. A request was submitted to its members for information on relevant activities, but none was received in time for consideration in this report.

Center for Substance Abuse Treatment as a sister agency, CMHS must address both treatment and prevention issues. Other major federal funding sources include the Office of National Drug Control Policy, MCHB, ED (including such initiatives as Safe and Drug-Free Schools[10]), and the Office of Juvenile Justice and Delinquency Prevention. ACF is the primary funder of Head Start and child welfare programs, and CDC is involved in suicide prevention programs and surveillance efforts.

In 2004, SAMHSA awarded $230 million over 5 years to 21 states for the creation of Strategic Prevention Frameworks (Substance Abuse and Mental Health Services Administration, 2004), an approach to planning and implementing prevention programs, broadly based on principles drawn from research. These funds are helping states to build the infrastructure and processes needed to promote healthy youth development, reduce risky behaviors, and prevent problem behaviors through community programs.

Although there are block grants for both mental health (Mental Health Services Block Grant) and substance abuse (Substance Abuse Prevention and Treatment Block Grant), only the substance abuse block grant includes a set-aside for prevention. States are mandated to use 20 percent of their block grant resources for universal, selective, and indicated prevention activities. In FY 2001, SAMHSA/CMHS awarded targeted capacity expansion grants for prevention and early intervention services, but the program has not been continued.

In 2006, Safe and Drug-Free Schools at ED appropriated $510 million for numerous programs targeting prevention of mental disorders and substance abuse. These programs focus on preventing illegal drug and alcohol use among youth and creating violence-free educational environments for both school- and college-age youth. Grants for the integration of Schools and Mental Health Systems aim to increase linkages between schools, mental health, and juvenile justice authorities to improve access to quality mental health services, including preventive services. ED also provides grants to assist local education authorities develop "innovative and effective" alcohol abuse prevention programs.

Increased concern about violence also led to the creation in 1999 of the Safe Schools/Healthy Students (SSHS) Program, a collaboration of HHS, ED, and Justice. Through this program, local education agencies receive three-year grants to work in partnership with local law enforcement and mental health agencies to develop a comprehensive approach to violence prevention that

---

[10]The Office of Safe and Drug-Free Schools administers several programs with preventive goals, including the Healthy Student Initiative, Governors' Grants, Grants to States to Improve Management of Drug and Violence Prevention Programs, State Grants, Prevention Models on College Campuses, Grants for School-based Student Drug Testing, Grants to Reduce Alcohol Abuse, and Grants to Prevent High-risk Drinking and Violent Behavior Among College Students (U.S. Department of Education).

includes safe school environments; violence, alcohol and drug, and mental health preventive services; early childhood services; and treatment services. Over 150 communities have been funded through this program.

SAMHSA also administers the majority of service grants aimed at preventing suicide through the Garrett Lee Smith Memorial Act Suicide Prevention Program, which provides grants to states and colleges and funds a technical resource center.

In FY 2008, SAMHSA announced a new grant program, Project Launch (Linking Actions for Unmet Needs in Children's Health), which is designed to promote the physical, emotional, social, and behavioral health of young children from birth to age 8. The grants will be provided to state or tribal governments for a wide range of early childhood service programs. The program is being implemented in collaboration with the Health Resources and Services Administration (HRSA).

The MCHB at HRSA continues to be active in encouraging integration of mental health and physical health concerns. For example, its Early Childhood Comprehensive Systems Grant Program includes "mental health and social-emotional development" as one of five core components. It administer the Healthy Start Program and several other programs aimed at improving the health and social-emotional functioning of young people.

ACF administers the Head Start and Child Abuse Prevention Programs and recently included prevention-related activities in a component of the Compassion Capital Fund. In addition to its involvement in the SSHS Progam, the Department of Justice, primarily through its Office of Juvenile Justice and Delinquency Prevention, operates multiple grant programs aimed at delinquency prevention, violence prevention, and truancy reduction. CDC conducts surveillance and funds coordinated school health programs aimed at integrating eight health components, including mental health and social services. Finally, the Office of National Drug Control Policy awards drug-free communities grants and administers a national antidrug media campaign.

Many federal prevention funds operate as competitive grants of limited duration. This can lead to problems, such as inadequate or interrupted funding, that impact the ability to sustain interventions (see Chapter 11).

Federal Coordination

HHS, ED, and Justice appear to have mechanisms in place to support the planning, implementation, and technical assistance associated with the SSHS Program (U.S. Government Accountability Office, 2007) and other targeted initiatives. However, there does not appear to be an obvious connection between ED's several programs and SAMHSA's Strategic Prevention Framework. Similarly, although there are multiple relevant interagency groups, including the Federal Executive Steering Committee on Mental Health, the Federal/National Partnership, which includes an integrating mental health and education and suicide prevention workgroup, the Coordinating Council on Juvenile Justice and Delinquency, an interagency coordinating group on underage drinking, the Department of Labor's Shared Youth Vision, and the White House–led helping America's Youth initiative, there is no apparent coordination among the groups or a clear sense of their distinct or complementary missions. Similarly, although there has long been an Office of Prevention Research in the Office of the Director at NIH, it has apparently limited linkage to activities at the various institutes or agencies involved in MEB disorders.

Both CDC and HRSA have established Mental Health Work Groups. However, there was no evidence that the two groups are aware of each other's activities, and it is not clear the extent to which these group have considered prevention or interact with the various other interagency groups.

State Investments

Some states also dedicate significant amounts of state resources to prevention. One example of significant state-level preventive mental health funding can be found in California, which passed its Mental Health Services Act in 2004. This act is funded by a 1 percent tax on personal incomes over $1 million and had generated $2.1 billion in additional revenues for mental health services through the end of FY 2006-2007, with an additional $1.5 billion expected in each of the next two fiscal years (California Department of Mental Health, 2008). As part of this initiative, California has recently completed expenditure and program planning guidelines for counties statewide to address mental health promotion and prevention for youth and their families (California Department of Mental Health, 2007). As of May 2008, over $300 million had been committed for prevention and early intervention[11] (California Department of Mental Health, 2008).

Another example is the Pennsylvania Commission on Crime and Delinquency's Research-Based Programs Initiative, which began funding replications of efficacious prevention programs a decade ago. In the late 1990s and early 2000s, 110 communities received state funding to supplement federal Title V funding to implement Communities That Care. Approximately two-thirds continued to operate four years after the initial implementation phase (Feinberg, Bontempo, and Greenberg, 2008). Even more communities have

---

[11]These funds would support efforts surrounding suicide prevention, stigma and discrimination reduction, ethnic and cultural disparity reduction, training and capacity building, evaluation, and student mental health.

been funded to implement research-based violence prevention or substance abuse prevention programs. The state has also established a technical assistance and training center to provide resources needed to facilitate quality implementation by communities.

In another example, Kentucky is devoting 25 percent of its Phase I Tobacco Settlement resources to an early childhood initiative that includes maternal and child health–related activities, voluntary home visitation, Healthy Start, and other developmentally oriented initiatives.[12] In late 2007, the state of Illinois announced that it would begin reimbursing community mental health providers for perinatal depression screening, which, if paired with interventions for the mother, could result in improved outcomes for her children. The state similarly accepts infants of mothers diagnosed with maternal depression into its early intervention program.

Some states are also making their own investments in early care and early childhood education services. For example, Illinois, Rhode Island, and North Carolina have each dedicated state resources to initiatives that include expanded child care, parenting, or prekindergarten programs (Mitchell and Alliance for Early Childhood Finance, 2005). In addition, most schools have various efforts in place to address the mental health needs of students, including universal interventions for all students, typically by patching together multiple funding streams (U.S. Government Accountability Office, 2007).

Networks of state and local agencies related to prevention of alcohol and drug abuse are better established than for mental health. For example, the National Association of State Alcohol and Drug Abuse Directors convenes the National Prevention Network, an organization of state-level agencies involved with alcohol and drug abuse prevention. A similar organization, Community Anti-Drug Coalitions of America, advances a community-level focus on drug and alcohol prevention. The National Association of State Mental Health Program Directors does not currently have a comparable prevention-oriented structure. However, other groups, such as Mental Health America, have been advocating at local, state, and national levels for expansion of prevention programs related to mental health.

Insurance

Health insurers, both public and private, also have the potential to fund preventive services for MEB disorders, although it is not clear to what extent this is currently happening. Given turnover in enrollees, private insurers may have little incentive to cover preventive services that yield long-term benefits.

---

[12]See http://www.kde.state.ky.us/KDE/Instructional+Resources/Early+Childhood+Development/KIDS+NOW+Initiative.htm for more information.

However, Dorfman and Smith (2002) reviewed preventive mental health and substance abuse programs and concluded that six types of preventive interventions would be appropriate for a managed care organization to deliver from both a cost-effective and feasibility perspective. These interventions include four programs that would benefit children and adolescents: prenatal and infancy home visits, smoking cessation counseling for pregnant smokers, targeted short-term mental health therapy, and brief counseling to reduce alcohol use. A combination of screening, brief intervention, referral, and treatment is one Medicaid-eligible service that includes early intervention for those at risk for developing substance abuse disorders.

SAMHSA recently reported the results of a study on barriers to and recommendations for reimbursement of mental health services in primary care settings, focusing on services for those with public insurance (Kautz, Mauch, and Smith, 2008). The report highlights a number of barriers that apply to both preventive and treatment services, including limitations on same-day billing for physical and mental health services, limitations on reimbursement for mental health services provided by primary care practitioners rather than mental health specialists, lack of reimbursement for collaborative care and case management, lack of reimbursement for services provided by nonphysician practitioners, and inadequate reimbursement for services in rural and urban settings. The report also specifically identifies the lack of reimbursement incentives for screening and for providing preventive mental health services as a priority barrier (Kautz, Mauch, and Smith, 2008).

Reimbursement for services is sometimes limited by the choices of state Medicaid offices, by local carriers of intermediaries' interpretations in processing claims, and by specific private insurance plans. Delivery of behavioral health services is frequently covered only if the services qualify as a "medical necessity," which may vary in definition in managed care contracts and may vary for different services and by different state Medicaid programs and private insurance plans (Kautz, Mauch, and Smith, 2008; Nitzkin and Smith, 2004). For preventive services, the combination of limited available billing codes and the limitations on what is interpreted to qualify as a reimbursable billed service can lead in practice to very restricted reimbursement for preventive services. This contributes to inadequate provision of preventive services by primary care practitioners or promotion of these services by health care systems (Nitzkin and Smith, 2004). In *Clinical Preventive Services in Substance Abuse and Mental Health Update: From Science to Services* (Nitzkin and Smith, 2004), SAMHSA provides more detailed suggestions for primary care physician reimbursement for preventive services.

There is also only limited reimbursement for mental health services, including preventive services, in schools. Schools can be reimbursed by

Medicaid for some mental health services provided to eligible students in special education as well as through school-based health centers. However, these centers can bill Medicaid for these services only if they are provided by enrolled Medicaid providers. Enrollment is not often supported by the administrative capacity of many of these centers, and available providers may not be eligible. In addition, a very small percentage of schools have school-based health centers. Most provide health services directly by school employees (e.g., nurses, psychologists) who can receive only limited Medicaid reimbursement through agreements that vary from state to state (Kautz, Mauch, and Smith, 2008). And 20 percent of public schools report Medicaid reimbursement as a funding source for preventive mental health services (Foster, Rollefson, et al., 2005).

Addressing these obstacles to adequate reimbursement from both private and public payers is one necessary step toward improving preventive services for MEB disorders in primary care and at the interface between primary care and the school system, two of the major entry points for children and families in need of these services.

Some of the identified barriers to reimbursement are amplified by misunderstanding or misinterpretation of covered services and reimbursement rules and could be addressed through clarification of and education about reimbursement policies and definitions, especially in cases in which interpretations at the state and local level may be narrower than federal law (Kautz, Mauch, and Smith, 2008). Some states have also taken advantage of both improved clarity and flexibility in designing Medicaid benefits using Medicaid waivers to achieve improved coverage for mental health services; these can serve as models for change in other states. Other reimbursement barriers would require an expansion of allowable coverage by both publicly and privately funded insurance to increase reimbursement for mental health services that include prevention and screening (Kautz, Mauch, and Smith, 2008; Nitzkin and Smith, 2004).

SYSTEMS THAT SUPPORT DELIVERY OF PREVENTIVE SERVICES

In addition to the provision of funding, federal, state, and local governments can support service delivery systems that provide preventive services by identifying effective interventions as well as by offering technical assistance to community coalitions or organizations.

Identifying Effective Interventions

Federal agencies have sponsored multiple efforts to assess the evidence available related to specific preventive intervention programs. Four federal programs that have analyzed information about preventive interventions are (1) SAMHSA's National Registry of Evidence-Based Programs and Practices (NREPP),[13] which focuses specifically on programs related to mental health and substance abuse; (2) the Department of Justice's Model Programs Guide; (3) the White House–sponsored Helping America's Youth system; and (4) ED's What Works Clearinghouse. All four list some programs related to prevention of MEB disorders.

Each system has independent processes for rating programs and uses different criteria. The Center for Study and Prevention of Violence compared the ratings assigned by 12 different review efforts; over one-third (34.5 percent) of the 298 programs listed were reviewed by more than one effort. The same program was often given different ratings by different systems; for example, one review assigned its highest rating and another its lowest for the same program.

The NREPP system is somewhat different from the others in that it does not assign an overall rating, but rather assigns a score of 0-4 on multiple criteria and multiple outcomes, leaving it to the user to determine their relevance. One innovative aspect of the system is the inclusion of criteria (implementation materials, training support, and quality assurance) related to readiness for dissemination. The Model Programs Guide of the Department of Justice lists 38 exemplary and 67 effective prevention programs, and NREPP lists 32 reviewed mental health promotion[14] and 30 reviewed substance abuse prevention programs.[15]

In addition to these federally sponsored systems, a number of private and state-level organizations have established online systems to identify effective programs. Blueprints for Violence Prevention (see Chapter 11) is one of the oldest efforts to identify and rate evidence-based violence prevention programs. California has established a clearinghouse for information on recommended child welfare programs, and other states having established more broad-based clearinghouses.

There have also been numerous published reviews, most funded by federal agencies, that identify recommended programs related to juvenile justice (Mendel, 2001; Sherman, Gottfredson, et al., 1997), school-based prevention interventions (Greenberg, Domitrovich, and Bumbarger, 2001; Mihalic and Aultman-Bettridge, 2004), community-based approaches (Communities That Care, 2004), drug abuse prevention (National Institute on Drug Abuse, 2003), youth violence prevention (U.S. Public Health

---

[13]NREPP began as the Model Programs initiative in the Center for Substance Abuse Prevention.

[14]NREPP does not include a category for prevention of mental disorders, so mental health promotion in this context combines the terms as used by the committee.

[15]NREPP's predecessor, Model Programs, identified 66 model and 37 effective programs (many of which are prevention programs). All of these programs had to re-reviewed to be included in NREPP.

Service, 2001c), and underage drinking (Spoth, Greenberg, and Turrisi, 2008). Programs are given various designations including "effective," "exemplary," "promising," "research-based," and "model." In addition, many federally funded technical assistance centers include lists of evidence-based or effective programs on their web pages, often drawing from these many resources.

Increasingly, federal agencies and programs are requiring that program funds be used exclusively for "evidence-based programs." Guidance of what might be considered evidence-based varies, but generally it includes, but is not limited to, inclusion of a program on one or more federal lists. ACF recently issued a request for proposals to support infrastructure for the delivery of evidence-based home visitation programs, specifically excluding evidence from pre-post designs and programs that did not sustain results after two years.[16]

The SSHS Program has a somewhat broader set of criteria, defining evidence-based practices or interventions as "approaches to prevention, behavioral intervention, and treatment that are validated by some form of documented scientific evidence to indicate their effectiveness. Programs, practices, and interventions that are based on tradition, convention, belief, or anecdotal evidence are not evidence-based" (Safe Schools/Healthy Students Initiative, 2009, p. 43).

SAMHSA's guidance to states in selecting interventions to be used under the Strategic Prevention Framework is even broader. In addition to inclusion on a federal list or registry or being reported with positive effects in a peer-reviewed journal, it states that effectiveness can be based on:

a. a solid theory or theoretical perspective that has been validated by research;
b. a documented body of knowledge generated from similar or related interventions with empirical evidence; and
c. a consensus among informed experts (key community prevention leaders, elders, or other respected leaders in indigenous cultures) regarding effectiveness based on a combination of theory, research, and practice experience.

The Society for Prevention Research (SPR) recommended standards for identifying effective prevention programs and policies in response to the proliferation of lists and guidelines. SPR proposed a tiered evidence standard with a basic standard for efficacious interventions, additional requirements for effective interventions, and a yet higher standard for determining that an intervention is ready for broad dissemination (Flay,

---

[16]See http://www.acf.hhs.gov/grants/open/HHS-2008-ACF-ACYF-CA-0130.html.

Biglan, et al., 2005). One of the 31 requirements for an intervention to be designated "effective" is evaluation in real-world conditions (Flay, Biglan, et al., 2005). The importance of this criterion was recently demonstrated by Hallfors, Pankratz, and Hartman (2007), who tested a drug abuse prevention intervention that was designated as a model program by SAMHSA (under the old CSAP system)[17] and as "research-based" by NIDA based on efficacy trial data. In a large, multisite effectiveness trial, they showed main effects that were either null or worse for the experimental group compared with the control group. They argue that small efficacy trials provide insufficient evidence for the selection of interventions at the community level (see also Chapter 10).

Linking Research and Services

Identifying strategies for effective implementation of evidence-based programs is a clear future research priority (see Chapter 11). NIH has adopted several efforts to facilitate this process from a research perspective. First, in response to a general lack of knowledge about how to disseminate and implement effective prevention programs, they are convening trans-NIH forums to prepare applicants for new grant programs on dissemination and implementation research that explore characteristics of communities, interventions, and system change that impact prevention outcomes in community settings. Ideally, researchers and community organizations will develop partnerships to move this next generation of research forward in a productive manner.

In addition, NIMH's agenda for facilitating prevention programs is laid out in the *Bridging Science and Service* report (National Institute of Mental Health, 2006a) and follow-up reports. It emphasizes linking its agenda on implementation research with ongoing funding of programs by other federal agencies that are responsible for service delivery, including SAMHSA and ED. It specifies that key research questions should focus on mechanisms for successful implementation, particularly with ethnic and minority populations.

Programs designed to fund services typically do not provide adequate funding for rigorous evaluations; when programs are evaluated, they typically do not include random assignment. Although both the SSHS Program and the Strategic Prevention Framework encourage evaluation, there is currently no national evaluation information available. SSHS has published a sample of data from local evaluations, with promising evidence of positive outcomes. These evaluations do not appear, however, in published scientific

---

[17]The program is being re-reviewed by NREPP, but it is unclear if this study will be included in the review.

literature. Improved formal linkages between service and research programs would help build the implementation knowledge base without redirecting service resources toward research and vice versa.

Technical Assistance and Clearinghouses

Federal agencies also provide support for a variety of activities aimed at building the capacity of states, communities, and organizations to provide services aimed at strengthening families, preventing youth risk factors, and designing systems of care. Federal agencies fund numerous technical assistance centers, often linked to specific grant programs (see Box 12-2). Many of the centers provide online guidance on program design, technical assistance and/or training on program design and implementation, and links to other resources. Unlike 1994, when there was "no federal clearinghouse for published information on prevention of mental disorders" (Institute of Medicine, 1994, p. 424), there is now a plethora of resource centers to provide information on preventive intervention. There appears to be no shortage of sources of information, although using them requires navigating through a maze of resources, and selection of the best program to match site variations and desired outcomes may be a daunting task.

In addition, through its Strategic Prevention Framework, SAMHSA aims to increase implementation of prevention and early intervention programs. Specific to substance abuse prevention, SAMHSA funds five Regional Centers for the Application of Prevention Technologies,[18] which provide training and technical assistance and offer a range of online resources through Prevention Pathways.[19] Technical assistance resources on the Communities That Care initiative (see Box 11-1) designed to help communities match evaluated programs with local risk and protective factors, are available on SAMHSA's Strategic Prevention Framework website.[20] SAMHSA's Suicide Prevention Resource Center provides training to strengthen suicide prevention networks, and most of the technical assistance centers provide some level of informal implementation training.

CREATING A TRAINED WORKFORCE

A well-trained workforce, an educated public, and an informed complement of policy makers and funders who will support prevention are all important components of success. For prevention of MEB disorders, the workforce must come from many disciplines, each of which should work

---

[18]See http://captus.samhsa.gov/home.cfm.
[19]See http://preventionpathways.samhsa.gov/.
[20]See http://ncadi.samhsa.gov/features/ctc/resources.aspx.

BOX 12-2
Federally Funded Technical Assistance Centers
with a Prevention or Promotion Focus

Center for Effective Collaboration and Practice (ED and HHS/SAMHSA/CMHS)
   http://cecp.air.org/center.asp
Center for Mental Health in Schools (HHS/HRSA/MCHB)
   http://smhp.psych.ucla.edu/overview.htm
Center for School Mental Health Analysis and Action (HHS/HRSA/MCHB)
   http://csmh.umaryland.edu/
Center on the Social and Emotional Foundations for Early Learning (HHS/ACF)
   http://www.vanderbilt.edu/csefel
Family Guide: Keeping Youth Mentally Healthy and Drug Free
   (HHS/SAMHSA/CSAP)
   http://www.family.samhsa.gov/
FRIENDS, the National Resource Center for Community-Based Child Abuse
   Prevention (HHS/ACF)
   http://www.friendsnrc.org.
National Center for Mental Health Promotion and Youth Violence Prevention
   (HHS/SAMHSA)
   http://www.promoteprevent.org
National Technical Assistance Center for Children's Mental Health (HHS/
   SAMHSA/CMHS and HHS/ACF/Children's Bureau)
   http://gucchd.georgetown.edu/programs/ta_center/index.html
National Youth Violence Prevention Resource Center (CDC and other federal
   partners)
   http://www.safeyouth.org
Suicide Prevention Resource Center (HHS/SAMHSA)
   http://www.sprc.org

NOTES: ACF = Administration for Children and Families, CDC = Centers for Disease Control and Prevention, CMHS = Center for Mental Health Services, CSAP = Center for Substance Abuse Prevention, ED = U.S. Department of Education, HHS = U.S. Department of Health and Human Services, HRSA = Health Resources and Services Administration, MCHB = Maternal and Child Health Bureau, SAMHSA = Substance Abuse and Mental Health Services Administration.

---

synergistically with the others. Training of neuroscientists, psychologists, sociologists, economists, systems engineers, and those in other basic science disciplines to carry out discovery efforts that will fuel new and better prevention interventions continues to be important (see also Chapter 5). Clinicians, including psychologists, social workers, nurses, and physicians, must be prepared to recognize risks and appropriately intervene within the scope of their clinical practice. Finally, teachers and others who work with children on a regular basis should have available training that enhances their knowledge, skills, and attitudes toward prevention of MEB disorders. Thus training and education not only require a broad effort, but also are extraordinarily complex and challenging.

The committee considers core aspects of training to include activities that enhance the knowledge, skills, attitudes, and experience of professionals who will carry out the various elements of programs addressing prevention of MEB disorders. Training must be directed to achieve research capabilities, teaching skills, and the capability to implement prevention programs as well as collect and analyze data on outcomes from such efforts.

The 1994 IOM report contained limited information on training activities in the areas of prevention science and prevention implementation, but it concluded that training needs and output were approximately in balance with workforce needs. It reported a total of 22 NIH-funded research trainee slots per year and estimated that there were no more than 500 professionals conducting prevention research related to MEB disorders. The report roughly estimated that there was a need for approximately 1,000 investigators in the field and proposed that numbers of trainees as well as support for training should gradually increase to match expected growth in this field of investigation.

Based on assessment of progress in prevention training since the 1994 IOM report, the current status of training efforts, and gaps to be bridged, the committee concludes that refinement, translation, and broad implementation of preventive interventions are likely to languish for another 14 years unless more extensive and robust training for both researchers and practitioners is realized.

There are no data about workforce numbers or training needs specifically directed to prevention of mental disorders and substance abuse. One difficulty arises from the fact that prevention science and prevention implementation are not distinct disciplines, but are embedded in related disciplines, such as psychology, psychiatry, social sciences, social work, nursing, and medical specialties. Neuroscience, epidemiology and biostatistics, developmental sciences, and education could be added to this list. This positioning of prevention sciences and prevention implementation should be viewed as a strength, but it also creates difficulty in estimating both need and response.

The committee concurs with the 1994 IOM report that prevention training and education should be multidisciplinary, both for research and implementation, and should be layered on the professional skills acquired in traditional training programs. Trainees must be prepared not only to conduct prevention research in their own specialty area, but also to collaborate with colleagues in related areas. Therefore, there is a need to coordinate and integrate training across many disciplines and across a spectrum of prevention functions. The complexity of prevention efforts calls for broad and coordinated organization of training as well as multidisciplinary funding mechanisms.

Overview of Training/Education Since 1994

Since the 1994 IOM report, membership in the Society for Prevention Research increased 450 percent from 125 in 1992 to 690 in 2005 (see http://www.preventionresearch.org/about.php, accessed February 8, 2008). A search of the SPR online membership database identified 339 members who reported mental health as a content area, 434 who identified drugs, and 401 who identified alcohol.[21] Other societies address specific areas in prevention research and program implementation (e.g., child abuse and neglect), but membership numbers do not capture those with a prevention orientation to MEB disorders.

One measure of training activity is the number of training grants awarded by NIH institutes for prevention training related to MEB disorders. Based on the committee's analysis of FY 2006 training grants[22] with either a major or minor focus on prevention:

- The number of individual training grants, or F series (n = 13), was nearly the same as in 1994 (n = 12). These awards were relatively evenly dispersed across the three institutes (five each by NIMH and NIDA, three by NIAAA).
- The number of institutional training grants (n = 29) grew substantially since 1994, when there were only five. Institutional prevention training grants addressing mental health were awarded to a variety of academic programs, including prevention science programs, schools of public health, and clinical psychology programs and departments of psychiatry, with a number mentioning opportunities for training across disciplines. NIMH funded a substantial majority of these institutional training awards (19 of 29). Nevertheless, institutional awards targeting some aspect of prevention made up less than 10 percent of all training awards from NIMH.
- The largest number (n = 69) of training awards targeting prevention of MEB disorders consisted of career development grants (K series). The majority of these (n = 60) included a major focus on prevention of MEB disorders, often along with nonprevention objectives. These grants represent a substantial investment in career develop-

---

[21]Members can report more than one content area.
[22]Abstracts of all FY 2006 grants listed in the NIH CRISP database were evaluated for proposed prevention-related research training and career development.

ment by the three institutes, particularly NIMH, which funded 40 of the 69 awards. It is unclear whether young professionals who receive prevention training early in their faculty careers sustain this research support as they advance academically. Data concerning the rate of conversion of K series (career development) prevention awards to R (research) awards are not readily available.

The NIMH, NIDA, and NIAAA prevention research centers mentioned above, as well as the methodology centers discussed in Chapter 10, undoubtedly also fund infrastructural elements important for research training. For example, the NIMH prevention research center at Arizona State University provides a long-standing (20-year) model of training in prevention research. It prepares both predoctoral and postdoctoral trainees in four phases of prevention research: (1) generative research involving theoretical models of development, (2) design of interventions, (3) experimental field trials to test theoretical models, and (4) dissemination or diffusion of interventions to improve mental health and substance use outcomes through work in interdisciplinary teams (Sandler and Chassin, 2002). Training mechanisms include recent directions, such as quantitative methods, cross-cultural research, integrative models and multidisciplinary approaches, and longitudinal research. By 2002, the program had had 29 predoctoral and 22 postdoctoral trainees. Of the predoctoral trainees, 16 had finished their doctoral degree and 11 are in tenure-track faculty positions. Of the postdoctoral trainees, 12 are in tenure-track positions and 5 in research positions at medical schools and research centers (Sandler and Chassin, 2002).

In the past, NIMH funded up to 11 institutional training grants in the area of psychiatric epidemiology, a pivotal discipline for prevention program planning. However, these numbers have dwindled in the last several years, with five current programs.[23]

Needs for prevention research and implementation capacity building have not been formally assessed. *Blueprint for Change: Research on Child and Adolescent Mental Health* (National Advisory Mental Health Council Workgroup on Child and Adolescent Mental Health Intervention Development and Deployment, 2001) called for greater research capacity to "take advantage of the promise of interdisciplinary research." It recommended the creation of Child and Adolescent Interdisciplinary Training Institutes to include basic behavioral and neuroscience, epidemiology, prevention, intervention development, health services, and health economics research,

---

[23]See http://www.psych.org/MainMenu/Research/ResearchTrainingandFunding/ResearchTraining Opportunities/PsychiatricEpidemiologyResearchTrainingPrograms/PsychiatricEpidemiologyTraining-ProgramDescriptions.aspx.

as well as training in methodology, statistics, and the range of service settings in which mental health care is delivered. The report recommended a national mentorship program and suggested that NIMH explore opportunities to partner with MCHB, AHRQ of HRSA, CMHS/SAMHSA, and CSAP/SAMHSA to create and fund research training activities. As in many other reports, the emphasis of the blueprint was on treatment, not prevention. That report did note that, whereas overall NIMH funding, including K awards, had increased impressively over the preceding decade, the percentage of funds allocated to individual and institutional training grants, particularly those addressing child mental health, had not kept pace.

An example of a broadly positioned training program is Project Mainstream (Multi-Agency Initiative on Substance Abuse Training and Education for America), which is administered by AMERSA (Association for Medical Education and Research in Substance Abuse) and funded by HRSA and SAMHSA.[24] The objectives of this project include the conduct of interdisciplinary faculty development programs and the creation of regional training networks as well as a national electronic communications resource to support faculty development in the area of substance abuse. This program has targeted training in 15 different health professions. The Project Mainstream strategic plan states that all graduating trainees should be competent in identifying and referring for assistance the children of parents with substance use disorders and advising communities about resources for effective substance use prevention programs, such as specialty-specific curricula and tools. Another goal of the strategic plan is to convene representatives of certification, accreditation, and licensure boards to consider how their organizations can contribute to substance use training through their requirements and testing processes. There is not a similar effort for multispecialty training in mental disorders identification, treatment, and prevention.

These data suggest that numbers of prevention science trainees have increased substantially since the 1994 IOM report. However, no conclusive statement can be made about the magnitude of growth in numbers of prevention scientists. It is likely that the numbers continue to fall short of needs and the opportunities to create, demonstrate efficacy of, and implement preventions that promise to reduce MEB disorders.

Current Training Efforts

Since 1994, when the focus of training was on prevention researchers, training and education needs have broadened. These now include other basic researchers who serve as discovery engines as well as a broad array

---

[24]See http://www.projectmainstream.net.

of implementers and an informed citizenry (including public policy makers and funders).

Prevention Research

As in 1994, the majority of prevention scientists are psychologists (Eddy, Smith, et al., 2005). Eddy, Smith, and colleagues (2005) noted "a common inclination" in the field to assess interventions through randomized controlled trials while highlighting an additional approach labeled collaborative community action research. This approach broadens research to include assessment of implementation and also considers quasi-experimental designs as important contributors to prevention science knowledge (Eddy, Smith, et al., 2005).

To explore how these prescriptions for prevention science training have influenced current training, Eddy, Smith, and colleagues (2005) surveyed 262 self-identified prevention scientists across the spectrum of trainees, early investigators, and established researchers in 13 content areas. Areas with the least knowledge, training, and preparedness were new or developing ones (compared with traditional areas), particularly the history of prevention research, funding for prevention research, and the conduct of economic analyses. Early career participants were considerably behind established researchers in the areas of design of preventive intervention trials and community collaboration.

The results suggested that a "learning as you go" or apprentice model prevails and may not be rapidly responsive to the emergence of new content areas. Recommendations for training experiences included testing of various training models, cross-site training opportunities, participation in protocols that are in different phases of development and involve different methodologies, and embedding more prevention science in traditional graduate curricula. For training of postdoctoral scientists, opportunities to standardize curricula and expectations for training outcomes will be limited. Although several efforts have attempted to attract underserved minority trainees into prevention science, success in this area has been limited (Eddy, Martinez, et al., 2002). Such efforts are needed to improve the cultural competence and sensitivity of teams studying risk factors in these populations.

A specific identified need is midcareer training for scientists who wish to switch to the prevention research field (Sandler and Chassin, 2002). Training and funding mechanisms to support these career changes have not been systematically implemented and represent an important future opportunity.

Neuroscience

Neuroscience has exploded over the last decade or two, across multiple disciplines. There is no shortage of scientists being trained or in early career development stages in neurophysiology, neurogenetics, neurotoxicology, molecular neurosciences, and central nervous system imaging. A substantial number are focusing their efforts on understanding the biology of cognition, emotional responses, brain development, and psychopathology. It is very difficult, however, to identify the array of laboratories that are asking questions about neurobiological systems directly relevant to risk factors or protective factors or to interventions for early symptoms that herald MEB disorders.

Numerous laboratories are identifying genes associated with mental disorders as well as gene–environment interactions and epigenetic mechanisms (see Chapter 5). Predictive and preventive use of genetic information represents an attractive target for basic and translational research. Opportunities to train in these settings are abundant. Similarly, young investigators are training in imaging centers that are attempting to identify structural or functional variations in the brain that predict MEB disorders. The potential for these studies to facilitate prevention in the future is broadly accepted. Ensuring that biological and psychosocial approaches to prevention converge will be an important objective of training (see Chapter 5).

Public Health

A master of public health (M.P.H.) degree or a doctoral degree (Ph.D., Dr.Ph.) from a school of public health can be an initial step toward a career in prevention science. The published accreditation criteria for schools of public health (Council on Education for Public Health, 2005) list social and behavior sciences as one of five areas of knowledge basic to public health. Often this translates to study of behaviors that influence health-related decisions on a population basis. Prevention components of educational curricula and research programs more often target physical diseases. Some schools of public health do have curricula in mental health epidemiology and programmatically tie such disciplines as epidemiology, economics, and political science to preventive interventions in such content areas as alcohol or tobacco use, adult depression, and child psychopathology (Perry, Albee, et al., 1996). Related areas of training include behavioral science, mental health promotion, and health policy. Although data are not available to allow quantification of the contribution of schools of public health to the workforce related to prevention of MEB disorders, these schools should prepare future leaders in mental health promotion and disorder prevention, whether in research, community services, or administration/policy.

Health Care Professionals

The observation that "the health care workforce [is] . . . not equipped uniformly and sufficiently in terms of knowledge and skills, cultural diversity and understanding, geographic distribution, and numbers to provide the access to and quality of services needed by consumers" (Institute of Medicine, 2006b, pp. 286-324) was made with reference to mental health and certainly holds true for prevention, which has historically taken a back seat to diagnosis and treatment. Compounding this shortcoming is the broad range of health professionals who are engaged in mental health and substance use efforts, trained apart using curricula that are not built on core competencies or interdisciplinary considerations. The potential for clinicians to contribute systematically to prevention of MEB disorders is substantial, but realizing this potential will require transformational changes on the part of training institutions, professional societies, regulatory bodies, and funders.

Physicians: Medical School. Although health promotion and disease prevention are addressed formally or informally in many medical schools, mental health promotion and prevention of MEB disorders are often neglected. Less than half of all U.S. medical schools specifically address prevention and health maintenance. For those schools, it is taught primarily in the first 2 years for an average of only 22 hours (Institute of Medicine, 2004). Prevention of mental disorders would occupy at most a small percentage of that time. Similarly, dedicated training in substance use is rarely offered. According to 1998-1999 data from the Liaison Committee on Medical Education, only 8 percent of medical schools had a required course on substance use (Haack and Adger, 2002). The current level of exposure of medical students to substance use issues does not give graduates the confidence to screen, assess, or provide needed interventions (Miller, Sheppard, et al., 2001).

The knowledge base, skills, and attitudes for graduates regarding prevention of MEB disorders are not systemically assessed. The IOM report *Improving Medical Education: Enhancing the Behavioral and Social Science Content of Medical School Curricula* (2004, p. 98) recommended "that the National Board of Medical Examiners increase behavioral and social science content on the US Medical Licensing Examination." Response to this recommendation would be a step in the right direction, but more specific attention to prevention and mental health promotion education is needed to prepare medical students for prevention activities related to MEB disorders.

Physicians: Residency. Postgraduate residency training in psychiatry; primary care specialties, such as pediatrics, internal medicine, and family medicine; preventive medicine; and in subspecialty training in such areas as behavioral and developmental pediatrics are particularly relevant to the prevention of MEB disorders among young people. However, there is no accredited pathway for subspecialty training of physicians in the prevention of MEB disorders.

Resident and subspecialty resident (fellow) experiences are dictated by the Accreditation Council for Graduate Medical Education (ACGME) program requirements and by the content specifications of the specialty and subspecialty certifying boards. Prevention research experiences for specialty and subspecialty residents are available to trainees, only if there are current research activities or interests in the environment in which they train.

Two programs of the Robert Wood Johnson Foundation have fostered prevention training: the highly competitive Clinical Scholars Program for postresidency training and the equally competitive Physician Faculty Scholars Program for assistant professors in an array of specialty areas. Both have funded scholars who have explored areas of prevention related to mental health. These programs are models for training that can attract future leaders to the area of prevention of MEB disorders.

ACGME requirements for psychiatry, pediatrics, and preventive medicine training pay little attention to prevention. For example:

- Psychiatry training requirements state that the didactic curriculum must include the fundamental principles of epidemiology, etiology, diagnosis, treatment, and prevention of all psychiatric disorders, including biological, psychosocial, sociocultural, and iatrogenic factors that affect the prevention, incidence, prevalence, long-term course, and treatment of psychiatric disorders. They state that the resident should "know how to advocate for the promotion of mental health and the prevention of disease." These are the only 2 sentences in 34 pages of requirements that directly address prevention of mental disorders and substance abuse; only eight hours on average are devoted to substance use health care in psychiatry residency (Isaacson, Fleming, et al., 2000).

- Pediatric residents must be instructed, during a required one-month block in development and behavioral pediatrics, in psychosocial screening techniques as well as approaches to the identification of the needs of children at risk, for example, in fragmented or substance abusing families or in foster care. As a component of their one-month experience in adolescent medicine, residents are expected to engage psychosocial issues, such as depression, eating disorders, and substance abuse. No mention is made of prevention. Residents are expected to know how to advocate for promotion of health and prevention of disease or injury, but with no specification of applications to behavioral disorders. Subspecialty residents in pediatrics are not formally trained to recognize chronic health disorders as risk factors for MEB disorders of youth.

- Requirements for training in preventive medicine[25] are largely silent with regard to prevention of MEB disorders. Core knowledge is expected to include "behavioral aspects of health," but the requirements do not otherwise address MEB disorders or their prevention. The certifying examination for preventive medicine does not specifically test knowledge or skills directed to prevention of MEB disorders. Drug use training in preventive medicine residency largely focuses on tobacco (Abrams, Saitz, and Sancet, 2003).

None of the medical specialty training requirements emphasize the need to be conversant with screening for risk or protective factors for mental disorders or to understand systems that are in place to manage risk as well as reinforce protective factors. The overall lack of attention to training related to prevention of MEB disorders contrasts with a consensus in the pediatric community that training for residents should be enhanced to prepare them for more knowledgeable, competent behavioral/mental health screening and care (American Academy of Pediatrics, 2001; American Academy of Pediatrics Task Force on Mental Health, in preparation). The American Board of Family Medicine (ABFM) has identified similar needs for their trainees (personal communication with Larry Green, ABFM board member, October 8, 2007).

Social Work

Master's-level social work training (the routine degree for practitioners) currently is provided by approximately 200 programs accredited by the Council on Social Work Education. Accreditation standards do not address substance use in general or prevention in this realm (Straussner and Senreich, 2002). Curriculum requirements emphasize content in human behavior, clinical diagnosis, treatment planning, and service delivery. Prevention frameworks and program examples are included in the Human Behavior and Social Environment course sequences required of all social work graduate curricula. While a 1996 report (Perry, Albee, et al., 1996) found that only 12 schools offered a course in prevention (not specifically prevention of MEB disorders), most schools of social work have elective courses in drug and alcohol abuse prevention, and many offer courses in mental health interventions, as well as child maltreatment prevention and treatment.

---

[25]Preventive medicine is a three-year training program for physicians that combines a year of clinical medicine and 24 months of academic and practicum training, leading to an M.P.H.

Since 1993, NIMH has funded a small number of social work programs to conduct research as well as provide special scholarships and coursework on prevention research for doctoral students, which has increased the supply of researchers trained in prevention research methods (Institute for the Advancement of Social Work Research, n.d.). Recently, NIMH launched other initiatives to enhance partnerships to integrate evidence-based mental health practices into social work education and research (Institute for the Advancement of Social Work Research, n.d.), but prevention research is a relatively small part of these initiatives.

Clinical Psychology. There are approximately 90,000 clinically trained psychologists in the United States, many of whom have training in child psychology. Training in prevention of MEB disorders is not standard for most master's- or doctoral-level curricula or for certification or licensure in school psychology. A 2003 report of a task force of the Society of Pediatric Psychology recommended 12 topic areas most important for training experiences of child psychologists. Three of these areas were prevention, family support, and health promotion (Spirito, Brown, et al., 2003). Similarly, in their call for redesign of clinical psychology graduate education, Snyder and Elliott make a case for focus on individual strengths (protective factors), and lifestyle or community-level influences on mental health. They conclude that prevention must be an essential feature of education curricula. They note that a few psychology training programs do stress reduction of risk factors, but they recommend that postdoctoral programs in clinical psychology increase their focus on prevention and health (Snyder and Elliott, 2005). The response to these recommendations will be important to monitor.

Similarly, psychologists typically receive little training or preparation for dealing with substance abuse. Half or more receive no didactic or practical training in substance use conditions according to a 1990s survey (Institute of Medicine, 2006b). Their clinical training, as for other health professionals, is focused on diagnosis and treatment. Certification of clinical competence is offered by the American Board of Professional Psychology. Licensure in some states requires written or oral evaluations of knowledge. Neither licensure nor certification assesses competence related to prevention of MEB disorders.

Community psychology, developmental psychology, and social psychology are other potential training pathways for a career in prevention research and program implementation, although none of these areas focuses exclusively or in major part on prevention. It is not uncommon for graduate students who wish to work in the area of prevention of MEB disorders to construct independent study programs (Perry, Albee, et al., 1996).

Nursing. Nursing education is generally completed in two (associate's degree) or four years (bachelor's degree; eligibility for licensure as a registered nurse). Increasing numbers of nursing students become nurse practitioners with advanced degrees, either a master's or a doctor of nursing practice. A number of nursing students are obtaining Ph.D.s, acquiring nursing research skills, and working in academic or research settings. Nursing school curricula stress prevention concepts, but most devote little time to prevention of MEB disorders. One effort has been the Nursing Child Assessment Satellite Training at the University of Washington, a national program to train nurses and other health care professionals to assess parent–child relationships in community settings.[26] Psychiatric nurses (more than 18,000; Institute of Medicine, 2006b) usually have added training or a graduate degree and are certified by the American Nurses Credentialing Center. There are more than 20 university-based master's degree programs in psychiatric nursing, many having specialty tracks specific to child and adolescent psychiatric nursing, and a certification process for child/adolescent psychiatric nursing. As with other health care professions, advanced training does not uniformly target prevention. However, there are innovative efforts, such as a 2008 HRSA award to the College of Nursing at Arizona State University for the multidisciplinary online training program called KySS (Keep Your Child/Yourself Safe, and Secure), focused on screening, identifying, and delivering evidence-based intervention for youth experiencing common MEB problems.[27] Prevention training related to MEB disorders in nursing is an important opportunity.

Substance Abuse and Mental Health Counseling. Substance abuse counselors and mental health counselors together comprise the largest group of mental health professionals. Numbers of mental health counselors alone approach 120,000, and half of the personnel delivering substance use treatment are substance abuse counselors (Institute of Medicine, 2006b). Coursework and practical experience requirements vary between these two groups, across state lines, and from program to program. Licensure or certification is required by some states, more for mental health than for substance abuse counselors. Requirements for coursework or practicum experience, when they are specified, do not include exposure or experience related to preventive aspects of MEB disorders (Kerwin, Walker-Smith, and Kirby, 2006). The content of continuing education is largely unspecified and does not require that preventive aspects of MEB disorders be addressed. While many states have certified preventionist positions in the area of substance abuse

---

[26]See http://www.ncast.org/index.html.
[27]See http://www.napnap.org/index.cfm?page=198&sec=221&ssec=499.

prevention, with criteria for certification specified, no comparable position exists in the mental health area.

Education Providers

Neither the core curriculum for a bachelor's degree nor the process for obtaining a teaching certificate anticipate that teachers will be prepared to recognize risk factors or detect early evidence of MEB disorders in their pupils. Coursework for education degree students includes descriptions of mental disorders (along with physical disorders and retardation), but it does not systematically include how to identify, intervene, or refer children at risk for MEB disorders. Special education trains teachers to recognize and work with children who have special needs that schools, by law, must address. Children with externalizing disorders (conduct, hyperactivity) are identified and directed to remedial programs when they are disruptive. Children with internalizing disorders (e.g., withdrawal, anxiety, depression) are often not identified for attention because they do not impose an added burden on the teacher or classroom. As federal mandates for testing and academic achievement have been strengthened, MEB issues have been relegated to lower priority status for teachers. Training in evidence-based behavior management techniques for teachers is essential for helping them to address the behavior problems that can develop into MEB disorders (Epstein, Atkins, et al., 2008).

The National Association of School Psychologists has 25,000 members and strongly encourages mental health promotion and prevention of disorders through a variety of programs. For example, Prevention, Crisis Intervention and Mental Health is 1 of 11 domains of the organization's continuing professional development program (NASP Professional Development; see http://www.nasponline.org, accessed September 29, 2008). However, the contribution of school psychologists has limitations as a result of school budget contractions. Except for a few schools that have adopted specific experimental or innovative universal or selective interventions, most schools do not prepare their staff to screen for risk factors, nor do they adopt universal measures to decrease risk or enhance protective factors (personal communication, Mary Boat, College of Education, University of Cincinnati). In many ways, this is an opportunity lost, but transformational changes will be needed in school systems to respond to this opportunity. Nevertheless, the school setting represents one of the best opportunities for prevention interventions, whether universal, selective, or indicated.

Preschools and day care centers (for children from birth to age 5) may be in the most advantageous position to observe young children and identify risks or early symptoms. However, preschool teachers often have less training than school teachers and are frequently unprepared to engage in activities that lead to identification and helpful intervention for mental, emotional, and behavioral problems.

Law and the Judicial System

While some individuals in the legal system appear to be aware and responsive to the needs of children, particularly those at risk for MEB disorders, children's needs are often secondary to other considerations. Such situations arise frequently when such issues as child custody and visitation are decided in cases of divorce, domestic violence, or child abuse and neglect. Recognition that these situations place children's mental health at risk should lead to decisions that consider, above all, the children's well-being. Enhanced mechanisms for informing lawyers, magistrates, and judges about the role they can play in the prevention of MEB disorders should be adopted, starting in law school.

Public Awareness and Public Policy

A pivotal effort must target the training of youth, their families, and the public to understand the importance of mitigating risks for MEB disorders. This universal approach should include policy makers and individuals who determine how public and private funds will be allocated in the attempt to improve mental health outcomes for children.

A public that is aware of the huge burden of MEB disorders, as well as the needs and opportunities for prevention, will be more likely to promote informed decision making about programmatic responses from both the private and the public sectors. Vehicles for dissemination of information include, first and foremost, the media, including opportunities to dispel the stigma associated with MEB disorders (see Chapter 8). Schools should also play a role, as should primary health care providers. Professional societies, as well as private and government agencies, should have major educational roles. Priorities have targeted diagnosis, treatment, and rehabilitation, perhaps at the expense of prevention efforts. Achieving the proper balance in the future will require informed discussions and decisions at the highest levels. Prevention often is not addressed because the public expects immediate return on its investment. Education should include compelling information about the real and potential benefits and cost reductions of successful prevention efforts. In particular, this information should be directed to public policy makers. Education and possibly publicly supported incentives must also target health care payers who currently often refuse reimbursement for prevention efforts.

CONCLUSIONS AND RECOMMENDATIONS

For the goals of prevention of MEB disorders to be achieved, the three elements of prevention program infrastructure in this chapter must be the focus of ongoing improvement efforts: innovation driven by funded research, a coordinated and effective delivery system, and enhancement of workforce quality and quantity.

Developing a Coordinated and Effective Delivery System

Numerous federal programs and resources fund and guide states and communities in their promotion and prevention efforts. Coordination across these efforts is limited and presents a barrier to large-scale implementation of best practices. Funding for programs and their evaluation is fragmented and inadequate to reach many youth in need. As communities increasingly are able to select programs from available lists of evidence-based approaches, the infrastructure to sort out how best to match program features with community needs and resources and to learn what constitutes the most effective match is often not in place.

Conclusion: Federal programs whose goals include the prevention of MEB disorders are not well coordinated, and there is little strategic synergy between research and service delivery.

Compounding the deficiencies of infrastructure are substantial barriers to implementation of prevention programs in potentially advantageous settings, such as day care, schools, and primary medical care. Too often programs are created de novo and require costly new infrastructure. Barriers such as funding or reimbursement of services can be addressed most effectively at a national or state level. Program funding often does not include expectations that demonstrably effective programs be implemented with fidelity or that outcomes of these programs be rigorously evaluated, and it does not typically support outcomes assessments.

Conclusion: There is a need for the development of systems (service sites and networks) that can implement evidence-based programs, test their effectiveness in real-world environments, and provide a funding stream for evidence-based prevention services.

Funding and infrastructure for substance abuse prevention interventions is more advanced than for prevention or promotion of mental health. There are no targeted funding streams for prevention in the mental health area.

Recommendation 12-1: Congress should establish a set-aside for prevention services and innovation in the Community Mental Health Services Block Grant, similar to the set-aside in the Substance Abuse Prevention and Treatment Block Grant.

Providing a set-aside with the Mental Health Services Block Grant could send a clear message that prevention is a priority and begin to help refocus the mental health system on prevention activities. This should be the first step in refocusing the mental health system to include a targeted focus on prevention and should be coupled with efforts across agencies to increase prevention funding, including collaborations between SAMHSA and the Centers for Medicaid and Medicare Services to address barriers to reimbursement of prevention services. At the same time, innovation in other service systems is also needed, ideally coupled with rigorous evaluation to continue to develop prevention systems. Resources for preventive services, however, often do not include sufficient evaluation resources.

Recommendation 12-2: The U.S. Departments of Health and Human Services, Education, and Justice should braid funding of research and practice so that the impact of programs and practices that are being funded by service agencies (e.g., the Substance Abuse and Mental Health Services Administration, the Office of Safe and Drug-Free Schools, the Office of Juvenile Justice and Delinquency Prevention) are experimentally evaluated through research funded by other agencies (e.g., the National Institutes of Health, the Institute of Education Sciences, the National Institute of Justice). This should include developing appropriate infrastructure through which evidence-based programs and practices can be delivered.

Models for implementing braided funding, which is supported by NIMH's *Bridging Science and Services* report (National Institute of Mental Health, 2006), could include joint requests for proposals or targeting research resources to existing service programs. One example of the latter approach is a recent request for applications from NIH that targeted research resources for research activities tied to grantees under SAMHSA's Comprehensive Community Mental Health Services Program for Children and Families.[28] Other federal programs, such as initiatives under SAMHSA's Strategic Prevention Framework, including the SSHS Program, could be similarly linked with NIH research resources.

Numerous preventive interventions are now available and being implemented by states and communities. However, efforts to expand these

---

[28]See http://grants.nih.gov/grants/guide/pa-files/PA-07-091.html.

interventions state-, county-, or locality-wide are needed to establish an infrastructure for the delivery of preventive interventions across systems of care.

> **Recommendation 12-3:** The U.S. Departments of Health and Human Services, Education, and Justice should fund states, counties, and local communities to implement and continuously improve evidence-based approaches to mental health promotion and prevention of MEB disorders in systems of care that work with young people and their families.

A dizzying array of technical assistance centers, online resources, and publications and guides is available. Prominent among them are efforts to identify effective programs. Differences across these efforts, particularly in the standards applied, make it difficult to understand the meaning of an assigned rating or to assess the expected results of a given program.

> **Recommendation 12-4:** Federal and state agencies should prioritize the use of evidence-based programs and promote the rigorous evaluation of prevention and promotion programs in a variety of settings in order to increase the knowledge base of what works, for whom, and under what conditions. The definition of evidence-based should be determined by applying established scientific criteria.

In applying scientific criteria, the agencies should consider the following standards:

- Evidence for efficacy or effectiveness of prevention and promotion programs should be based on designs that provide significant confidence in the results. The highest level of confidence is provided by multiple, well-conducted randomized experimental trials, and their combined inferences should be used in most cases. Single trials that randomize individuals, places (e.g., schools), or time (e.g., wait-list or some time-series designs) can all contribute to this type of strong evidence for examining intervention impact.
- When evaluations with such experimental designs are not available, evidence for efficacy or effectiveness cannot be considered definitive, even if based on the next strongest designs, including those with at least one matched comparison. Designs that have no control group (e.g., pre-post comparisons) are even weaker.
- Programs that have widespread community support as meeting community needs should be subject to experimental evaluations before being considered evidence-based.

- Priority should be given to programs with evidence of effectiveness in real-world environments, reasonable cost, and manuals or other materials available to guide implementation with a high level of fidelity.

Also key to these efforts will be education of the public about the need for prevention efforts and the benefits that can be achieved. An informed and supportive public is needed to adopt and advocate for effective prevention of MEB disorders and promotion of better mental health outcomes.

Research

Although the volume of prevention research and evidence for successful intervention efforts has grown substantially since 1994, there are rapidly expanding needs for more and better research. In contrast to the need and opportunity, funding for studies of preventive interventions for MEB disorders and their implementation has taken a back seat to funding of studies directed to the diagnosis and treatment of behavioral disorders. In addition, no single agency (federal or private) has prioritized research funding directed to the prevention of MEB disorders or is driving prevention research efforts in a coordinated way.

Conclusion: Federal agencies responsible for funding mental health research have prioritized studies of treatment over prevention.

Several NIH institutes (NIMH, NICHD, NIDA, NIAAA, AHRQ) contribute substantially but focus largely on a single disorder. Coordinated funding by NIH institutes and other agencies is not visible. This paucity of prospective, collaborative funding makes it particularly difficult to generate an integrated, comprehensive approach to innovative prevention research. Funding mechanisms for stimulating research at the intersection of basic science and the development and implementation of new and better preventive interventions are needed now and will be increasingly critical in the future. Basic research in neurobiology, psychology, sociology, economics, and related fields should be supported to fuel the creation of novel strategies for prevention and to promote collaborative, multidisciplinary translational research to document the effectiveness of these strategies (see also Recommendations 5-2 and 5-3).

Recommendation 12-5: The National Institutes of Health and other federal agencies should increase funding for research on prevention and promotion strategies that reduce multiple MEB disorders and that strengthen accomplishment of age-appropriate developmental tasks. High priority should be given to increasing collaboration and joint funding across institutes and across federal agencies that are responsible for separate but developmentally related outcomes (e.g., mental health, substance use, school success, contact with the justice system).

To date there is relatively little cofunding of prevention research across NIH institutes. Such efforts may be discouraged if each institute is not given sufficient recognition of its support on a cofunded grant. Given the importance of looking at comprehensive outcomes that are the purview of specific institutes and the current fiscal limitations for NIH research, it may be necessary to offer additional incentives for institutes to cofund important prevention research. The new policy at NIH that acknowledges the important contributions of multiple investigators is a model that could also be used at the institute level to acknowledge the contributions of multiple agencies providing cofunding.

Training

Training in prevention research, whether basic, epidemiological, translational, or implementation, is not responsive to ongoing opportunity or needs. Workforce numbers remain insufficient to carry out research and service programs targeted to prevention of MEB disorders. The complexity of prevention efforts calls for more coordinated training in multidisciplinary settings. More and better investigators are needed in all areas, particularly in the field of implementation sciences. Recruitment of future leaders should be enhanced by attracting the most talented young investigators to prevention research, through NIH-supported multidisciplinary training programs. As discussed in Chapter 5, coordination among researchers from diverse disciplines, such as developmental neuroscience, developmental psychopathology and prevention science, as well as collaboration across institutions are needed to integrate expanding knowledge from these fields.

Prevention training is neglected for a broad array of health professionals (doctors, nurses, psychologists, social workers) and for teachers as well as other school personnel, for whom prevention should be a priority issue. When mental health or substance abuse is included in a training curriculum, it tends to focus on diagnosis and treatment. Similarly, prevention and promotion content tends to emphasize general health over mental health concerns. Refinement and broad implementation of prevention interventions are likely to languish unless more extensive and robust training is realized.

Conclusion: Most training programs in major disciplines, such as medicine, education, psychology, social work, and public health, do not include core components on the prevention of MEB disorders of young people, including how to identify and manage the risks and preclinical symptoms of these disorders.

Recommendation 12-6: Training programs for relevant health (including mental health), education, and social work professionals should include prevention of MEB disorders and promotion of mental, emotional, and behavioral health. National certifying and accrediting bodies for training should set relevant standards using available evidence on identifying and managing risks and preclinical symptoms of MEB disorders.

Recommendation 12-7: The U.S. Departments of Health and Human Services, Education, and Justice should convene a national conference on training in prevention and promotion to (1) set guidelines for model prevention research and practice training programs and (2) contribute to the development of training standards for certifying and accrediting training programs in specific disciplines, such as health (including mental health), education, and social work.

Recommendation 12-8: Once guidelines have been developed, the U.S. Departments of Health and Human Services, Education, and Justice should set aside funds for competitive prevention training grants to support development and dissemination of model interdisciplinary training programs. Training should span creation, implementation, and evaluation of effective preventive approaches.

Training models should be applied in both research contexts involving multiple disciplines and multidisciplinary approaches to training providers that work with young people.

13

Toward an Improved
Approach to Prevention

The preceding chapters described the substantial scientific progress in the conceptualization, design, assessment, and evaluation of preventive intervention approaches for children, youth, and families since the 1994 Institute of Medicine (IOM) report *Reducing Risks for Mental Disorders: Frontiers for Preventive Intervention Research*. There has been laudable progress in the science of mental health promotion and prevention of mental, emotional, and behavioral (MEB) disorders. It is now evident that the incidence of some of these disorders, such as depression, can be significantly reduced. There is also evidence to support multiple approaches aimed at strengthening individual, family, and community competencies that have been causally linked to mental, emotional, and behavioral health, either by reducing malleable risk factors for disorders or enhancing protective factors. We call on the nation to put this knowledge into practice. At the same time, as discussed in earlier chapters, we have identified significant gaps in current knowledge and key areas in which more research and infrastructure changes are needed to fully release the potential to significantly reduce MEB disorders among young people.

The promise of preventing MEB disorders, evident in the research over the past several decades, has prompted numerous federal agencies and stakeholder organizations to encourage grantees and community organizations to adopt evidence-based interventions. The National Institutes of Health (NIH) and other agencies have funded multiple parallel research projects. It is now time for a coordinated, strategic approach that brings together the range of resources, provides consistent advice to communities, and strategically aligns research priorities to needs. As discussed in the preceding chapter, although there are a number of interagency efforts, they tend to be focused on a single program or an isolated issue related to prevention rather than on a holistic vision. Historically, prevention has received far less attention than treatment in either mental health or physical health. A fundamental paradigm shift needs to occur. The substantial progress in prevention science summarized in this report calls for the adoption of a prevention perspective and a resolve to test and determine the most promising application of specific evidence-based preventive approaches.

> **Recommendation 13-1:** The federal government should make the healthy mental, emotional, and behavioral development of young people a national priority, establish public goals for the prevention of specific MEB disorders and for the promotion of healthy development among young people, and provide needed research and service resources to achieve these aims.

Accomplishing this will require a more systematic approach at multiple levels—national, state, and local—and continued progress in prevention research.

A NEW NATIONAL DISCOURSE

The 1994 IOM report strongly recommended the creation of a mechanism to coordinate research and services across federal departments, suggesting the creation of a national scientific council as one model, possibly under an office in the White House. A variety of national-level groups (New Freedom Commission on Mental Health, 2003; U.S. Public Health Service, 2000) have concurred in saying that the nation should consider a strong, broad-based public health infrastructure to both monitor and deploy resources in mental and physical health care.

Current federal policy, research, and practice relevant to prevention of MEB disorders are fragmented across a wide variety of agencies. Research on prevention (and treatment) is organized to address individual disorders and problems. However, evidence that common risk factors lead to multiple interrelated disorders and problems, coupled with significant evidence on possible approaches to mitigating these factors, calls for a concerted strategic, national effort to coordinate research, policy, and practice aimed at preventing MEB disorders and promoting healthy development. This effort would build on the significant evidence currently available and continue to be informed by new research as it emerges.

> **Recommendation 13-2:** The White House should create an ongoing mechanism involving federal agencies, stakeholders (including profes-

sional associations), and key researchers to develop and implement a strategic approach to the promotion of mental, emotional, and behavioral coordinating and health and the prevention of MEB disorders and related problem behaviors in young people. The U.S. Departments of Health and Human Services, Education, and Justice should be accountable for coordinating and aligning their resources, programs, and initiatives with this strategic approach and for encouraging their state and local counterparts to do the same.

One of the first tasks would be to establish specific, measurable goals for the next 10 years (see Recommendation 13-1) and a strategy to support the accomplishment of goals. In establishing goals, consideration should be given to the prevalence of disorders, costs associated with those disorders, and the strength of the evidence that the disorder is preventable. Promising areas include the prevention of depression, substance abuse, and conduct disorder. Existing surveys provide data on substance use and adolescent (ages 12-17) depression. The Federal Interagency Forum on Child and Family Statistics has recently added an indicator related to the prevalence of depression among youth in its Key National Indicators of Well-Being report and includes indicators of alcohol and drug use. The forum has also identified the need for measures of positive behaviors.[1] This could serve as a starting point. Similarly, consideration should be given to the approaches that both promote healthy development and have the greatest potential to affect multiple disorders, such as those aimed at strengthening families.

In developing the strategy, priority should be placed on educating the public on the potential to improve support of the nation's young people, including efforts to reduce the stigma associated with mental, emotional, and behavioral problems, and on engaging relevant professional and intergovernmental organizations in a coordinated approach to improving support systems for young people and their families. Development of the strategy would have multiple components:

- Identify and evaluate all federal programs and policies to determine which ones should be recommended to states and communities based on an agreed standard of evidence; these programs should be given highest priority for dissemination.
- Create networks of prevention delivery programs involving schools, primary health care, behavioral health care, and other community-based programs that are sites for investigation and innovation

---

[1]See http://www.childstats.gov.

for both family-centered preventive intervention and individual-centered intervention.

- Explore the possibility of set-asides or targeted funding for promotion and prevention activities, similar to the set-aside proposed for the Mental Health Services Block Grant (see Recommendation 12-1).
- Consult with leading researchers, major stakeholder and professional organizations, and constituency groups in developing priorities, goals, and a shared action agenda.
- Coordinate with relevant foundations to identify priority partnerships aimed at better understanding the implementation of evidence-based programs, possibly through the Child Mental Health Foundations and Agencies network, a collaborative of public and private agencies and foundations interested in issues of child development and public policy.
- Coordinate with NIH on the development of a 10-year research agenda (see Recommendation 13-5) and plan, organize, and support further research, led by NIH:
  — To further examine the impact of programs and policies to determine the extent to which they prevent the development of problems, promote mental health, or both. That research should assess the impact of interventions on multiple disorders and problems.
  — To experimentally evaluate strategies for getting effective programs and policies widely and effectively adopted.
- Oversee development of approaches to monitor the prevalence of disorders and key risk and protective factors, as well as relevant service use across a range of delivery systems (see Recommendations 2-1 and 2-2).
- Identify specific opportunities to braid the funding of research and practice so that the impact of programs and practices that are being funded by service agencies, such as the Substance Abuse and Mental Health Services Administration (SAMHSA), are experimentally evaluated through research funded by such agencies as NIH or the Institute of Education Sciences (IES) (see Recommendation 12-2).
- Consider the potential to develop a standardized system to measure core promotion and prevention outcomes that could be used and adapted by states and communities across the country to monitor performance, potentially building on existing community monitoring systems.
- Oversee the development and implementation of consistent, rigorous standards of evidence for endorsement of prevention programs (see Recommendation 12-4).

Both service and research components of the relevant agencies should be involved. These include, in the U.S. Department of Health and Human Services, NIH, SAMHSA, the Health Resources and Services Administration, the Administration for Children and Families, the Centers for Medicare and Medicaid Services, the Centers for Disease Control and Prevention, and the Office of the Assistant Secretary for Planning and Evaluation; in the U.S. Department of Education, IES and Safe Schools; and in the U.S. Department of Justice, the Office of Juvenile Justice and Delinquency Prevention and the National Institute of Justice. The need for high-level coordination across multiple agencies, the broad implications of healthy development for multiple components of society, and the significant cost associated with MEB disorders call for ongoing White House involvement. The White House has played a leadership role in other related issues, such as violence against women, mental health policy (the New Freedom Commission), strengthening youth, and drug control policy. A new, ongoing interagency mechanism focused on the emotional and behavioral health of young people could build on and extend the current White House effort to help America's youth. This current effort, a "nationwide effort to raise awareness about the challenges facing our youth, particularly at-risk boys, and to motivate caring adults to connect with youth in three key areas: family, school, and community,"[2] already recognizes many of the core findings outlined in this report.

The specific mechanism could take many forms, including a new White House office, an ongoing commission, or a White House–led strategic coordinating group. Regardless of the form it takes, it should have adequate authority to direct agency resources in a coordinated manner, facilitate a paradigm shift that emphasizes promotion and prevention, and have a long-term mandate.

Just as there have been significant advances in prevention science in the past 15 years, it is highly likely that there will be considerable progress in the next 15 years with the development of new, more refined prevention strategies. The nation should have a mechanism in place to benefit from rapid deployment of these advances. The creation of an ongoing strategic mechanism to coordinate federal efforts will facilitate consideration of how these advances are best applied. A major need for the immediate future is to systematically study how to effectively translate these strategies to broad-based prevention programs and to identify mechanisms for federal support of community and state efforts. The time is ripe for interventions to be delivered and tested in primary care, in the mental health care sector, in schools, in community organizations, and in families.

Mental health efforts are often fragmented and of uneven quality for

---

[2] See http://www.helpingamericasyouth.gov/whatishay.cfm.

children, youth, and families, as they are for adults (Institute of Medicine, 2006b) and for physical health care (Institute of Medicine, 2001). In the long run, consideration needs to be given to an effective, broad-based, strong public health network that can provide adequate data to monitor progress and support the delivery of high-quality preventive services focused on mental and physical health in a variety of sectors. Linked services for the promotion of mental and physical health can respond to the growing recognition that mental health is dependent on good physical health and vice versa.

The committee was struck by the pervasive role played by poverty in development of a range of MEB disorders and related problems. Similarly, the health care system in the United States, which limits access to and quality of care for many of the most poor and disenfranchised, complicates effective prevention. National attention should be paid to narrowing income and health care disparities as a fundamental part of the promotion of mental health and prevention of MEB disorders.

DEVELOPING STATE AND LOCAL SYSTEMS

Prevention science has identified the major malleable risk factors for the development of most MEB disorders and related problems. The number of efficacy trials and the experimental and statistical methods needed to make reliable conclusions have exploded since 1994. Numerous interventions have been tested in two or more randomized controlled trials, and several have been tested in multiple U.S. communities or implemented nationwide in European countries.

The inability of the mental health care system to respond to the demands for treatment is well documented. Many young people receive treatment in systems outside the formal mental health care system, such as schools, primary medical care, child welfare, and criminal justice. Not all cases of MEB disorder can be prevented, but a concerted effort to determine the proportion of such disorders that can be prevented is now possible. Shifting the focus toward prevention may help alleviate pressures on treatment resources; this would need to be empirically tested through community- or statewide implementation of prevention.

The mental, emotional, and behavioral health of young people cannot, and should not, be the responsibility of the mental health care system alone. Improvements or potential savings from effective prevention inherently benefit systems other than, or in addition to, the system implementing an intervention. Similarly, the failure of one system involved in a young person's life can have costs for another. For example, there is evidence that improving social and emotional functioning improves academic outcomes. Interventions involving both families and schools seem to have a high level of success. Increasingly, parents are bringing their children to physicians' offices with behavioral concerns. Schools and primary care settings may be less stigmatizing for children and families and may enable exploration of emotional and behavioral health issues more openly than a mental health setting.

Successes in other areas, such as prevention of smoking, suggest that approaches that involve complementary components at multiple levels are needed. Involving multiple community systems has the potential to leverage resources and implement approaches that support young people throughout their development rather than only in a particular grade or a particular school.

Multiple federal programs have required state and local grantees to implement evidence-based programs. This has both raised awareness regarding evidence-based programs and created a missed opportunity to learn about effective implementation and how adaptation of programs to local circumstances might affect outcomes. This information is needed not only at the national level, but also to inform the community on progress, determine changes needed, and sustain interest in community-wide efforts. Creating systems that support the implementation of preventive interventions, allow their continuous improvement, and facilitate the introduction of new approaches, while evaluating results, should complement national research and planning efforts.

Recommendation 13-3: States and communities should develop networked systems to apply resources to the promotion of mental health and prevention of MEB disorders among their young people. These systems should involve individuals, families, schools, justice systems, health care systems, and relevant community-based programs. Such approaches should build on available evidence-based programs and involve local evaluators to assess the implementation process of individual programs or policies and to measure community-wide outcomes.

Both the identification of problems and resources and the development of solutions will vary by community. However, monitoring systems, a key component of public health, should be integral to any state or community-wide system in order to track the incidence and prevalence of MEB disorders as well as key risk and protective factors and provide information needed to guide efforts. Many states are implementing monitoring systems similar to available national surveys, such as Monitoring the Future, the Youth Risk Behavior Survey, and the National Household Survey of Drug Use and Health (Mrazek, Biglan, and Hawkins, 2004; Boles, Biglan, and Smolkowski, 2006). These surveys provide estimates of substance use and, in some cases, data on adolescents' self-reported antisocial behavior and high-risk sexual behavior. States and communities need to develop monitoring systems that are capable of providing data on other targeted disorders. In addition, these systems can be used to mobilize support for community-based prevention efforts. For example, annual data on adolescent depression could be used to motivate support for the implementation of evidence-based depression preventions. This requires, however, that data be summarized and delivered to key target audiences in a timely, clear, and useful manner. Web-based systems for delivering this information show great promise (Mrazek, Biglan, and Hawkins, 2004). Ideally, a template for a community monitoring system would be developed at the national level and available to all communities, and the national system recommended by the committee (see Chapter 2) would adopt use of unique identifiers to enable use by state and local networks.

MONITORING, FUNDING, AND TRAINING

National and state systems will have to be supported by adequate monitoring systems, funding, and trained personnel. In addition, rigorous standards must be developed and implemented to provide clear guidance to states and communities on the readiness for implementation of specific interventions. The committee's recommendations call for action in each of these areas by federal agencies and by relevant training programs.

- **Monitoring system.** There is a need to develop approaches to report on the prevalence of disorders and key risk and protective factors and to report on the utilization of mental health care services across multiple service systems that work with young people (see Chapter 2).
- **Standards.** Federal and state agencies need to identify and prioritize the use of evidence-based programs by applying scientific criteria to assess programs (see Chapter 12).
- **Funding.** Federal agencies need to increase resources to states and local communities to implement approaches to prevention, ideally partnered with research funding, targeted to communities with greatest need (see Chapters 8, 11, and 12).
- **Training.** Guidelines, model training programs, and accreditation standards are needed for training both researchers and practitioners on prevention of MEB disorders and promotion of mental health. Research training programs that facilitate creation of multidisciplinary training teams will advance translational prevention research efforts aimed at integrating developmental neuroscience and preventive intervention research (see Chapters 5 and 12).

REFINING AND EXPANDING PREVENTION RESEARCH

Substantial progress has been made since the 1994 IOM report in identifying mechanisms to affect risk or protective factors for MEB disorders, developing specific approaches to affect those factors, and strategies to prevent specific disorders, such as depression and substance abuse. However, despite the high prevalence of MEB disorders and the promise apparent from prevention research, research on prevention has not received attention or funding commensurate to that of treatment research.

> **Recommendation 13-4:** Federal agencies and foundations funding research on the prevention of MEB disorders should establish parity between research on preventive interventions and treatment interventions.

Multiple federal agencies, across several departments, fund research related to prevention. Research priorities differ across agencies, making it difficult to systematically identify and address new research needs. Continued progress over the next decade and the nation's ability to reduce the prevalence of disorders will require that efforts to implement what is currently known are married with rigorous efforts to address gaps in research knowledge.

> **Recommendation 13-5:** The National Institutes of Health, with input from other funders of prevention research, should develop a comprehensive 10-year research plan targeting the promotion of mental health and prevention of both single and comorbid MEB disorders. This plan should consider current needs, opportunities for cross-disciplinary and multi-institute research, support for the necessary research infrastructure, and establishment of a mechanism for assessing and reporting progress against 10-year goals.

Several specific recommendations related to gaps in research knowledge have been identified throughout the report and should be considered in development of this plan:

- **Screening.** Approaches needed to develop and test models for screening in school and primary care settings (see Chapter 8).
- **Intervention effectiveness.** Development of new and more effective interventions, as well as research aimed at replicating findings with a range of target populations and demonstrating outcomes over time, ideally across developmental phases (see Chapters 7 and 10).

- **Multi-institute collaborations.** Collaborative funding of interventions that target risk factors common to multiple disorders and assess multiple outcomes (see Chapters 4 and 12).
- **Cultural relevance.** Research on how interventions developed with one cultural or ethnic group work with other groups (see Chapter 11).
- **Economic analyses.** Need for guidelines, measures, and funding for economic analyses (see Chapter 9).
- **Dissemination and implementation.** Methodologies and strategies for dissemination and implementation of preventive interventions, including research on (1) state- and community-wide implementation, (2) alternative approaches to implementation that vary such factors as type of provider or training, (3) potential strategies for use of the mass media and Internet, and (4) identification of program components that might facilitate implementation (see Chapter 11).
- **Competencies.** Need for improved understanding of etiology and development of competencies, their protective role, and development of measurement tools (see Chapter 4).
- **Neuroscience and prevention.** Approaches to linking findings from brain research and research on gene–environment interactions with intervention research, to test hypotheses related to epigenetics and neuroscience, and development of guidelines on ethics of using individually identifiable information (see Chapter 5).
- **Gaps in current research.** Interventions for such groups as young adults and young people with chronic health problems, in such settings as primary care, comprehensive interventions, and approaches to addressing poverty (see Chapters 6 and 7).

To assist in the implementation of a prevention research agenda and to help distinguish prevention research from treatment research, this report calls on the prevention community to adopt a definition of prevention that focuses on populations that do not currently have a disorder, including three levels of intervention: *universal* (for all), *selective* (for groups or individuals at greater than average risk), and *indicated* (for high-risk individuals with specific phenotypes or early symptoms of a disorder). However, it also calls on the prevention community to embrace mental health promotion as within the spectrum of mental health research. In addition, prevention researchers are advised to broaden the focus of their research to include consideration of cost-effectiveness and the impact of interventions on multiple outcomes.

ENVISIONING THE FUTURE

The scientific foundation has been created for the nation to begin to create a society in which young people arrive at adulthood with the skills, interests, assets, and health habits needed to live healthy, happy, and productive lives in caring relationships with others. Implementation of the recommendations of this report will move it firmly in the direction of such a society.

This movement can be guided by a vision of what families, schools, neighborhoods, health care providers, and community organizations could be like. There would be a well-organized system of organizations, programs, and policies to ensure strong families and schools and nurturing neighborhoods. Young people would have access to high-quality, well-administered schools, access to health care and other community services, and healthy environments, activities, and food. The system would include the following elements specific to prevention:

1. Factors shown to improve the physical and mental health of children and their caregivers are explicitly addressed by the systems that provide services to them. Responsibility for and investment in interventions affecting children's development and long-term futures is shared by multiple service systems, including education, child welfare, primary care, and mental health.

2. Families and children have ready access to the best available evidence-based preventive interventions, delivered in their own communities in a culturally competent and respectful (nonstigmatizing) way.

3. Preventive interventions are provided as a routine component of school, health, and community service systems, reducing stigma to a minimum.

4. A well-organized public health monitoring system is in place at the national and community levels to track the incidence and prevalence of MEB disorders in young people and used to appropriately direct resources as well as to monitor the cost and impact of prevention and treatment efforts.

5. Services are coordinated and integrated with multiple points of entry for children and their families (e.g., through schools, health care settings, and community-based organizations, such as youth centers and churches).

6. As further new discoveries, interventions, or adaptations occur, including such innovations as the use of the Internet for preventive purposes, these are incorporated into already existing networks for the delivery of services.

7. Families are informed that they have access to resources when they need them without barriers of culture, cost, or type of service.
8. Families and communities are partners in the development and implementation of preventive interventions and learn to manage their access and utilization of prevention services.
9. The development and application of appropriate preventive intervention strategies contribute to narrowing rather than widening health disparities.
10. Teachers, child care workers, health care providers, and other professionals who work with young people are routinely trained on approaches to support the behavioral and emotional health of young people and the prevention of MEB disorders.

The type of system envisioned above, which routinely provides universal interventions that support healthy development for all and systematically identifies groups and individuals at greater risk to provide them with specific services, could result in very different outcomes for the nation's young people. Table 13-1 illustrates what a system might look like at various developmental phases.

International Perspectives

The committee was impressed with evidence showing that some of the prevention advances being suggested for the United States are already in place in other developed nations. A comprehensive review of international policies and programs is outside the scope of this report. However, a brief discussion and a few examples illustrate that our recommendations are not merely utopian dreams, but rather a call for the nation to make available to children and families the types of services and initiatives that are already being implemented in other countries.

Europe as a whole is working toward a comprehensive strategy on mental health, with a strong focus on mental health promotion and the prevention of MEB disorders (Jané-Llopis and McDaid, 2005). As this process unfolds, it could inform how the United States should integrate prevention into systems at the federal, state, and local levels while taking into account the distinct needs of different communities. At the World Health Organization Ministerial Conference on Mental Health in 2005, member states of the European Region endorsed a European Action Plan for Mental Health that includes the promotion of mental health and prevention of mental illness (World Health Organization, 2005). In support of the implementation of the action plan, the European Commission produced a Green Paper on Mental Health. This document outlined a framework to increase the coherence of health and nonhealth policies in support of mental

TABLE 13-1 Examples of Potential Components of a Prevention System That Supports Developmental Phases

Developmental Stage	In the Absence of Interventions	Illustrative Intervention Opportunities
Conception, pregnancy, postpartum	High risk of postpartum depression	Pregnant women screened routinely for risk factors and provided needed interventions, such as mood management training, home visitation, and nutritional counseling to prevent maternal depression during child's critical developmental stages
	Baby at risk for problems of attachment, later preschool or school problems, or later depression if mother is depressed	Well-baby visits to screen and intervene for developmental problems, abnormal feeding patterns, interactions with mother or other caretaker
Infancy	Infant at risk for abnormal development	Screening is offered for age-appropriate behaviors and evidence of normal brain development
	Early behavioral difficulties increase risk for later bonding problems, negative patterns of parent-child interactions	On-time remedial interventions are offered, such as parent training and referral to a developmental specialist
Preschool years	Child does not receive early cognitive stimulation	Caregivers are encouraged to read to their children
	Child does not learn self-efficacy, prosocial skills, or appropriate school behaviors	In-home and out-of-home enrichment experiences such as early childhood education are offered for the child to build skills needed for school and social success
		Families receive needed parenting support to foster nurturing relationships
Primary school	Child has difficulty establishing positive relationships with peers, caregivers, or teachers	Families and schools increase nurturance and decrease punitive experiences
	Child does not experience early successes	Children learn skills to enhance school performance and manage problem behaviors

continued

TABLE 13-1 Continued

Developmental Stage	In the Absence of Interventions	Illustrative Intervention Opportunities
Middle school	Early adolescent engages in risky behaviors, such as smoking, using alcohol or other drugs, delinquency, or risky sexual behavior	Families and schools provide high-level reinforcement for prosocial behavior
	Early adolescent experiences few academic successes and bonds with deviant peers	Young people at risk due to academic or peer-interaction problems are identified and provided with individual or family intervention options
High school	Adolescent lacks self-esteem, has limited academic success, engages in antisocial behaviors, and does not develop positive health habits	Family- and school-focused programs shape attitudes and behaviors around substance abuse, delinquency, and sexual behaviors and provide self-identity and coping skills
	Depression, conduct disorder, and substance abuse increase	Adolescents are routinely screened for early signs of depression and other MEB disorders, with appropriate interventions provided
Young adulthood	Young adult flounders in transition to independence, including continued education, employment, marriage, and childrearing	Community programs support decisions about education, work and relationships, and model parenting skills, including constructive parent–child communication
	Young adults struggle with readiness to have and to parent children	Interventions are available in college, the workplace, and community settings as needed to reduce obstacles to raising a family, including academic, job-related, and marital difficulties

health at the level of member states and communities (Commission of the European Communities, 2005). The green paper launched a process that included consultation with relevant European institutions, governments, health professionals, and stakeholders in the research community and other civic sectors (Commission of the European Communities, 2005). These deliberations on mental health include a strong emphasis on mental health promotion and prevention of mental illness.

To work toward developing a comprehensive strategy to address promotion and prevention in mental health, 29 European countries have formed the European Network for Mental Health Promotion and Mental Disorder Prevention. The aim of the network is to serve as an information resource to disseminate evidence-based knowledge and tools and to develop integrated approaches to training, policy, and implementation (Jané-Llopis and Anderson, 2006). Individual countries have linked their prevention programs to the shared policies of the European Union. This includes an emphasis on prenatal programs and a healthy start in life, along with early education programs, which are generally more developed and available than in the United States (Jané-Llopis and Anderson, 2006). In addition, many countries are working to integrate mental health promotion and prevention efforts both with the systems that address physical health and with antipoverty programs, recognizing that poverty is a major factor in the development of MEB disorders (Jané-Llopis and Anderson, 2005).

Many European countries experience challenges to translating this interest in promotion and prevention into action; these challenges are similar to those described in this report, including financing, infrastructure, and implementation support (Jané-Llopis and Anderson, 2006). However, there are also notable successes in nationwide implementation and comprehensive national approaches in Europe and elsewhere that offer promising models from which lessons can potentially be learned.

Some countries have undertaken nationwide or widespread implementation of specific evidence-based programs. For example, Parent Management Training, a program originally developed in the United States, has been adapted in Norway and implemented nationwide through the creation of a national implementation and research center that coordinates training for providers, supervision, consultation, and research in support of implementation with strong partnership at the regional and local levels (Ogden, Forgatch, et al., 2005).

Australia has launched a National Mental Health Promotion, Prevention, and Early Intervention Action Plan (Commonwealth Department of Health and Aged Care, 2000) as part of a multiyear effort to position mental heath as a new strategic direction. It includes the implementation of multiple policies and programs as part of a national effort. As a component of a national initiative on depression, the Triple P Program (a multilevel parenting program; see Chapter 6) was tested on a population level in multiple Australian communities. It demonstrated significant reductions in the number of children with recognizable and borderline behavioral and emotional problems and the number of parents who reported depression, stress, and coercive parenting, although reductions were modest (Sanders, Ralph, et al., 2008).

The Netherlands has a comprehensive national infrastructure for health promotion and prevention that includes public health, mental health, and addiction. This infrastructure includes mechanisms that support research and dissemination of evidence-based programs and involves multiple sectors, such as the health system, the justice system, and schools. It is supported by a specialized professional workforce of trained health promoters and prevention workers, about half of whom are primarily or partly focused on mental health (Jané-Llopis and Anderson, 2006). One of the areas of priority is the care of children of mentally ill parents. The Netherlands, as well as Finland, have implemented country-wide systems to support the children of mentally ill parents in their health care systems (see Box 13-1).

Scotland launched the National Programme for Improving Mental Health and Well Being in 2001. The key aims include raising awareness and promoting mental health and well-being, eliminating stigma and discrimination, preventing suicide, and promoting and supporting recovery from mental illness. The priority areas include, among others, the mental health of infants, children, and young people. The national program includes campaigns; research, evaluation, and training initiatives; monitoring; partnerships; and implementation support at the national level as well as services and partnerships at the local level (Scottish Executive, 2003). It is guided by a National Advisory Council made up of a range of stakeholders from the public and private sectors in a variety of settings, including schools, prisons, and the health system (Jané-Llopis and Anderson, 2006). Information on Scotland's progress is available at http://www.wellscotland.info/index.html.

Systematic attempts to affect the entire population have great value in public health, and integrative models in Europe and other countries may offer efficient approaches to supporting the development of young people, although empirical evidence to date appears to be lacking. Although these models still need more comprehensive study, as the United States moves forward with prevention, federal, state, and local governments should look for evidence-based progress in other countries and applicable lessons learned that can be adapted to systems here.

CONCLUDING THOUGHTS

The gap between what is known and what is being done is far too large. It can be addressed only by continuing to refine the science and by a strong commitment to develop the infrastructure and put in place systems that allow for equitable delivery of preventive interventions on a population-based, large-scale basis. The United States needs to build on the extensive

BOX 13-1
Health System–Based Approaches to Prevention
in the Netherlands and Finland

The Netherlands and Finland have both developed system-wide approaches that initially focused on children of depressed parents and now include prevention work with children of parents with mental illness.

The Netherlands

The Netherlands began in the 1970s to develop a network of prevention and health promotion teams. These teams were placed in multiple health sectors (e.g., public health, mental health, addiction clinics) and supported by prevention-oriented national institutes and national research centers. The work is part of a national health policy that allots about 5-10 percent of the budgets of community mental health centers for prevention of mental disorders.

The experience has been that having preventionists certified to do preventive care has made a difference. It also facilitates the adoption and dissemination of evidence-based programs when they become available and application of continuous quality improvement processes. Preventionists have a network in which they collaborate with research institutes. This structure enables a constant interplay between research and practice. It also has provided a vital infrastructure through which to deliver preventive services. Preventive care for children of the mentally ill is an integral part of the mental health and primary health care system.

Care of children of parents with mental illness is one of five mental health priority areas. To make care of children of mentally ill parents a regular part of the systems of care (not an isolated activity), adults with mental illness are routinely asked if they have children. If children are present, the family automatically qualifies for services. Parents and children receive informal home visits and are offered an array of services, including play and talk groups, information support groups, online websites, brochures, videos, school-based education, a buddy system for children and for parents, home-based mother–baby interventions, and parent training. Delivery of services is accompanied by extensive postgraduate training for providers. Many of the practitioners have been educated in Dutch academic and training programs that first focus on prevention, health education, and health promotion.

Finland

In Finland, under the leadership of Tytti Solantaus, a nationwide program has been developed effectively in a stepwise fashion starting in 2001. The Finnish Child Welfare Act states that if a parent is identified as receiving treatment, the needs of children should be addressed. Before 2001, there had not been a systematic program to do so. The initiative began with the Efficient Family Program, the aim of which is building care of patients' children into routine practice, with every parent receiving support. This was deliberately conceived as a change from an

continued

BOX 13-1 Continued

individual- and treatment-centered program to a family- and prevention-centered one. Mass media campaigns, national and local conferences, and seminars were offered, and the clinics' leadership and the clinicians were eager to learn. Training began with extensive training of master trainers, who then trained many others.

Over time, a decision was made to implement a series of interventions. This included the Family Talk Intervention (see Box 7-3), a 1-2 session intervention using a book for parents, the Let's Talk About Children discussion, peer groups, and family courses for parents and children. In addition, clinicians or adults (including parents) responsible for children could request a network meeting attended by all professionals involved in the care of a child to devise a coordinated plan. Health help booklets were also provided. This was combined with an extensive campaign to address postpartum depression. Implementation was accompanied by evaluations, with a randomized trial comparing the Family Talk Intervention with the Let's Talk About Children discussion under way.

Based on research showing that nurses, doctors, psychologists, social workers, and therapists can master the Let's Talk About Children discussion, the Finnish system now requires that each of these professionals be responsible for initiating child preventive services when working with mentally ill parents.

In this approach, prevention services in the Finnish system are not segregated, but rather routinely included in the work of all clinicians. At the end of 2006, there were 650 fully trained professionals and 80 qualified trainers in a country of 5 million. The work, which began with parental depression, has been extended to drug and alcohol problems, parents with cancer, and other severe physical illnesses. The specific example of children of mentally ill parents takes place against the larger backdrop of Finland's long tradition of adapting evidence-based preventive interventions in health and mental health nationwide. Their system is set up to accommodate new interventions as they become available.

SOURCES: Beardslee, Hosman, et al. (2005); Solantaus and Toikka (2006); Toikka and Solantaus (2006).

research now available by addressing gaps in the available research and developing a shared vision and strategy for applying the knowledge at hand.

When IOM's report *Reducing Risks for Mental Disorders: Frontiers for Preventive Intervention Research* was published in 1994, the majority of available studies were efficacy studies, with a few addressing the effectiveness of interventions. The report called on the field to continue to develop rigorous efficacy and effectiveness evaluations while at the same time moving further toward the final stage in the proposed prevention research cycle to "facilitate large scale implementation and ongoing evaluation of the preventive intervention program in the community." It is now clear, however, that achieving community ownership and implementation of science-based preventive interventions is not only an issue of dissemination of information about effective interventions, but also a matter of empirically evaluating strategies achieving effective adoption, implementation, and maintenance of evidence-based preventive interventions. The next major milestone will be the translation of existing knowledge into population-wide reductions in the incidence and prevalence of emotional and behavioral problems. One of the areas of greatest need is to develop strategies and outcome measures to ensure that high-quality evidence-based approaches are successfully adapted for use in a broad array of different cultural, ethnic, and linguistic settings. As research on development and implementation of specific interventions continues, states and communities need to also continuously refine effective interventions and implementation approaches.

Similarly, while there has been sustained research over the past 15 years, we recommend attention to areas that have heretofore been neglected, such as effectiveness in real-world situations, cost-effectiveness, integration of genetics and neuroscience with intervention research, and the careful monitoring of rates of disorder and present risk factors to assess whether population-based improvements can be achieved. Without adequate surveillance, what the burden of disorder is for the society or where best to direct national resources will not be fully known.

References

Abbott, R.D., O'Donnell, J., Hawkins, J.D., Hill, K.G., Kosterman, R., and Catalano, R.F. (1998). Changing teaching practices to promote achievement and bonding to school. *American Journal of Orthopsychiatry, 68*(4), 542-552.

Abrams, W.T., Saitz, R., and Sancet, J.H. (2003). Education of preventive medicine residents: Alcohol, tobacco and other drug abuse. *American Journal of Preventive Medicine, 24,* 101-105.

Abramson, L.Y., Alloy, L.B., Hankin, B.L., Haeffel, G.J., MacCoon, D.G., and Gibb, B.E. (2002). Cognitive vulnerability-stress models of depression in a self-regulatory and psychobiological context. In I.H. Gotlib and C.L. Hammen (Eds.), *Handbook of Depression* (pp. 268-294). New York: Guildford Press.

Adams, C.D., and Drabman, R.S. (1995). Improving morning interactions: Beat-the-buzzer with a boy having multiple handicaps. *Child and Family Behavior Therapy, 17,* 13-26.

Adcock, R.A., Thangavel, A., Whitfield-Gabrieli, S., Knutson, B., and Gabrieli, J.D.E. (2006). Reward-motivated learning: Mesolimbic activation precedes memory formation. *Neuron, 50*(3), 507-517.

Adelman, H., and Taylor, L. (2000). Moving prevention from the fringes into the fabric of school improvement. *Journal of Educational and Psychological Consultation, 11,* 7-36.

Administration for Children and Families. (2005). *Head Start Impact Study: First-Year Findings.* Washington, DC: U.S. Department of Health and Human Services.

Administration for Children and Families. (2006). *FACES Findings: New Research on Head Start Outcomes and Program Quality.* Washington, DC: U.S. Department of Health and Human Services.

Administration for Children and Families. (2007). *Preliminary Findings from the Early Head Start Prekindergarten Follow-up.* Washington, DC: U.S. Department of Health and Human Services.

Agnew, Z.K., Bhakoo, K.K., and Puri, B.K. (2007). The human mirror system: A motor resonance theory of mind-reading. *Brain Research Reviews, 54*(2), 286-293.

Akirav, I., and Maroun, M. (2007). The role of the medial prefrontal cortex-amygdala circuit in stress effects on the extinction of fear. *Neural Plasticity,* Art. ID 30873, 11 pp.

Albert, P., and Brown, C.H. (1990). The design of a panel study under an alternating Poisson process assumption. *Biometrics, 47*, 921-932.

Alcohol Research and Health. (2000). Prenatal exposure to alcohol. *Alcohol Research & Health, 24*(1), 32-41. Available: http://pubs.niaaa.nih.gov/publications/arh24-1/32-41.pdf [accessed March 2009].

Alper, J. (2002). The nurse home visitation program. In S.L. Isaacs and J.R. Knickman (Eds.), *To Improve Health and Health Care Volume V: The Robert Wood Johnson Anthology* (pp. 3-22). San Francisco, CA: Jossey-Bass.

Amat, J.A., Bansal, R., Whiteman, R., Haggerty, R., Royal, J., and Peterson, B.S. (2008). Correlates of intellectual ability with morphology of the hippocampus and amygdala in healthy adults. *Brain and Cognition, 66*(2), 105-114.

Amato, P.R. (1996). Explaining the intergenerational transmission of divorce. *Journal of Marriage and the Family, 58*(3), 628-640.

Amato, P.R. (2000). The consequences of divorce for adults and children. *Journal of Marriage and the Family, 62*(4), 1269-1287.

Amato, P.R. (2001). Children of divorce in the 1990s: An update of the Amato and Keith (1991) meta-analysis. *Journal of Family Psychology, 15*(3), 355-370.

Amato, P.R., and Keith, B. (1991a). Parental divorce and the well-being of children: A meta-analysis. *Psychological Bulletin, 110*(1), 26-46.

Amato, P.R., and Keith, B. (1991b). Parental divorce and adult well-being: A meta-analysis. *Journal of Marriage and the Family, 53*, 43-58.

Amato, P.R., and Sobolewski, J.M. (2001). The effects of divorce and marital discord on adult children's psychological well-being. *American Sociological Review, 66*, 900-921.

American Academy of Pediatrics. (2001). Policy statement: The new morbidity revisited: A renewed commitment to the psychosocial aspects of pediatric care. Committee on Psychosocial Aspects of Child and Family Health. *Pediatrics, 108*(5), 1227-1230.

American Academy of Pediatrics Task Force on Mental Health. (in preparation). *Policy Statement, The Future of Pediatrics: Mental Health Competencies for the Care of Children and Adolescents in Primary Care Settings.* Elk Grove, IL.

American Academy of Pediatrics Task Force on Violence. (1999). The role of the pediatrician in youth violence prevention in clinical practice and at the community level. *Pediatrics, 103*(1), 173-181.

American Psychiatric Association. (1994). *Diagnostic and Statistical Manual of Mental Disorders* (4th ed.). Washington, DC: Author.

American Psychiatric Association. (2004). Practice guideline for the treatment of patients with acute stress disorder and posttraumatic stress disorder. *American Journal of Psychiatry, 161*(Nov. Suppl.), 3-31.

Anda, R.F., Brown, D.W., Felitti, V.J., Bremner, J.D., Dube, S.R., and Giles, W.H. (2007). Adverse childhood experiences and prescribed psychotropic medications in adults. *American Journal of Preventive Medicine, 32*, 389-394.

Anderson, L.M., Shinn, C., Fullilove, M.T., Scrimshaw, S.C., Fielding, J.E., Normand, J., Carande-Kulis, V.G., and the Task Force on Community Preventive Services. (2003). The effectiveness of early childhood development programs: A systematic review. *American Journal of Preventive Medicine, 24*(3S), 32-46.

Andrews, D.W., and Dishion, T.J. (1995). The adolescent transitions program for high-risk teens and their parents: Toward a school-based intervention. *Education and Treatment of Children, 18*(4), 478-499.

Angold, A., and Costello, E.J. (2001). The epidemiology of depression in children and adolescents. In I. Goodyer (Ed.), *The Depressed Child and Adolescent: Developmental and Clinical Perspectives* (2nd ed., pp. 143-178). New York: Cambridge University Press.

Angold, A., Costello, E.J., and Erkanli, A. (1999). Comorbidity. *Journal of Child Psychology and Psychiatry and Allied Disciplines, 40*(1), 57-87.

Angold, A., Erkanli, A., Farmer, E.M.Z., Fairbank, J.A., Burns, B.J., Keeler, G., and Costello, E.J. (2002). Psychiatric disorder, impairment, and service use in rural African American and white youth. *Archives of General Psychiatry, 59*, 893-901.

Angrist, J.D., Imbens, G.W., and Rubin, D.B. (1996). Identification of causal effects using instrumental variables. *Journal of the American Statistical Association, 91*, 444-455.

Aos, S., Lieb, R., Mayfiel, J., Miller, M., and Pennucci, A. (2004). *Benefits and Costs of Prevention and Early Intervention Programs for Youth.* (No. 04-07-3901). Olympia: Washington State Institute for Public Policy.

Appleton, K.M., Hayward, R.C., Gunnell, D., Peters, T.J., Rogers, P.J., Kessler, D., and Ness, A.R. (2006). Effects of n–3 long-chain polyunsaturated fatty acids on depressed mood: Systematic review of published trials. *American Journal of Clinical Nutrition, 84*(6), 1308-1316.

Apter, A., Pauls, D.L., Bleich, A., Zohar, A.H., Kron, S., Ratzoni, G., Dycian, A., Kotler, M., Weizman, A., Gadot, N., and Cohen, D. (1993). An epidemiologic study of Gilles de la Tourette's syndrome in Israel. *Archives of General Psychiatry, 50*(9), 734-738.

Armstrong, T.D., and Costello E.J. (2002). Community studies on adolescent substance use, abuse, or dependence and psychiatric comorbidity. *Journal of Consulting and Clinical Psychology, 70*, 1224-1239.

Arnett, J.J. (2000). Emerging adulthood: A theory of development from the late teens through the twenties. *American Psychologist, 55*, 469-480.

Arnold, A.P. (2004). Sex chromosomes and brain gender. *Nature Reviews Neuroscience, 5*(9), 701-708.

Arnold, A.P., and Breedlove, S.M. (1985). Organizational and activational effects of sex steroids on brain and behavior: A reanalysis. *Hormones and Behavior, 19*(4), 469-498.

Arseneault, L., Moffitt, T.E., Caspi, A., Taylor, P.J., and Silva, P.A. (2000). Mental disorders and violence in a total birth cohort: Results from the Dunedin study. *Archives of General Psychiatry, 57*, 979-986.

Ary, D.V., Duncan, T.E., Biglan, A., Metzler, C.W., Noell, J.W., and Smolkowski, K. (1999). Development of adolescent problem behavior. *Journal of Abnormal Child Psychology, 27*(2), 141-150.

Aseltine, Jr., R.H., and DeMartino, R. (2004). An outcome evaluation of the SOS suicide prevention program. *American Journal of Public Health, 94*(3), 446-451.

Asparouhov, T., and Muthén, B.O. (2007). Multilevel mixture models. In G.R. Hancock and K.M. Samuelsen (Eds.), *Advances in Latent Variable Mixture Models.* Charlotte, NC: Information Age.

Atallah, H.E., Frank, M.J., and O'Reilly, R.C. (2004). Hippocampus, cortex, and basal ganglia: Insights from computational models of complementary learning systems. *Neurobiology of Learning and Memory, 82*(3), 253-267.

Atkins, M.S., Graczyk, P.A., Frazier, S.L., and Abdul-Adil, J. (2003). Toward a new model for promoting urban children's mental health. *School Psychology Review, 32*, 503-514.

Atkins, M.S., Frazier, S.L., Birman, D., Abdul Adil, J., Jackson, M., Graczyk, P.A., Talbott, E., Farmer, D.A., Bell, C.C., and McKay, M.M. (2006). School-based mental health services for children living in high poverty urban communities. *Administration and Policy in Mental Health and Mental Health Services Research, 33*(2), 146-159.

Austin, J., and Honer, W. (2005). The potential impact of genetic counseling for mental illness. *Clinical Genetics, 67*(2), 134-142.

Ayoola, A., Brewer, J., and Nettleman, M. (2006). Epidemiology and prevention of unintended pregnancy in adolescents. *Primary Care: Clinics in Office Practice, 33*, 391-403.

Bakermans-Kranenburg, M.J., and van Ijzendoorn, M.H. (2007). Research review: Genetic vulnerability or differential susceptibility in child development: The case of attachment. *Journal of Child Psychology and Psychiatry, 48*(12), 1160-1173.

Bakermans-Kranenburg, M.J., van IJzendoorn, M.H., and Juffer, F. (2003). Less is more: Meta-analyses of sensitivity and attachment interventions in early childhood. *Psychological Bulletin, 129,* 195-215.

Bandura, A. (2006). Going global with social cognitive theory: From prospect to paydirt. In S.I. Donaldson, D.E. Berger, and K. Pezdek (Eds.), *The Rise of Applied Psychology: New Frontiers and Rewarding Careers* (pp. 53-70). Mahwah, NJ: Lawrence Erlbaum.

Banken, J.A. (2004). Drug abuse trends among youth in the United States. *Annals of the New York Academy of Sciences, 1025,* 465-471.

Baptiste, D.R., Bhana, A., Petersen, I., McKay, M., Voisin, D., Bell, C.C., and Martinez, D.D. (2006). Community collaborative youth-focused HIV/AIDS prevention in South Africa and Trinidad: Preliminary findings. *Journal of Pediatric Psychology, 31*(9), 905-916.

Baptiste, D.R., Blachman, D., Cappella, E., Dew, D., Dixon, K., Bell, C.C., Coleman, D., and Coleman, I. (2007). Transferring a university-led HIV/AIDS prevention initiative to a community agency. In M.M. McKay and R.L. Paikoff (Eds.), *Community Collaborative Partnerships: The Foundation for HIV Prevention Research Efforts* (pp. 269-293). Binghamton, NY: Haworth Press.

Barak, A., Hen, L., Boniel-Nissim, M., and Shapira, N. (2008). A comprehensive review and a meta-analysis of the effectiveness of internet-based psychotherapeutic interventions. *Journal of Technology in Human Services, 26*(2/4), 109-160.

Barbarin, O. (2007). Mental health screening of preschool children: Validity and reliability of ABLE. *American Journal of Orthopsychiatry, 77*(3), 402-418.

Barkley, R.A., Cook, E.H., Diamond, A., Zametkin, A., Thapar, A., Teeter, A., et al. (2002). International consensus statement on ADHD-January 2002. *Clinical Child and Family Psychology Review, 5*(2), 89-111.

Barlow, J., Coren, E., and Stewart-Brown, S. (2002). Meta-analysis of the effectiveness of parenting programmes in improving maternal psychosocial health. *British Journal of General Practice, 52,* 223-233.

Barnard, J., Frangakis, C., Hill, J., and Rubin, D.B. (2002). School choice in New York City: A Bayesian analysis of an imperfect randomized experiment. In C. Gatsonis, R.E. Kass, B. Carlin, A. Carriquiry, A. Gelman, I. Verdinelli, and M. West (Eds.), *Case Studies in Bayesian Statistics* (pp. 3-98). New York: Springer-Verlag.

Barnard, J., Frangakis, C.E., Hill, J.L., and Rubin, D.B. (2003). Principal stratification approach to broken randomized experiments: A case study of school choice vouchers in New York City. *Journal of the American Statistical Association, 98,* 299-323.

Barnett, W.S., and Masse, L.N. (2006). Comparative benefit-cost analysis of the Abecedarian program and its policy implications. *Economics of Education Review, 26,* 113-125.

Barrera, A.Z., Torres, L.D., and Muñoz, R.F. (2007). Prevention of depression: The state of the science at the beginning of the 21st century. *International Review of Psychiatry, 19*(6), 655-670.

Barrera, M., Jr., Biglan, A., Taylor, T.K., Gunn, B.K., Smolkowski, K., Black, C., Ary, D.V., and Fowler, R.C. (2002). Early elementary school intervention to reduce conduct problems: A randomized trial with Hispanic and non-Hispanic children. *Prevention Science, 3,* 83-94.

Barrett, P.M. (1998). Evaluation of cognitive-behavioral group treatments for childhood anxiety disorders. *Journal of Clinical Child Psychology, 27,* 459-468.

Barrett, P.M., and Turner, C. (2001). Prevention of anxiety symptoms in primary school children: Preliminary results from a universal school-based trial. *The British Journal of Clinical Psychology, 40*(Pt.4), 399-410.

Barrett, P.M., Dadds, M.R., and Rapee, R.M. (1996). Family treatment of childhood anxiety: A controlled trial. *Journal of Consulting and Clinical Psychology, 64*(27), 333-342.

Barrett, P.M., Lowry-Webster, H., and Turner, C. (2000). *FRIENDS Program for Children: Group Leaders Manual.* Brisbane: Australian Academic Press.

Barrett, P.M., Lock, S., and Farrell, L.J. (2005). Developmental differences in universal preventive intervention for child anxiety. *Clinical Child Psychology and Psychiatry, 10*(4), 539-555.

Barrett, P.M., Farrell, L.J., Ollendick, T.H., and Dadds, M. (2006). Long-term outcomes of an Australian universal prevention trial of anxiety and depression symptoms in children and youth: An evaluation of the FRIENDS Program. *Journal of Clinical Child and Adolescent Psychology, 35*(3), 403-411.

Baxter, M.G., and Murray, E.A. (2002). The amygdala and reward. *Nature Reviews Neuroscience, 3*(7), 563-573.

Bear, M.F., Dolen, G., Osterweil, E., and Nagarajan, N. (2008). Fragile X: Translation in action. *Neuropsychopharmacology, 33*(1), 84-87.

Beardslee, W.R., and Podorefsky, D. (1988). Resilient adolescents whose parents have serious affective and other psychiatric disorders: The importance of self-understanding and relationships. *American Journal of Psychiatry, 145*(1), 63-69. [Reprinted in Chess, S., Thomas, A., and Hertzig, M.E. (Eds.). (1990). *Annual Progress in Child Psychiatry and Child Development.* New York: Bruner-Miesels.]

Beardslee, W.R., Salt, P., Versage, E.M., Gladstone, T.R.G., Wright, E.J., and Rothberg, P.C. (1997). Sustained change in parents receiving preventive interventions for families with depression. *American Journal of Psychiatry, 154*(4), 510-515.

Beardslee, W.R., Versage, E.M., Wright, E.J., Salt, P.C., Rothberg, P.C., Drezner, K., and Gladstone, R.G. (1997). Examination of preventive interventions for families with depression: Evidence of change. *Development and Psychopathology, 9*, 109-130.

Beardslee, W.R., Wright, E.J., Salt, P., Drezner, K., Gladstone, T.R.G., Versage, E.M., and Rothberg, P.C. (1997). Examination of children's responses to two preventive intervention strategies over time. *Journal of the American Academy of Child and Adolescent Psychiatry, 36*(2), 196-204.

Beardslee, W.R., Versage, E.M., and Gladstone, T.R.G. (1998). Children of affectively ill parents: A review of the past 10 years. *Journal of the American Academy of Child and Adolescent Psychiatry, 37*, 1134-1141.

Beardslee, W.R., Gladstone, T.R., Wright, E.J., and Cooper, A.B. (2003). A family-based approach to the prevention of depressive symptoms in children at risk: Evidence of parental and child change. *Pediatrics, 112*(2), e119-e131.

Beardslee, W.R., Hosman, C., Solantaus, T., van Doesum, K., and Cowling, V. (2005). Children of mentally ill parents: An opportunity for effective prevention all too often neglected. In C. Hosman, E. Jané-Llopis, and S. Saxena (Eds.), *Prevention of Mental Disorders: Effective Interventions and Policy Options* (Chapter 8). Oxford, England: Oxford University Press.

Beardslee, W.R., Wright, E.J., Gladstone, T.R.G., and Forbes, P. (2008). Long-term effects from a randomized trial of two public health preventive interventions for parental depression. *Journal of Family Psychology, 21*(4), 703-713.

Beardslee, W.R., Ayoub, C., Avery, M.W., and Watts, C.L. (in press). Family connections: Helping Early Head Start/Head Start staff and parents make sense of mental health challenges. Submitted to *Zero to Three Journal.*

Becker, L.E., Armstrong, D.L., Chan, F., and Wood, M.M. (1984). Dendritic development in human occipital cortical neurons. *Brain Research, 315*(1), 117-124.

Beelmann, A., and Losel, F. (2006). Child social skills training in developmental crime prevention: Effects on antisocial behavior and social competence. *Psicothema, 18*(3), 603-610.

Belfield, C.R., Nores, M., Barnett, S., and Schweinhart, L. (2006). The high/scope Perry preschool program: Cost-benefit analysis using data from the age-40 follow up. *Journal of Human Resources, 41*(1), 162-190.

Bell, C.C. (2004). *The Sanity of Survival: Reflections on Community Mental Health and Wellness.* Chicago, IL: Third World Press.

Bell, C.C. (2005). Cultural sensitivity is essential: Perspective. *Clinical Psychiatry News, 33*(5), 64.

Bell, C.C., and Jenkins, E.J. (1991). Traumatic stress and children. *Journal of Health Care for the Poor and Underserved, 2*(1), 175-188.

Bell, C.C., Gamm, S., Vallas, P., and Jackson, P. (2001). Strategies for the prevention of youth violence in Chicago public schools. In M. Shafii and S. Shafii (Eds.), *School Violence: Assessment, Management, Prevention* (pp. 251-272). Washington, DC: American Psychiatric Press.

Bell, C.C., Flay, B., and Paikoff, R. (2002). Strategies for health behavioral change. In J. Chunn (Ed.), *The Health Behavioral Change Imperative: Theory, Education, and Practice in Diverse Populations* (pp. 17-40). New York: Kluwer Academic/Plenum.

Bell, C.C., Bhana, A., McKay, M.M., and Petersen, I. (2007). A commentary on the triadic theory of influence as a guide for adapting HIV prevention programs for new contexts and populations: The CHAMP-South Africa story. In M.M. McKay and R.L. Paikoff (Eds.), *Community Collaborative Partnerships: The Foundation for HIV Prevention Research Efforts* (pp. 243-261). Binghamton, NY: Haworth Press.

Bell, C.C., Bhana, A., Petersen, I., McKay, M.M., Gibbons, R., Bannon, W., and Amatya, A. (2008). Building protective factors to offset sexually risky behaviors among black youths: A randomized control trial. *Journal of the National Medical Association, 100*(8), 936-944.

Bengi-Arslan, L., Verhulst, F.C., van der Ende, J., and Erol, N. (1997). Understanding childhood (problem) behaviors from a cultural perspective: Comparison of problem behaviors and competencies in Turkish immigrant, Turkish, and Dutch children. *Social Psychiatry and Psychiatric Epidemiology, 32*, 477-484.

Benton, J.P., Christopher, A.N., and Walter, M.I. (2007). Death anxiety as a function of aging anxiety. *Death Studies, 31*(4), 337-350.

Berends, M., Bodilly, S.J., and Kirby, S.N. (2002). *Facing the Challenges of Whole-School Reform: New American Schools After a Decade.* Santa Monica, CA: RAND.

Berger, R., Pat-Horenczyk, R., and Gelkopf, M. (2007). School-based intervention for prevention and treatment of elementary-students' terror-related distress in Israel: A quasi-randomized controlled trial. *Journal of Traumatic Stress 20*(4), 541-551.

Berkson, J. (1946). Limitations of the application of fourfold table analysis to hospital data. *Biometrics Bulletin, 2*, 47-52.

Bernal, G., Bonilla, J., and Bellido, C. (1995). Ecological validity and cultural sensitivity for outcome research: Issues for the cultural adaptation and development of psychosocial treatments with Hispanics. *Journal of Abnormal Child Psychology, 23*(1), 67-82.

Bhana, A., Petersen, I., Mason, A., Mahintsho, Z., Bell, C.C., and McKay, M.M. (2004). Children and youth at risk: Adaptation and pilot study of the CHAMP (Amaqhawe) programme in South Africa. *African Journal of AIDS Research, 3*(1), 33-41.

Biederman, J., Rosenbaum, J.F., Bolduc-Murphy, E.A., Faraone, S.V., Chaloff, J., Hirshfeld, D.R., and Kagan, J. (1993). A 3-year follow-up of children with and without behavioral inhibition. *Journal of the American Academy of Child and Adolescent Psychiatry, 32*, 814-821.

Bienvenu, O., and Ginsburg, G.S. (2007). Prevention of anxiety disorders. *International Journal of Psychiatry, 19*(6), 647-654.

Bierer, L.M., Yehuda, R., Schmeidler, J., Mitropoulou, V., New, A.S., Silverman, J.M., et al. (2003). Abuse and neglect in childhood: Relationship to personality disorder diagnoses. *CNS Spectrums, 8*(10), 737-754.

Bierman, K.L., Bruschi, C., Domitrovich, C., Fang, G.F., Miller-Johnson, S., and the Conduct Problems Prevention Research Group. (2004). Early disruptive behaviors associated with emerging antisocial behaviors among girls. In M. Putallaz and K.L. Bierman (Eds.), *Aggression, Antisocial Behavior, and Violence Among Girls* (pp. 137-161). New York: Guilford Press.

Bierman, K.L., Nix, R.L., Maples, J.J., Murphy, S.A., and the Conduct Problems Prevention Research Group. (2006). Examining the use of clinical judgment in the context of an adaptive intervention design: The fast track prevention program. *Journal of Consulting and Clinical Psychology, 74*, 468-481.

Biglan, A. (2004). Contextualism and the development of effective prevention practices. *Prevention Science, 5*, 15-21.

Biglan, A., and Taylor T. (2000). Why have we been more successful in reducing tobacco use than violent crime? *American Journal of Community Psychology, 28*(3), 269-302.

Biglan, A., Metzler, C.W., Wirt, R., Ary, D., Noell, J., Ochs, L.L., French, C., and Hood, D. (1990). Social and behavioral factors associated with high-risk sexual behavior among adolescents. *Journal of Behavioral Medicine, 13*(3), 245-261.

Biglan, A., Metzler, C.W., and Ary, D.V. (1994). Increasing the prevalence of successful children: The case for community intervention research. *The Behavior Analyst, 17*, 335-351.

Biglan, A., Ary, D., Koehn, V., Levings, D., Smith, S., Wright, Z., James, L., and Henderson, J. (1996). Mobilizing positive reinforcement in communities to reduce youth access to tobacco. *American Journal of Community Psychology, 24*(5), 625-638.

Biglan, A., Ary, D.V., Smolkowski, K., Duncan, T.E., and Black, C. (2000). A randomized controlled trial of a community intervention to prevent adolescent tobacco use. *Tobacco Control, 9*, 24-32.

Biglan, A., Brennan, P.A., Foster, S.L., and Holder, H.D. (2004). *Helping Adolescents at Risk: Prevention of Multiple Problem Behaviors.* New York: Guilford Press.

Biglan, A., Hayes, S.C., and Pistorello, J. (2008). Acceptance and commitment: Implications for prevention science. *Prevention Science, 9*, 139-152.

Bird, H.R., Canino, G.J., Davies, M., Zhang, H., Ramirez, R., and Lahey, B.B. (2001). Prevalence and correlates of antisocial behaviors among three ethnic groups. *Journal of Abnormal Child Psychology, 29*, 465-478.

Bittner, A., Egger, H.L., Erkanli, A., Costello, E.J., Foley, D.L., and Angold, A. (2007). What do childhood anxiety disorders predict? *Journal of Child Psychology and Psychiatry, 48*(12), 1174-1183.

Blair, C. (2002). School readiness: Integrating cognition and emotion in a neurobiological conceptualization of children's functioning at school entry. *American Psychologist, 57*(2), 111-127.

Bleichrodt, H., and Quiggin, J. (1999). Life-cycle preferences over consumption and health: When is cost-effectiveness analysis equivalent to cost-benefit analysis? *Journal of Health Economics, 18*, 681-708.

Blenkiron, P. (2001). Coping with depression: A pilot study to assess the efficacy of a self-help audio cassette. *British Journal of General Practice, 51*, 366-370.

Block, J., Block, J.H., and Gjerde, P.F. (1988). Parental functioning and the home environment in families of divorce: Prospective and concurrent analyses. *Journal of the American Academy of Child and Adolescent Psychiatry, 27*(2), 207-213.

Block, J.H. (1984). Making school learning activities more playlike: Flow and mastery learning. *Elementary School Journal, 85,* 65-75.

Bloom, H.S. (1984). Accounting for no-shows in experimental evaluation designs. *Evaluation Review, 8,* 225-246.

Blumberg, H.P., Leung, H.C., Skudlarski, P., Lacadie, C.M., Fredericks, C.A., Harris, B.C., Charney, D.S., Gore, J.C., Krystal, J.H., and Peterson, B.S. (2003). A functional magnetic resonance imaging study of bipolar disorder: State- and trait-related dysfunction in ventral prefrontal cortices. *Archives of General Psychiatry, 60*(6), 601-609.

Blumberg, H.P., Martin, A., Kaufman, J., Leung, H.C., Skudlarski, P., Lacadie, C., Fulbright, R.K., Gore, J.C., Charney, D.S., Krystal, J.H., and Peterson, B.S. (2003). Frontostriatal abnormalities in adolescents with bipolar disorder: Preliminary observations from functional MRI. *American Journal of Psychiatry, 160*(7), 1345-1347.

Bögels, S.M., and Brechman-Toussaint, M.L. (2006). Family issues in child anxiety: Attachment, family functioning, parental rearing and beliefs. *Clinical Psychology Review, Special Issue: Anxiety of Childhood and Adolescence: Challenges and Opportunities,* 26(7), 834-856.

Boles, S., Biglan, A., and Smolkowski, K. (2006). Relationships among negative and positive behaviors in adolescence. *Journal of Adolescence, 29,* 33-52.

Bolger, K., and Patterson, C. (2003). Sequelae of child maltreatment. In S.S. Luthar (Ed.), *Resilience and Vulnerability: Adaptation in the Context of Childhood Adversities* (pp. 156-181). New York: Cambridge University Press.

Boris, N.W., Ou, A.C., and Singh, R. (2005). Preventing post-traumatic stress disorder after mass exposure to violence. *Biosecurity and Bioterrorism: Biodefense Strategy, Practice and Science, 3*(2), 154-163.

Borowsky, S.J., Rubenstein, L.V., Meredith, L.S., Camp, P., Jackson-Triche, M.E., and Wells, K.B. (2000). Who is at risk of nondetection of mental health problems in primary care? *Journal of General Internal Medicine, 15,* 381-388.

Botvin, G.J. (1986). Substance abuse prevention research: Recent developments and future directions. *Journal of School Health, 56,* 369-374.

Botvin, G.J. (1996). *Life Skills Training: Promoting Health and Personal Development.* Princeton, NJ: Princeton Health Press.

Botvin, G.J. (2000). *Life Skills Training.* Princeton, NJ: Princeton Health Press.

Botvin, G.J. (2004). Advancing prevention science and practice: Challenges, critical issues, and future directions. *Prevention Science, 5,* 69-72.

Botvin, G.J., and Griffin, K.W. (2004). Life skills training: Empirical finding and future directions. *Journal of Primary Prevention, 25,* 211-232.

Botvin, G.J., Baker, E., Dusenbury, L., Tortu, S., and Botvin, E.M. (1990). Preventing adolescent drug abuse through a multimodal cognitive-behavioral approach: Results of a 3-year study. *Journal of Consulting and Clinical Psychology, 58*(4), 437-446.

Botvin, G.J., Baker, E., Dusenbury, L., Tortun, S., and Botvin, E.M. (1992). Preventing adolescent drug abuse thrugh a multimodal cognitive-behavioral approach: Results of a 3-year study. *Journal of Consulting and Clinical Psychology, 58*(4) 437-446.

Botvin, G.J., Schinke, S.P., Epstein, J.A., and Diaz, T. (1994). Effectiveness of culturally focused and generic skills training approaches to alcohol and drug abuse prevention among minority youths. *Psychology of Addictive Behaviors, 8,* 116-127.

Botvin, G.J., Baker, E., Dusenbury, L., Botvin, E.M., and Diaz, T. (1995). Long-term follow-up results of a randomized drug abuse prevention trial in a white middle-class population. *Journal of the American Medical Association, 273*(14), 1106-1112.

Botvin, G.J., Schinke, S.P., Epstein, J.A., Diaz, T., and Botvin, E.M. (1995). Effectiveness of culturally-focused and generic skills training approaches to alcohol and drug abuse prevention among minority adolescents: Two-year follow-up results. *Psychology of Addictive Behaviors, 9,* 183-194.

Botvin, G.J., Mihalic, S.F., and Grotpeter, J.K. (1998). Life skills training. In D.S. Elliot (Ed.), *Blueprints for Violence Prevention*. Boulder, CO: Center for the Study and Prevention of Violence.

Botvin, G.J., Griffin, K.W., Diaz, T., Scheier, L.M., Williams, C., and Epstein, J.A. (2000). Preventing illicit drug use in adolescents: Long-term follow-up data from a randomized control trial of a school population. *Addictive Behaviors, 25*(5), 769-774.

Botvin, G.J., Griffin, K.W., Diaz, T., and Ifill-Williams, M. (2001). Drug abuse prevention among minority adolescents: Posttest and one-year follow-up of a school-based prevention intervention. *Prevention Science, 2*, 1-13.

Botvin, G.J., Griffin, K.W., and Nichols, T.R. (2006). Preventing youth violence and delinquency through a universal school-based prevention approach. *Prevention Science, 7*, 403-408.

Bourgeois, J.P., Goldman-Rakic, P.S., and Rakic, P. (1994). Synaptogenesis in the prefrontal cortex of rhesus monkeys. *Cerebral Cortex, 4*(1), 78-96.

Boushey, H., Brocht, C., Gundersen, B., and Bernstein, J. (2001). *Hardships in America: The Real Story of Working Families*. Washington, DC: Economic Policy Institute.

Bower, P., Richards, D., and Lovell, K. (2001). The clinical and cost-effectiveness of self-help treatments for anxiety and depressive disorders in primary care: A systematic review. *British Journal General Practice, 51*, 838-845.

Boyce, W.T., Frank, E., Jensen, P.S., Kessler, R.C., Nelson, C.A., Steinberg, L., and the MacArthur Foundation Research Network on Psychopathology and Development. (1998). Social context in developmental psychopathology: Recommendations for future research from the MacArthur network on psychopathology and development. *Development and Psychopathology, 10*(2), 143-164.

Boyd, S.D. (2008). Everything you wanted to know about small RNA but were afraid to ask. *Laboratory Investigation, 88*(6), 569-578.

Bramlett, M.D., and Mosher, W.D. (2002). *Cohabitation, Marriage, Divorce, and Remarriage in the United States*. Vital and Health Statistics, Series 23, No. 22. Washington, DC: U.S. Department of Health and Human Services. Available: http://www.cdc.gov/nchs/data/series/sr_23/sr23_022.pdf [accessed April 2009].

Braun, J.M., Kahn, R.S., Froehlich, T., Auinger, P., and Lanphear, B.P. (2006). Exposures to environmental toxicants and attention deficit hyperactivity disorder in U.S. children. *Environmental Health Perspectives, 114*(12), 1904-1909.

Braun, J.M., Froehlich, T.E., Daniels, J.L., Dietrich, K.N., Hornung, R., Auinger, P., and Lanphear, B.P. (2008). Association of environmental toxicants and conduct disorders in U.S. children. *Environmental Health Perspectives, 116*(7), 956-962.

Braver, S.L., and Smith, M.C. (1996). Maximizing both internal and external validity in longitudinal true experiments with voluntary treatments: The "combined modified" design. *Evaluation and Program Planning, 19*, 287-300.

Braver, S.L., Griffin, W.A., and Cookston, J.T. (2005). Prevention programs for divorced nonresident fathers. *Family Court Review, 43*, 81-96.

Bremner, J.D., Elzinga, B., Schmahl, C., and Vermetten, E. (2008). Structural and functional plasticity of the human brain in posttraumatic stress disorder. *Progress in Brain Research, 167*, 171-186.

Brennan, P.A., Grekin, E.R., Mortensen, E.L., and Mednick, S.A. (2002). Maternal smoking during pregnancy and offspring criminal arrest and hospitalization for substance abuse: A test of gender specific relationships. *American Journal of Psychiatry, 159*, 48-54.

Breslow, L. (1999). From disease prevention to health promotion. *Journal of the American Medical Association, 281*, 1030-1033.

Bridges, L.J., Margie, N.G., and Zaff, J.F. (2001). *Background for Community-Level Work on Emotional Well-Being in Adolescence: Reviewing the Literature on Contributing Factors*. Washington, DC: Child Trends.

Bridging Work Group. (2005). Bridging the gap between research and practice in bereavement: Report from the Center for the Advancement of Health. *Death Studies, 29*, 1-30.

Briggs-Gown, M.J., Horwitz, S.M., Schwab-Stone, M.E., Leventhal, J.M., and Leaf, P.J. (2000). Mental health in pediatric settings: Distribution of disorders and factors related to service use. *Journal of the American Academy of Child and Adolescent Psychiatry, 39*(7), 841-849.

Brody, G.H., Dorsey, S., Forehand, R., and Armistead, L. (2002). Unique and protective contributions of parenting and classroom processes to the adjustment of African American children living in single-parent families. *Child Development, 73*(1), 274-286.

Brody, G.H., Murry, V.M., Gerrard, M., Gibbons, F.X., McNair, L., Brown, A.C., Wills, T.A., Molgaard, V., Spoth, R.L., Luo, Z., and Chen, Y.F. (2006a). The Strong African American Families (SAAF) Program: Prevention of youths' high-risk behavior and a test of a model of change. *Journal of Family Psychology, 20*(1), 1-11.

Brody, G.H., Murry, V.M., Kogan, S.M., Gerrard, M., Gibbons, F.X., Molgaard, V., Brown, A.C., Anderson, T., Chen, Y.-F., Luo, Z., and Wills, T.A. (2006b). The Strong African American Families Program: A cluster-randomized prevention trial of long-term effects and a mediational model. *Journal of Consulting and Clinical Psychology, 74*(2), 356-366.

Brody, G.H., Kogan, S.M., Chen, Y.F., and McBride, M.V. (2008). Long-term effects of the Strong African American Families Program on youths' conduct problems. *Journal of Adolescent Health, 43*(5), 474-481.

Bromet, E.J., and Fennig, S. (1999). Epidemiology and natural history of schizophrenia. *Biological Psychiatry, 46*, 871-881.

Bronfenbrenner, U. (1979). *The Ecology of Human Development: Experiments by Nature and Design.* Cambridge, MA: Harvard University Press.

Bronfenbrenner, U. (1986). Ecology of the family as a context for human development research. *Developmental Psychology, 22*, 723-742.

Bronfenbrenner, U., and Morris, P.A. (1998). The ecology of developmental process. In R.M. Lerner (Ed.), *Handbook of Child Psychology, Volume 1: The Theoretical Models of Human Development* (5th ed., pp. 993-1028). New York: Wiley.

Brook, J.S., Cohen, P., Whiteman, M., and Gordon, A.S. (1992). Psychosocial risk factors in the transition from moderate to heavy use or abuse of drugs. In R.W. Pickens and M. Glantz (Eds.), *Vulnerability to Drug Abuse* (pp. 359-388). Washington, DC: American Psychological Association.

Brooks-Gunn, J., and Duncan, G.J. (1997). The effects of poverty on children. *Children and Poverty, 7*(2), 55-71.

Brotanek, J.M., Halterman J.S., Auinger P., Flores G., and Weitzman M. (2005). Iron-deficiency, prolonged bottle feeding, and racial/ethnic disparities in young children. *Archives of Pediatric Adolescent Medicine, 159,* 1038-1042.

Brotman, M.A., Kassem, L., Reising, M.M., Guyer, A.E., Dickstein, D.P., and Rich, B.A. (2007). Parental diagnoses in youth with narrow phenotype bipolar disorder or severe mood dysregulation. *American Journal of Psychiatry, 164,* 1238-1241.

Brotman, M.A., Rich, B.A., Schmajuk, M., Reising, M., Monk, C.S., and Dickstein, D.P. (2007). Attention bias to threat faces in children with bipolar disorder and comorbid lifetime anxiety disorders. *Biological Psychiatry, 61,* 819-821.

Brown, C.H. (1993a). Analyzing preventive trials with generalized additive models. *American Journal of Community Psychology, 21,* 635-664.

Brown, C.H. (1993b). Statistical methods for preventive trials in mental health. *Statistical Medicine, 12*(3-4), 289-300.

Brown, C.H. (2003). Design principles and their application in preventive field trials. In W.J. Bukoski and Z. Sloboda (Eds.), *Handbook of Drug Abuse Prevention: Theory, Science, and Practice,* (pp. 523-540). New York: Plenum Press.

Brown, C.H., and Faraone, S.V. (2004). Prevention of schizophrenia and psychotic behavior: Definitions and methodologic issues. In W.S. Stone, S.V. Faraone, and M.T. Tsuang (Eds.), *Early Clinical Intervention and Prevention in Schizophrenia* (pp. 255-284). New York: Humana Press.

Brown, C.H., and Liao, J. (1999). Principles for designing randomized preventive trials in mental health: An emerging developmental epidemiology paradigm. *American Journal of Community Psychology, 27*(5), 673-710.

Brown, C.H., Berndt, D., Brinales, J.M., Zong, X., and Bhagwat, D. (2000). Evaluating the evidence of effectiveness for preventive interventions: Using a registry system to influence policy through science. *Addictive Behaviors, 25*, 955-964.

Brown, C.H., Indurkhya, A., and Kellam, S.G. (2000). Power calculations for data missing by design with application to a follow-up study of exposure and attention. *Journal of the American Statistical Association, 95*, 383-395.

Brown, C.H., Wyman, P.A., Guo, J., and Peña, J. (2006). Dynamic wait-listed designs for randomized trials: New designs for prevention of youth suicide. *Clinical Trials, 3*, 259-271.

Brown, C.H., Guo, J., Singer, T., Downes, K., and Brinales, J.M. (2007). Examining the effects of school-based drug prevention programs on drug use in rural settings: Methodology and initial findings. *Journal of Rural Health, 23*(Suppl.1), 29-36.

Brown, C.H., Wyman, P.A., Brinales, J.M., and Gibbons, R.D. (2007). The role of randomized trials in testing interventions for the prevention of youth suicide. *International Review of Psychiatry, 19*(6), 617-631.

Brown, C.H., Costigan, T., and Kendziora, K. (2008). Data analytic frameworks: Analysis of variance, latent growth, and hierarchical models. In A. Nezu and C. Nezu (Eds.), *Evidence-Based Outcome Research: A Practical Guide to Conducting Randomized Clinical Trials for Psychosocial Intervention* (pp. 285-313). London, England: Oxford University Press.

Brown, C.H., Wang, W., and Sandler, I. (2008). Examining how context changes intervention impact: The use of effect sizes in multilevel mixture meta-analysis. *Child Development Perspectives, 2*, 198-205.

Brown, C.H., Wang, W., Kellam, S.G., Muthén, B.O., Petras, H., Toyinbo, P., Poduska, J., Ialongo, N., Wyman, P.A., Chamberlain, P., Sloboda, Z., MacKinnon, D.P., Windham, A., and Prevention Science and Methodology Group. (2008). Methods for testing theory and evaluating impact in randomized field trials: Intent-to-treat analyses for integrating the perspectives of person, place, and time. *Drug and Alcohol Dependence, 95*, S74-S104.

Brown, E.C., Catalano, R.F., Fleming, C.B., Haggerty, K.P., and Abbott, R.D. (2005). Adolescent substance use outcomes in the Raising Healthy Children Project: A two-part latent growth curve analysis. *Journal of Consulting and Clinical Psychology, 73*(4), 699-710.

Brown, L.K., DiClemente, R.J., and Park, T. (1992). Predictors of condom use in sexually active adolescents. *Journal of Adolescent Health, 13*(8), 651-657.

Bruel-Jungerman, E., Davis, S., Rampon, C., and Laroche, S. (2006). Long-term potentiation enhances neurogenesis in the adult dentate gyrus. *Journal of Neuroscience, 26*(22), 5888-5893.

Bryant, R.A., and Guthrie, R.M. (2005). Maladaptive appraisals as a risk factor for posttraumatic stress: A study of trainee firefighters. *Psychological Science, 16*(10), 749-752.

Bryde, J.F. (1971). *Modern Indian Psychology*. Vermillion, SD: Dakota Press.

Buchanan, C.M., Maccoby, E.E., and Dornbusch, S.M. (1991). Caught between parents: Adolescents' experience in divorced homes. *Child Development, 62*(5), 1008-1029.

Bugental, D.B., Ellerson, P.C., Lin, E.K., Rainey, B., Kokotovic, A., and O'Hara, N. (2002). A cognitive approach to child abuse prevention. *Journal of Family Psychology, 16*(3), 243-258.

Bumpass, L., and Lu, H.-H. (2000). Trends in cohabitation and implications for children's family contexts in the United States. *Population Studies, 54,* 29-41.

Burns, B., and Hoagwood, K. (Eds.). (2002). *Community Treatment for Youth: Evidence-Based Interventions for Severe Emotional and Behavioral Disorders.* New York: Oxford University Press.

Burns, B.J., Costello, E.J., Angold, A., Tweed, D., Stangl, D., Farmer, E.M.Z., and Erkanli, A. (1995). Children's mental health service use across service sectors. *Health Affairs, 14*(3), 147-159.

Busch, S.H., and Barry, C.L. (2007). Mental health disorders in childhood: Assessing the burden on families. *Health Affairs, 26*(4), 1088-1095.

Bushman, B.J., and Huesmann L.R. (2006). Short-term and long-term effects of violent media on aggression in children and adults. *Archives of Pediatric Adolescent Medicine, 160,* 348-352.

Bussing, R., Zima, B.T., Perwien, A.R., Belin, T.R., and Widawski, M. (1998). Children in special education programs: Attention deficit hyperactivity disorder, use of services, and unmet needs. *American Journal of Public Health, 88*(6), 880-886.

California Department of Mental Health. (2005). *Frequently Asked Questions: General Information about the Mental Health Services Act.* Available: http://www.cchealth.org/groups/mental_health/mhsa/pdf/faq_general_2005_02.pdf [accessed August 2008].

California Department of Mental Health. (2007). *The Mental Health Services Act (MHSA) Prevention and Early Intervention Component—Proposed Three-Year Program and Expenditure Plan Guidelines, Fiscal Years 2007-08 and 2008-09.* DHM Information Notice No. 07-19. Available: http://www.dmh.ca.gov/DMHDocs/docs/notices07/07_19_Notice.pdf [accessed August 2008].

California Department of Mental Health. (2008). *Mental Health Services Act Progress Report.* Available: http://www.dmh.ca.gov/Prop_63/MHSA/Publications/docs/ProgressReports/MHSA_Progress_July2008.pdf [accessed August 2008].

Cameron, H.A., and McKay, R.D. (2001). Adult neurogenesis produces a large pool of new granule cells in the dentate gyrus. *Journal of Comparative Neurology, 435*(4), 406-417.

Cameron, J.L (2007). *The Importance of Early Life Experience on Lifelong Emotion Regulation.* Presentation at the meeting of the Committee on Prevention of Mental Disorders and Substance Abuse Among Children, Youth, and Young Adults, December 6-7, Washington, DC. Available: http://www.bocyf.org/cameron_presentation.pdf [accessed February 2009].

Canfield, R.L., Henderson, C.R., Cory-Slechta, D.A., Cox, C., Jusko, T.A., and Lanphear, B.P. (2003). Intellectual impairment in children with blood lead concentration below 10 microg per deciliter. *New England Journal of Medicine, 348,* 1517-1526.

Canino, I.A., and Spurlock, J. (1994). *Culturally Diverse Children and Adolescents: Assessment, Diagnosis, and Treatment.* New York: Guilford Press.

Cannon, M., and Clarke, M.C. (2005a). Epidemiology and risk factors. *Psychiatry, 4*(10), 7-10.

Cannon, M., and Clarke, M.C. (2005b). Risk for schizophrenia: Broadening the concepts, pushing back the boundaries. *Schizophrenia Research, 79*(1), 5-13.

Cantor-Graae, E. (2007). The contribution of social factors to the development of schizophrenia: A review of recent findings. *The Canadian Journal of Psychiatry/La Revue Canadienne de Psychiatrie, 52*(5), 277-286.

Caplan, G. (1964). *Principles of Prevention Psychiatry.* Oxford, England: Basic Books.

Cardemil, E.V., Reivich, K.J., and Seligman, M.E.P. (2002). The prevention of depressive symptoms in low-income minority middle school students. *Prevention and Treatment, 5*(1), Art. D8.

Cardemil, E.V., Reivich, K.J., Beevers, C.G., Seligman, M.E.P., and James, J. (2007). The prevention of depressive symptoms in low-income, minority children: Two-year follow up. *Behaviour Research and Therapy, 45*(2), 313-327.

Cardinal, R.N., Parkinson, J.A., Hall, J., and Everitt, B.J. (2002). Emotion and motivation: The role of the amygdala, ventral striatum, and prefrontal cortex. *Neuroscience and Biobehavioral Reviews, 26*(3), 321-352.

Carey, K.B., Carey, M.P., Maisto, S.A., and Henson, J.M. (2006). Brief motivational interventions for heavy college drinkers: A randomized controlled trial. *Journal of Consulting and Clinical Psychology, 74*, 943-954.

Carey, K.B., Scott-Sheldon, L.A.J., Carey, M.P., and DeMartini, K.E.S. (2007). Individual-level interventions to reduce college student drinking: A meta-analytic review. *Additive Behaviors, 32*, 2469-2494.

Carlin, J.B., Wolfe, R., Brown, C.H., and Gelman, A. (2001). A case study on the choice, interpretation, and checking of multilevel models for longitudinal, binary outcomes. *Biostatistics, 2*, 397-416.

Caspi, A., and Moffitt, T.E. (2006). Gene-environment interactions in psychiatry: Joining forces with neuroscience. *Nature Reviews Neuroscience, 7*(7), 583-590.

Caspi, A., Taylor, A., Moffit, T.E., and Plomin, R. (2000). Neighborhood deprivation affects children's mental health: Environmental risks identified in a genetic design. *Psychological Science, 11*(4), 338-342.

Caspi, A., McClay, J., Moffitt, T.E., Mill, J., Martin, J., Craig, I.W., Taylor, A., and Poulton, R. (2002). Role of genotype in the cycle of violence in maltreated children. *Science, 297*(5582), 851-854.

Caspi, A., Sugden, K., Moffitt, T.E., Taylor, A., Craig, I.W., Harrington, H., McClay, J., Mill, J., Martin, J., Braithwaite, A., and Poulton, R. (2003). Influence of life stress on depression: Moderation by a polymorphism in the 5-HTT gene. *Science, 301*(5631), 386-389.

Castellanos, F.X., Lee, P.P., Sharp, W., Jeffries, N.O., Greenstein, D.K., Clasen, L.S., Blumenthal, J.D., James, R.S., Ebens, C.L., Walter, J.M., Zijdenbos, A., Evans, A.C., Giedd, J.N., and Rapoport, J.L. (2002). Developmental trajectories of brain volume abnormalities in children and adolescents with attention-deficit/hyperactivity disorder. *Journal of the American Medical Association, 288*(14), 1740-1748.

Castonguay, A., Levesque, S., and Robitaille, R. (2001). Glial cells as active partners in synaptic functions. *Progress in Brain Research, 132*, 227-240.

Castro, F.G., Barrera, M., and Martinez, C.R. (2004). The cultural adaptation of prevention interventions: Resolving tensions between fidelity and fit. *Prevention Science, 5*, 41-45.

Catalano, R.F., Berglund, M.L., Ryan, J.A.M., Lonczak, H.S., and Hawkins, J.D. (2002). Positive youth development in the United States: Research findings on evaluations of positive youth development programs. *Prevention and Treatment, 5*(1), Art. D15.

Catalano, R.F., Hawkins, J.D., Berglund, L., Pollard, J.A., and Arthur, M.W. (2002). Prevention science and positive youth development: Competitive or cooperative frameworks? *Journal of Adolescent Health, 31*, 230-239.

Catalano, R.F., Mazza, J.J., Harachi, T.W., Abbott, R.D., Haggerty, K.P., and Fleming, C.B. (2003). Raising healthy children through enhancing social development in elementary school: Results after 1.5 years. *Journal of School Psychology, 41*(2), 143-164.

Catalano, R.F., Berglund, M.L., Ryan, J.A.M., Lonczak, H.S., and Hawkins, J.D. (2004). Positive youth development in the United States: Research findings on evaluations of positive youth development programs. *Annals of the American Academy of Political and Social Science, 591*, 98-124.

Celentano, D.D., Bond, K.C., Lyles, C.M., Eiumtrakul, S., Go, V.F., Beyrer, C., Chiangmai, C., Nelson, K.E., Khamboonruang, C., and Vaddhanaphuti, C. (2000). Preventive intervention to reduce sexually transmitted infections: A field trial in the Royal Thai Army. *Archives of Internal Medicine, 160,* 535-540.

Center for the Study and Prevention of Violence, University of Colorado. (2007). *Blueprints for Violence Prevention, Program Matrix.* Available: http://www.colorado.edu/cspv/blueprints/matrixfiles/matrix.pdf [accessed August 2008].

Center on the Developing Child. (2007). *A Science-based Framework for Early Childhood Policy: Using Evidence to Improve Outcomes in Learning, Health, and Behaviors for Vulnerable Children.* Available: http://www.developingchild.harvard.edu/content/downloads/Policy_Framework.pdf [accessed August 2008].

Centers for Disease Control and Prevention. (2006). *Advancing the Nation's Health: A Guide to Public Health Research, 2006-2015.* Atlanta, GA: Author. Available: http://www.cdc.gov/od/science/PHResearch/cdcra/AdvancingTheNationsHealth.pdf [accessed May 2009].

Centers for Disease Control and Prevention. (2007). The effectiveness of universal school-based programs for the prevention of violent and aggressive behavior: A report on recommendations of the Task Force on Community Preventive Services. *Morbidity and Mortality Weekly Report, 56*(RR-7), 1-16.

Centers for Disease Control and Prevention. (2009). *Guide to Community Preventive Services: Preventing Excessive Alcohol Use.* Available: http://thecommunityguide.org/alcohol/index.html [accessed February 2009].

Cerel, J., Fristad, M.A., Verducci, J., Weller, R.A., and Welle, E.B. (2006). Childhood bereavement: Pychopathology in the 2 years postparental death. *Journal of the American Academy of Child and Adolescent Psychiatry, 45,* 681-690.

Chahrour, M., and Zoghbi, H.Y. (2007). The story of Rett syndrome: From clinic to neurobiology. *Neuron, 56*(3), 422-437.

Chamberlain, P. (1990). Comparative evaluation of specialized foster care for seriously delinquent youths: A first step. *Community Alternatives: International Journal of Family Care, 2,* 21-36.

Chamberlain, P., Price, J.M., Reid, J.B., Landsverk, J., Fisher, P.A., and Stoolmiller, M. (2006). Who disrupts from placement in foster and kinship care? *Child Abuse and Neglect, 30,* 409-424.

Chamberlain, P., Price, J., Leve, L.D., Laurent, H., Landsverk, J., and Reid, J.B. (2008). Prevention of behavior problems for children in foster care: Outcomes and mediation effects. *Prevention Science, 9*(1), 17-27.

Chamberlain, P., Saldana, L., Brown, H., and Leve, L.D. (in press). Implementation of multidimensional treatment foster care in California: A randomized control trial of an evidence-based practice. In M. Roberts-DeGennaro and S.J. Fogel (Eds.), *Empirically Supported Interventions for Community and Organizational Change.* Chicago, IL: Lyceum.

Chambers, D.A. (2008). Advancing the science of implementation: A workshop summary. *Administration and Policy in Mental Health and Mental Health Services Research, 35*(1-2), 3-10.

Champagne, F.A. (2008). Epigenetic mechanisms and the transgenerational effects of maternal care. *Frontiers in Neuroendocrinology, 29*(3), 386-397.

Chang, S., Bray, S.M., Li, Z., Zarnescu, D.C., He, C., Jin, P., and Warren, S.T. (2008). Identification of small molecules rescuing fragile X syndrome phenotypes in Drosophila. *Nature Chemical Biology, 4*(4), 256-263.

Changeaux, J.P., and Danchin, A. (1976). Selective stabilisation of developing synapses as a mechanism for the specification of neuronal networks. *Nature, 264*(5588), 705-712.

Chao, H.T., Zoghbi, H.Y., and Rosenmund, C. (2007). MeCP2 controls excitatory synaptic strength by regulating glutamatergic synapse number. *Neuron, 56*(1), 58-65.

Chase-Lansdale, P.L., Cherlin, A.J., and Kiernan, K.E. (1995). The long-term effects of parental divorce on the mental health of young adults: A developmental perspective. *Child Development, 66*(6), 1614-1634.

Chemtob, C.M., Nakashima, J.P., and Hamada, R.S. (2002). Psychosocial intervention for postdisaster trauma symptoms in elementary school children: A controlled community field study. *Archives of Pediatric and Adolescent Medicine, 156*, 211-216.

Chervin, R.D., Hedger Archbold, K., Dillon, J.E., Pituch, K.J., Panahi, P. Dahl, R.E., and Guilleminault, C. (2002). Associations between symptoms of inattention, hyperactivity, restless legs, and periodic leg movements, *Sleep, 25*, 213-218.

Child Welfare League of America. (2007). *CWLA Standards of Excellence for Health Care Services for Children in Out-of-Home Care.* Washington, DC: Author.

Chilton, J.K. (2006). Molecular mechanisms of axon guidance. *Developmental Biology, 292*(1), 13-24.

Chinman, M., Hannah, G., Wandersman, A., Ebener, P., Hunter, S.G., Imm, P., and Sheldon, J. (2005). Developing a community science research agenda for building community capacity. *American Journal of Community Psychology, 35*, 143-158.

Chou, C.-P., Bentler, P.M., and Pentz, M.A. (1998). Comparisons of two statistical approaches to study growth curves: The multilevel model and the latent curve analysis. *Structural Equation Modeling, 5*, 247-266.

Christakis, D.A., Zimmerman, F.J., DiGiuseppe, D.L., and McCarty, C.A. (2004). Early television exposure and subsequent attentional problems in children. *Pediatrics, 113*, 708-713.

Christensen, H., and Griffiths, K.M. (2002). The prevention of depression using the Internet. *Medical Journal of Australia, 177*, S122-S125.

Christie, B.R., and Cameron, H.A. (2006). Neurogenesis in the adult hippocampus. *Hippocampus, 16*(3), 199-207.

Chung, H., Park, Y., and Lanza, S.T. (2005). Latent transition analysis with covariates: Pubertal timing and substance use behaviors in adolescent females. *Statistics in Medicine, 24*(18), 2895-2910.

Chung, H., Walls, T., and Park, Y. (2007). A latent transition model with logistic regression. *Psychometrika, 72*(3), 413-435.

Cialdini, R.B. (1993). *Influence: Science and Practice* (3rd ed.). New York: HarperCollins College.

Cicchetti, D., and Toth, S.L. (1992). The role of developmental theory in prevention and intervention. *Development and Psychopathology, 4*, 489-493.

Cicchetti, D., and Toth, S.L. (1998). The development of depression in children and adolescents. *American Psychologist, 53*(2), 221-241.

Cicchetti, D., Rappaport, J., Sandler, I., and Weissberg, R.P. (Eds.). (2000). *The Promotion of Wellness in Children and Adolescents.* Washington, DC: CWLA Press.

Clark, C., Rodgers, B., Caldwell, T., Power, C., and Stansfeld, S. (2007). Childhood and adulthood psychological ill health as predictors of midlife affective and anxiety disorders: The 1958 British birth cohort. *Archives of General Psychiatry, 64*(6), 668-678.

Clarke, G.N., Hawkins, W.E., Murphy, M., Sheeber, L.B., Lewinsohn, P.M., and Seeley, J.R. (1995). Targeted prevention of unipolar depressive disorder in an at-risk sample of high school adolescents: A randomized trial of a group cognitive intervention. *Journal of the American Academy of Child and Adolescent Psychiatry, 34*, 312-321.

Clarke, G.N., Hornbrook, M., Lynch, F., Polen, M., Gale, J., Beardslee, W., O'Connor, E., and Seeley, J. (2001). A randomized trial of a group cognitive intervention for preventing depression in adolescent offspring of depressed parents. *Archives of General Psychiatry, 58*(12), 1127-1134.

Coate, D., and Grossman, M. (1988). Effects of alcoholic beverage prices and legal drinking ages on youth alcohol use. *Journal of Law and Economics, 31*(1), 145-171.

Cohen, J.A., Kelleher, K.J., and Mannarino, A.P. (2008). Identifying, treating, and referring traumatized children: The role of pediatric providers. *Archives of Pediatric and Adolescent Medicine, 162*(5), 447-452.

Cohen, P., Brook, J.S., Cohen, J. Velez, C.N., and Garcia, M. (1990). Common and uncommon pathways to adolescent psychopathology and problem behavior, In L.N. Robins and M. Rutter (Eds.), *Straight and Devious Pathways from Childhood* (pp. 242-258). New York: Cambridge University Press.

Coie, J.D., Watt, N.F., West, S.G., Hawkins, D.J., Asarnow, J.R., Markman, H.J., Ramey, S.L., Shure, M.B., and Long, B. (1993). The science of prevention: A conceptual framework and some directions for a national research program. *American Psychologist, 48,* 1013-1022.

Cole, D.A., and Maxwell, S.E. (2003). Testing mediational models with longitudinal data: Questions and tips in the use of structural equation modeling. *Journal of Abnormal Psychology, 112*(4), 558-577.

Collaborative for Academic, Social, and Emotional Learning. (2003). *Safe and Sound: An Educational Leader's Guide to Evidence-Based Social and Emotional Learning Programs.* Available: http://www.casel.org/downloads/Safe%20and%20Sound/1A_Safe_and_Sound. pdf [accessed August 2008].

Collins, L.M., Graham, J.W., Rousculp, S.S., Fidler, P.L., Pan, J., and Hansen, W.B. (1994). Latent transition analysis and how it can address prevention research questions. In L.M. Collins and L. Seitz (Eds.), *Advances in Data Analysis for Prevention Research.* National Institute on Drug Abuse Research Monograph Series 142, NIH Pub. No. 94-3599. Rockville, MD: National Institutes of Health.

Collins, L.M., Hyatt, S.L., and Graham, J.W. (2000). LTA as a way of testing models of stage-sequential change in longitudinal data. In T.D. Little, K.U. Schnabel, and J. Baumert (Eds.), *Modeling Longitudinal and Multiple-Group Data: Practical Issues, Applied Approaches, and Specific Examples* (pp. 147-161). Hillsdale, NJ: Lawrence Erlbaum.

Collins, L.M., Murphy, S.A., and Bierman, K.L. (2004). A conceptual framework for adaptive preventive interventions. *Prevention Science, 5*(3), 185-196.

Collins, L.M., Murphy, S.A., and Strecher, V. (2007). The multiphase optimization strategy (MOST) and the sequential multiple assignment randomized trial (SMART): New methods for more potent e-health interventions. *American Journal of Preventive Medicine, 32,* s112-s118.

Collishaw, S., Maughan, B., Goodman, R., and Pickles, A. (2004). Time trends in adolescent mental health. *Journal of Child Psychology and Psychiatry, 45,* 1350-1362.

Commission of the European Communities. (2005). *Improving the Mental Health of the Population: Towards a Strategy on Mental Health for the European Union.* A green paper. Brussels, Belgium: Health and Consumer Protection Directorate, European Commission.

Commission on Positive Youth Development. (2005). The positive perspective on youth development. In D.W. Evans, E.B. Foa, R.E. Gur, H. Hendin, C.P. O'Brien, M.E.P. Seligman, and B.T. Walsh (Eds.), *Treating and Preventing Adolescent Mental Health Disorders: What We Know and What We Don't Know* (pp. 497-527). New York: Oxford University Press.

Commonwealth Department of Health and Aged Care. (2000). *National Action Plan for Promotion, Prevention and Early Intervention for Mental Health.* Canberra, Australia: Mental Health and Special Programs Branch.

Communities That Care. (2004). *Communities That Care Prevention Strategies: A Research Guide to What Works.* Washington, DC: U.S. Department of Health and Human Services.

Compton, M.T. (2004). Considering schizophrenia from a prevention perspective. *American Journal of Preventive Medicine, 26*, 178-185.

Conduct Problems Prevention Research Group. (1992). A developmental and clinical model for the prevention of conduct disorders: The fast track program. *Development and Psychopathology, 4*, 509-527.

Conduct Problems Prevention Research Group. (1999a). Initial impact of the fast track prevention trial for conduct problems: I. The high-risk sample. *Journal of Consulting and Clinical Psychology, 67*, 631-647.

Conduct Problems Prevention Research Group. (1999b). Initial impact of the fast track prevention trial for conduct problems: II. Classroom effects. *Journal of Consulting and Clinical Psychology, 67*, 648-657.

Conduct Problems Prevention Research Group. (2007). Fast track randomized controlled trial to prevent externalizing psychiatric disorders: Findings from grades 3 to 9. *Journal of the American Academy of Child and Adolescent Psychiatry, 46*(10), 1250-1262.

Conger, R.D., Ge, X., Elder, G.H., Jr., Lorenz, F.O., and Simons, R.L. (1994). Economic stress, coercive family process, and developmental problems of adolescents. *Child Development, 65*(2), 541-561.

Connell, A.M., Dishion, T.J., Yasui, M., and Kavanagh, K. (2007). An adaptive approach to family intervention: Linking engagement in family-centered intervention to reductions in adolescent problem behavior. *Journal of Consulting and Clinical Psychology, 75*(4), 568-579.

Cook, T.D., and Campbell, D.T. (1979). *Quasi-Experimentation. Design and Analysis Issues for Field Settings.* Boston: Houghton Mifflin.

Cook, T.D., and Wong, V.C. (2007). The warrant for universal pre-K: Can several thin reeds make a strong policy boat? *Social Policy Report, XXI*(3), 14-15.

Cooke, B., Hegstrom, C.D., Villeneuve, L.S., and Breedlove, S.M. (1998). Sexual differentiation of the vertebrate brain: Principles and mechanisms. *Frontiers in Neuroendocrinology, 19*(4), 323-362.

Cooley, M.R., Boyd, R.C., and Grados, J.J. (2004). Feasibility of an anxiety preventive intervention for community violence exposed African-American children. *Journal of Primary Prevention, 25*(1), 105-123.

Cooper, S., Valleley, R.J., Polaha, J., Begeny, J., and Evans, J.H. (2006). Running out of time: Physician management of behavioral health concerns in rural pediatric primary care. *Pediatrics, 118*, e132-e138.

Copeland, W.E., Miller-Johnson, S., Keeler, G., Angold, A., and Costello, E.J. (2007) Childhood psychiatric disorders and young adult crime: A prospective, population-based study. *American Journal of Psychiatry, 164*, 1668-1675.

Corbin, J. (2007). Reactive attachment disorder: A biopsychosocial disturbance of attachment. *Child and Adolescent Social Work Journal, 24*(6), 539-552.

Corrigan, P.W., and Wassel, A. (2008). Understanding and influencing the stigma of mental illness. *Journal of Psychosocial Nursing and Mental Health Services, 46*, 42-48.

Costello, E.J., Angold, A., Burns, B.J., Stangl, D.K., Tweed, D.L, Erkanli, A., and Worthman, C.M. (1996). *The Great Smoky Mountains Study of Youth: Goals, Design, Methods, and the Prevalence of DSM-III-R Disorders.* Unpublished manuscript, Developmental Epidemiology Program, Duke University Medical Center, Durham, NC, and the Department of Anthropology, Emory University, Atlanta, GA.

Costello, E.J., Keeler, G.P., and Angold, A. (2001). Poverty, race/ethnicity and psychiatric disorder: A study of rural children. *American Journal of Public Health, 91*, 1494-1498.

Costello, E.J., Compton, S.N., Keeler, G., and Angold, A. (2003). Relationships between poverty and psychopathology: A natural experiment. *Journal of the American Medical Association, 290*, 2023-2029.

Costello, E.J., Mustillo, S., Erkanli, A., Keeler, G., and Angold, A. (2003). Prevalence and development of psychiatric disorders in childhood and adolescence. *Archives of General Psychiatry, 60*(8), 837-844.

Costello, E.J., Egger, H.L., and Angold, A. (2004). Developmental epidemiology of anxiety disorders. In T.H. Ollendick and J.S. March (Eds.), *Phobic and Anxiety Disorders in Children and Adolescents: A Clinician's Guide to Effective Psychosocial and Pharmacological Interventions* (pp. 61-91). New York: Oxford University Press.

Costello, E.J., Mustillo, S., Keeler, G., and Angold, A. (2004). Prevalence of psychiatric disorders in childhood and adolescence. In L.B. Lubotsky, J. Petrila, and K. Hennessy (Eds.), *Mental Health Services: A Public Health Perspective* (pp. 111-128). New York: Oxford University Press.

Costello, E.J., Erkanli, A., and Angold, A. (2006). Is there an epidemic of child or adolescent depression? *Journal of Child Psychology and Psychiatry, 47*, 1263-1271.

Costello, E.J., Foley, D.L., and Angold, A. (2006). 10-year research update review: The epidemiology of child and adolescent psychiatric disorders: II. Developmental epidemiology. *Journal of the American Academy of Child and Adolescent Psychiatry, 45*(1), 8-25.

Costello, E.J., Copeland, W., Cowell, A., and Keeler, G. (2007). Service costs of caring for adolescents with mental illness in a rural community, 1993-2000. *The American Journal of Psychiatry, 164*(1), 36-42.

Council on Education for Public Health. (2005). *Accreditation Criteria: Public Health Programs.* Available: http://www.ceph.org/files/public/PHP-Criteria-2005.SO5.pdf [accessed April 2009].

Courchesne, E., Yeung-Courchesne, R., Press, G.A., Hesselink, J.R., and Jernigan, T.L. (1988). Hypoplasia of cerebellar vermal lobules VI and VII in autism. *New England Journal of Medicine, 318*(21), 1349-1354.

Couzin, J. (2008). Science and commerce: Gene tests for psychiatric risk polarize researchers. *Science, 319*(5861), 274-277.

Cowen, E.L. (1977). Baby-steps toward primary prevention. *American Journal of Community Psychology, 5*, 1-22.

Cowen, E.L. (1980). The wooing of primary prevention. *American Journal of Community Psychology, 8*, 258-284.

Cowen, E.L. (2000). Psychological wellness: Some hopes for the future. In D. Cicchetti, J. Rappaport, I.N. Sandler, and R.P. Weissberg (Eds.), *The Promotion of Wellness in Children and Adolescents* (pp. 477-503). Washington, DC: Child Welfare League of America.

Cox, J., and Holden, J. (2003). The origins and development of the Edinburgh postnatal depression scale. In *Perinatal Mental Health: A Guide to the Edinburgh Postnatal Depression Scale* (pp. 15-20). London, England: Gaskell.

Craft, L.L., Freund, K.M., Culpepper, L., and Perna, F.M. (2008). Intervention study of exercise for depressive symptoms in women. *Journal of Women's Health, 16*, 1499-1509.

Craske, M.G., and Zucker, B.G. (2001). Prevention of anxiety disorders: A model for intervention. *Applied and Preventive Psychology, 10*(3), 155-175.

Crews, S.D., Bender, H., Cook, C.R., Gersham, F.M., Kern, L., and Vanderwood, M. (2007). Risk and protective factors of emotional and/or behavioral disorders in children and adolescents: A mega-analytic synthesis. *Behavioral Disorders, 32*(2), 64-77.

Cryan, J.F., and Holmes, A. (2005). The ascent of mouse: Advances in modeling human depression and anxiety. *Nature Reviews Drug Discovery, 4*(9), 775-790.

Cuijpers, P. (2002). Peer-led and adult-led school drug prevention: A meta-analytic comparison. *Journal of Drug Education, 32*, 107-119.

Cuijpers, P., van Straten, A., Smit F., Mihalopoulos C., and Beekman A. (2008). Preventing the onset of depressive disorders: A meta-analytic review of psychological interventions. *American Journal of Psychiatry, 165*(10), 1272-1280.

Cunha, F., and Heckman, J. (2007). The technology of skill formation. *American Economic Review, 97*, 31-47.

Curran, P.J., and Muthén, B.O. (1999). The application of latent curve analysis to testing developmental theories in intervention research. *American Journal of Community Psychology, 27*, 567-595.

Currier, J.M., Holland, J.M, and Neimeyer, R.A. (2007). The effectiveness of bereavement interventions with children: A meta-analytic review of controlled outcome research. *Journal of Clinical Child and Adolescent Psychology, 36*(2), 253-259.

Curtis, C.E., and Luby, J.L. (2008). Depression and social functioning in preschool children with chronic medical conditions. *Journal of Pediatrics, 153*(3), 408-413.

Cutuli, J.J., Chaplin, T.M., Gillham, J.E., Reivich, K., and Seligman, M.E.P. (2006). Preventing co-occurring depression symptoms in adolescents with conduct problems: The Penn resiliency program. *Annals of the New York Academy of Sciences, 1094*, 282-286.

Dadds, M.R., Spence, S.H., Holland, D.E., Barrett, P.M., and Laurens, K.R. (1997). Prevention and early intervention for anxiety disorders: A controlled trial. *Journal of Consulting and Clinical Psychology, 65*, 627-635.

Dagne, G.A., Howe, G., Brown, C.H., and Muthén, B.O. (2002). Hierarchical modeling of sequential behavioral data: An empirical Bayesian approach. *Psychological Methods, 7*(2), 262-280.

Dagne, G.A., Brown, C.H., and Howe, G.W. (2003). Bayesian hierarchical modeling of heterogeneity in multiple contingency tables: An application to behavioral observation data. *Journal of Educational and Behavioral Statistics, 28*, 339-352.

Dagne, G.A., Brown, C.H., and Howe, G.W. (2007). Hierarchical modeling of sequential behavioral data: Log-linear extensions to study complex association patterns in mediation models. *Psychological Methods, 12*(3), 298-316.

Dallman, P.R., Siimes, M.A., and Steckel, A. (1980). Iron deficiency in infancy and childhood. *American Journal of Clinical Nutrition, 33*, 86-118.

Dancause, N., Barbay, S., Frost, S.B., Plautz, E.J., Chen, D., Zoubina, E.V., Stowe, A.M., and Nudo, R.J. (2005). Extensive cortical rewiring after brain injury. *Journal of Neuroscience, 25*(44), 10167-10179.

Dane, A.V., and Schneider, B.H. (1998). Program integrity in primary and early secondary prevention: Are implementation effects out of control? *Clinical Psychology Review, 18*, 23-45.

D'Angelo, E.J., Llerena-Quinn, R., Shapiro, R., Colon, F., Gallagher, K., and Beardslee, W.R. (in press). Adaptation of the preventive intervention program for depression for use with Latino families. Submitted to *Family Process*.

Dapretto, M., Davies, M.S., Pfeifer, J.H., Scott, A.A., Sigman, M., Bookheimer, S.Y., and Iacoboni, M. (2006). Understanding emotions in others: Mirror neuron dysfunction in children with autism spectrum disorders. *Nature Neuroscience, 9*(1), 28-30.

Daum, I., Schugens, M.M., Ackermann, H., Lutzenberger, W., Dichgans, J., and Birbaumer, N. (1993). Classical conditioning after cerebellar lesions in humans. *Behavioral Neuroscience, 107*(5), 748-756.

Davies, P., Walker., A., and Grimshaw, J. (2003). Theories of behaviour change in studies of guideline implementation. *Proceedings of the British Psychological Society, 11*, 120.

Davies, P.T., Sturge-Apple, M.L., Cicchetti, D., and Cummings, E.M. (2007). The role of child adrenocortical functioning in pathways between interparental conflict and child maladjustment. *Developmental Psychology, 43*, 918-930.

Davies, W., and Wilkinson, L.S. (2006). It is not all hormones: Alternative explanations for sexual differentiation of the brain. *Brain Researcher, 1126*(1), 36-45.

Davies, W., Isles, A.R., and Wilkinson, L.S. (2001). Imprinted genes and mental dysfunction. *Annals of Medicine, 33*(6), 428-436.

Davis, C.H., MacKinnon, D.P., Schultz, A., and Sandler, I. (2003). Cumulative risk and population attributable fraction in prevention. *Journal of Clinical Child and Adolescent Psychology, 32*, 228-235.

Davis, M.K., and Gidycz, C.A. (2000). Child sexual abuse prevention programs: A meta-analysis. *Journal of Clinical Child Psychology, 29*(2), 257-265.

de Graaf-Peters, V.B., and Hadders-Algra, M. (2006). Ontogeny of the human central nervous system: What is happening when? *Early Human Development, 82*(4), 257-266.

DeGarmo, D.S., and Forgatch, M.S. (2005). Early development of delinquency in divorced families: Evaluating a randomized preventive intervention trial. *Developmental Science, 8*, 229-239.

DeGarmo, D.S., Patterson, G.R., and Forgatch, M.S. (2004). How do outcomes in a specified parent training intervention maintain or wane over time. *Prevention Science, 5*(2), 73-89.

Demirtas, H., and Schafer, J.L. (2003). On the performance of random-coefficient pattern-mixture models for nonignorable nonresponse. *Statistics in Medicine, 22*(16), 2553-2575.

Dempster, A.P., Laird, N.M., and Rubin, D.B. (1977). Maximum likelihood from incomplete data via the EM algorithm. *Journal of the Royal Statistical Society, B, 39*, 1-38.

Derzon, J.H., and Lipsey, M.W. (2002). A meta-analysis of the effectiveness of mass-communication for changing substance-use knowledge, attitudes, and behavior. In W.D. Crano and M. Burgoon (Eds.), *Mass Media and Drug Prevention: Classic and Contemporary Theories and Research* (pp. 231-258). Mahwah, NJ: Lawrence Erlbaum.

Derzon, J.H., Sale, E., Springer, J.F., and Brounstein, P. (2005). Estimating intervention effectiveness: Synthetic projection of field evaluation results. *Journal of Primary Prevention, 26*(4), 321-343.

D'Esposito, M. (2007). From cognitive to neural models of working memory. *Philosophical Transactions of the Royal Society of London, 362*(1481), 761-772.

Detrait, E.R., George, T.M., Etchevers, H.C., Gilbert, J.R., Vekemans, M., and Speer, M.C. (2005). Human neural tube defects: Developmental biology, epidemiology, and genetics. *Neurotoxicology and Teratology, 27*(3), 515-524.

Devoe, J.F., Peter, K., Kaufman, P., Ruddy, S.A., Miller, A.K., Planty, M., Snyder, T.D., and Rand, M.R. (2003). *Indicators of School Crime and Safety: 2003.* (NCES 2004-004/NCJ 201257). Washington, DC: U.S. Departments of Education and Justice.

Diamond, A., Barnett, W.S., Thomas, J., and Munro, S. (2007). Preschool program improves cognitive control. *Science, 318*, 1387-1388.

DiCenso, A., Guyatt, G., Willan, A., and Griffith, L. (2002). Interventions to reduce unintended pregnancies among adolescents: Systematic review of randomised controlled trials. *British Medical Journal, 324*, 1426-1430.

Diego, M.A., Field, T.M., and Sanders, C.E. (2003). Academic performance, popularity, and depression predict adolescent substance use. *Adolescence, 38*(149), 35-43.

Dierssen, M., and Ramakers, G.J.A. (2006). Dendritic pathology in mental retardation: From molecular genetics to neurobiology. *Genes, Brain and Behavior, 50*(Suppl. 2), 48-60.

Dilorio, C., Resnicow, K., Denzmore, P., Rogers-Tillman, G., Wang, D.T., Dudley, W.N., Lipana, J., and Van Marter, D.F. (2000). Keepin' It R.E.A.L.! A mother-adolescent HIV prevention program. In W. Pequegnat and J. Szapocznik (Eds.), *Working with Families in the Era of AIDS* (pp. 113-132). Thousand Oaks, CA: Sage.

Dilorio, C., Pluha, E., and Belcher, L. (2003). Parent-child communication about sexuality: A review of the literature from 1980-2001. *Journal of HIV/AIDS Prevention and Education in Adolescents and Children, 5,* 7-31.

Dilorio, C., McCarty, F., and Denzmore, P. (2006a). An exploration of social cognitive theory mediators of father-son communication about sex. *Journal of Pediatric Psychology, 31*(9), 917-927.

Dilorio, C., McCarty, F., Resnicow, K., Lehr, S., and Denzmore, P. (2006b). REAL Men: A group-randomized trial of an HIV prevention intervention for adolescent boys. *American Journal of Public Health, 97,* 1084-1089. [Erratum, *American Journal of Public Health, 97,* 1350.]

Dilorio, C., Resnicow, K., McCarty, F., De, A.K., Dudley, W.N., Wang, D.T., and Denzmore, P. (2006). Keepin' It R.E.A.L.! Results of a mother-adolescent HIV prevention program. *Nursing Research, 55,* 43-51.

Dishion, T.J. (2000). Cross-setting consistency in early adolescent psychopathology: Deviant friendships and problem behavior sequelae. *Journal of Personality, 68,* 1109-1126.

Dishion, T.J., and Andrews, D.W. (1995). Preventing escalation in problem behaviors with high-risk young adolescents: Immediate and 1-year outcomes. *Journal of Consulting and Clinical Psychology, 63,* 538-548.

Dishion, T.J., and Kavanagh, K. (2003). *Intervening in Adolescent Problem Behavior: A Family-Centered Approach.* New York: Guilford Press.

Dishion, T.J., and Stormshak, E. (2007). *Intervening in Children's Lives: An Ecological, Family-Centered Approach to Mental Health Care.* Washington, DC: APA Books.

Dishion, T.J., Spracklen, K.M., Andrews, D.W., and Patterson, G.R. (1996). Deviancy training in male adolescent friendships. *Behavior Therapy, 27,* 373-390.

Dishion, T.J., McCord, J., and Poulin, F. (1999). When interventions harm: Peer groups and problem behavior. *American Psychologist, 54,* 755-764.

Dishion, T.J., Burraston, B., and Poulin, F. (2001). Peer group dynamics associated with iatrogenic effects in group interventions with high-risk young adolescents. In C. Erdley and D.W. Nangle (Eds.), *Damon's New Directions in Child Development: The Role of Friendship in Psychological Adjustment* (pp. 79-92). San Francisco: Jossey-Bass.

Dishion, T.J., Kavanagh, K., Schneiger, A., Nelson, S., and Kaufman, N. (2002). Preventing early adolescent substance use: A family-centered strategy for public middle school. In R.L. Spoth, K. Kavanagh., and T.J. Dishion (Eds.), Universal family-centered prevention strategies: Current findings and critical issues for public health impact [Special Issue], *Prevention Science, 3*(3), 191-201.

Dishion, T.J., Kavanagh, K., Veltman, M., McCartney, T., Soberman, L., and Stomshak, E. (2003). *Family Management Curriculum V. 2.0: Leader's Guide.* Eugene, OR: Child and Family Center.

Divac, I., Rosvold, H.E., and Szwarcbart, M.K. (1967). Behavioral effects of selective ablation of the caudate nucleus. *Journal of Comparative Physiology and Psychology, 63*(2), 184-190.

Dobrez, D., Lo Sasso, A., Holl, J., Shalowitz, M., Leon, S., and Budetti, P. (2001). Estimating the cost of developmental and behavioral screening of preschool children in pediatric practice. *Pediatrics, 108,* 913-920.

Dolan, L.J., Kellam S.G., Brown, C.H., Werthamer-Larsson, L., Rebok, G.W., Mayer, L.S., Laudolff, J., Turkkan, J.S., Ford, C., and Wheeler, L. (1993). The short-term impact of two classroom-based preventive intervention trials on aggressive and shy behaviors and poor achievement. *Journal of Applied Developmental Psychology, 14,* 317-345.

Dolen, G., Osterweil, E., Rao, B.S., Smith, G.B., Auerbach, B.D., Chattarji, S., and Bear, M.F. (2007). Correction of fragile X syndrome in mice. *Neuron, 56*(6), 955-962.

Domitrovich, C., and Greenberg, M.T. (2000). The study of implementation: Current finding from effective programs for school-aged children. *Journal of Educational and Psychological Consultation, 11*, 193-221.

Donenberg, G., Bryant, F., Emerson, E., Wilson, H., and Pasch, K. (2003). Tracing the roots of early sexual debut among adolescents in psychiatric care. *Journal of the American Academy of Child and Adolescent Psychiatry, 42*, 594-608.

Donovan, C.L., and Spence, S.H. (2000). Prevention of childhood anxiety disorders. *Clinical Psychology Review, 20*(4), 509-531.

Dorfman, S.L., and Smith, S.A. (2002). Preventive mental health and substance abuse programs and services in managed care. *The Journal of Behavioral Health Services and Research, 29*(3), 233-258.

Dowsett, S.M., and Livesey, D.J. (2000). The development of inhibitory control in preschool children: Effects of "executive skills" training. *Developmental Psychobiology, 36*(2), 161-174.

Doyon, J., and Benali, H. (2005). Reorganization and plasticity in the adult brain during learning of motor skills. *Current Opinion in Neurobiology, 15*(2), 161-167.

Dryfoos, J. (1990). *Adolescents at Risk: Prevalence and Prevention.* New York: Oxford University Press.

Dubrow, N.F., and Garbarino, J. (1989). Living in the war zone: Mothers and young children in a public housing development. *Child Welfare, 68*(1), 3-20.

Duggan, A., McFarlane, E., Fuddy, L., Burrell, L., Higman, S.M., Windham, A., and Sia, C. (2004). Randomized trial of a statewide home visiting program: Impact in preventing child abuse and neglect. *Child Abuse and Neglect, 28*, 597-622.

Dumka, L.E., Mauricio, A.M., and Gonzales, N.A. (2007). Research partnerships with schools to implement prevention programs for Mexican origin families. *Journal of Primary Prevention, 28*(5), 403-420.

DuMont, K., Mitchell-Herzfeld, S., Greene, R., Lee, E., Lowenfels, A., Rodriguez, M., and Dorabawila, V. (2008). Healthy families New York (HFNY) randomized trial: Effects on early child abuse and neglect. *Child Abuse and Neglect, 32*(3), 295-315.

Durlak, J.A. (1998). Why program implementation is important. *Journal of Prevention and Intervention in the Community, 17*, 5-18.

Durlak, J.A., and Wells, A.M. (1997). Primary prevention mental health programs for children and adolescents: A meta-analytic review. *American Journal of Community Psychology, 25*, 115-152.

Durlak, J.A., and Wells, A.M. (1998). Evaluation of indicated preventive intervention (secondary prevention) mental health programs for children and adolescents. *American Journal of Community Psychology, 26*, 775-802.

Durlak, J.A., Weissberg, R.P., Taylor, R.D., and Dymnicki, A.B. (2007). *The Effects of School-Based Social and Emotional Learning: A Meta-analytic Review.* Unpublished manuscript, Loyola University, Chicago, IL.

Dykman, R., and Casey, P. (2003). Behavioral and cognitive status in school-aged children with a history of failure to thrive during early childhood. *Clinical Pediatrics, 40*, 63-70.

Dzewaltowski, D.A., Estabrooks, P.A., Klesges, L.M., Bull, S., and Glasgow, R.E. (2004). Behavior change intervention research in community settings: How generalizable are the results? *Health Promotion International, 19*(2), 235-245.

Eaton, W.O., and Enns, L.R. (1986). Sex differences in human motor activity level. *Psychological Bulletin, 100*(1), 19-28.

Eccles, J.S. (1996). The power and difficulty of university-community collaboration. *Journal of Research on Adolescence, 6*, 81-86.

Eccles, J.S., and Harold, R.D. (1996). Family involvement in children's and adolescents' schooling. In A. Bloom and J.F. Bunn (Eds.), *Family-School Links: How Do They Affect Educational Outcomes?* (pp. 3-34). Mahwah, NJ: Lawrence Erlbaum.

Eccles, J.S., Midgley, C., Wigfield, A., Buchanan, C.M., Reuman, D., Flanagan, C., and MacIver, D. (1993). Development during adolescence: The impact of stage-environment fit on young adolescents' experiences in schools and in families. *American Psychologist, 48*, 90-101.

Eddy, J.M., Reid, J.B., and Fetrow, R.A. (2000). An elementary school-based prevention program targeting modifiable antecedents of youth delinquency and violence: Linking the interests of families and teachers (LIFT). *Journal of Emotional and Behavioral Disorders, 8*, 165-186.

Eddy, J.M., Martinez, C., Morgan-Lopez, A., Smith, P., and Fisher, P.A. (2002). Diversifying the ranks of prevention scientists through a community collaborative approach to education. *Prevention and Treatment, 5*(1).

Eddy, J.M., Smith, P., Brown, C.H., and Reid, J.B. (2005). A survey of prevention science training: Implications for educating the next generation. *Prevention Science, 6*, 59-71.

Education Commission of the States. (2001). *A Closer Look: State Policy Trends in Three Key Areas of the Bush Education Plan—Testing, Accountability, and School Choice.* Denver, CO: Author.

Edwards, V.J., Holden, G.W., Anda, R.F., and Felitti, V.J. (2003). Experiencing multiple forms of childhood maltreatment and adult mental health: Results from the adverse childhood experiences (ACE) study. *American Journal of Psychiatry, 160*(8), 1453-1460.

Egger, H.L., and Angold, A. (2006). Common emotional and behavioral disorders in preschool children: Presentation, nosology, and epidemiology. *Journal of Child Psychiatry and Psychology, 47*, 313-337.

Egger, H.L., Erkanli, A., Keeler, G., Potts, E., Walter, B., and Angold, A. (2006). The test-retest reliability of the preschool age psychiatric assessment (PAPA). *Journal of the American Academy of Child and Adolescent Psychiatry, 45*, 538-549.

Eichenbaum, H. (2000). A cortical-hippocampal system for declarative memory. *Nature Reviews Neuroscience, 1*(1), 41-50.

Eisenberg, D., and Neighbors, K. (2007). *Economics of Preventing Mental Disorders and Substance Abuse Among Young People.* Paper commissioned by the Committee on Prevention of Mental Disorders and Substance Abuse Among Children, Youth, and Young Adults: Research Advances and Promising Interventions, Board on Children, Youth, and Families, National Research Council and Institute of Medicine, Washington, DC.

Eisenberg, N., Fabes, R.A., Guthrie, I.K., Murphy, B.C., Maszk, P., Holmgren, R., and Suh, K. (1996). The relations of regulation and emotionality to problem behavior in elementary school children. *Development and Psychopathology, 8*, 141-162.

Elias, M.J., Zins, J.E., Weissberg, K.S., Greenberg, M.T., Haynes, N.M., Kessler, R., Schwab-Stone, M.E., and Shriver, T.P. (1997). *Promoting Social and Emotional Learning: Guidelines for Educators.* Alexandria, VA: Association for Supervision and Curriculum Development.

Ellickson, P.L., and Bell, R.M. (1990). Drug prevention in junior high: A multisite longitudinal test. *Science, 247*, 1299-1305.

Ellickson, P.L., Bell, R.M., and McGuigan, K. (1993). Preventing adolescent drug use: Long-term results of a junior high program. *American Journal of Public Health, 83*(6), 856-861.

Ellickson, P.L., McCaffrey, D.F., Ghosh-Dastidar, B., and Longshore, D.L. (2003). New inroads in preventing adolescent drug use: Results from a large-scale trial of Project ALERT in middle schools. *Adolescent Health, 93*(1), 1830-1836.

Elliott, D.S., and Mihalic, S. (2004). Issues in disseminating and replicating effective prevention programs. *Prevention Science, 5*(1), 47-53.

Elliott, R., Dolan, R.J., and Frith, C.D. (2000). Dissociable functions in the medial and lateral orbitofrontal cortex: Evidence from human neuroimaging studies. *Cerebral Cortex, 10*(3), 308-317.

Elliott, S.A., Leverton, T.J., Sanjack, M., Turner, H., Cowmeadow, P., Hopkins, J., and Bushnell, D. (2000). Promoting mental health after childbirth: A controlled trial of primary prevention of postnatal depression. *British Journal of Clinical Psychology, 39,* 223-241.

Elliott, S.N., and Busse, R.T. (2004). Assessment and evaluation of students' behavior and intervention outcomes: The utility of rating scale methods. In R.B. Rutherford, M.M. Quinn, and S.P. Mathur (Eds.), *Handbook of Research in Emotional and Behavioral Disorders* (pp. 123-142). New York: Guilford Press.

Elliott, S.N., Huai, N., and Roach, A. (2007). Universal and early screening for educational difficulties: Current and future approaches. *Journal of School Psychology, 45,* 137-161.

Else-Quest, N.M., Hyde, J.S., Goldsmith, H.H., and Van Hulle, C.A. (2006). Gender differences in temperament: A meta-analysis. *Psychological Bulletin, 132*(1), 33-72.

Embry, D.D. (2002). The good behavior game: A best practice candidate as a universal behavioral vaccine. *Clinical Child and Family Psychology Review, 5,* 273-297.

Embry, D.D. (2004). Community-based prevention using simple, low-cost, evidence-based kernels and behavior vaccines. *Journal of Community Psychology, 32,* 575-591.

Emery, R.E., Sbarra, D., and Grover, T. (2005). Divorce mediation: Research and reflections. *Family Court Review, Special Issue on Prevention: Research, Policy, and Evidence-Based Practice, 43,* 22-37.

Ennett, S.T., Ringwalt, C.L., Thorne, J., Rohrbach, L.A., Vincus, A., Simons-Rudolph, A., and Jones, S. (2003). A comparison of current practice in school-based substance use prevention programs with meta-analysis findings. *Prevention Science, 4,* 1-14.

Ensminger, M.E., Kellam, S.G., and Rubin, B.R. (1983). School and family origins of delinquency: Comparisons by sex. In K.T. Van Dusen and S.A. Mednick (Eds.), *Prospective Studies of Crime and Delinquency* (pp. 73-97). Boston: Kluwer-Nijhoff.

Ensminger, M.E., Brown, C.H., and Kellam, S.G. (1984). Social control as an explanation of sex differences in substance use among adolescents. NIDA Research Monograph: Problems of Drug Dependence, 1983. *Proceedings of the 45th Annual Scientific Meeting of the College on Problems of Drug Dependence, 49,* 296-304.

Epps, S.R., and Huston, A.C. (2007). Effects of a poverty intervention policy demonstration on parenting and child social competence: A test of the direction of effects. *Social Science Quarterly, 88*(2), 344-365.

Epstein, J.L. (1991). Effects of teacher practices of parent involvement on student achievement in reading and math. In S. Silvern (Ed.), *Literacy Through Family, Community, and School Interaction* (pp. 261-276). Greenwich, CT: JAI.

Epstein, M., Atkins, M., Cullinan, D., Kutash, K., and Weaver, R. (2008). *Reducing Behavior Problems in the Elementary School Classroom: A Practice Guide.* (NCEE #2008-012). Washington, DC: Institute of Education Sciences, U.S. Department of Education.

Erickson, M., Sroufe, L.A., and Egeland, B. (1985). The relationship of quality of attachment and behavior problems in preschool in a high-risk sample. In I. Bretherton and E. Waters (Eds.), *Growing Points in Attachment Theory and Research. Monographs of the Society for Research in Child Development* (1-2, Serial No. 209). Chicago, IL: University of Chicago Press.

Erikson, E.H. (1968). *Identity: Youth and Crisis.* New York: Norton.

Eriksson, P.S., Perfilieva, E., Bjork-Eriksson, T., Alborn, A.M., Nordborg, C., Peterson, D.A., and Gage, F.H. (1998). Neurogenesis in the adult human hippocampus. *Nature Medicine, 4*(11), 1313-1317.

Erlenmeyer-Kimling, L., Rock, D., Roberts, S.A., Janal, M., Kestenbaum, C., Cornblatt, B., Adamo, U.H., and Gottesman, I.I. (2000). Attention, memory, and motor skills as childhood predictors of schizophrenia-related psychoses: The New York high risk project. *American Journal of Psychiatry, 57,* 1416-1422.

Ettner, S.L., Frank, R.G., and Kessler, R.C. (1997). The impact of psychiatric disorders on labor market outcomes. *Industrial and Labor Relations Review, 51*(1), 64-81.

Evans, J.P. (2007). Health care in the age of genetic medicine. *Journal of the American Medical Association, 298*(22), 2670-2672.

Eyberg, S.M., Funderburk, B.W., Hembree-Kigin, T.L., McNeil, C.B., Querido, J.G., and Hood, K.K. (2001). Parent-child interaction therapy with behavior problem children. *Child and Family Behavior Therapy, 23*(4), 1-20.

Fagan, A.A., and Mihalic, S. (2003). Strategies for enhancing the adoption of school-based prevention programs: Lessons learned from the blueprints for violence prevention replications of the life skills training program. *Journal of Community Psychology, 31*, 235-253.

Faggiano, F., Vigna-Taglianti, F.D., Versino, E., Zambon, A., Borraccino, A., and Lemma, P. (2005). School-based prevention for illicit drug use. *Cochrane Database of Systematic Reviews*, Art. No. CD003020.

Fantuzzo, J., Sutton-Smith, B., Atkins, M., Stevenson, H., Coolahan, K., Weiss, A., and Manz, P. (1996). Community-based resilient peer treatment of withdrawn maltreated preschool children. *Journal of Consulting and Clinical Psychology, 64*(6), 1377-1386.

Faraone, S.V., and Tsuang, M.T. (1985). Quantitative models of the genetic transmission of schizophrenia. *Psychological Bulletin, 98*, 41-66.

Faraone, S.V., Biederman, J., Chen, W.J., Milberger, S., Warburton, R.M., and Tsuang, M.T. (1995). Genetic heterogeneity in attention deficit hyperactivity disorder: Gender, psychiatric comorbidity and maternal ADHD. *Journal of Abnormal Psychology, 104*, 334-345.

Faraone, S.V., Kremen, W.S., Lyons, M.J., Pepple, J.R., Seidman, L.J., and Tsuang, M.T. (1995). Diagnostic accuracy and linkage analysis: How useful are schizophrenia spectrum phenotypes? *American Journal of Psychiatry, 152*, 1286-1290.

Faraone, S.V., Seidman, L.J., Kremen, W.S., Pepple, J.R., Lyons, M.J., and Tsuang, M.T. (1995). Neuropsychological functioning among the nonpsychotic relatives of schizophrenic patients: A diagnostic efficiency analysis. *Journal of Abnormal Psychology, 104*, 286-304.

Faraone, S.V., Brown, C.H., Glatt, S.J., and Tsuang, M.T. (2002). Preventing schizophrenia and psychotic behaviour: Definitions and methodological issues. *Canadian Journal of Psychiatry, 47*(6), 527-537.

Farmer, E.M.Z., Burns, B., Phillips, S., Angold, A., and Costello, E. (2003). Pathways into and through mental health services for children and adolescents. *Psychiatric Services, 54*, 60-66.

Farmer, J.E., and Peterson, L. (1995). Injury risk factors in children with attention deficit hyperactivity disorder. *Health Psychology, 14*(4), 325-332.

Farrelly, M.C., Healton, C.G., Davis, K.C., Messeri, P., Hersey, J.C., and Haviland, M.L. (2002). Getting to the truth: Evaluating national tobacco countermarketing campaigns. *American Journal of Public Health, 92*(6), 901-907.

Farrelly, M.C., Davis, K.C., Yarsevich, J.M., Haviland, M.L., Hersey, J., Girlando, M.E., and Healton, C.G. (2006). American Legacy Foundation, getting to the truth: Assessing youths' reactions to the truth and "Think. Don't smoke" tobacco countermarketing campaigns. *Tobacco Control: Surveys and Program Evaluations from Outside UCSF*. Paper FLR9. Available: http://repositories.cdlib.org/context/tc/article/1205/type/pdf/viewcontent/ [accessed April 2009].

Farrington, D.P., and Welsh, B.C. (2006). *Saving Children from a Life of Crime: Early Risk Factors and Effective Interventions*. New York: Oxford University Press.

Feinberg, M.E., Ridenour, T.A., and Greenberg, M.T. (2007). Aggregating indices of risk and protection for adolescent behavior problems: The Communities That Care youth survey. *Journal of Adolescent Health, 40*, 506-513.

Feinberg, M.T., Bontempo, D., and Greenberg, M.T. (2008). Predictors and levels of sustainability of community prevention coalitions. *American Journal of Preventive Medicine, 34,* 495-501.

Felitti, V.J., Anda, R.F., Nordenberg, D., Williamson, D.F., Spitz, A.M., Edwards, V., Koss, M.P., and Marks, J.S. (1998). The relationship of adult health status to childhood abuse and household dysfunction. *American Journal of Preventive Medicine, 14,* 245-258.

Felner, R.D., Brand, S., Adan, A.M., Mulhall, P.F., Flowers, N., Sartain, B., and Du Bois, D.L. (1993). Restructuring the ecology of the school as an approach to prevention during school transitions: Longitudinal follow-ups and extensions of the school transitional environment project (STEP). *Prevention in Human Services, 10*(2), 103-136.

Fenton, W.S. (2000). Depression, suicide, and suicide prevention in schizophrenia. *Suicide Life-Threatening Behavior, 30,* 34-49.

Fergusson, D.M., and Horwood, L.J. (2003). Resilience to childhood adversity: Results of a 21-year study. In S.S. Luthar (Ed.), *Resilience and Vulnerability: Adaptation in the Context of Childhood Adversities* (pp. 130-155). New York: Cambridge University Press.

Fergusson, D.M., Woodward, L.J., and Horwood, L.J. (1998). Maternal smoking during pregnancy and psychiatric adjustment in late adolescence. *Archives of General Psychiatry, 55*(8), 721-727.

Fergusson, D.M., Boden, J.M., and Horwood, J. (2007). Exposure to single parenthood in childhood and later mental health, educational, economic, and criminal behavior outcomes. *Archives of General Psychiatry, 64,* 1089-1095.

Fichtenberg, C.M., and Glantz, S.A. (2002). Effect of smoke-free workplaces on smoking behaviour: Systematic review. *British Medical Journal, 325,* 188-195.

Field, A.E., Javaras, K.M., Aneja, P., Kitos, N., Camargo, Jr., C.A., Taylor, C.B., and Laird, N.M. (2008). Family, peer, and media predictors of becoming eating disordered. *Archives of Pediatric and Adolescent Medicine, 162*(6), 574-579.

Finnegan, L.P., and Kandall, S.R. (1997). Maternal and neonatal effects of alcohol and drugs. In J.H. Lowinson, P. Ruiz, R.B. Millman, and J.G. Langrod (Eds.), *Substance Abuse: A Comprehensive Textbook* (3rd ed., pp. 513-534). Baltimore: Williams and Wilkins.

Fischer, A., Sananbenesi, F., Wang, X., Dobbin, M., and Tsai, L.H. (2007). Recovery of learning and memory is associated with chromatin remodeling. *Nature, 447*(7141), 178-182.

Fish, E.W., Shahrokh, D., Bagot, R., Caldji, C., Bredy, T., Szyf, M., and Meaney, M.J. (2004). Epigenetic programming of stress responses through variations in maternal care. *Annals of the New York Academy of Sciences, 1036,* 167-180.

Fishbein, D. (2000). The importance of neurobiological research to the prevention of psychopathology. *Prevention Science, 1*(2), 89-106.

Fisher, P.A., and Chamberlain, P. (2000). Multidimensional treatment foster care: A program for intensive parenting, family support, and skill building. *Journal of Emotional and Behavioral Disorders, 8*(3), 155-164.

Fisher, P.A., Gunnar, M.R., Chamberlain, P., and Reid, J.B. (2000). Preventive interventions for maltreated preschoolers: Impact on children's behavior, neuroendocrine activity, and foster parent functioning. *Journal of the American Academy of Child and Adolescent Psychiatry, 39,* 1356-1364.

Fisher, P.A., Burraston, B., and Pears, K. (2005). The early intervention foster care program: Permanent placement outcomes from a randomized trial. *Child Maltreatment, 10*(1), 61-71.

Fisher, P.A., Stoolmiller, M., Gunnar, M.R., and Burraston, B.O. (2007). Effects of a therapeutic intervention for foster preschoolers on diurnal cortisol activity. *Psychoneuroendocrinology, 32,* 892-905.

Fixsen, D.L., Naoom, S.F., Blase, K.A., Friedman, R.M., and Wallace, F. (2005). *Implementation Research: A Synthesis of the Literature*. (FMHI Publication #231). Tampa: University of South Florida, Louis de la Parte Florida Mental Health Institute.

Flay, B.R. (1986). Efficacy and effectiveness trials (and other phases of research) in the development of health promotion programs. *Preventive Medicine, 15*(5), 451-474.

Flay, B.R., Graumlich, S., Segawa, E., Burns, J., Amuwo, S., Bell, C.C., Campbell, R., Cowell, J., Cooksey, J., Dancy, B., Hedeker, D., Jagers, R., Levy, S.R., Paikoff, R., Punwani, I., and Weisberg, R. (2004). The ABAN AYA youth project: Effects of comprehensive prevention programs on high-risk behaviors among inner city African American youth, a randomized trial. *Archives of Pediatrics and Adolescent Medicine, 158*(4), 377-384.

Flay, B.R., Biglan, A., Boruch, R.F., Castro, F.G., Gottfredson, D., Kellam, S., Moscicki, E.K., Schinke, S., Valentine, J.C., and Ji, P. (2005). Standards of evidence: Criteria for efficacy, effectiveness and dissemination. *Prevention Science, 6*(3), 151-175.

Fleishman, J.L. (2007). *The Foundation: A Great American Secret*. New York: Public Affairs Books.

Fletcher, J., and Wolfe, B. (2008). Child mental health and human capital accumulation: The case of ADHD revisited. *Journal of Health Economics, 27*(3), 794-800.

Florez, J.C. (2008). The genetics of type 2 diabetes: A realistic appraisal circa 2008. *Journal of Clinical Endocrinology and Metabolism, 93*(12), 4633-4642.

Flynn, J.T., Schiffman, J., Feuer, W., and Corona, A. (1998). The therapy of amblyopia: An analysis of the results of amblyopia therapy utilizing the pooled data of published studies. *Transactions of the American Ophthalmological Society, 96*, 431-450.

Folkman, S., Lazarus, R.S., Dunkel-Schetter, C., DeLongis, A., and Gruen, R.J. (1986). Dynamics of a stressful encounter: Cognitive appraisal, coping, and encounter outcomes. *Journal of Personality and Social Psychology, 50*(5), 992-1003.

Fombonne, E. (2005). Epidemiology of autistic disorder and other pervasive developmental disorder. *Journal of Clinical Psychiatry, 66*, 3-8.

Food and Drug Administration. (1998). Guidance on statistical principles for clinical trial. *Federal Register, 63*(179), 49583-49598.

Forgatch, M.S., and DeGarmo, D.S. (1999). Parenting through change: An effective prevention program for single mothers. *Journal of Consulting and Clinical Psychology, 67*, 711-724.

Forgatch, M.S., and Martinez, C.R. (1999). Parent management training: A program linking basic research and practical application. *Parent Management Training, 36*, 923-937.

Forgatch, M.S., DeGarmo, D.S., and Beldavs, Z. (2005). An efficacious theory-based intervention for stepfamilies. *Behavior Therapy, 36*, 357-365.

Forgatch, M., Beldavs, Z., Patterson, G., and DeGarmo, D. (2008). From coercion to positive parenting: Putting divorced mothers in charge of change. In M. Kerr, H. Stattin, and R.C.M.E. Engels (Eds.), *What Can Parents Do? New Insights into the Role of Parents in Adolescent Problem Behavior* (pp. 191-209). London, England: Wiley.

Forrest, C.B., Glade, G.B., Baker, A.E., Bocian, A.B., Kang, M., and Starfield, B. (1999). The pediatric primary-specialty care interface: How pediatricians refer children and adolescents to specialty care. *Archives of Pediatrics and Adolescent Medicine, 153*(7), 705-714.

Fortin, N.J., Agster, K.L., and Eichenbaum, H.B. (2002). Critical role of the hippocampus in memory for sequences of events. *Nature Neuroscience, 5*(5), 458-462.

Foster, E.M., Dodge, K.A., and Jones, D. (2003). Issues in the economic evaluation of prevention programs. *Applied Developmental Science, 7*(2), 76-86.

Foster, E.M., Jones, D.E., and Conduct Problems Research Group. (2005). The high costs of aggression: Public expenditures resulting from conduct disorder. *American Journal of Public Health, 25*(9), 1767-1772.

Foster, E.M., Jones, D., and Conduct Problems Prevention Research Group. (2006). Can a costly intervention be cost-effective?: An analysis of violence prevention. *Archives of General Psychiatry, 63*(11), 1284.

Foster, E.M., Johnson-Shelton, D., and Taylor, T.K. (2007). Measuring time costs in interventions designed to reduce behavior problems among children and youth. *American Journal of Community Psychology, 40*(1-2), 64-81.

Foster, E.M., Porter, M., Ayers, T., Kaplan, D., and Sandler, I. (2007). Estimating the costs of preventive interventions. *Evaluation Review, 31*(3), 261-286.

Foster, S., Rollefson, M., Doksum, T., Noonan, D., and Robinson, G. (2005). *School Mental Health Services in the United States, 2002-2003.* (DHHS Publication No. SMA 05-4068). Rockville, MD: Center for Mental Health Services, Substance Abuse and Mental Health Services Administration.

Fox, D.P., Gottfredson, D.C., Kumpfer, K.L., and and Beatty, P.D. (2004). Challenges in disseminating model programs: A qualitative analysis of the strengthening WDC families project. *Clinical Child and Family Psychology Review, 7*(3), 165-176.

Foxcroft, D.R., Ireland, D., Lowe, G., and Breen, R. (2002). Primary prevention for alcohol misuse in young people. *Cochrane Database of Systematic Reviews, 3,* Art. No. CD003024.

Francis, D.R. (2009). *The Earned Income Tax Credit Raises Employment.* National Bureau of Economic Research. Available: http://www.nber.org/cgi-bin/printit?uri=/digest/aug06/w11729.html [accessed April 2009].

Frangakis, C.E., and Rubin, D.B. (1999). Addressing complications of intention-to-treat analysis in the combined presence of all-or-none treatment-noncompliance and subsequent missing outcomes. *Biometrika, 86,* 365-379.

Frangakis, C.E., and Rubin, D.B. (2002). Principal stratification in causal inference. *Biometrics, 58,* 21-29.

Franklin, C., Grant, D., Corcoran, J., Miller, P.O., and Bultman, L. (1997). Effectiveness of prevention programs for adolescent pregnancy: A meta-analysis. *Journal of Marriage and the Family, 59,* 551-567.

Freeman, M.P., Hibbeln, J.R., Wisner, K.L., Davis, J.M., Mischoulon, D., Peet, M., Keck, Jr., P.E., Marangell, L.B., Richardson, A.J., Lake, J., and Stoll, A.L. (2006). Omega-3 fatty acids: Evidence basis for treatment and future research in psychiatry. *Journal of Clinical Psychiatry, 67*(12), 1954-1967.

Friedman, L.M., Furberg, C.D., and DeMets, D.L. (1998). *Fundamentals of Clinical Trials* (3rd ed.). St. Louis, MO: Mosby-Year Book.

Fruntes, V., and Limosin, F. (2008). Schizophrenia and viral infection during neurodevelopment: A pathogenesis model? *Medical Science Monitor, 14*(6), RA71-RA77.

Fruzzetti, A.E., Shenk, C., and Hoffman, P.D. (2005). Family interaction and the development of borderline personality disorder: A transactional model. *Development and Psychopathology, 17*(4), 1007-1030.

Fullilove, M.T., and Fullilove III, R.E. (1993). Understanding sexual behaviors and drug use among African Americans: A case study of issues for survey research. In D.G. Ostrow and R.C. Kessler (Eds.), *Methodological Issues in AIDS Behavioral Research* (pp. 117-132). New York: Plenum Press.

Fullilove, R.E., Green, L., and Fullilove, M.T. (2000). The family to family program: A structural intervention with implications for the prevention of HIV/AIDS and other community epidemics. *AIDS, 14*(Suppl. 1), S63-S67.

Furstenberg, F.F., and Teitler, J.O. (1994). Reconsidering the effects of marital disruption: What happens to children of divorce in early adulthood? *Journal of Family Issues, 15*(2), 173-190.

Furstenberg, F.F., Jr., Kennedy, S., McCloyd, V.C., Rumbaut, R.G., and Settersten, R.A., Jr. (2003). *Between Adolescence and Adulthood: Expectations About the Timing of Adulthood.* Available: http://www.transad.pop.upenn.edu/downloads/between.pdf [accessed August 2008].

Gafni, A. (1997). Willingness-to-pay (WTP) in the context of an economic evaluation of health-care programs: Theory and practice. *The American Journal of Managed Care, 3,* 521-532.

Galbraith, J., Ricardo, I., Stanton, B., Black, M., Feigelman, S., and Kaljee, L. (1996). Challenges and rewards of involving community in research: An overview of the "Focus on Kids" HIV risk reduction program. *Health Education Quarterly, 23,* 383-394.

Gao, Y., Yan, C.H., Tian, Y., Wang, Y., Xie, H.F., Zhou, X., Yu, X.D., Yu, X.G., Tong, S., Zhou, Q.X., and Shen, X.M. (2007). Prenatal exposure to mercury and neurobehavioral development of neonates in Zhoushan City, China. *Environmental Research, 105*(3), 390-399.

Garber, J. (2006). Depression in children and adolescents: Linking risk research and prevention. *American Journal of Prevention Medicine, 31*(6, Suppl. 1), S104-S125.

Garber, J., and Flynn, C. (2001). Vulnerability to depression in childhood and adolescence. In R.E. Ingram and J.M. Price (Eds.), *Vulnerability to Psychopathology: Risk Across the Lifespan* (pp. 175-225). New York: Guilford Press.

Garber, J., Clarke, G.N., Brent, D.A., Beardslee, W.R., Weersing, R., Gladstone, T.R.G., Debar, L., D'Angelo, E.J., and Hollon, S. (2007). *Preventing Depression in At-Risk Adolescents: Rationale, Design, and Preliminary Results.* Paper presented at Symposium 48, AACAP 54th Annual Meeting, Boston, MA.

Garber, J., Clarke, G.N., Weersing, V.R., Beardslee, W.R., Brent, D.A., Gladstone, T.R.G., DeBar, L.L., Lynch, F.L., D'Angelo, E., Hollon, S.D., Shamseddeen, W., and Iyengar, S. (in press). Prevention of depression in at-risk adolescents: A randomized controlled trial. Submitted to *Journal of the American Medical Association.*

Gardner, F., Burton, J., and Klimes, I. (2006). Randomised controlled trial of a parenting intervention in the voluntary sector for reducing child conduct problems: Outcomes and mechanisms of change. *Journal of Child Psychology and Psychiatry, 47,* 1123-1132.

Gates, S., McCambridge, J., Smith, L.A., and Foxcroft, D.R. (2006). Interventions for prevention of drug use by young people delivered in non-school settings. *Cochrane Database of Systematic Reviews, 1,* Art. No. CD005030.

Gaviria, A., and Raphael, S. (2001). School-based peer effects and juvenile behavior. *The Review of Economics and Statistics, 83*(2), 257-268.

Gaynes, B.N., Gavin, N., Meltzer-Brody, S., Lohr, K.N., Swinson, T., Gartlehner, G., Brody, S., and Miller, W.C. (2005). *Perinatal Depression: Prevalence, Screening Accuracy, and Screening Outcomes.* (Evidence Report/Technology Assessment No. 119, AHRQ Pub. No. 05-E006-2.) Rockville, MD: Agency for Healthcare Research and Quality. Available: http://www.ncbi.nlm.nih.gov/books/bv.fcgi?rid=hstat1a.chapter.86039 [accessed March 2009].

Geddes, J.R., and Lawrie, S.M. (1995). Obstetric complications and schizophrenia: A meta-analysis. *British Journal of Psychiatry, 167,* 786-793.

Geeraert, L., Noortgate, W.V.D., Grietens, H., and Onghena, P. (2004). The effects of early prevention programs for families with young children at risk for physical child abuse and neglect: A meta-analysis. *Child Maltreatment, 9*(3), 277-291.

Gega, L., Marks, I., and Mataix-Cols, D. (2004). Computer-aided CBT self-help for anxiety and depressive disorders: Experience of a London clinic and future directions. *Journal of Clinical Psychology, 60*(2), 147-167.

Gendry Meresse, I., Zilbovicius, M., Boddaert, N., Robel, L., Philippe, A., Sfaello, I., Laurier, L., Brunelle, F., Samson, Y., Mouren, M., and Chabane, N. (2005). Autism severity and temporal lobe functional abnormalities. *Annals of Neurology, 58*(3), 466-469.

Geresten, J.C., Beals, J., and Kallgren, C.A. (1991). Epidemiology and preventive interventions: Parental death in childhood as a case example. *American Journal of Community Psychology, 19*, 481-500.

Gershoff, E. (2003). *Low Income and the Development of America's Kindergartners.* New York: National Center for Children in Poverty.

Gershoff, E.T., and Aber, J.L. (2006). Neighborhoods and schools: Contexts and consequences for the mental health and risk behaviors of children and youth. In L. Balter and C. Tamis-LeMonda (Eds.), *Child Psychology: A Handbook of Contemporary Issues* (2nd ed., pp. 611-645). New York: Psychology Press/Taylor & Francis.

Gershoff, E.T., Aber, J.L., and Raver, C.C. (2003). Child poverty in the U.S.: An evidence-based conceptual framework for programs and policies. In R.M. Lerner, F. Jacobs, and D. Wertleib (Eds.), *Handbook of Applied Developmental Science: Promoting Positive Child, Adolescent, and Family Development through Research, Policies, and Programs* (vol. 2, pp. 81-136). Thousand Oaks, CA: Sage.

Gershoff, E.T., Pedersen, S., Ware, A., and Aber, J.L. (2004). Violence exposure and parenting impacts on behavior problems and risk behaviors in multilevel neighborhood context. In E. Gershoff (Chair), *Advances in Measurement, Trajectory, and Multilevel Analyses of Violence Exposure and Adolescent Problem Behaviors and Achievement.* Paper presented at the biennial meeting of the Society for Research in Adolescence, Baltimore, MD.

Gersten, J.C., Beals, J., and Kallgren, C.A. (1991). Epidemiology and preventive interventions: Parental death in childhood as a case example. *American Journal of Community Psychology, 19*(4), 481-500.

Gervais, H., Belin, P., Boddaert, N., Leboyer, M., Coez, A., Sfaello, I., Barthélémy, C., Brunelle, F., Samson, Y., and Zilbovicius, M. (2004). Abnormal cortical voice processing in autism. *Nature Reviews Neuroscience, 7*(8), 801-802.

Ghashghaei, H.T., Lai, C., and Anton, E.S. (2007). Neuronal migration in the adult brain: Are we there yet? *Nature Reviews Neuroscience, 8*(2), 141-151.

Ghosh-Dastidar, B., Longshore, D.L., Ellickson, P.L., and McCaffrey, D.F. (2004). Modifying pro-drug risk factors in adolescents: Results from project ALERT. *Health Education and Behavior, 31*(3), 318-334.

Giacometti, E., Luikenhuis, S., Beard, C., and Jaenisch, R. (2007). Partial rescue of MeCP2 deficiency by postnatal activation of MeCP2. *Proceedings of the National Academy of Sciences, 104*(6), 1931-1936.

Giaconia, R.M., Reinherz, H.Z., Silverman, A.B., Pakiz, B., Frost, A.K., and Cohen, E. (1995). Traumas and posttraumatic stress disorder in a community population of older adolescents. *Journal of the American Academy of Child and Adolescent Psychiatry, 34*, 1369-1380.

Gibbons, R.D., Hedeker, D., Waternaux, C., and Davis, J.M. (1988). Random regression models: A comprehensive approach to the analysis of longitudinal psychiatric data. *Psychopharmacology Bulletin, 24*, 438-443.

Gibbons, R.D., Hur, K., Bhaumik, D.K., and Bell, C.C. (2007). Profiling of county-level foster care placements using random-effects Poisson regression models. *Health Services and Outcomes Research Methodology, 7*(3-4), 97-108.

Giedd, J.N., Blumenthal, J., Jeffries, N.O., Castellanos, F.X., Liu, H., Zijdenbos, A., Paus, T., Evans, A.C., and Rapoport, J.L. (1999). Brain development during childhood and adolescence: A longitudinal MRI study. *Nature Neuroscience, 2*, 861-863.

Gillham, J.E., Reivich, K.J., Jaycox, L.H., and Seligman, M.E.P. (1995). Prevention of depressive symptoms in schoolchildren: Two-year follow up. *Psychological Science, 6*(6), 343-351.

Gillham, J.E., Hamilton, J., Freres, D.R., Patton, K., and Gallop, R. (2006). Preventing depression among early adolescents in the primary care setting: A randomized controlled trial of the Penn resiliency program. *Journal of Abnormal Child Psychology, 34*(2), 203-219.

Gillham, J.E., Reivich, K.J., Freres, D.R., Lascher, M., Litzinger, S., Shatte, A., and Seligman, M.E.P. (2006). School-based prevention of depression and anxiety symptoms in early adolescence: A pilot of a parent intervention component. *School Psychology Quarterly, 21*(3), 323-348.

Gillham, J.E., Brunwasser, S.M., and Freres, D.R. (2007). Preventing depression in early adolescence: The Penn resiliency program. In J.R.Z. Abela and B.L. Hankin (Eds.), *Depression in Children and Adolescents: Causes, Treatment and Prevention* (pp. 309-332). New York: Guilford Press.

Gillham, J.E., Reivich, K.J., Freres, D.R., Chaplin, T.M., Shatte, A.J., Samuels, B., Elkon, A.G.L., Litzinger, S., Lascher, M., Gallop, R., and Seligman, M.E.P. (2007). School-based prevention of depressive symptoms: A randomized controlled study of the effectiveness and specificity of the Penn resiliency program. *Journal of Consulting and Clinical Psychology, 75*(1), 9-19.

Gilliam, W.S. (2005). *Pre-Kindergarteners Left Behind: Expulsion Rates in State Pre-Kindergarten Systems.* New Haven, CT: Yale University Child Study Center.

Gilliam, W.S., and Shahar, G. (2006). Pre-kindergarten expulsion and suspension: Rates and predictors in one state. *Infants and Young Children, 19*(3), 228-245.

Gilliam, W.S., and Zigler, E.F. (2001). A critical meta-analysis of all impact evaluations of state-funded preschool from 1977 to 1998: Implications for policy, service delivery, and program evaluation. *Early Childhood Research Quarterly, 15,* 441-473.

Gilman, S.E., Kawachi, I., Fitzmaurice, G.M., and Buka, S.L. (2002). Socioeconomic status in childhood and the lifetime risk of major depression. *International Journal of Epidemiology, 31,* 359-367.

Gilman, S.E., Kawachi, I., Fitzmaurice, M., and Buka, S.L. (2003). Socioeconomic status, family disruption, and residential stability in childhood: Relation to onset, recurrence, and remission of major depression. *Psychological Medicine, 33,* 1341-1355.

Gladstone, T.R.G., and Beardslee, W.R. (in press). The prevention of depression in children and adolescents: A review. Submitted to *Canadian Journal of Psychiatry.*

Glascoe, F.P. (2000). Early detection of developmental and behavioral problems. *Pediatrics in Review, 21,* 272-280.

Glasgow, R.E., Vogt, T.M., and Boles, S.M. (1999). Evaluating the public health impact of health promotion interventions: The RE-AIM framework. *American Journal of Public Health, 89,* 1322-1327.

Glasgow, R.E., Klesges, L.M., Dzewaltowski, D.A., Bull, S.S., and Estabrooks, P. (2004). The future of health behavior change research: What is needed to improve translation of research into health promotion practice? *Annals of Behavioral Medicine, 27*(1), 3-12.

Glied, S., and Cuellar, A. (2003). Trends and issues in child and adolescent mental health. *Health Affairs, 22*(5), 39-50.

Glied, S., and Pine, D.S. (2002). Consequences and correlates of adolescent depression. *Archives of Pediatrics and Adolescent Medicine, 156*(10), 1009-1014.

Gliner, J.A., and Morgan, G.A. (2000). *Research Methods in Applied Settings.* Mahwah, NJ: Lawrence Erlbaum.

Glisson, C. (2002). The organizational context of children's mental health services. *Clinical Child and Family Psychology Review, 5,* 233-253.

Glisson, C., and James, L.R. (2002). The cross-level effects of culture and climate in human service teams. *Journal of Organizational Behavior, 23,* 767-794.

Glisson, C., Dukes, D., and Green, P. (2006). The effects of the ARC organizational intervention on caseworker turnover, climate, and culture in children's service systems. *Child Abuse and Neglect, 30*(8), 855-880.

Glover, T., and Albers, C. (2007). Considerations for evaluating universal screening assessments. *Journal of School Psychology, 45*(2), 117-135.

Goark, C.J., and McCall, R.B. (1996). Building successful university–community human service agency collaborations. In C.D. Fisher, J.P. Murray, and I.E. Sigel (Eds.), *Applied Developmental Science: Graduate Training for Diverse Disciplines and Educational Settings* (pp. 28-49). Norwood, NJ: Ablex.

Gold, M., Russell, L., Siegel, J., and Weinstein, M. (Eds.). (1996). *Cost-Effectiveness in Health and Medicine.* London, England: Oxford University Press.

Goldman, D., Oroszi, G., and Ducci, F. (2005). The genetics of addictions: Uncovering the genes. *Nature Reviews Genetics, 6*(7), 521-532.

Goldman-Rakic, P. (1987). Circuitry of primate prefrontal cortex and regulation of behavior by representational memory. In V. Mountcastle, F. Plum, and S. Geiger (Eds.), *Handbook of Physiology: The Nervous System* (pp. 373-416). Bethesda, MD: American Physiological Society.

Goldscheider, F., and Goldscheider, C. (1993). Effects of childhood family structure on leaving and returning home. *Journal of Marriage and the Family, 60*(3), 745-756.

Goldstone, A.P. (2004). Prader-Willi syndrome: Advances in genetics, pathophysiology, and treatment. *Trends in Endocrinology and Metabolism, 15*(1), 12-20.

Golier, J.A., Yehuda, R., Bierer, L.M., Mitropoulou, V., New, A.S., Schmeidler, J., Silverman, J.M., and Siever, L.J. (2003). The relationship of borderline personality disorder to posttraumatic stress disorder and traumatic events. *American Journal of Psychiatry, 160*(11), 2018-2024.

Gomby, D.S. (1999). Home visiting: Recent program evaluations—analysis and recommendations. *The Future of Children, 9,* 4-26.

Gonzales, N., Cauce, A.M., Friedman, R., and Mason, C. (1996). Family, peer, and neighborhood influences on academic achievement among African American adolescents: One-year prospective effects. *American Journal of Community Psychology, 24,* 365-387.

Goodman, M., New, A., and Siever, L. (2004). Trauma, genes, and the neurobiology of personality disorders. *Annals of the New York Academy of Sciences, 1032,* 104-116.

Goodman, S.H., and Gotlib, I.H. (1999). Risk for psychopathology on the children of depressed parents: A developmental approach to the understanding of mechanisms. *Psychological Review, 106,* 458-490.

Goodyer, I.M., and Altham, P.M.E. (1991). Lifetime exit events and recent social and family adversities in anxious and depressed school-age children and adolescents—II. *Journal of Affective Disorders, 21*(4), 229-238.

Gordon, R. (1983). An operational classification of disease prevention. *Public Health Reports, 98,* 107-109.

Gorman-Smith, D., and Tolan, P. (1998). The role of exposure to community violence and developmental problems among inner-city youth. *Development and Psychopathology, 10*(1), 101-116.

Gormley, W.T., Gayer, T., and Phillips, D. (2005). The effects of universal pre-k on cognitive development. *Developmental Psychology, 41*(6), 872-884.

Gothelf, D. (2007). Preface. *Special Edition, Child and Adolescent Psychiatric Clinics of North America, 16,* xvii-xx.

Gottesman, I.I. (1991). *Schizophrenia Genesis: The Origins of Madness.* New York: H. Freeman.

Gottesman, I.I., and Gould, T.D. (2003). The endophenotype concept in psychiatry: Etymology and strategic intentions. *American Journal of Psychiatry, 160*(4), 636-645.

Gottfredson, D.C., and Gottfredson, G.D. (2002). Quality of school-based prevention programs: Results from a national survey. *Journal of Research on Crime and Delinquency, 39*(1), 3-35.

Gottfredson, D.C., and Wilson, D.B. (2003). Characteristics of effective school-based substance abuse prevention. *Prevention Science, 4*(1), 27-38.

Gottlieb, G., and Blair, C. (2004). How early experience matters in intellectual development in the case of poverty. *Prevention Science, 5*(4), 245-252.

Gould, E. (2007). How widespread is adult neurogenesis in mammals? *Nature Reviews Neuroscience, 8*(6), 481-488.

Gould, M., Jamieson, P., and Romer, D. (2003). Media contagion and suicide among the young. *American Behavioral Scientist, 46*(9), 1269-1284.

Graham, J.W. (2003). Adding missing-data relevant variables to FIML-based structural equation models. *Structural Equation Modeling, 10*(1), 80-100.

Graham, J.W., Cumsille, P.E., and Elek-Fisk, E. (2003). Methods for handling missing data. In J.A. Schinka and W.F. Velicer (Eds.), *Research Methods in Psychology* (vol. 2, pp. 87-114). Hoboken, NJ: Wiley.

Grant, B.F., and Dawson, D.F. (1997). Age of onset of alcohol use and its association with DSM IV alcohol abuse and dependence: Results from the national longitudinal alcohol epidemiologic survey. *Journal of Substance Abuse, 9*, 103-110.

Grant, K.E., Compas, B.E., Stuhlmacher, A.F., Thurm, A.E., McMahon, S.D., and Haplpert, J.A. (2003). Stressors and child and adolescent psychopathology: Moving from markers to mechanisms of risk. *Psychological Bulletin, 129*, 447-466.

Grant, K.E., Compas, B.E., Thurm, A.E., McMahon, S.D., Gipson, P.Y., and Campbell, A.J. (2006). Stressors and child and adolescent psychopathology: Evidence of moderating and mediating effects. *Clinical Psychology Reviews, 26*, 257-283.

Green, L.W. (2007). Translation 2 research: The road less traveled. *American Journal of Preventive Medicine, 33*, 137-138.

Greenberg, M.T. (2004). Current and future challenges in school-based prevention: The researcher perspective. *Prevention Science, 5*, 5-13.

Greenberg, M.T. (2006). Promoting resilience in children and youth: Preventive interventions and their interface with neuroscience. *Annals of the New York Academy of Sciences, 1094*, 139-150.

Greenberg, M.T., and Kusche, C.A. (1998). Preventive intervention for school-aged deaf children: The PATHS curriculum. *Journal of Deaf Studies and Deaf Education, 3*, 49-63.

Greenberg, M.T., and Weissberg, R. (2001). In the name of prevention: Commentary on "Priorities for prevention research at NIMH." *Prevention and Treatment, 4*, Art. 25.

Greenberg, M.T., Kusche, C.A., Cook, E.T., and Quamma, J.P. (1995). Promoting emotional competence in school-aged children: The effects of the PATHS curriculum. *Development and Psychopathology, 7*, 117-136.

Greenberg, M.T., Domitrovich, C.E., and Bumbarger, B. (2000). *Preventing Mental Disorders in School-aged Children: A Review of the Effectiveness of Prevention Programs* (revised). State College, PA: College of Health and Human Development, Pennsylvania State University.

Greenberg, M.T., Domitrovich, C.E., and Bumbarger, B. (2001). The prevention of mental disorders in school-aged children: Current state of the field. *Prevention and Treatment, 4*(1), 1-62.

Greenberg, M.T., Weissberg, R.P., O'Brien, M.U., Zins, J.E., Fredericks, L., Resnik, H., and Elias, M.J. (2003). Enhancing school-based prevention and youth development through coordinated social, emotional, and academic learning. *American Psychologist, 58*, 466-474.

Greenberg, M.T., Domitrovich, C.E., Graczyk, P.A., and Zins, J.E. (2006). *The Study of Implementation in School-based Prevention Research: Implications for Theory, Research, and Practice.* Rockville, MD: Center for Mental Health Services, Substance Abuse and Mental Health Services Administration.

Greenberg, M.T., Feinberg, M.E., Meyer-Chilenski, S., Spoth, R.L., and Redmond, C. (2007). Community and team member factors that influence the early phase functioning of community prevention teams: The PROSPER project. *Journal of Primary Prevention, 28,* 485-504.

Greenwald, P.E., and Cullen, J.W. (1985). The new emphasis in cancer control. *Journal of the National Cancer Institute, 74,* 543-551.

Greenwood, C.R. (1991a). Classwide peer tutoring: Longitudinal effects on the reading, language, and mathematics achievement of at-risk students. *Journal of Reading, Writing, and Learning Disabilities International, 7,* 105-123.

Greenwood, C.R. (1991b). Longitudinal analysis of time, engagement, and achievement in at-risk versus nonrisk students. *Exceptional Children, 57,* 521-535.

Gregory, A.M., and Eley, T.C. (2007). Genetic influences on anxiety in children: What we've learned and where we're heading. *Clinical Child and Family Psychology Review, 10,* 199-212.

Gregory, A.M., Caspi, A., Moffitt, T.E., Koenen, K., Eley, T.C., and Poulton, R. (2007). Juvenile mental health histories of adults with anxiety disorders. *American Journal of Psychiatry, 164*(2), 301-308.

Griffin, K.W., Scheier, L.M., Botvin, G.J., and Diaz, T. (2001). Protective role of personal competence skills in adolescent substance use: Psychological well-being as a mediating factor. *Psychology of Addictive Behaviors, 15*(3), 194-203.

Gross, D., Fogg, L., Webster-Stratton, C., Garvey, C., Julion, W., and Grady, J. (2003). Parent training of toddlers in day care in low-income urban communities. *Journal of Consulting and Clinical Psychology, 71,* 261-278.

Grossman, J.P., and Tierney, J.P. (1998). Does mentoring work?: An impact study of Big Brothers/Big Sisters. *Evaluation Review, 22,* 403-426.

Gruber, E., DiClemente, R.J., Anderson, M.M., and Lodico, M. (1996). Early drinking onset and its association with alcohol use and problem behavior in late adolescence. *Preventive Medicine, 25,* 293-300.

Grupp-Phelan, J., Wade, T.J., Pickup, T., Ho, M.L., Lucas, C.P., Brewer, D.E., and Kelleher, K.J. (2007). Mental health problems in children and caregivers in the emergency department setting. *Journal of Developmental and Behavioral Pediatrics, 28,* 16-21.

Grych, J.H., and Fincham, F.D. (1992). Interventions for children of divorce: Toward greater integration of research and action. *Psychological Bulletin, 111,* 434-454.

Guerrini, R., and Filippi, T. (2005). Neuronal migration disorders, genetics, and epileptogenesis. *Journal of Child Neurology, 20*(4), 287-299.

Guevara, J.P., Rothbard, A., Shera, D., Zhao, H., Forrest, C.B., Kelleher, K., and Schwarz, D. (2007). Correlates of behavioral care management strategies used by primary care pediatric providers. *Ambulatory Pediatrics, 7*(2), 160-166.

Gunnar, M.R. (2001). Effects of early deprivation: Findings from orphanage-reared infants and children. In C.A. Nelson and M. Luciana (Eds.), *Handbook of Developmental Cognitive Neuroscience* (pp. 617-629). Cambridge: Massachusetts Institute of Technology.

Gunnar, M.R., Morison, S.J., Chisholm, K., and Schuder, M. (2001). Salivary cortisol levels in children adopted from Romanian orphanages. *Development and Psychopathology, 13*(3), 611-628.

Gupta, R., Stringer, B., and Meakin, A. (1990). A study to access the effectiveness of home-based reinforcement in a secondary school: Some preliminary findings. *Association of Educational Psychologists Journal, 5,* 197.

Gutman, L.M., and Sameroff, A.J. (2004). Continuities in depression from adolescence to young adulthood: Contrasting ecological influences. *Development and Psychopathology, 16,* 967-984.

Gutman, L.M., McLoyd, V.C., and Tokoyawa, T. (2005). Financial strain, neighborhood stress, parenting behaviors, and adolescent adjustment in urban African American families. *Journal of Research on Adolescence, 15,* 425-449.

Guy, J., Gan, J., Selfridge, J., Cobb, S., and Bird, A. (2007). Reversal of neurological defects in a mouse model of Rett syndrome. *Science, 315*(5815), 1143-1147.

Haack, M.R., and Adger, H. (Eds.). (2002). *Strategic Plan for Interdisciplinary Faculty Development: Arming the Nation's Health Professional Workforce for a New Approach to Substance Use Disorders.* Dordrecht, the Netherlands: Kluwer Academic/Plenum.

Haas, G.L., Garratt, L.S., and Sweeney, J.A. (1998). Delay to first antipsychotic medication in schizophrenia: Impact on symptomatology and clinical course of illness. *Journal of Psychiatric Research, 32*(3-4), 151-159.

Hahn, R., Fuqua-Whitley, D., Wethington, H., Lowy, J., Crosby, A., Fullilove, M., Johnson, R., Liberman, A., Moscicki, E., Price, L., Snyder, S., Tuma, F., Cory, S., Stone, G., Mukhopadhaya, K., Chattopadhyay, S., and Dahlberg, L. (2007). Effectiveness of universal school-based programs to prevent violent and aggressive behavior: A systematic review. *American Journal of Preventive Medicine, 33,* S114-S129.

Haine, R.A., Sandler, I.N., Wolchik, S.A., Tein, J.-Y., and Dawson-McClure, S.R. (2003). Changing the legacy of divorce: Evidence from prevention programs and future directions. *Family Relations, 52,* 397-405.

Hall, G., and Hord, S. (2001). *Implementing Change: Patterns, Principles, and Potholes.* Needham Heights, MA: Allyn and Bacon.

Hallfors, D., and Godette, D. (2002). Will the "principles of effectiveness" improve prevention practice? Early findings from a diffusion study. *Health Education Research, 17*(4), 461-470.

Hallfors, D., Pankratz, M., and Hartman, S. (2007). Does federal policy support the use of scientific evidence in school-based prevention programs? *Prevention Science, 8,* 75-81.

Hammen, C., and Brennan, P.A. (2003). Severity, chronicity, and timing of maternal depression and risk for adolescent offspring diagnoses as a community sample. *Archives of General Psychiatry, 60,* 253-258.

Hammen, C., and Rudolph, K.D. (2003). Child mood disorders. In E.J. Mash and R.A. Barkley (Eds.), *Child Psychopathology* (2nd ed., pp. 233-278). New York: Guilford Press.

Hammitt, J. (2002). QALYs versus WTP. *Risk Analysis, 22*(5), 985-1001.

Harachi, T.W., Fleming, C.B., White, H.R., Ensminger, M.E., Abbott, R.D., Catalano, R.F., and Haggerty, K.P. (2006). Aggressive behavior among girls and boys during middle childhood: Predictors and sequelae of trajectory group membership. *Aggressive Behavior, 32,* 279-293.

Harman, J.S., Childs, G.E., and Kelleher, K.J. (2000). Mental health care utilization and expenditures by children in foster care. *Archives of Pediatrics and Adolescent Medicine, 154*(11), 1114-1117.

Harris, B., Huckle, P., Thomas, R., Johns, S., and Fund, H. (1989). The use of rating scales to identify post-natal depression. *British Journal of Psychiatry, 154,* 813-817.

Harwood, H. (2000). *Updating Estimates of the Economic Costs of Alcohol Abuse in the United States: Estimates, Updated Methods, and Data.* Report prepared for the National Institute on Drug Abuse and the National Institute on Alcohol Abuse and Alcoholism, National Institutes of Health, NIH Pub. No. 98-4327. Rockville, MD: National Institutes of Health.

Harwood, H., Ameen, A., Denmead, G., Englert, E., Fountain, D., and Livermore, G. (2000). *The Economic Costs of Mental Illness, 1992.* Rockville, MD: National Institutes of Health.

Haskins, R., Wulczyn, F., and Webb, M.B., (Eds.). (2007). *Child Protection: Using Research to Improve Policy and Practice.* Washington, DC: Brookings Institution Press.

Hatch, J., Moss, N., Saran, A., Presley-Cantrell, L., and Mallory, C. (1993). Community research: Partnership in black communities. *American Journal of Preventive Medicine, 9*(Suppl. 6), 27-31.

Hatten, M.E. (1993). The role of migration in central nervous system neuronal development. *Current Opinion in Neurobiology, 3*(1), 38-44.

Hawkins, J.D. (2006). Science, social work, prevention: Finding the intersections. *Social Work Research, 30,* 137-152.

Hawkins, J.D., and Catalano, R.F., Jr. (1992). *Communities That Care.* San Francisco, CA: Jossey-Bass.

Hawkins, J.D., Catalano, R.F., and Miller, J.Y. (1992). Risk and protective factors for alcohol and other drug problems in adolescence and early adulthood: Implications for substance abuse prevention. *Psychological Bulletin, 112,* 64-105.

Hawkins, J.D., Kosterman, R., Catalano, R.F., Hill, K.G., and Abbott, R.D. (2005). Promoting positive adult functioning through social development intervention in childhood: Long-term effects from the Seattle social development project. *Archives of Pediatrics and Adolescent Medicine, 159,* 25-31.

Hawkins, J.D., Brown, E.C., Oesterle, S., Arthur, M.W., Abbott, R.D., and Catalano, R.F. (2008). Early effects of Communities That Care on targeted risks and initiation of delinquent behavior and substance use. *Journal of Adolescent Health, 43,* 15-22.

Hawkins, J.D., Kosterman, R., Catalano, R.F., Hill, K.G., and Abbott, R.D. (2008). Effects of social development intervention in childhood 15 years later. *Archives of Pediatric and Adolescent Medicine, 162,* 1133-1141.

Hawkins, J.D., Oesterle, S., Brown, E.C., Arthur, M.W., Abbott, R.D., Fagan, A.A., and Catalano, R.F. (in press). Results of a type 2 translational research trial to prevent adolescent drug use and delinquency: A test of Communities That Care. Submitted to *Archives of Pediatric and Adolescent Medicine.*

Hayes, S.C. (2004). Acceptance and commitment therapy, relational frame theory, and the third wave of behavioral and cognitive therapies. *Behavior Therapy, 35,* 639-665.

Hayes, S.C., Luoma, J.B., Bond, F.W., Masuda, A., and Lillis, J. (2006). Acceptance and commitment therapy: Model, processes, and outcomes. *Behaviour Research and Therapy, 44,* 1-25.

Head Start Quality Research Consortium. (2003). *Head Start FACES: A Whole-Child Perspective on Program Performance.* Washington, DC: U.S. Department of Health and Human Services.

Heckman, J.J. (1999). *Policies to Foster Human Development.* Working paper 7288. Cambridge, MA: National Bureau of Economic Research.

Heckman, J.J. (2007). Economics of health and mortality special feature: The economics, technology, and neuroscience of human capability formation. *Proceedings of the National Academy of Sciences, 104*(33), 13250.

Heiervang, E.M., Stormark, K., Lundervold, A.J., Heimann, M., Goodman, R., Posserud, M., Ullebo, A.K., Plessen, K., Bjelland, I., Lie, S., and Gillberg, C. (2007). Psychiatric disorders in Norwegian 8- to 10-year-olds: An epidemiological survey of prevalence, risk factors, and service use. *Journal of the American Academy of Child and Adolescent Psychiatry, 46,* 438-447.

Heiervang, E., Goodman, A., and Goodman, R. (2008). The Nordic advantage in child mental health: Separating health differences from reporting style in a cross-cultural comparison of psychopathology. *Journal of Child Psychology and Psychiatry, 49,* 678-685.

Heller, K. (2001). Prevention research priorities: Forward movement and backward steps in the NAMHC workgroup recommendations. *Prevention and Treatment, 4*(1), Art. ID 22c.

Henggeler, S.W., Brondino, M.J., Melton, G.B., Scherer, D.G., and Hanley, J.H. (1997). Multisystemic therapy with violent and chronic juvenile offenders and their families: The role of treatment fidelity in successful dissemination. *Journal of Consulting and Clinical Psychology, 65*(5), 821-833.

Henggeler, S.W., Clingempeel, W.G., Brondino, M.J., and Pickrel, S. (2002). Four-year follow up of multisystemic therapy with substance-abusing and substance-dependent juvenile offenders. *Journal of the American Academy of Child and Adolescent Psychiatry, 41*(7), 868-874.

Henry J. Kaiser Family Foundation. (2007). *State Coverage Initiatives for Children.* The Kaiser Commission on Medicaid and the Uninsured. Available: http://www.kff.org/uninsured/kcmu051607oth.cfm [accessed August 2008].

Herrmann, M., King, K., and Weitzman, M. (2008). Prenatal tobacco smoke and postnatal secondhand smoke exposure and child neurodevelopment. *Current Opinion in Pediatrics, 20*(2), 184-190.

Hetherington, E.M. (1999). Should we stay together for the sake of the children? In E.M. Hetherington (Ed.), *Coping with Divorce, Single Parenting, and Remarriage: A Risk and Resiliency Perspective* (pp. 93-116). Mahwah, NJ: Lawrence Erlbaum.

Hibbeln, J. (2002). Seafood consumption, the DHA content of mother's milk, and the prevalence of postpartum depression: A cross-national, ecological analysis. *Journal of Affective Disorders, 69*(1-3), 15-29.

Hibbeln, J., Davis, J., Steer, C., Emmett, P., Rogers, I., Williams, C., and Golding, J. (2007). Maternal seafood consumption in pregnancy and neurodevelopmental outcomes in childhood (ALSPAC study): An observational cohort study. *The Lancet, 369*, 578-585.

Hihara, S., Notoya, T., Tanaka, M., Ichinose, S., Ojima, H., Obayashi, S., Fujii, N., and Iriki, A. (2006). Extension of corticocortical afferents into the anterior bank of the intraparietal sulcus by tool-use training in adult monkeys. *Neuropsychologia, 44*(13), 2636-2646.

Hill, M.K., and Sahhar, M. (2006). Genetic counselling for psychiatric disorders. *Medical Journal of Australia, 185*(9), 507-510.

Hines, M. (2003). Sex steroids and human behavior: Prenatal androgen exposure and sex-typical play behavior in children. *Annals of the New York Academy of Sciences, 1007*, 272-282.

Hingson, R., McGovern, T., Howland, J., and Heeren, T. (1996). Reducing alcohol-impaired driving in Massachusetts: The saving lives program. *American Journal of Public Health, 86*, 791-797.

Hinshaw, S.P. (1992). Externalizing behavior problems and academic underachievement in childhood and adolescence: Causal relationships and underlying mechanisms. *Psychological Bulletin, 111*(1), 127-155.

Hirano, K., Imbens, G.W., Rubin, D.B., and Zhou, X. (2000). Assessing the effect of an influenza vaccine in an encouragement design. *Biostatistics, 1*, 69-88.

Hirayama, S., Hamazaki, T., and Terasawa, K. (2004). Effect of docosahexaenoic acid-containing food administration on symptoms of attention-deficit/hyperactivity disorder: A placebo-controlled double-blind study. *European Journal of Clinical Nutrition, 58*, 467-473.

Hirth, R.A., Chernew, M.E., Miller, E., Fendrick, A.M., and Weissert, W.G. (2000). Willingness to pay for a quality-adjusted life year: In search of a standard. *Medical Decision Making, 20*(3), 332-342.

Hoagwood, K.E., and Koretz, D. (1996). Embedding prevention services within systems of care: Strengthening the nexus for children. *Applied and Preventive Psychology, 5*, 225-234.

Hoagwood, K.E., and Olin, S. (2002). The NIMH blueprint for change report: Research priorities in child and adolescent mental health. *Journal of American Academy of Child and Adolescent Psychiatry, 41*(7), 760-767.

Hoagwood, K.E., Burns, B.J., Kiser, L., Ringeisen, H., and Schoenwald, S.K. (2001). Evidence-based practice in child and adolescent mental health services. *Psychiatric Services, 52*(9), 1179-1189.

Hoagwood, K.E., Olin, S.S., Kerker, B.D., Kratochwill, T.R., Crowe, M., and Saka, N. (2007). Empirically based school interventions target at academic and mental health functioning. *Journal of Emotional and Behavioral Disorders, 15*, 66-94.

Hoath, F.E., and Sanders, M.R. (2002). A feasibility study of enhanced group Triple P-Positive Parenting Program for parents of children with attention-deficit/hyperactivity disorder. *Behaviour Change, 19*, 191-206.

Hofer, M.A. (1994). Hidden regulators in attachment, separation, and loss. *Monographs of the Society for Research in Child Development, 59*(2-3), 192-207.

Hofer, M.A. (1996). On the nature and consequences of early loss. *Psychosom Medicine, 58*(6), 570-581.

Hoffman, J.P., and Johnson, R.A. (1998). A national portrait of family structure and adolescent drug use. *Journal of Marriage and the Family, 60*(3), 633-645.

Holder, H.D., Saltz, R.F., Grube, J.W., Voas, R.B., Gruenewald, P.J., and Treno, A.J. (1997). A community prevention trial to reduce alcohol-involved accidental injury and death: Overview. *Addiction, 92*(Suppl. 2), 155-171.

Holland, P.C., and Gallagher, M. (1999). Amygdala circuitry in attentional and representational processes. *Trends in Cognitive Science, 3*(2), 65-73.

Holland, P.W. (1986). Statistics and causal inference. *Journal of the American Statistical Association, 81*, 945-960.

Hollon, S.D., Muñoz, R.F., Barlow, D.H., Beardslee, W.R., Bell, C.C., Bernal, G., Clarke, G.N., Franciosi, L.P., Kazdin, A.E., Kohn, L., Linehan, M.M., Markowitz, J.C., Miklowitz, D.J., Persons, J.B., Niederehe, G., and Sommers, D. (2002). Psychosocial intervention development for the prevention and treatment of depression: Promoting innovation and increasing access. *Biological Psychiatry, 52*, 610-630.

Horowitz, J.L., and Garber, J. (2006). The prevention of depressive symptoms in children and adolescents: A meta-analytic review. *Journal of Consulting and Clinical Psychology, 74*(3), 401-415.

Horowitz, S., Leaf, P., Leventhal, J., Forsyth, B., and Speechley, K. (1992). Identification and management of psychosocial and developmental problems in community-based, primary care pediatric practices. *Pediatrics, 89*(3), 480-485.

Hosman, C., Jané-Llopis, E., and Saxena, S. (Eds.). (2005). *Prevention of Mental Disorders: Effective Interventions and Policy Options.* Geneva, Switzerland: World Health Organization.

Howe, G.W., Reiss, D., and Yuh, J. (2002). Can prevention trials test theories of etiology? *Development and Psychopathology, 14*, 673-694.

Howe, G.W., Dagne, G., and Brown, C.H. (2005). Multilevel methods for modeling observed sequences of family interaction. *Journal of Family Process, 19*, 72-85.

Hu, T. (2006). An international review of the national cost estimates of mental illness, 1990-2003. *Journal of Mental Health Policy and Economics, 9*(1), 3-13.

Hudson, J.L., and Rapee, R.M. (2001). Parent-child interactions and anxiety disorders: An observational study. *Behaviour Research and Therapy, 39*, 1411-1427.

Hudson, J.L., Flannery-Schroeder, E., and Kendall, P.C. (2004). Primary prevention of anxiety disorders. In J.A. Dozois and K.S. Dobson (Eds.), *The Prevention of Anxiety and Depression: Theory, Research, and Practice* (pp. 101-130). Washington, DC: American Psychological Association.

Huesmann, L.R., Moise-Titus, J., Podolski, C.L., and Eron, L.D. (2003). Longitudinal relations between childhood exposure to TV violence and their aggressive and violent behavior in young adulthood: 1977-1992. *Developmental Psychology, 39*, 201-221.

Huisman, T.A., Martin, E., Kubik-Huch, R., and Marincek, B. (2002). Fetal magnetic resonance imaging of the brain: Technical considerations and normal brain development. *European Journal of Radiology, 12*(8), 1941-1951.

Hussey, J., Chang, J.J., and Kotch, J.B. (2006). Child maltreatment in the United States: Prevalence, risk factors, and adolescent health consequences. *Pediatrics, 118*(3), 933-942.

Huston, A.C., Duncan, G.J., McLoyd, V.C., Crosby, D.A., Ripke, M.N., Weisner, T.S., and Eldred, C.A. (2005). Impacts on children of a policy to promote employment and reduce poverty for low-income parents: New hope after five years. *Developmental Psychology, 41*(6), 902-918.

Hutchings, J., Bywater, T., Daley, D., Gardner, F., Whitaker, C., Jones, K., Eames, C., and Edwards, R.T. (2007). Parenting intervention in sure start services for children at risk of developing conduct disorder: Pragmatic randomised controlled trial. *British Medical Journal, 334*, 678-684.

Hutchinson, M.K., and Cooney, T.M. (1998). Patterns of parent-teen sexual risk communication: Implications for intervention. *Family Relations, 47*(2), 185-194.

Huttenlocher, P.R. (1984). Synapse elimination and plasticity in developing human cerebral cortex. *American Journal of Mental Deficiency, 88*(5), 488-496.

Huttenlocher, P.R. (1990). Morphometric study of human cerebral cortex development. *Neuropsychologia, 28*(6), 517-527.

Huttenlocher, P.R., and Dabholkar, A.S. (1997). Regional differences in synaptogenesis in human cerebral cortex. *Journal of Comparative Neurology, 387*(2), 167-178.

Hutton, J.B. (1983). How to decrease problem behavior at school by rewarding desirable behavior at home. *Pointer, 27,* 25.

Hwang, M.S., Yeagley, K.L., and Petosa, R. (2004). A meta-analysis of adolescent psychosocial smoking prevention programs published between 1978 and 1997 in the United States. *Health Education and Behavior, 31*(6), 702-719.

Iacoboni, M., and Dapretto, M. (2006). The mirror neuron system and the consequences of its dysfunction. *Nature Reviews Neuroscience, 7*(12), 942-951.

Ialongo, N.S., Werthamer, L., Kellam, S.G., Brown, C.H., Wang, S., and Lin, Y. (1999). Proximal impact of two first-grade preventive interventions on the early risk behaviors for later substance abuse, depression, and antisocial behavior. *American Journal of Community Psychology, 27*(5), 599-641.

Ialongo, N.S., Rogosch, F.A., Cichetti, S.L., Buckley, J., Petras, H., and Neiderhiser, J. (2006). A developmental psychopathology approach to the prevention of mental health disorders. In D. Cicchetti and D.J. Cohen (Eds.), *Developmental Psychopathology: Theory and Method* (pp. 968-1018). New York: Wiley.

Innis, S.M. (2008). Dietary omega-3 fatty acids and the developing brain. *Brain Research, 1237,* 35-43.

Innocenti, G.M. (1981). Growth and reshaping of axons in the establishment of visual callosal connections. *Science, 212*(4496), 824-827.

Inoue, K., and Lupski, J.R. (2003). Genetics and genomics of behavioral and psychiatric disorders. *Current Opinion in Genetics and Development, 13*(3), 303-309.

Insel, T.R. (2008). From prevention to preemption: A paradigm shift in psychiatry. *Psychiatric Times, 25*(9). Available: http://www.psychiatrictimes.com/display/article/10168/1171240 [accessed March 2009].

Insel, T.R., and Young, L.J. (2001). The neurobiology of attachment. *Nature Reviews Neuroscience, 2*(2), 129-136.

Institute for the Advancement of Social Work Research. (n.d.). *NIMH Funded Social Work Research Development Center: 1993 through 2005*. Available: http://www.charityadvantage. com/iaswr/NIMH%20Funded%20Centers%201993-2005.doc [accessed August 2008].

Institute for the Advancement of Social Work Research. (2007). *Partnerships to Integrate Evidence-Based Mental Health Practices into Social Work Education and Research*. Report from symposium sponsored by the National Institute of Mental Health, April 12, Washington, DC: Author. Available: http://www.charityadvantage.com/iaswr/ EvidenceBasedPracticeFinal.pdf [accessed August 2008].

Institute of Medicine. (1994). *Reducing Risks for Mental Disorders: Frontiers for Preventive Intervention Research*. P.J. Mrazek and R.J. Haggerty (Eds.), Committee on Prevention of Mental Disorders, Division of Biobehavorial Sciences and Mental Disorders. Washington, DC: National Academy Press.

Institute of Medicine. (1998). *Bridging the Gap Between Practice and Research: Forging Partnerships with Community-based Drug and Alcohol Treatment*. S. Lamb, M.R. Greenlick, and D. McCarty (Eds.), Committee on Community-Based Drug Treatment, Division of Neuroscience and Behavioral Health. Washington, DC: National Academy Press.

Institute of Medicine. (2001) *Crossing the Quality Chasm: A New Health System for the 21st Century*. Committee on Quality of Health Care in America. Washington, DC: National Academy Press.

Institute of Medicine. (2002). *Reducing Suicide: A National Imperative*. S.K. Goldsmith, T.C. Pellman, A.M. Kleinman, and W.E. Bunney (Eds.), Committee on Pathophysiology and Prevention of Adolescent and Adult Suicide. Washington, DC: National Academy Press.

Institute of Medicine. (2004). *Improving Medical Education: Enhancing the Behavioral and Social Science Content of Medical School Curricula*. P.A. Cuff and N.A. Vanselow (Eds.), Committee on Behavioral and Social Sciences in Medical School Curricula, Board on Neuroscience and Behavioral Health. Washington, DC: The National Academies Press.

Institute of Medicine. (2006a). *Genes, Behavior, and the Social Environment: Moving Beyond the Nature/Nurture Debate*. L.M. Hernandez and D.G. Blazer (Eds.), Committee on Assessing Interactions Among Social, Behavioral, and Genetic Factors in Health, Board on Health Sciences Policy. Washington, DC: The National Academies Press.

Institute of Medicine. (2006b). *Improving the Quality of Health Care for Mental and Substance-Use Conditions: Quality Chasm Series*. Committee on Crossing the Quality Chasm: Adaptation to Mental Health and Addictive Disorders, Board on Health Care Services. Washington, DC: The National Academies Press.

Institute of Medicine. (2006c). *Sleep Disorders and Sleep Deprivation: An Unmet Public Health Problem*. H.R. Colten and B.M. Altevogt (Eds.), Committee on Sleep Medicine and Research, Board on Health Sciences Policy. Washington, DC: The National Academies Press.

Institute of Medicine. (2007a). *Advancing Quality Improvement Research: Challenges and Opportunities, Workshop Summary*. S. Chao (Rapporteur), Forum on the Science of Health Care Quality Improvement and Implementation, Board on Health Care Services. Washington, DC: The National Academies Press.

Institute of Medicine. (2007b). *Ending the Tobacco Problem: A Blueprint for the Nation*. R.J. Bonnie, K. Stratton, and R.B. Wallace (Eds.), Committee on Reducing Tobacco Use: Strategies, Barriers, and Consequences, Board on Population Health and Public Health Practice. Washington, DC: The National Academies Press.

Institute of Medicine. (2007c). *Preterm Birth: Cause, Consequences, and Prevention*. Committee on Understanding Premature Birth and Assuring Healthy Outcomes, Board on Health Sciences Policy. Washington, DC: The National Academies Press.

Institute of Medicine. (2007d). *The State of Quality Improvement and Implementation Research: Expert Views, Workshop Summary.* S. Chao (Rapporteur), Forum on the Science of Health Care Quality Improvement and Implementation, Board on Health Care Services. Washington, DC: The National Academies Press.

International Schizophrenia Consortium. (2008). Rare chromosomal deletions and duplications increase risk of schizophrenia. *Nature, 455*(7210), 237-241.

Ireland, J.L., Sanders, M.R., and Markie-Dadds, C. (2003). The impact of parent training on marital functioning: A comparison of two group versions of the Triple P-Positive Parenting Program for parents of children with early-onset conduct problems. *Behavioural and Cognitive Psychotherapy, 31,* 127-142.

Iriki, A. (2006). The neural origins and implications of imitation, mirror neurons, and tool use. *Current Opinion in Neurobiology, 16*(6), 660-667.

Irvine, A.B., Biglan, A., Smolkowski, K., Metzler, C.W., and Ary, D.V. (1999). The effectiveness of a parenting skills program for parents in middle school students in small communities. *Journal of Consulting and Clinical Psychology, 67*(6), 811-825.

Isaacson, J.H., Fleming, M., Kraus, M., Kahn, R., and Mundt, M. (2000). A national survey of training in substance use disorders in residency programs. *Journal of Studies on Alcohol and Drugs, 61,* 912-915.

Isohanni, M., Moilanen, I., and Rantakallio, P. (1991). Determinants of teenage smoking, with special reference to nonstandard family background. *British Journal of Addiction, 86,* 391-398.

Israel, B.A., Schulz, A.J., Parker, E.A., and Becker, A.B. (1998). Review of community-based research: Assessing partnership approaches to improve public health. *Annual Review of Public Health, 19,* 173-202.

Israel, B.A., Schulz, A.J., Parker, E.A., Becker, A.B., Allen, A.J., and Guzman, J.R. (2003). Critical issues in developing, following community-based participatory research principles. In M. Minkler and N. Wallerstein (Eds.), *Community-based Participatory Research for Health* (pp. 53-76). San Francisco, CA: Jossey-Bass.

Itomura, M., Hamazaki, K., Sawazaki, S., Kobayashi, M., Terasawa, K., Watanabe, S., and Hamazaki, T. (2005). The effect of fish oil on physical aggression in school children: A randomized, double-blind, placebo-controlled trial. *Journal of Nutritional Biochemistry, 16,* 163-171.

Jaccard, J., Dittus, P.J., and Gordon, V.V. (1998). Parent-adolescent congruency in reports of adolescents' sexual behavior and in communication about sexual behavior. *Child Development, 69*(1), 247-261.

Jacobsen, T. (1999). Effects of postpartum disorders on parenting and on offspring. In L.J. Miller (Ed.), *Postpartum Mood Disorders* (pp. 119-139). Washington, DC: American Psychiatric Press.

Jaffee, S.R., and Price, T.S. (2007). Gene-environment correlations: A review of the evidence and implications for prevention of mental illness. *Molecular Psychiatry, 12*(5), 432-442.

Jaffee, S.R., Harrington, H., Cohen, P., and Moffitt, T.E. (2005). Cumulative prevalence of psychiatric disorder in youths. *Journal of the American Academy of Child and Adolescent Psychiatry, 44*(5), 406-407.

Jané-Llopis, E., and Anderson, P. (2005). *Mental Health Promotion and Mental Disorder Prevention. A Policy for Europe.* Nijmegen, the Netherlands: Radboud University Nijmegen.

Jané-Llopis, E., and Anderson, P. (Eds.). (2006). *Mental Health Promotion and Mental Disorder Prevention Across European Member States: A Collection of Country Stories.* Luxembourg: European Communities.

Jané-Llopis, E., and McDaid, D. (2005). Promoting mental health in Europe: A timely oppor-tunity. *Eurohealth, 11*(4), 9-10.

Jané-Llopis, E., Hosman, C., Jenkins, R., and Anderson, P. (2003). Predictors of efficacy in depression prevention programmes: Meta-analysis. *British Journal of Psychiatry, 183,* 384-397.

Jaycox, L.H., Reivich, K.J., Gillham, J., and Seligman, M.E.P. (1994). Prevention of depressive symptoms in school children. *Behaviour Research and Therapy, 3*(8), 801-816.

Jemmott, J.B., Jemmott, L.S., Braverman, P.K., and Fong, G.T. (2005). HIV/STD risk reduction interventions for African American and Latino adolescent girls at an adolescent medicine clinic: A randomized controlled trial. *Archives of Pediatric Adolescence Medicine, 159,* 440-449.

Jenkins, E.J., and Bell, C.C. (1994). Violence exposure, psychological distress and high risk behaviors among inner-city high school students. In S. Friedman (Ed.), *Anxiety Disorders in African-Americans* (pp. 76-88). New York: Springer.

Jenkins, E.J., and Bell, C.C. (1997). Exposure and response to community violence among children and adolescents. In J. Osofsky (Ed.), *Children in a Violent Society* (pp. 9-31). New York: Guilford Press.

Jenkins, W.M., Merzenich, M.M., Ochs, M.T., Allard, T., and Guic-Robles, E. (1990). Func-tional reorganization of primary somatosensory cortex in adult owl monkeys after behav-iorally controlled tactile stimulation. *Journal of Neurophysiology, 63*(1), 82-104.

Jensen, P.S., Hoagwood, K., and Trickett, E. (1999). Ivory tower or earthen trenches? Com-munity collaborations to foster real-world research. *Journal of Applied Developmental Science, 3,* 206-212.

Jensen, P., Bornemann, T., Costello, E.J., Friedman, R., Kessler, R., Spencer, S., and Goldman, E. (2006). *The Warning Signs Project: A Toolkit to Help Parents, Educators and Health Professionals Identify Children at Behavioral and Emotional Risk.* New York: Center for the Advancement of Children's Mental Health at Columbia University. Available: http://www.thereachinstitute.net/documents/warning%20signs%20toolkit%20final.doc [accessed August 2008].

Jo, B. (2002). Estimation of intervention effects with noncompliance: Alternative model speci-fications. *Journal of Educational and Behavioral Statistics, 27*(4), 385-409.

Jo, B., and Muthén, B.O. (2001). Modeling of intervention effects with noncompliance: A latent variable approach for randomized trials. In G.A. Marcoulides and R.E. Schumacker (Eds.), *New Developments and Techniques in Structural Equation Modeling* (pp. 57-87). Hillsdale, NJ: Lawrence Erlbaum.

Jo, B., Asparouhov, T., Muthén, B.O., Ialongo, N., and Brown, C.H. (in press). Cluster ran-domized trials with treatment noncompliance. Submitted to *Psychological Methods.*

Joel, D. (2006). Current animal models of obsessive compulsive disorder: A critical review. *Progress in Neuro-Psychopharmacology and Biological Psychiatry, 30*(3), 374-388.

Johansen-Berg, H. (2007). Structural plasticity: Rewiring the brain. *Current Biology, 17*(4), R141-R144.

Johnson, C.A., Pentz, M.A., Weber, M.D., Dwyer, J.H., Baer, N., MacKinnon, D.P., Hanson, W.B., and Flay, B.R. (1990). Relative effectiveness of comprehensive community pro-gramming for drug abuse prevention with high-risk and low-risk adolescents. *Journal of Consulting and Clinical Psychology, 58,* 447-456.

Johnson, C.P., Myers, S.M., and the American Academy of Pediatrics Council on Children with Disabilities. (2007). Identification and evaluation of children with autism spectrum disorders. *Pediatrics, 120,* 1183-1215.

Johnson, J.G., Cohen, P., Chen, H., Kasen, S., and Brook, J.S. (2006). Parenting behaviors associated with risk for offspring personality disorder during adulthood. *Archives of General Psychiatry, 63*(5), 579-587.

Johnson, K., and Theberge, S. (2007). *Local Systems Development.* New York: National Center for Children in Poverty. Available: http://www.nccp.org/publications/pub_758. html [accessed May 2009].

Jones, J., Lopez, A., and Wilson, M. (2003). Congenital toxoplasmosis. *American Family Physician, 67*(10), 2131-2138.

Joober, R., Sengupta, S., and Boksa, P. (2005). Genetics of developmental psychiatric disorders: Pathways to discovery. *Journal of Psychiatry and Neuroscience, 30*(5), 349-354.

Judd, C.M., Kenny, D.A., and McClelland, G.H. (2001). Estimating and testing mediation and moderation in within-subject designs. *Psychological Methods, 6*(2), 115-134.

Judge David L. Bazelon Center for Mental Health Law. (2009). *An Evaluation of State EPSDT Screening Tools.* Issue Paper #3. Available: http://www.bazelon.org/issues/managedcare/ moreresources/epsdtfactsheet.htm [accessed March 2009].

Kaffman, A., and Meaney, M.J. (2007). Neurodevelopmental sequelae of postnatal maternal care in rodents: Clinical and research implications of molecular insights. *Journal of Child Psychology and Psychiatry, 48*(3-4), 224-244.

Kahn, R.S., Khoury, J., Nichols, W.C., and Lanphear, B.P. (2003). Role of dopamine transporter genotype and maternal prenatal smoking in childhood hyperactive-impulsive, inattentive, and oppositional behaviors. *Journal of Pediatrics, 143*(1), 104-110.

Kahn, R.S., Brandt, D., and Whitaker, R.C. (2004). Combined effect of mothers' and fathers' mental health symptoms on children's behavioral and emotional well-being. *Archives of Pediatrics and Adolescent Medicine, 158*(8), 721-729.

Kalivas, P.W., and O'Brien, C. (2008). Drug addiction as a pathology of staged neuroplasticity. *Neuropsychopharmacology, 33*(1), 166-180.

Kalivas, P.W., Peters, J., and Knackstedt, L. (2006). Animal models and brain circuits in drug addiction. *Molecular Interventions, 6*(6), 339-344.

Kaltiala-Heino, R., Rimpela, M., Rantanen, P., and Rimpela, A. (2000). Bullying at school: An indicator of adolescents at risk for mental disorders. *Journal of Adolescence, 23,* 661-674.

Kam, C.M., Greenberg, M.T., and Wells, C. (2003). Examining the role of implementation quality in school-based prevention using the PATHS Curriculum. *Prevention Science, 4,* 55-63.

Kam, C.M., Greenberg, M.T., and Kusche, C.A. (2004). Sustained effects of the PATHS curriculum on the social and psychological adjustment of children in special education. *Journal of Emotional and Behavioral Disorders, 12,* 66-78.

Kaminski, J.W., Valle, L.A., Filene, J.H., and Boyle, C.L. (2008). A meta-analytic review of components associated with parent training program effectiveness. *Journal of Abnormal Child Psychology, 36,* 567-589.

Kandel, D.B., Johnson, J.G., Bird, H.R., Weissman, M.M., Goodman, S.H., Lahey, B.B., Regier, D.A., and Schwab-Stone, M.E. (1999). Psychiatric comorbidity among adolescents with substance use disorders: Findings from the MECA study. *Journal of the American Academy of Child and Adolescent Psychiatry, 38*(6), 693-699.

Kandel, E.R. (2001). The molecular biology of memory storage: A dialogue between genes and synapses. *Science, 294*(5544), 1030-1038.

Kandel, E.R., Schwartz, J.H., and Jessell, T.M. (2000). *Principles of Neural Science* (4th ed.). Stamford, CT: Appleton and Lange.

Kanof, M.E. (2003). *Youth Illicit Drug Use Prevention: DARE Long-Term Evaluations and Federal Efforts to Identify Effective Programs.* Washington, DC: General Accounting Office.

Karoly, L.A., Kilburn, M.R., and Cannon, J.S. (2005). *Early Childhood Interventions: Proven Results, Future Promise.* Santa Monica, CA: RAND.

Kaslow, N.J., Abramson, L., and Collins, M.H. (2000). A developmental psychopathology perspective on the cognitive components of child and adolescent depression. In A.J. Sameroff, M. Lewis, and S.M. Miller (Eds.), *Handbook of Developmental Psychopathology* (2nd ed., pp. 491-510). New York: Kluwer/Plenum.

Kataoka, S.H., Zhang, L., and Wells, K. (2002). Unmet need for mental health care among U.S. children: Variation by ethnicity and insurance status. *American Journal of Psychiatry, 159,* 1548-1555.

Kauer, J.A., and Malenka, R.C. (2007). Synaptic plasticity and addiction. *Nature Reviews Neuroscience, 8*(11), 844-858.

Kautz, C., Mauch, D., and Smith, S.A. (2008). *Reimbursement of Mental Health Services in Primary Care Settings.* (HHS Pub. No. SMA-08-4324). Rockville, MD: Center for Mental Health Services, Substance Abuse and Mental Health Services Administration.

Kaye, N., and Rosenthal, J. (2008, February). *Improving the Delivery of Health Care That Supports Young Children's Healthy Mental Development: Update on Accomplishments and Lessons from a Five-State Consortium.* New York: The Commonwealth Fund.

Kaye, N., May, J., and Abrams, M. (2006, December). *State Policy Options to Improve Delivery of Child Development Services: Strategies from the Eight ABCD States.* New York: The Commonwealth Fund.

Keenan, K., Shaw, D., Delliquadri, E., Giovannelli, J., and Walsh, B. (1998). Evidence for the continuity of early problem behaviors: Application of a developmental model. *Journal of Abnormal Child Psychology, 26,* 441-452.

Kellam, S.G. (1990). Developmental epidemiological framework for family research on depression and aggression. In G.R. Patterson (Ed.), *Depression and Aggression in Family Interaction* (pp. 11-48). Hillsdale, NJ: Lawrence Erlbaum.

Kellam, S.G. (2000). Community and institutional partnerships for school violence prevention. In *Preventing School Violence: Plenary Papers of the 1999 Conference on Criminal Justice Research and Evaluation: Enhancing Policy and Practice Through Research* (vol 2, pp. 1-217). Washington, DC: National Institute of Justice.

Kellam, S.G., and Anthony, J.C. (1998). Targeting early antecedents to prevent tobacco smoking: Findings from an epidemiologically based randomized field trial. *American Journal of Public Health, 88,* 1490-1495.

Kellam, S.G., and Langevin, D.J. (2003). A framework for understanding "evidence" in prevention research and programs. *Prevention Science, 4*(3), 137-153.

Kellam, S.G., and Rebok, G.W. (1992). Building developmental and etiological theory through epidemiologically based preventive intervention trials. In J. McCord and R.E. Tremblay (Eds.), *Preventing Antisocial Behavior: Interventions from Birth Through Adolescence* (pp. 162-195). New York: Guilford Press.

Kellam, S.G., Branch, J.D., Agrawal, K.C., and Ensminger, M.E. (1975). *Mental Health and Going to School: The Woodlawn Program of Assessment, Early Intervention, and Evaluation.* Chicago, IL: University of Chicago Press.

Kellam, S.G., Brown, C.H., Rubin, B.R., and Ensminger, M.E. (1983). Paths leading to teenage psychiatric symptoms and substance use: Developmental epidemiological studies in Woodlawn. In S.B. Guze, F.J. Earls, and J.E. Barrett (Eds.), *Childhood Psychopathology and Development* (pp. 17-51). New York: Raven.

Kellam, S.G., Werthamer-Larsson, L., Dolan, L.J., Brown, C.H., Mayer, L.S., Rebok, G.W., Anthony, J.C., Landolff, J., and Edelsohn, G. (1991). Developmental epidemiologically based preventive trials: Baseline modeling of early target behaviors and depressive symptoms. *American Journal of Community Psychology, 19,* 563-584.

Kellam, S.G., Rebok, G.W., Ialongo, N.S., and Mayer, L.S. (1994). The course and malleability of aggressive behavior from early first grade into middle school: Results of a developmental epidemiologically based preventive trial. *Journal of Child Psychology, 35,* 259-281.

Kellam, S.G., Ling, X., Merisca, R., Brown, C.H., and Ialongo, N. (1998). The effect of the level of aggression in the first grade classroom on the course and malleability of aggressive behavior into middle school. *Development and Psychopathology, 10,* 165-185.

Kellam, S.G., Koretz, D., and Moscicki, E.K. (1999). Core elements of developmental epidemiologically based prevention research. *American Journal of Community Psychology 27,* 463-482.

Kellam, S.G., Brown, C.H., Poduska, J.M., Ialongo, N.S., Wang, W., Toyinbo, P., Petras, H., Ford, C., Windham, A., and Wilcox, H.C. (2008). Effects of a universal classroom behavior management program in first and second grades on young adult behavioral, psychiatric, and social outcomes. *Drug and Alcohol Dependence, 95*(Suppl. 1), S5-S28.

Kelleher, K.J., McInerny, T.K., Gardner, W.P., Childs, G.E., and Wasserman, R.C. (2000). Increasing identification of psychosocial problems: 1979-1996. *Pediatrics, 105*(6), 1313-1321.

Kelley, M.L., Carper, L.B., Witt, J.C., and Elliott, S.N. (1988). Home-based reinforcement procedures. In S.N. Elliott, F. Gresham, and J.C. Witt (Eds.), *Handbook of Behavior Therapy in Education* (p. 419). New York: Plenum Press.

Kelly, J.A., St. Lawrence, J.S., Diaz, Y.E., Stevenson, L.Y., Hauth, A.C., Brasfield, T.L., Kalichman, S.C., Smith, J.E., and Andrew, M.E. (1991). HIV risk behavior reduction following intervention with key opinion leaders of population: An experimental analysis. *American Journal of Public Health, 81*(2), 168-171.

Kelly, J.B., and Emery, R.E. (2003). Children's adjustment following divorce: Risk and resilience perspective. *Family Relations, 52,* 352-362.

Kelly, R.H., Zatzick, D.F., and Anders, T.F. (2001). The detection and treatment of psychiatric disorders and substance use among pregnant women cared for in obstetrics. *American Journal of Psychiatry, 158,* 213-219.

Kelly, R.H., Russo, J., Holt, V.L., Danielsen, B.H., Zatzick, D.F., Walker, E., and Katon, W. (2002). Psychiatric and substance use disorders as risk factors for low birth weight and preterm delivery. *Obstetrics and Gynecology, 10,* 297-304.

Kemper, K.J., and Kelleher, K.J. (1996). Family psychosocial screening: Instruments and techniques. *Ambulatory Child Health, 1,* 325-339.

Kemper, K., and Shannon, S. (2007). Complementary and alternative medicine therapies to promote healthy mood. *Pediatric Clinics of North America, 54*(6), 901-926.

Kempermann, G., Kuhn, H.G., and Gage, F.H. (1997). More hippocampal neurons in adult mice living in an enriched environment. *Nature, 386*(6624), 493-495.

Kendall, P.C. (1994). Treating anxiety disorders in children: Results of a randomized clinical trial. *Journal of Consulting and Clinical Psychology, 62,* 100-110.

Kendall, P.C. (2000). *Cognitive-Behavioral Therapy for Anxious Children: Therapist Manual* (2nd ed.). Ardmore, PA: Workbook.

Kendall, P.C., Safford, S., Flannery-Schroeder, E., and Webb, A. (2004). Child anxiety treatment: Outcomes in adolescence and impact on substance use and depression at 7.4-year follow up. *Journal of Consulting and Clinical Psychology, 72,* 276-287.

Kendler, K.S. (1983). Overview: A current perspective on twin studies of schizophrenia. *American Journal of Psychiatry, 140,* 1413-1425.

Kendler, K.S. (2000). Schizophrenia: Genetics. In B.J. Sadock, V.A. Kaplan (Eds.), *Comprehensive Textbook of Psychiatry* (pp. 1147-1159). Philadelphia: Lippincott, Williams and Wilkins.

Kendler, K.S. (2005). "A gene for . . .": The nature of gene action in psychiatric disorders. *American Journal of Psychiatry, 162*(7), 1243-1252.

Kendler, K.S., Gardner, C.O., and Prescott, C.A. (2002). Toward a comprehensive developmental model for major depression in women. *American Journal of Psychiatry, 159*(7), 1133-1145.

Kennedy, D.P., Redcay, E., and Courchesne, E. (2006). Failing to deactivate: Resting functional abnormalities in autism. *Proceedings of the National Academy of Sciences, 103*(21), 8275-8280.

Kerwin, M.E., Walker-Smith, K., and Kirby, K.C. (2006). Comparative analysis of state requirements for the training of substance abuse and mental health counselors. *Journal of Substance Abuse Treatment, 30*(3), 173-181.

Kessler, R.C. (1994). The national comorbidity survey of the United States. *International Review of Psychiatry, 6,* 365-376.

Kessler, R.C., Sonnega, A., Bromet, E., Hughes, M., and Nelson, C.B. (1995). Posttraumatic stress disorder in the national comorbidity survey. *Archives of General Psychiatry, 52,* 1048-1060.

Kessler, R.C., Anthony, J.C., Blazer, D.G., Bromet, E., Eaton, W.W., and Kendler, K. (1997). The U.S. national comorbidity survey: Overview and future directions. *Epidemiological Psychiatry Society, 6,* 4-16.

Kessler, R.C., Davis, C.G., and Kendler, K.S. (1997). Childhood adversity and adult psychiatric disorder in the U.S. national comorbidity survey. *Psychological Medicine, 27,* 1101-1119.

Kessler, R.C., Ormel, J., Demler, O., and Stang, P.E. (2003). Comorbid mental disorders account for the role impairment of commonly occurring chronic physical disorders: Results from the national comorbidity survey. *Journal of Occupational and Environmental Medicine, 45*(12), 1257-1266.

Kessler, R.C., Berglund, P., Demler, O., Jin, R., Merikangas, K.R., and Walters, E.E. (2005). Lifetime prevalence and age-of-onset distributions of DSM-IV disorders in the national comorbidity survey replication. *Archives of General Psychiatry, 62*(6), 593-602.

Kessler, R.C., Chiu, W.T., Demler, O., and Walters, E.E. (2005). Prevalence, severity, and comorbidity of 12-month DSM-IV disorders in the national comorbidity survey replication. *Archives of General Psychiatry, 62*(6), 617-627.

Kessler, R.C., Gruber, M., Hettema, J.M., Hwang, I., Sampson, N., and Yonkers, K.A. (2007). Co-morbid major depression and generalized anxiety disorders in the national comorbidity survey follow-up. *Psychological Medicine, 38,* 365-374.

Kessler, R.C., Heeringa, S., Lakoma, M., Petukhova, M., Rupp, A., Schoenbaum, M., Wang, P., and Zaslavsky, A. (2008). Individual and societal effects of mental disorders on earnings in the United States: Results from the National Comorbidity Survey Replication. *American Journal of Psychiatry, 165*(6), 703-711.

Kessler, R.C., Pecora, P.J., Williams, J., Hiripi, E., O'Brien, K., English, D., White, J., Zerbe, J.R., Downs, A.C., Plotnick, R., Hwang, I., and Sampson, N.A. (2008). The effects of enhanced foster care on the long-term physical and mental health of foster care alumni. *Archives of General Psychiatry, 65*(6), 625-633.

Kibar, Z., Capra, V., and Gros, P. (2007). Toward understanding the genetic basis of neural tube defects. *Clinical Genetics, 71*(4), 295-310.

Kim-Cohen, J., Caspi, A., Moffitt, T., Harrington, H., Milne, B., and Poulton, R. (2003). Prior juvenile diagnoses in adults with mental disorder: Developmental follow-back of a prospective-longitudinal cohort. *Archives of General Psychiatry, 60,* 709-717.

Kim-Cohen, J., Caspi, A., Taylor, A., Williams, B., Newcombe, R., Craig, I.W., and Moffitt, T. (2006). MAOA, maltreatment, and gene-environment interaction predicting children's mental health: New evidence and a meta-analysis. *Molecular Psychiatry, 11*(10), 903-913.

King, V., and Sobolewski, J.M. (2006). Nonresident fathers' contributions to adolescent well-being. *Journal of Marriage and Family, 68,* 537-557.

Knickmeyer, R.C., and Baron-Cohen, S. (2006). Fetal testosterone and sex differences. *Early Human Development, 82*(12), 755-760.

Knitzer, J. (2007). Putting knowledge into policy: Toward an infant-toddler policy agenda. *Infant Mental Health Journal, 28,* 237-245.

Knitzer, J., and Lefkowitz, J. (2006). *Helping the Most Vulnerable Infants, Toddlers, and Their Families.* New York: National Center for Children in Poverty, Columbia University.

Knowlton, B.J., Squire, L.R., and Gluck, M.A. (1994). Probabilistic classification learning in amnesia. *Learning and Memory, 1,* 106-120.

Kolevzon, A., Gross, R., and Reichenberg, A. (2007). Prenatal and perinatal risk factors for autism: A review and integration of findings. *Archives of Pediatrics and Adolescent Medicine, 161*(4), 326-333.

Komro, K.A., Perry, C.L., Veblen-Mortenson, S., Farbakhsh, K., Toomey, T.L., Stigler, M.H., Jones-Webb, R., Kugler, K.C., Pasch, K.E., and Williams, C.L. (2008). Outcomes from a randomized controlled trial of a multicomponent alcohol use preventive intervention for urban youth: Project Northland Chicago. *Addiction, 103*(4), 606-618.

Kondrat, M.E., Greene, G.J., and Winbush, G.B. (2002). Using benchmarking research to locate agency best practices for African American clients. *Administration and Policy in Mental Health, 29*(6), 495-518.

Kornack, D.R., and Rakic, P. (1995). Radial and horizontal deployment of clonally related cells in the primate neocortex: Relationship to distinct mitotic lineages. *Neuron, 15*(2), 311-321.

Koroloff, N.M., Elliott, D.J., Koren, P.E., and Friesen, B.J. (1994). Connecting low-income families to mental health services: The role of the family associate. *Journal of Emotional and Behavioral Disorders, 2*(4), 240-246.

Kouzarides, T. (2007). Chromatin modifications and their function. *Cell, 128*(4), 693-705.

Kraag, G., Zeegers, M.P., Kok, G., Hosman, C., and Abu-Saad, H.H. (2006). School programs targeting stress management in children and adolescents: A meta-analysis. *Journal of School Psychology, 44*(6), 449-472.

Krabbendam, L., and van Os, J. (2005). Schizophrenia and urbanicity: A major environmental influence—conditional on genetic risk. *Schizophrenia Bulletin, 31*(4), 795-799.

Kraemer, H.C., Kazdin, A.E., Offord, D.R., Kessler, R.C., Jensen, P.S., and Kupfer, D.J. (1997). Coming to terms with terms of risk. *Archives of General Psychiatry, 54*(4), 327-343.

Kraemer, H.C., Mintz, J., Noda, A., Tinklenberg, J., and Yesavage, J.A. (2006). Caution regarding the use of pilot studies to guide power calculations for study proposals. *Archives of General Psychiatry, 63*(5), 484-489.

Kramer, M.S. (2008). Effects of prolonged and exclusive breastfeeding on childhood behavior and maternal adjustment: Evidence from a large randomized trial–Reply. *Pediatrics, 122*(2), 474-475.

Kramer, M.S., Aboud, F., Mironova, E., and colleagues for the Promotion of Breastfeeding Intervention Trial (PROBIT) Study Group. (2008). Breastfeeding and child cognitive development: New evidence from a large randomized trial. *Archives of General Psychiatry, 65*(5), 578-584.

Krauss, B.J., Goldsamt, L., Bula, E., and Sember, R. (1997). The white researcher in the multicultural community: Lessons in HIV prevention education learned in the field. *Journal of Health Education, 28,* S67-S71.

Krauss, B.J., Tiffany, J., and Goldsamt, L. (1997). Research notes: Parent and pre-adolescent training for HIV prevention in a high seroprevalence neighborhood. *AIDS/STD Health Promotion Exchange, 1,* 10-12.

Krauss, B.J., Godfrey, C., Yee, D., Goldsamt, L., Tiffany, J., Almeyda, L., Davis, W.R., Bula, E., Reardon, D., Jones, Y., DeJesus, J., Pride, J., Gracia, E., Pierre-Louis, M., Rivera, C., Trouche, E., Daniels, T., O'Day, J., and Velez, R. (2000). Saving our children from a silent epidemic: The PATH program for parents and preadolescents. In W. Pequegnat and J. Szapocznik (Eds.), *Working with Family in the Era of AIDS* (pp. 89-112). Thousand Oaks, CA: Sage.

Krauss, B.J., Godfrey, C.C., O'Day, J., and Freidin, E. (2006). Hugging my uncle: The impact of parent training on children's comfort interacting with persons with HIV. *Journal of Pediatric Psychology, 31*(9), 891-904.

Krauss, B.J., McGinniss, S., O'Day, J., Hodorek, S., Bournea, M., and Kaplan, R. (2007). *Delaying Tactics: Parent HIV Education as a Protective Factor for Early Sexual Debut.* Poster presented at National Institute of Mental Health International Conference on the Role of Families in Preventing and Adapting to HIV/AIDS, San Francisco, CA.

Kuehn, B.M. (2008). Asthma linked to psychiatric disorders. *Journal of the American Medical Association, 299*(2), 158-160.

Kumar, A., Choi, K.H., Renthal, W., Tsankova, N.M., Theobald, D.E., Truong, H.T., Russo, S.J., LaPlant, Q., Sasaki, T.S., Whistler, K.N., Neve, R.L., Self, D.W., and Nestler, E.J. (2005). Chromatin remodeling is a key mechanism underlying cocaine-induced plasticity in striatum. *Neuron, 48*(2), 303-314.

Kumpfer, K.L., Alvarado, R., Smith, P., and Bellamy, N. (2002). Cultural sensitivity and adaptation in family-based prevention interventions. *Prevention Science, 3*(3), 241-246.

Kunugi, H., Nanko, S., and Murray, R.M. (2001). Obstetric complications and schizophrenia: Prenatal underdevelopment and subsequent neurodevelopmental impairment. *British Journal of Psychiatry, 40*(Suppl.), S25-S29.

Kusche, C.A., and Greenberg, M.T. (1994). *The PATHS Curriculum.* Seattle, WA: Developmental Research and Programs.

Kusche, C.A., Cook, E.T., and Greenberg, M.T. (1993). Neuropsychological and cognitive functioning in children with anxiety, externalizing, and comorbid psychopathology. *Journal of Clinical Child Psychology, 22*, 172-195.

Kwok, O.-M., Haine, R., Sandler, I.N., Ayers, T.S., and Wolchik, S.A. (2005). Positive parenting as a mediator of the relations between parental psychological distress and mental health problems of parentally bereaved children. *Journal of Clinical Child and Adolescent Psychology, 34*, 261-272.

La Greca, A., and Silverman, W. (2002). Children experiencing disasters: Definitions, reactions, and predictors of outcomes. In A. La Greca, W. Silverman, E. Vernberg, and M. Roberts (Eds.) *Helping Children Cope with Disasters and Terrorism* (pp. 11-33). Washington, DC: American Psychological Association.

LaFromboise, T.D. (1995). Zuni life skills development curriculum: Description and evaluation of a suicide prevention program. *Journal of Counseling Psychology, 42*(4), 479-486.

LaFromboise, T.D. (1996). *American Indian Life Skills Development Curriculum.* Madison: University of Wisconsin Press.

LaFromboise, T.D., and Howard-Pitney, B. (1993). The Zuni life skills development curriculum: A collaborative approach to curriculum development. *American Indian and Alaska Native Mental Health Research: The Journal of the National Center, 4*, 98-121.

LaFromboise, T.D., and Lewis, H.A. (2008). The Zuni life skills development program: A school/community-based suicide prevention. *Suicide and Life-Threatening Behavior, 38*(3), 343-353.

LaFromboise, T.D., Coleman, H.L.K., and Hernandez, A. (1991). Development and factor structure of the cross-cultural counseling inventory-revised. *Professional Psychology: Research and Practice, 22*, 380-388.

Lalande, M., and Calciano, M.A. (2007). Molecular epigenetics of Angelman syndrome. *Cellular and Molecular Sciences, 64*(7-8), 947-960.

Lamberg, L. (2003). Programs target youth violence prevention. *Journal of the American Medical Association, 290*, 585-586.

Lantz, P.M., Jacobson, P.D., Warner, K.E., Wasserman, J., Pollack, H.A., Berson, J., and Ahlstrom, A. (2000). Investing in youth tobacco control: A review of smoking prevention and control strategies. *Tobacco Control, 9*(1), 47-63.

Lanza, S.T., Collins, L.M., Schafer, J.L., and Flaherty, B.P. (2005). Using data augmentation to obtain standard errors and conduct hypothesis tests in latent class and latent transition analysis. *Psychological Methods, 10*(1), 84-100.

Larimer, M.E., Kilmer, J.R., and Lee, C.M. (2005). College student drug prevention: A review of individually oriented prevention strategies. *Journal of Drug Issues, 35*(2), 431-456.

LaRocco-Cockburn, A., Melville, J., Bell, M., and Katon, W. (2003). Depression screening attitudes and practices among obstetrician-gynecologists. *Obstetrics and Gynecology, 101,* 892-898.

Larun, L., Nordheim, L.V., Ekeland, E., Hagen, K.B., and Heian, F. (2006). Exercise in prevention and treatment of anxiety and depression among children and young people. *Cochrane Database of Systematic Reviews, 3,* Art. No. CD004691.

Last, C.G., Hersen, M., Kazdin, A.E., Francis, G., and Grubb, H.J. (1987). Psychiatric illness in the mothers of anxious children. *American Journal of Psychiatry, 144,* 1580-1583.

Lau, J.Y., and Eley, T.C. (2008). Disentangling gene-environment correlations and interactions on adolescent depressive symptoms. *Journal of Child Psychology and Psychiatry, 49*(2), 142-150.

Layne, C.M., Saltzman, W.R., Poppleton, L., Burlinggame, G.M., Pasalic, A., Durakovic, E., Music, M., Compara, N., Dapo, N., Arslanagic, B., Steinberg, A.M., and Pynoos, R.S. (2008). Effectiveness of a school-based psychotherapy program for war-exposed adolescents: A randomized controlled trial. *Journal of the American Academy of Child and Adolescent Psychiatry, 47*(9), 1048-1062.

Lee, C.M., Picard, M., and Bain, M.D. (1994). A methodological and substantive review of intervention outcome studies for families undergoing divorce. *Journal of Family Psychology, 8,* 3-15.

Lee, J.A., and Lupski, J.R. (2006). Genomic rearrangements and gene copy-number alterations as a cause of nervous system disorders. *Neuron, 52*(1), 103-121.

Leland, N.L., and Barth, R.P. (1993). Characteristics of adolescents who have attempted to avoid HIV and who have communicated with their parents about sex. *Journal of Adolescent Research, 8,* 58-76.

Lenzer, J. (2004). Bush's plan to screen for mental health meets opposition in Illinois. *British Medical Journal, 329*(7474), 1065.

Leucht, S., Pitschel-Walz, G., Abraham, D., and Kissling, W. (1999). Efficacy and extrapyramidal side-effects of the new antipsychotics olanzapine, quetiapine, risperidone, and sertindole compared to conventional antipsychotics and placebo. A meta-analysis of randomized controlled trials. *Schizophrenia Research, 35,* 51-68.

Leung, H.C., Skudlarski, P., Gatenby, J.C., Peterson, B.S., and Gore, J.C. (2000). An event-related functional MRI study of the stroop color word interference task. *Cerebral Cortex, 10*(6), 552-560.

Leung, M.M., Sanders, M.R., Leung, S., Mak, R., and Lau, J. (2003). An outcome evaluation of the implementation of the Triple P-Positive Parenting Program in Hong Kong. *Family Process, 42,* 531-544.

Levenson, J.M., and Sweatt, J.D. (2005). Epigenetic mechanisms in memory formation. *Nature Reviews Neuroscience, 6*(2), 108-118.

Levenson, J.M., and Sweatt, J.D. (2006). Epigenetic mechanisms: A common theme in vertebrate and invertebrate memory formation. *Cellular and Molecular Life Sciences, 63*(9), 1009-1016.

Levenson, J.M., Roth, T.L., Lubin, F.D., Miller, C.A., Huang, I.C., Desai, P., Malone, L.M., and Sweatt, J.D. (2006). Evidence that DNA (cytosine-5) methyltransferase regulates synaptic plasticity in the hippocampus. *Journal of Biological Chemistry, 281*(23), 15763-15773.

Leventhal, T., and Brooks-Gunn, J. (2003). Moving on up: Neighborhood effects on children and families. In M.H. Bornstein and R.H. Bradley (Eds.), *Socioeconomic Status, Parenting, and Child Development* (pp. 209-230). Mahwah, NJ: Lawrence Erlbaum.

Levinson, D.F. (2006). The genetics of depression: A review. *Biological Psychiatry, 60*(2), 84-92.

Levinson, D.J. (1978). *Seasons of a Man's Life*. New York: Knopf.

Levitt, J.M., and Jensen, P.S. (2004). *Minimum Standards for Selecting Behavioral Health Screening Tools*. New York: Columbia University.

Levitt, J., Saka, N., Romanelli, L., and Hoagwood, K. (2007). Early identification of mental health problems in schools: The status of instrumentation. *Journal of School Psychology, 45*(2), 163-191.

Levitt, P. (2003). Structural and functional maturation of the developing primate brain. *Journal of Pediatrics, 143*(Suppl. 4), S35-S45.

Lewinsohn, P.M., and Essau, C.A. (2002). Depression in adolescents. In I.H. Gotlib and C.L. Hammen (Eds.), *Handbook of Depression* (pp. 541-559). New York: Guilford Press.

Lewinsohn, P.M., Munoz, R.F., Youngren, M.A., and Ziess, A.M. (1986). *Control Your Depression*. New York: Simon and Schuster.

Lewinsohn, P.M., Rohde, P., and Seeley, J.R. (1998). Major depressive disorder in older adolescents: Prevalence, risk factors, and clinical implications. *Clinical Psychology Review, 18*, 765-794.

Lewis, D.A. (2002). The human brain revisited: Opportunities and challenges in postmortem studies of psychiatric disorders. *Neuropsychopharmacology, 26*(2), 143-154.

Lewis, D.A., and Levitt, P. (2002). Schizophrenia as a disorder of neurodevelopment. *Annual Review of Neuroscience, 25*(1), 409.

Li, X., Feigelman, S., and Stanton, B. (2000). Perceived parental monitoring and health risk behaviors among urban low-income African American children and adolescents. *Journal of Adolescent Health, 27*, 43-48.

Libby, A.M., Brent, D.A., Morrato, E.H., Orton, H.D., Allen, R., and Valuck, R.J. (2007). Decline in treatment of pediatric depression after FDA advisory on risk of suicidality with SSRIs. *American Journal of Psychiatry, 164*(6), 884.

Liberzon, I., and Sripada, C.S. (2008). The functional neuroanatomy of PTSD: A critical review. *Progress in Brain Research, 167*, 151-169.

Lieb, K., Zanarini, M.C., Schmahl, C., Linehan, M.M., and Bohus, M. (2004). Borderline personality disorder. *Lancet, 364*(9432), 453-461.

Lieberman, J.A., Perkins, D., Belger, A., Chakos, M., Jarskog, F., Boteva, K., and Gilmore, J. (2001). The early stages of schizophrenia: Speculations on pathogenesis, pathophysiology, and therapeutic approaches. *Biological Psychiatry, 50*(11), 884-897.

Lilienfeld, S. (2003). Comorbidity between and within childhood externalizing and internalizing disorders: Reflections and directions. *Journal of Abnormal Child Psychology, 31*, 285-291.

Lin, K.K., Sandler, I.N., Ayers, T.S., Wolchik, S.A., and Luecken, L.J. (2004). Resilience in parentally bereaved children and adolescents seeking preventive services. *Journal of Clinical Child and Adolescent Psychology, 33*(4), 673-683.

Lin, P.Y., and Su, K.P. (2007). A meta-analytic review of double-blind, placebo-controlled trials of antidepressant efficacy of omega-3 fatty acids. *Journal of Clinical Psychiatry, 68*(7), 1056-1061.

Linares, L.O., Montalto, D., Li, M., and Oza, V.S. (2006). A promising parenting intervention in foster care. *Journal of Consulting and Clinical Psychology, 74*, 32-41.

Linehan, M.M., Goodstein, J.L., Nielsen, S.L., and Chiles, J.A. (1983). Reasons for staying alive when you are thinking of killing yourself: The reasons for living inventory. *Journal of Consulting and Clinical Psychology, 51*, 276-286.

Lipsey, M.W., and Derzon, J.H. (1998). Predictors of violent or serious delinquency in adolescence and early adulthood: A synthesis of longitudinal research. In R. Loeber and D.P. Farrington (Eds.), *Serious and Violent Juvenile Offenders* (pp. 86-104). Thousand Oaks, CA: Sage.

Liston, C., Watts, R., Tottenham, N., Davidson, M.C., Niogi, S., Ulug, A.M., and Casey, B.J. (2006). Frontostriatal microstructure modulates efficient recruitment of cognitive control. *Cerebral Cortex*, 16(4), 553-560.

Little, R.J., and Yau, L.H.Y. (1996). Intent-to-treat analysis for longitudinal studies with dropouts. *Biometrics*, 52, 1324-1333.

Lledo, P.M., Alonso, M., and Grubb, M.S. (2006). Adult neurogenesis and functional plasticity in neuronal circuits. *Nature Reviews Neuroscience*, 7(3), 179-193.

Lochman, J.E., and Conduct Problems Prevention Research Group. (1995). Screening of child behavior problems for prevention programs at school entry. *Journal of Consulting and Clinical Psychology*, 63, 549-559.

Lochman, J.E., and van-den-Steenhoven, A. (2002). Family-based approaches to substance abuse prevention. *Journal of Primary Prevention*, 23, 49-114.

Lochman, J.E., and Wells, K. (1996). A social-cognitive intervention with aggressive children: Prevention effects and contextual implementation issues. In R.D. Peters and R.J. McMahon (Eds.), *Preventing Childhood Disorders, Substance Abuse and Delinquency* (pp. 111-143). Thousand Oaks, CA: Sage

Loebel, A.D., Lieberman, J.A., Alvir, M.J., Mayerhoff, D.I., Geisler, S.H., and Szymanski, S.R. (1992). Duration of psychosis and outcome in first-episode schizophrenia. *American Journal of Psychiatry*, 149(9), 1183-1188.

Loeber, R., Wei, E., Stouthamer-Loeber, M., Huizinga, D., and Thornberry, T.P. (1999). Behavioral antecedents to serious and violent offending: Joint analyses from the Denver youth survey, Pittsburgh youth study, and the Rochester youth development study. *Studies on Crime and Crime Prevention*, 8, 245-263.

Loeber, R., Farrington, D.P., Stouthamer-Loeber, M., Moffitt, T., Caspi, A., White, H., Wei, E.H., and Beyers, J. (2003). The development of male offending: Key findings from fourteen years of the Pittsburgh youth study. In T.P. Thornberry and M.D. Krohn (Eds.), *Taking Stock of Delinquency: An Overview of Findings from Contemporary Longitudinal Studies* (pp. 93-136). New York: Kluwer Academic/Plenum.

Logan, C.G., and Grafton, S.T. (1995). Functional anatomy of human eyeblink conditioning determined with regional cerebral glucose metabolism and positron-emission tomography. *Proceedings of the National Academy of Sciences*, 92(16), 7500-7504.

Longshore, D., Ellickson, P.L., McCaffrey, D.F., and St. Clair, P.A. (2007). School-based drug prevention among at-risk adolescents: Effects of ALERT plus. *Health Education and Behavior*, 34(4), 651-668.

Lopez-Leon, S., Janssens, A.C., Gonzalez-Zuloeta Ladd, A.M., Del-Favero, J., Claes, S.J., Oostra, B.A., and van Duijn, C.M. (2008). Meta-analyses of genetic studies on major depressive disorder. *Molecular Psychiatry*, 13(8), 772-785.

Los Angeles Unified School District. (2007). *Discipline Foundation Policy: School-Wide Positive Behavior Support*. (BUL-3638.0). Los Angeles: Student Health and Human Services. Available: http://notebook.lausd.net/pls/ptl/docs/PAGE/CA_LAUSD/FLDR_ORGANIZATIONS/STUDENT_HEALTH_HUMAN_SERVICES/SHHS/DISCIPLINE_POLICY/BUL-3638.0.PDF [accessed May 2009].

Love, J.M., Kisker, E.E., Ross, C.M., Schochet, P.Z., Brooks-Gunn, J., Paulsell, D., et al. (2002). *Making a Difference in the Lives of Infants and Toddlers and Their Families: The Impacts of Early Head Start. Volume I: Final Technical Report*. Princeton, NJ: Mathematica Policy Research.

Lowry-Webster, H.M., Barrett, P.M., and Dadds, M. (2001). A universal prevention trial of anxiety and depressive symptomatology in childhood: Preliminary data from an Australian study. *Behaviour Change, 18*(1), 36-50.

Lozoff, B., Jimenez, E., Hagen, J., Mollen, E., and Wolf, A.W. (2000). Poorer behavioral and developmental outcome more than 10 years after treatment for iron deficiency in infancy. *Pediatrics, 105*(4), E51.

Ludwig, J., and Miller, M. (2005). Interpreting the WIC debate. *Journal of Policy Analysis and Management, 24*(4), 691-701.

Ludwig, J., and Miller, D.L. (2007). Does Head Start improve children's life chances? Evidence from a regression discontinuity design. *Quarterly Journal of Economics, 122*, 159-208.

Ludwig, J., and Phillips, D. (2007). *The Benefits and Costs of Head Start.* NBER working paper No. W12973. Cambridge, MA: National Bureau of Economic Research.

Lundahl, B.W., Nimer, J., and Parsons, B. (2006). Preventing child abuse: A meta-analysis of parent training programs. *Research on Social Work Practice, 16*, 251-262.

Luria, A.R. (1980). *Higher Cortical Functions in Man.* New York: Basic Books.

Luthar, S.S. (1999). *Poverty and Children's Adjustment. Developmental Clinical Psychology and Psychiatry Series* (vol. 41). Thousand Oaks, CA: Sage.

Luthar, S.S. (2003). *Resilience and Vulnerability: Adaptation in the Context of Childhood Adversities.* New York: Cambridge University Press.

Luthar, S.S., and Cicchetti, D. (2000). The construct of resilience: Implications for interventions and social policies. *Development and Psychopathology, 12*, 857-885.

Luthar, S.S., and Lantendresse, S.J. (2005). Comparable "risks" at the socioeconomic status extremes: Pre-adolescents' perceptions of parenting. *Development and Psychopathology, 17*, 207-230.

Lynch, F.L., Hornbrook, M., Clarke, G.N., Perrin, N., Polen, M.R., O'Connor, E., and Dickerson, J. (2005). Cost-effectiveness of an intervention to prevent depression in at-risk teens. *Archives of General Psychiatry, 62*(11), 1241-1248.

Lyons, D.E., Santos, L.R., and Keil, F.C. (2006). Reflections of other minds: How primate social cognition can inform the function of mirror neurons. *Current Opinion in Neurobiology, 16*(2), 230-234.

MacKinnon, D.P. (2008). *Introduction to Statistical Mediation Analysis.* Mahwah, NJ: Lawrence Erlbaum.

MacKinnon, D.P., and Dwyer, J.H. (1993). Estimating mediated effects in prevention studies. *Evaluation Review, 17*, 144-158.

MacKinnon, D.P., Weber, M.D., and Pentz, M.A. (1989). How do school-based drug prevention programs work and for whom? *Drugs and Society, 3*, 125-143.

MacKinnon, D.P., Lockwood, C.M., Hoffman, J.M., West, S.G., and Sheets, V. (2002). A comparison of methods to test mediation and other intervening variable effects. *Psychological Methods, 7*, 83-104.

MacKinnon, D.P., Lockwood, C.M., Brown, C.H., and Hoffman, J.M. (2007). The intermediate endpoint effect in logistic and probit regression. *Clinical Trials, 4*, 499-513.

MacLeod, J., and Nelson, G. (2000). Programs for the promotion of family wellness and the prevention of child maltreatment: A meta-analytic review. *Child Abuse and Neglect, 24*(9), 1127–1149.

Madison, S., McKay, M.M., and the CHAMP Collaborative Board. (1998). *Parents on the Move.* Funded grant proposal, Center for Urban Educational Research and Development (CUERD). Available from M.M. McKay, Mount Sinai Hospital, NY.

Madison, S., McKay, M.M., Paikoff, R., and Bell, C.C. (2000). Basic research and community collaboration: Necessary ingredients for the development of a family-based HIV prevention program. *AIDS Education and Prevention, 12*(4), 281-298.

Madon, T., Hofman, K.J., Kupfer, L., and Glass, R.I. (2007). Public health: Implementation science. *Science, 318*(5857), 1728-1729.

Maekikyroe, T., Sauvola, A., Moring, J., Veijola, J., Nieminen, P., Jarvelin, M.-R., and Isohanni, M. (1998). Hospital-treated psychiatric disorders in adults with a single-parent and two-parent family background: A 28-year follow-up of the 1966 Northern Finland birth cohort. *Family Process, 37*(3), 335-344.

Maestas, N., and Gaillot, S. (2008). *An Outcome Evaluation of the Spirituality for Kids Program, Technical Report.* Santa Monica, CA: RAND.

Magnuson, K., Ruhm, C., and Waldfogel, J. (2007). The persistence of preschool effects: Do subsequent classroom experiences matter? *Early Childhood Research Quarterly, 22*(1), 18-38.

Mahieu, G., Denis, S., Lovialle, M., and Vancassel, S. (2008). Synergistic effects of stress and omega-3 fatty acid deprivation on emotional response and brain lipid composition in adult rats. *Prostaglandins Leukot Essent Fatty Acids, 78,* 391-401.

Maier, H., and Lachman, M.E. (2000). Consequences of early parental loss and separation for health and well-being in midlife. *International Journal of Behavioral Development, 24*(2), 183-189.

Manassis, K., Mendlowitz, S.L., Scapillato, D., Avery, D., Fiksenbaum, L., Freire, M., Monga, S., and Owens, M. (2002). Group and individual cognitive-behavioral therapy for childhood anxiety disorders: A randomized trial. *Journal of the American Academy of Child and Adolescent Psychiatry, 41,* 1423-1430.

Mark, T.L., Coffey, R.M., Vandivort-Warren, R., Harwood, H.J., King, E.C., and MHSA Spending Estimates Team. (2005). U.S. spending for mental health and substance abuse treatment, 1991-2001. *Health Affairs,* Suppl. Web Exclusives, W5-133-W5-142.

Marks, I.M., Cavanagh, K., and Gega, L. (2007). *Hands-on Help: Computer-Aided Psychotherapy.* Florence, NY: Taylor and Francis.

Marsh, R., Alexander, G.M., Packard, M.G., Zhu, H., Wingard, J.C., Quackenbush, G., and Peterson, B.S. (2004). Habit learning in Tourette syndrome: A translational neuroscience approach to a developmental psychopathology. *Archives of General Psychiatry, 61*(12), 1259-1268.

Marsh, R., Zhu, H., Schultz, R.T., Quackenbush, G., Royal, J., Skudlarski, P., and Peterson, B.S. (2006). A developmental fMRI study of self-regulatory control. *Human Brain Mapping, 27*(11), 848-863.

Marsh, R., Zhu, H., Wang, Z., Skudlarski, P., and Peterson, B.S. (2007). A developmental fMRI study of self-regulatory control in Tourette's syndrome. *American Journal of Psychiatry, 164*(6), 955-966.

Marsh, R., Gerber, A.J., and Peterson, B.S. (2008). Neuroimaging studies of normal brain development and their relevance for understanding childhood neuropsychiatric disorders. *Journal of the American Academy of Child and Adolescent Psychiatry, 47*(11), 1233-1251.

Marsh, R., Gerber, A.J., Steinglass, J.E., O'Leary, K.G., Walsh, B.T., and Peterson, B.S. (2009). Deficient activity in the neural systems that mediate self-regulator control in Bulimia Nervosa. *Archives of General Psychiatry, 66*(1), 51-63.

Marshall, C.R., Noor, A., Vincent, J.B., Lionel, A.C., Feuk, L., Skaug, J., et al. (2008). Structural variation of chromosomes in autism spectrum disorder. *American Journal of Human Genetics, 82*(2), 477-488.

Marshall, M., Lewis, S., Lockwood, A., Drake, R., Jones, P., and Croudace, T. (2005). Association between duration of untreated psychosis and outcome in cohorts of first-episode patients: A systematic review. *Archives of General Psychiatry, 62,* 975-983.

Martin, A.J., and Sanders, M.R. (2003). Balancing work and family: A controlled evaluation of the Triple P-Positive Parenting Program as a work-site intervention. *Child and Adolescent Mental Health, 8,* 161-169.

Martinez, C.R., Jr., and Forgatch, M.S. (2001). Preventing problems with boy's noncompliance: Effects of a parent training intervention for divorcing mothers. *Journal of Consulting and Clinical Psychology, 69,* 416-428.

Maryland Governor's Office of Crime Control and Prevention. (2003). *Maryland Blueprints.* Available: http://www.jhsph.edu/preventyouthviolence/Resources/blueprints.sect1.pdf and http://www.jhsph.edu/preventyouthviolence/Resources/blueprints.sect2.pdf [accessed August 2008].

Masi, R., and Cooper, J. (2006). *Children's Mental Health Facts for Policymakers.* New York: National Center for Children in Poverty. Available: http://www.nccp.org/publications/pub_687.html [accessed August 2008].

Masten, A.S. (2001). Ordinary magic: Resilience processes in development. *American Psychologist, 56,* 227-238.

Masten, A.S. (2004). Regulatory processes, risk, and resilience in adolescent development. *Annals of the New York Academy of Sciences, 1021,* 310-319.

Masten, A.S. (2006). Developmental psychopathology: Pathways to the future. *International Journal of Behavior Disorders, 30,* 47-54.

Masten, A.S., and Coatsworth, J.D. (1995). Competence, resilience, and psychopathology. In D. Cicchetti and D.J. Cohen (Eds.), *Developmental Psychopathology: Risk, Disorder, and Adaptation* (vol. 2, pp. 715-752). New York: Wiley.

Masten, A.S., Roisman, G.I., Long, J.D., Burt, K.B., Obradovic, J., Riley, J.R., Boelcke-Stennes, K., and Tellegen, A. (2005). Developmental cascades: Linking academic achievement and externalizing and internalizing symptoms over 20 years. *Developmental Psychology, 41*(5), 733-746.

Masten, A.S., Burt, K., and Coatsworth, J.D. (2006). Competence and psycho-pathology in development. In D. Cicchetti and D.J. Cohen, (Eds.), *Developmental Psychopathology Risk, Disorder, and Adaptation* (vol. 3, pp. 696-738). New York: Wiley.

Masten, A.S., Obradovic, J., and Burt, K.B. (2006). Resilience in emerging adulthood: Developmental perspectives on continuity and transformation. In J.J. Arnett and J.L. Tanner (Eds.), *Emerging Adults in America: Coming of Age in the 21st Century* (pp. 173-190). Washington, DC: American Psychological Association.

Masten, A.S., Faden, V.B., Zucker, R.A., and Spear, L.P. (2008). Underage drinking: A developmental framework. *Pediatrics, 121*(Suppl. 4), S235-S251.

Mathalon, D.H., Sullivan, E.V., Lim, K.O., and Pfefferbaum, A. (2001). Progressive brain volume changes and the clinical course of schizophrenia in men: A longitudinal magnetic resonance imaging study. *Archives of General Psychiatry, 58*(2), 148-157.

Maton, K., Schellenbach, C., Leadbeater, B., and Solarz, A. (Eds.). (2004). *Investing in Children, Youth, Families, and Communities: Strengths-Based Public Policies.* Washington, DC: American Psychological Association.

May, P.A., Sena, P., Hurt, L., and DeBruyn, L.M. (2005). Outcome evaluation of a public health approach to suicide prevention in an American Indian tribal nation. *American Journal of Public Health, 95*(7), 1238-1244.

Mayer, G.R. (1995). Preventing antisocial behavior in the schools. *Journal of Applied Behavior Analysis, 28*(4), 467-478.

Mayes, L.C., and Suchman, N. (2006). Developmental pathways to substance abuse. In D. Cicchetti and D. Cohen (Eds.), *Developmental Psychopathology: Risk, Disorder, and Adaptation* (vol. 3, pp. 599-619). New York: Wiley.

McBride, C.K., Baptiste, D., Paikoff, R.L., Madison-Boyd, S., Coleman, D., and Bell, C.C. (2007). Family-based HIV preventive intervention: Child-level results from the CHAMP family program. In M.M. McKay and R.L. Paikoff (Eds.), *Community Collaborative Partnerships: The Foundation for HIV Prevention Research Efforts* (pp. 203-220). Binghamton, NY: Haworth Press.

McCabe, S.E. (2008). Screening for drug abuse among medical and nonmedical users of prescription drugs in a probability sample of college students. *Archives of Pediatric and Adolescent Medicine, 162*(3), 225-231.

McCain, A.P., and Kelley, M.L. (1993). Managing the classroom behavior of an ADHD preschooler: The efficacy of a school-home note intervention. *Child and Family Behavior Therapy, 15,* 33.

McCann, J.C., and Ames, B.N. (2008). Is there convincing biological or behavioral evidence linking vitamin D deficiency to brain dysfunction? *The Journal of the Federation of American Societies for Experimental Biology, 22,* 982-1001.

McCartney, K., and Rosenthal, R. (2000). Effect size, practical importance, and social policy for children. *Child Development, 71,* 173-180.

McCauley, E., Katon, W., Russo, J., Richardson, L., and Lozano, P. (2007). Impact of anxiety and depression on functional impairment in adolescents with asthma. *General Hospital Psychiatry, 29*(3), 214-222.

McClure, E.B., and Pine, D.S. (2006). Social anxiety and emotion regulation: A model for developmental psychopathology perspectives on anxiety disorders. In D. Cicchetti and D.J. Cohen (Eds.), *Developmental Psychopathology: Risk, Disorder, and Adaptation* (vol. 3, pp. 470-502). New York: Wiley.

McCormick, A., McKay, M.M., Wilson, M., McKinney, L., Paikoff, R., Bell, C., Baptiste, D., Coleman, D., Gillming, G., Madison, S., and Scott, R. (2000). Involving families in an urban HIV prevention intervention: How community collaboration addresses barriers to participation. *AIDS Education and Prevention, 12*(4), 299-307.

McDermott, B.M., Mamum, A.A., Najman, J.M., Williams, G.M., O'Callaghan, M.J., and Bor, W. (2008). Preschool children perceived by mother as irregular eaters. *Journal of Developmental Behavioral Pediatrics, 29,* 197-205.

McFarlane, W.R. (2007). Prevention of schizophrenia. In *Report to the Institute of Medicine.* Washington, DC: The National Academies Press.

McGaugh, J.L. (2004). The amygdala modulates the consolidation of memories of emotionally arousing experiences. *Annual Review of Neuroscience, 27,* 1-28.

McGlashan, T.H., and Hoffman, R.E. (2000). Schizophrenia as a disorder of developmentally reduced synaptic connectivity. *Archives of General Psychiatry, 57*(7), 637-648.

McGlashan, T.H., Addington, J., Cannon, T., Heinimaa, M., McGorry, P., O'Brien, M., Penn, D., Perkins, D., Salokangas, R.K., Walsh, B., Woods, S.W., and Yung, A. (2007). Recruitment and treatment practices for help-seeking "prodromal" patients. *Schizophrenic Bulletin, 33*(3), 715-726.

McGorry, P.D., Yung, A.R., Phillips, L.J., Yuen, H.P., Francey, S., Cosgrave, E.M., Germano, D., Bravin, J., McDonald, T., Blair, A., Adlard, S., and Jackson, H. (2002). Randomized controlled trial of interventions designed to reduce the risk of progression to first-episode psychosis in a clinical sample with subthreshold symptoms. *Archives of General Psychiatry, 59*(10), 921-928.

McKay, A., Fisher, W., Maticka-Tyndale, E., and Barrett, M. (2001). Adolescent sexual health education: Does it work? Can it work better? An analysis of recent research and media reports. *Canadian Journal of Human Sexuality, 10,* 127-135.

McKay, M.M., and Paikoff, R.L. (Eds.). (2007). *Community Collaborative Partnerships: The Foundation for HIV Prevention Research Efforts.* Binghamton, NY: Haworth Press.

McKay, M.M., Baptiste, D., Coleman, D., Madison, S., Paikoff, R., and Scott, R. (2000). Preventing HIV risk exposure in urban communities: The CHAMP family program. In W. Pequegnat and J. Szapocznik (Eds.), *Working with Families in the Era of HIV/AIDS* (pp. 67-87). Thousand Oaks, CA: Sage.

McKay, M.M., Chasse, K.T., Paikoff, R., McKinney, L.D., Baptiste, D., Coleman, D., Madison, S., and Bell, C.C. (2004). Family-level impact of the CHAMP family program: A community collaborative effort to support urban families and reduce youth HIV risk exposure. *Family Process, 43*(1), 79-93.

McKay, M.M., Bannon, W.M., Rodriquez, J., and Chasse, K.T. (2007). Understanding African American youth HIV knowledge: Exploring the role of racial socialization and family communication about "hard to talk about topics." In M.M. McKay and R.L. Paikoff (Eds.), *Community Collaborative Partnerships: The Foundation for HIV Prevention Research Efforts* (pp. 79-98). Binghamton, NY: Haworth Press.

McKay, M.M., Block, M., Mellins, C., Traube, D.E., Brackis-Cott, E., Minott, D., Miranda, C., Petterson, J., and Abrams, E.J. (2007). Adapting a family-based HIV prevention program for HIV-infected preadolescents and their families. *Social Work in Mental Health, 5*(3/4), 355-378.

McKay, M.M., Hibbert, R., Lawrence, R., Miranda, A., Paikoff, R., Bell, C.C., Madison-Boyd, S., Baptiste, D., Coleman, D., Pinto, R.M., and Bannon, W.M. (2007). Creating mechanisms for meaningful collaboration between members of urban communities and university-based HIV prevention researchers. In M.M. McKay and R.L. Paikoff (Eds.), *Community Collaborative Partnerships: The Foundation for HIV Prevention Research Efforts* (pp. 147-168). Binghamton, NY: Haworth Press.

McKiernan, K.A., Kaufman, J.N., Kucera-Thompson, J., and Binder, J.R. (2003). A parametric manipulation of factors affecting task-induced deactivation in functional neuroimaging. *Journal of Cognitive Neuroscience, 15*(3), 394-408.

McKinney, W.T. (2001). Overview of the past contributions of animal models and their changing place in psychiatry. *Seminars in Clinical Neuropsychiatry, 6*(1), 68-78.

McLanahan, S.S. (1999). Father absence and the welfare of children. In E.M. Hetherington (Ed.), *Coping with Divorce, Single Parenting, and Remarriage: A Risk and Resiliency Perspective* (pp. 117-146). Mahwah, NJ: Lawrence Erlbaum.

McLaughlin, A.E., Campbell, F.A., Pungello, E.P., and Skinner, M. (2007). Depressive symptoms in young adults: The influences of the early home environment and early educational child care. *Child Development, 78*(3), 746-756.

McLoyd, V.C. (1990). The impact of economic hardship on Black families and children: Psychological distress, parenting, and socioemotional development. *Child Development, 61*(2), 311-345.

McMahon, S.D., Grant, K.E., Compas, B.E., Thurm, A.E., and Ey, S. (2003). Stress and psychopathology in children and adolescents: Is there evidence of specificity? *Journal of Child Psychology and Psychiatry and the Allied Disciplines: Annual Research Review, 44*, 107-133.

Mehnert, A., and Koch, U. (2007). Prevalence of acute and post-traumatic stress disorder and comorbid mental disorders in breast cancer patients during primary cancer care: A prospective study. *Psycho-Oncology, 16*, 181-188.

Meier, D., and Woods, G. (Eds.). (2004). *Many Children Left Behind: How the No Child Left Behind Act Is Damaging Our Children and Our Schools*. Boston: Beacon Press.

Meisels, S.J., and Atkins-Burnett, S. (2005). *Developmental Screening in Early Childhood: A Guide (5th ed.)*. Washington, DC: National Association for the Education of Young Children.

Melhem, N.M., Walker, M., Moritz, G., and Brent, D.A. (2008). Antecendents and sequelae of sudden parental death in offspring and surviving caregivers. *Archives of Pediatrics and Adolescent Medicine, 162*(5), 403-410.

Mendel, R.A. (2001). *Less Hype, More Help: Reducing Juvenile Crime, What Works and What Doesn't.* Washington, DC: American Youth Policy Forum.

Mendelsohn, A.L., Dreyer, B.P., Flynn, V., Tomopoulos, S., Rovira, I., Tineo, W., Pebenito, C., Torres, C., Torres, H., and Nixon, A.F. (2005). Use of videotaped interactions during pediatric well-child care to promote child development: A randomized, controlled trial. *Journal of Developmental and Behavioral Pediatrics, 26*, 34-41.

Mendlowitz, S.L., Manassis, K., Bradley, S., Scapillato, D., Miezitis, S., and Shaw, B. (1999). Cognitive behavioral group treatments in childhood anxiety disorders: The role of parental involvement. *Journal of the American Academy of Child and Adolescent Psychiatry, 38*, 1223-1229.

Merry, S.N., and Spence, S.H. (2007). Attempting to prevent depression in youth: A systematic review of the evidence. *Early Intervention in Psychiatry, 1*, 128-137.

Merzenich, M.M., Nelson, R.J., Stryker, M.P., Cynader, M.S., Schoppmann, A., and Zook, J.M. (1984). Somatosensory cortical map changes following digit amputation in adult monkeys. *Journal of Comparative Neurology, 224*(4), 591-605.

Meyer, U., Yee, B.K., and Feldon, J. (2007). The neurodevelopmental impact of prenatal infections at different times of pregnancy: The earlier the worse? *Neuroscientist, 13*(3), 241-256.

Michaud, C.M., McKenna, M.T., Begg, S., Tomijima, N., Majmudar, M., Bulzacchelli, M.T., Ebrahim, S., Ezzati, M., Salomon, J.A., Kreiser, J.G., Hogan, M., and Murray, C.J.L. (2006). The burden of disease and injury in the United States, 1996. *Population Health Metrics, 4*, 11.

Michel, A.E., and Garey, L.J. (1984). The development of dendritic spines in the human visual cortex. *Human Neurobiology, 3*(4), 223-227.

Mihalic, S., and Aultman-Bettridge, T. (2004). A guide to effective school-based prevention programs. In W.L. Tulk (Ed.), *School Crime and Policing.* Englewood Cliffs, NJ: Prentice Hall.

Mihalic, S., and Irwin, K. (2003). From research to real world settings: Factors influencing the successful replication of model programs. *Youth Violence and Juvenile Justice, 1*, 307-329.

Mihalic, S., Ballard, D., Michalski, A., Tortorice, J., Cunningham, L., and Argamaso, S. (2002). *Blueprints for Violence Prevention, Violence Initiative: Final Process Evaluation Report.* Boulder, CO: Center for the Study and Prevention of Violence, Institute of Behavioral Science, University of Colorado.

Miller, B.C., Norton, M.C., Curtis, T., Hill, E.J., Schwaneveldt, P., and Young, M.H. (1997). The timing of sexual intercourse among adolescents: Family, peer, and other antecedents. *Youth and Society, 29*(1), 54-83.

Miller, K.S., Forehand, R., and Kotchick, B.A. (1999). Adolescent sexual behavior in two ethnic minority samples: The role of family variables. *Journal of Marriage and the Family, 61*, 85-98.

Miller, N.S., Sheppard, L.M., Colenda, C.C., and Magen, J. (2001). Why physicians are unprepared to treat patients who have alcohol and drug-related disorders. *Academic Medicine, 76*, 410-418.

Miller, R.L., and Shinn, M. (2005). Learning from communities: Overcoming difficulties in dissemination of prevention and promotion efforts. *American Journal of Community Psychology, 35*, 169-183.

Miller, T. (2004). The social costs of adolescent problem behavior. In A. Biglan, P. Brennan, S. Foster, and H. Holder (Eds.), *Helping Adolescents at Risk: Prevention of Multiple Problem Behaviors* (pp. 31-56). New York: Guilford Press.

Mills, C., Stephan, S.H., Moore, E., Weist, M.D., Daly, B.P., and Edwards, M. (2006). The President's New Freedom Commission: Capitalizing on opportunities to advance school-based mental health services. *Clinical Child and Family Psychology Review, 9,* 149-161.

Minkler, M. (2004). Ethical challenges for the "outside" researcher in community-based participatory research. *Health Education and Behavior, 31*(6), 684-697.

Mirsky, A.F., Yardley, S.L., Jones, B.P., Walsh, D., and Kendler, K.S. (1995). Analysis of the attention deficit in schizophrenia: A study of patients and their relatives in Ireland. *Journal of Psychiatric Research, 29*(1), 23-42.

Mishkin, M., and Manning, F.J. (1978). Nonspatial memory after selective prefrontal lesions in monkeys. *Brain Research, 143*(2), 313-323.

Mitchell, A., and Alliance for Early Childhood Finance. (2005). *Success Stories: State Investment in Early Care and Education in Illinois, North Carolina and Rhode Island.* Raleigh, NC: Smart Start's National Technical Assistance Center.

Mitchell, R.E., Florin, P., and Stevenson, J.F. (2002) Supporting community-based prevention and health promotion initiatives: Developing effective technical assistance systems. *Health Education and Behavior, 29*(5), 620-639.

Moffatt, M.F. (2008). Genes in asthma: New genes and new ways. *Current Opinion in Allergy and Clinical Immunology, 8,* 411-417.

Moffitt, T.E., Caspi, A., Rutter, M., and Silva, P.A. (2001). *Sex Differences in Antisocial Behaviour: Conduct Disorder, Delinquency, and Violence in the Dunedin Longitudinal Study.* New York: Cambridge University Press.

Molnar, B.E., Buka, S.L., and Kessler, R.C. (2001). Child sexual abuse and subsequent psychopathology: Results from the national comorbidity survey. *American Journal of Public Health, 91*(5), 753-760.

Monk, C.S., Webb, S.J., and Nelson, C.A. (2001). Prenatal neurobiological development: Molecular mechanisms and anatomical change. *Developmental Neuropsychology, 19*(2), 211-236.

Moreno, C., Laje, G., Blanco, C., Jiang, H., Schmidt, A.B., and Olfson, M. (2007). National trends in the outpatient diagnosis and treatment of bipolar disorder in youth. *Archives of General Psychiatry, 64,* 1032-1039.

Moriceau, S., and Sullivan, R.M. (2005). Neurobiology of infant attachment. *Developmental Psychobiology, 47*(3), 230-242.

Moriceau, S., and Sullivan, R.M. (2006). Maternal presence serves as a switch between learning fear and attraction in infancy. *Nature Neuroscience, 9*(8), 1004-1006.

Morris, P., Duncan, G., and Clark-Kauffman, E. (2005). Child well-being in an era of welfare reform: The sensitivity of transitions in development to policy change. *Developmental Psychology, 41,* 919-932.

Moser, M.B., and Moser, E.I. (1998). Functional differentiation in the hippocampus. *Hippocampus, 8*(6), 608-619.

Moy, S.S., and Nadler, J.J. (2008). Advances in behavioral genetics: Mouse models of autism. *Molecular Psychiatry, 13*(1), 4-26.

Mrazek, P.J., and Hall, M. (1997). A policy perspective on prevention. *American Journal of Community Psychology, 25*(2), 221-226.

Mrazek, P.J., Biglan, A., and Hawkins, J.D. (2004). *Community-Monitoring Systems: Tracking and Improving the Well-being of America's Children and Adolescents.* Falls Church, VA: Society for Prevention Research. Available: http://www.preventionresearch.org/CMSbook.pdf [accessed August 2008].

Mrzljak, L., Uylings, H.B., Kostovic, I., and van Eden, C.G. (1992). Prenatal development of neurons in the human prefrontal cortex. II. A quantitative Golgi study. *Journal of Comparative Neurology, 316*(4), 485-496.

Muhle, R., Trentacoste, S.V., and Rapin, I. (2004). The genetics of autism. *Pediatrics, 113*(5), e472-e486.

Muñoz, R.F., and Ying, Y.W. (1993). *The Prevention of Depression: Research and Practice.* Baltimore, MD: Johns Hopkins University Press.

Muñoz, R.F., Glish, M., Soo-Hoo, T., and Robertson, J.L. (1982). The San Francisco mood survey project: Preliminary work toward the prevention of depression. *American Journal of Community Psychology, 10*, 317-329.

Muñoz, R.F., Mrazek, P.J., and Haggerty, R.J. (1996). Institute of Medicine report on prevention of mental disorders: Summary and commentary. *American Psychologist, 51*, 1116-1122.

Muñoz, R.F., Lenert, L.L., Delucchi, K., Stoddard, J., Pérez, J.E., Penilla, C., and Pérez-Stable, E.J. (2006). Toward evidence-based Internet interventions: A Spanish/English web site for international smoking cessation trials. *Nicotine and Tobacco Research, 8*, 77-87.

Muñoz, R.F., Le, H.N., Clarke, G.N., Barrera, A.Z., and Torres, L.D. (2008). Preventing first onset and recurrence of major depressive episodes. In I.H. Gotlib and C.L. Hammen (Eds.). *Handbook of Depression* (2nd ed., pp. 533-553). New York: Guilford Press.

Murcia, C.L., Gulden, F., and Herrup, K. (2005). A question of balance: A proposal for new mouse models of autism. *International Journal of Developmental Neuroscience, 23*(2-3), 265-275.

Muris, P. (2006). The pathogenesis of childhood anxiety disorders: Considerations from a developmental psychopathology perspective. *International Journal of Behavioral Development, 30*(1), 5-11.

Muris, P., and Merckelbach, H. (1998). Perceived parental rearing: Behavior and anxiety disorder symptoms in normal children. *Personality and Individual Differences, 25*, 1199-1206.

Murphy, S.A. (2003). Optimal dynamic treatment regimes (with discussion). *Journal of the Royal Statistical Society, Series B, 65*, 331-366.

Murphy, S.A. (2005). An experimental design for the development of adaptive treatment strategies. *Statistics in Medicine, 24*(10), 1455-1481.

Murphy, S.A., van der Laan, M.J., Robins, J.M., and Conduct Problems Prevention Research Group. (2001). Marginal mean models for dynamic regimes. *Journal of the American Statistical Association, 96*, 1410-1423.

Murphy, S.A., Collins, L.M., and Rush, A.J. (2007). Customizing treatment to the patient: Adaptive treatment strategies. *Drug and Alcohol Dependence, 88*(2), s1-s72.

Murphy, S.A., Lynch, K.G., McKay, J.R., Oslin, D., and TenHave, T. (2007). Developing adaptive treatment strategies in substance abuse research. *Drug and Alcohol Dependence, 88*(2), s24-s30.

Murray, D.M. (1998). *Design and Analysis of Group-Randomized Trials.* New York: Oxford University Press.

Murray, L., and Carothers, A.D. (1990). The validation of the Edinburgh post-natal depression scale on a community sample. *British Journal of Psychiatry, 157*, 288-290.

Murry, V.M., and Brody, G.H. (2004). Partnering with community stakeholders: Engaging rural American families in basic research and the Strong African American Families Preventive Intervention Program. *Journal of Marital and Family Therapy, 30*(3), 271-283.

Murry, V.M., Brody, G.H., McNair, L.D., Luo, Z., Gibbons, F.X., Gerrard, M., and Wills, T.A. (2005). Parental involvement promotes rural African American youths' self-pride and sexual self-concepts. *Journal of Marriage and Family, 67*(3), 627-642.

Muthén, B.O. (1991). Analysis of longitudinal data using latent variable models with varying parameters. In L. Collins and J. Horn (Eds.), *Best Methods for the Analysis of Change: Recent Advances, Unanswered Questions, Future Directions* (pp. 1-17). Washington, DC: American Psychological Association.

Muthén, B.O. (1997). Latent variable modeling with longitudinal and multilevel data. In A. Raftery (Ed.), *Sociological Methodology* (pp. 453-480). Boston: Blackwell.

Muthén, B.O. (2007). Latent variable hybrids: Overview of old and new models. In G.R. Hancock and K.M. Samuelsen (Eds.), *Advances in Latent Variable Mixture Models* (pp. 1-24). Charlotte, NC: Information Age.

Muthén, B.O., and Asparouhov, T. (2006). Growth mixture analysis: Models with non-Gaussian random effects. In G. Fitzmaurice, M. Davidian, G. Verbeke, and G. Molenberghs (Eds.), *Advances in Longitudinal Data Analysis*. London, England: Chapman and Hall/CRC Press.

Muthén, B.O., and Curran, P. (1997). General longitudinal modeling of individual differences in experimental designs: A latent variable framework for analysis and power estimation. *Psychological Methods, 2*, 371-402.

Muthén, B.O., and Masyn, K. (2005). Discrete-time survival mixture analysis. *Journal of Educational and Behavioral Statistics, 30*(1), 27-58.

Muthén, L.K., and Muthén, B.O. (2007). *Mplus: Statistical Analysis with Latent Variables: User's Guide, Version 5.1*. Los Angeles: Muthén and Muthén.

Muthén, B.O., and Shedden, K. (1999). Finite mixture modeling with mixture outcomes using the EM algorithm. *Biometrics, 55*, 463-469.

Muthén, B.O., Brown, C.H., Masyn, K., Jo, B., Khoo, S.T., Yang, C.C., Wang, C.P., Kellam, S.G., and Carlin, J.B. (2002). General growth mixture modeling for randomized preventive interventions. *Biostatistics, 3*, 459-475.

Muthén, B.O., Jo, B., and Brown, C.H. (2003). Assessment of treatment effects using latent variable modeling: Comment on the Barnard, Frangakis, Hill and Rubin article—Principal stratification approach to broken randomized experiments: A case study of school choice vouchers in New York City. *Journal of the American Statistical Association, 98*, 311-314.

Myers, K.M., and Davis, M. (2007). Mechanisms of fear extinction. *Molecular Psychiatry, 12*(2), 120-150.

Mytton, J., DiGuiseppi, C., Gough, D., Taylor, R., and Logan, S. (2006). School-based secondary prevention programmes for preventing violence. *Cochrane Database of Systematic Reviews, 3*, Art. No. CD004606.

Nagin, D.S., and Land, K.C. (1993). Age, criminal careers, and population heterogeneity: Specification and estimation of a nonparametric, mixed Poisson model. *Criminology, 31*, 327-362.

Najaka, S.S., Gottfredson, D.C., and Wilson, D.B. (2001). A meta-analytic inquiry into the relationship between selected risk factors and problem behavior. *Prevention Science, 2*, 257-271.

Natale, M., Gur, R.E., and Gur, R.C. (1983). Hemispheric asymmetries in processing emotional expressions. *Neuropsychologia, 21*, 555-565.

National Advisory Mental Health Council Workgroup on Child and Adolescent Mental Health Intervention Development and Deployment. (2001). *Blueprint for Change: Research on Child and Adolescent Mental Health*. Bethesda, MD: National Institute of Mental Health.

National Advisory Mental Health Council Workgroup on Mental Disorders Prevention Research. (1998). *Priorities for Prevention Research at NIMH*. (NIH Publication No. 98-4321). Bethesda, MD: National Institute of Mental Health.

National Center on Addiction and Substance Abuse at Columbia University. (2004). *Criminal Neglect: Substance Abuse, Juvenile Justice and the Children Left Behind.* Available: http://www.casacolumbia.org/absolutenm/articlefiles/379-Criminal%20Neglect.pdf [accessed August 2008].

National Institute of Mental Health. (1999). *Mental Health: A Report of the Surgeon General.* Bethesda, MD: Author.

National Institute of Mental Health. (2002). *Dissemination and Implementation Research in Mental Health.* Available: http://grants.nih.gov/grants/guide/pa-files/pa-02-131.html [accessed August 2008].

National Institute of Mental Health. (2003). *Breaking Ground, Breaking Through: The Strategic Plan for Mood Disorders Research.* Available: http://www.nimh.nih.gov/about/strategic-planning-reports/breaking-ground-breaking-through--the-strategic-plan-for-mood-disorders-research.pdf [accessed August 2008].

National Institute of Mental Health. (2006a). *Bridging Science and Service: A Report by the National Advisory Mental Health Council's Clinical Treatment and Services Research Workgroup.* Bethesda, MD: Author. Available: http://www.ti-gr.com/Resources/Publication%20Materials/NIMH-Bridging%20Science%20and%20Service.pdf [accessed April 2009].

National Institute of Mental Health. (2006b). *The Road Ahead: Research Partnerships to Transform Services.* Available: http://www.nimh.nih.gov/about/advisory-boards-and-groups/namhc/reports/road-aHead.pdf [accessed August 2008].

National Institute on Alcohol Abuse and Alcoholism. (2002). *How to Reduce High-Risk College Drinking: Use Proven Strategies, Fill Research Gaps.* Final report of the Panel on Prevention and Treatment. Rockville, MD: National Institutes of Health.

National Institute on Drug Abuse. (1997). *Preventing Drug Use Among Children and Adolescents: A Research-Based Guide for Parents, Educators, and Community Leaders* (1st ed.). Rockville, MD: National Institutes of Health.

National Institute on Drug Abuse. (2003). *Preventing Drug Use Among Children and Adolescents: A Research-Based Guide for Parents, Educators, and Community Leaders* (2nd ed.). Rockville, MD: National Institutes of Health.

National Institutes of Health. (2006). *NIH Seeks Input on Proposed Repository for Genetic Information* (press release, August 30). Available: http://www.nih.gov/news/pr/aug2006/od-30.htm [accessed February 2009].

National Research Council. (2002). *Minority Students in Special and Gifted Education.* M.S. Donovan and C.T. Cross (Eds.), Committee on Minority Representation in Special Education, Division of Behavioral and Social Sciences and Education. Washington, DC: National Academy Press.

National Research Council and Institute of Medicine. (2000). *From Neurons to Neighborhoods: The Science of Early Childhood Development.* J.P. Shonkoff and D.A. Phillips (Eds.), Committee on Integrating the Science of Early Childhood Development, Board on Children, Youth, and Families. Washington, DC: National Academy Press.

National Research Council and Institute of Medicine. (2001). *Juvenile Crime, Juvenile Justice.* J. McCord, C.S. Widom, and N.A. Crowell (Eds.), Panel on Juvenile Crime: Prevention, Treatment, and Control, Committee on Law and Justice, and Board on Children, Youth, and Families. Washington, DC: National Academy Press.

National Research Council and Institute of Medicine. (2002). *Community Programs to Promote Youth Development.* J. Eccles and J.A. Gootman (Eds.), Committee on Community-Level Programs for Youth, Board on Children, Youth, and Families. Washington, DC: National Academy Press.

National Research Council and Institute of Medicine. (2003). *Engaging Schools: Fostering High School Students' Motivation to Learn.* Committee on Increasing High School Students' Engagement and Motivation to Learn, Board on Children, Youth, and Families. Washington, DC: The National Academies Press.

National Research Council and Institute of Medicine. (2004a). *Children's Health, the Nation's Wealth: Assessing and Improving Child Health.* Committee on Evaluation of Children's Health, Board on Children, Youth, and Families, Division of Behavioral and Social Sciences and Education. Washington, DC: The National Academies Press.

National Research Council and Institute of Medicine. (2004b). *Reducing Underage Drinking: A Collective Responsibility.* R.J. Bonnie and M.E. O'Connell (Eds.), Committee on Developing a Strategy to Reduce and Prevent Underage Drinking, Board on Children, Youth, and Families. Washington, DC: The National Academies Press.

Neal, J., Altman, K., and Burritt, N. (2003). *South Carolina Toolkit for Evidence-Based Prevention Programs and Strategies.* Available: http://www.daodas.state.sc.us/documents/ToolkitSection1.pdf [accessed May 2009].

Nelson III, C.A., Zeanah, C.H., Fox, N.A., Marshall, P.J., Smyke, A.T., and Guthrie, D. (2007). Cognitive recovery in socially deprived young children: The Bucharest early intervention project. *Science, 318*(5858), 1937-1940.

Nelson, G., Westhues, A., and MacLeod, J. (2003). A meta-analysis of longitudinal research on preschool prevention programs for children. *Prevention and Treatment,* 6, Art. 31. Available: http://journals.apa.org/prevention/volume6/toc-dec18-03.html [accessed February 2009].

Neumann, M.S., and Sogolow, E.D. (2000). Replicating effective programs: HIV/AIDS prevention technology transfer. *AIDS Education and Prevention, 1*(Suppl. A), 35-48.

Nevada State Department of Education. (1998). *Nevada School-Based Substance Abuse and Violence Prevention Programs: An Examination of Effectiveness, 1997-1998.* Carson City: Author.

New Freedom Commission on Mental Health. (2003). *Achieving the Promise: Transforming Mental Health Care in America. Final Report.* (DHHS Pub. No. SMA-03-3832). Rockville, MD: U.S. Department of Health and Human Services.

Newman, B., Mu, H., Butler, L.M., Millikan, R.C., Moorman, P.G., and King, M.C. (1998). Frequency of breast cancer attributable to BRCA1 in a population-based series of American women. *Journal of the American Medical Association, 279*(12), 915-921.

Newton, M., and Ciliska, D. (2005). *Innovations in the Prevention of Eating Disorders: A Systematic Review of Web-based Interventions.* Edmonton, Alberta, Canada: Margaret Wright Scott Research Day, University of Alberta.

Newton, S.S., and Duman, R.S. (2006). Chromatin remodeling: A novel mechanism of psychotropic drug action. *Molecular Pharmacology, 70*(2), 440-443.

Neyman, J. (1990). On the application of probability theory to agricultural experiments. Essay on principles. Section 9. *Statistical Science, 5*(4), 465-472. [Translated and edited by D.M. Dabrowska and T.P. Speed from the Polish original, which appeared in Roczniki Nauk Rolniczych Tom X (1923) 1-51, *Annals of Agricultural Sciences.*]

Nicholls, R.D., and Knepper, J.L. (2001). Genome organization, function, and imprinting in Prader-Willi and Angelman syndromes. *Annual Reviews in Genomics and Human Genetics, 2,* 153-175.

Nitzkin, J., and Smith, S.A. (2004). *Clinical Preventive Services in Substance Abuse and Mental Health Update: From Science to Services.* (HHS Pub. No. SMA-04-3906). Rockville, MD: Center for Mental Health Services, Substance Abuse and Mental Health Services Administration.

Noble, M., McLennan, D., and Whitworth, A. (2009). *Tracking Neighbourhoods: The Economic Deprivation Index 2008.* Social Disadvantage Research Centre, University of Oxford. Available: http://www.communities.gov.uk/documents/communities/pdf/1126154.pdf [accessed April 2009].

Noll, J.G., Trickett, P.K., Harris, W.W., and Putnam, F.W. (2009). The cumulative burden borne by offspring whose mothers were sexually abused as children. *Journal of Interpersonal Violence, 24*(3), 424-449.

Ochsner, K.N., and Gross, J.J. (2005). The cognitive control of emotion. *Trends in Cognitive Sciences, 9*(5), 242-249.

Ochsner, K.N., Bunge, S.A., Gross, J.J., and Gabrieli, J.D. (2002). Rethinking feelings: An fMRI study of the cognitive regulation of emotion. *Journal of Cognitive Neuroscience, 14*(8), 1215-1229.

O'Connor, T.G., and Cameron, J.L. (2006). Translating research findings on early experience to prevention: Animal and human evidence on early attachment relationships. *American Journal of Preventive Medicine, 31*(6 Suppl. 1), S175-S181.

O'Connor, T.G., Marvin, R.S., Rutter, M., Olrick, J.T., and Britner, P.A. (2003). Child-parent attachment following early institutional deprivation. *Development and Psychopathology, 15*(1), 19-38.

Office of Juvenile Justice and Delinquency Prevention. (n.d.). *Title V Training and Technical Assistance Programs for State and Local Governments: Effective and Promising Programs Guide.* Washington, DC: Office of Justice Programs, U.S. Department of Justice.

Office of National Drug Control Policy. (2001). *The Economic Costs of Drug Abuse in the United States, 1992-1998.* (No. NCJ-100636). Washington, DC: Executive Office of the President.

Office of National Drug Control Policy. (2004). *The Economic Costs of Drug Abuse in the United States: 1992-2002.* Pub. No. 207303. Washington, DC: Executive Office of the President.

Ogden, T., and Amlund-Hagen, K. (2006). Multisystemic therapy of serious behavior problems in youth: Sustainability of therapy effectiveness two years after intake. *Child and Adolescent Mental Health, 11,* 142-149.

Ogden, T., Forgatch, M.S., Askeland, E., Patterson, G.R., and Bullock, B.M. (2005). Implementation of parent management training at the national level: The case of Norway. *Journal of Social Work Practice, 19*(3), 319-331.

O'Hara, M.W., and Swain, A.M. (1996). Rates and risk of postpartum depression: A meta-analysis. *International Review of Psychiatry, 8,* 37-54.

Olchowski, A., Foster, E.M., and Webster-Stratton, C. (2007). Implementing behavioral intervention components in a cost-effective manner: Analysis of the incredible years program. *Journal of Early and Intensive Behavior Intervention, 3*(4), 284-304.

Olds, D.L. (2002). Prenatal and infancy home visiting by nurses: From randomized trials to community replication. *Prevention Science, 3,* 153.

Olds, D.L. (2006). The nurse-family partnership: An evidence-based preventive intervention. *Infant Mental Health Journal, 27,* 5-25.

Olds, D.L., Henderson, C.R., Cole, R., Eckenrode, J., Kitzman, H., Luckey, D., Pettitt, L., Sidora, K., Morris, P., and Powers, J. (1998). Long-term effects of nurse home visitation on children's criminal and antisocial behavior: 15-year follow-up of a randomized controlled trial. *Journal of the American Medical Association, 280*(14), 1238-1244.

Olds, D.L., Robinson, J., O'Brien, R., Luckey, D.W., Petit, L.M., Henderson, C.R., Ng, R.N., Korfmacher, J., Hiatt, S., and Talmi, A. (2002). Home visiting by nurses and by paraprofessionals: A randomized controlled trial. *Pediatrics, 110*(3), 486-496.

Olds, D.L., Hill, P.L., O'Brien, R., Racine, D., and Moritz, P. (2003). Taking preventive intervention to scale: The nurse-family partnership. *Cognitive and Behavioral Practice, 10*(4), 278-290.

Olds, D.L., Robinson, J., Pettitt, L., Luckey, D.W., Holmberg, J., Ng, R.K., Isacks, K., Sheff, K., and Henderson, C.R. (2004). Effects of home visits by paraprofessionals and by nurses: Age 4 follow-up results of a randomized trial. *Pediatrics, 114*(6), 1560-1568.

Olsen, M.K, and Schafer, J.L. (2001). A two-part random effects model for semicontinuous longitudinal data. *Journal of the American Statistical Association, 96*, 730-745.

Olweus, D. (1991). Bully/victim problems among school children: Basic facts and effects of a school-based intervention program. In D.J. Pepler and K.H. Rubin (Eds.), *The Development and Treatment of Childhood Aggression* (pp. 411-448). Hillsdale, NJ: Lawrence Erlbaum.

Olweus, D. (2004). The Olweus bullying prevention programme: Design and implementation issues and a new national initiative in Norway. In P.K. Smith, D. Pepler, and K. Rigby (Eds.), *Bullying in Schools: How Successful Can Interventions Be?* (pp. 13-36). Cambridge, England: Cambridge University Press.

Olweus, D. (2005). A useful evaluation design and effects of the Olweus bullying prevention program. *Psychology, Crime, and Law, 11*(4), 389-402.

Olweus, D., Limber, S.P., and Mihalic, S. (1999). *The Bullying Prevention Program: Blueprints for Violence Prevention.* Boulder, CO: Center for the Study and Prevention of Violence.

Ong, S.H., Wickramaratne, P., Tang, M., and Weissman, M.M. (2006). Early childhood sleep and eating problems as predictors of adolescent and adult mood and anxiety disorders. *Journal of Affective Disorders, 96*, 1-8.

Oosterlaan, J., and Sergeant, J.A. (1998). Effects of reward and response cost on response inhibition in AD/HD, disruptive, anxious, and normal children. *Journal of Abnormal Child Psychology, 26*(3), 161-174.

Orr, S.K., and Bazinet, R.P. (2008). The emerging role of docosahexaenoic acid in neuroinflammation. *Current Opinion in Investigational Drugs, 9*, 735-743.

Orwin, R., Cadell, D., and Chu, A. (2006). *Evaluation of the National Youth Anti-Drug Media Campaign: 2004 Report of Findings.* Washington, DC: Westat.

Orwin, R., Cadell, D., Chu, A., Kalton, G., Maklan, D., Morin, C., Piesse, A., Sridharan, S., Steele, D., Taylor, K., and Tracy, E. (2006). *Evaluation of the National Youth Anti-Drug Media Campaign: 2004 Report of Findings, Executive Summary.* Delivered to National Institute on Drug Abuse, Rockville, MD. Available: http://www.nida.nih.gov/DESPR/Westat/NSPY2004Report/ExecSumVolume.pdf [accessed February 2009].

Osher, D., Dwyer, K., and Jackson, S. (2002). *Safe, Supportive, and Successful Schools, Step by Step.* Rockville, MD: U.S. Department of Health and Human Services.

O'Tuathaigh, C.M., Babovic, D., O'Meara, G., Clifford, J.J., Croke, D.T., and Waddington, J.L. (2007). Susceptibility genes for schizophrenia: Characterization of mutant mouse models at the level of phenotypic behavior. *Neuroscience and Behavioral Reviews, 31*(1), 60-78.

Owen, M.J., O'Donovan, M.C., and Harrison, P.J. (2005). Schizophrenia: A genetic disorder of the synapse? Glutamatergic synapses might be the site of primary abnormalities. *British Medical Journal, 330*(7484), 158-159.

Packard, M.G., and Knowlton, B.J. (2002). Learning and memory functions of the basal ganglia. *Annual Review of Neuroscience, 25*, 563-593.

Paikoff, R.L. (1995). Early heterosexual debut: Situations of sexual possibilities during the transition to adolescence. *American Journal of Orthopsychiatry, 65*(3), 389-401.

Paikoff, R.L., Parfenoff, S.H., Williams, S.A., McCormick, A., Greenwood, G.L., and Hombeck, G.N. (1997). Parenting, parent-child relationships, and sexual possibility situations among African American pre-adolescents: Preliminary findings and implications for HIV prevention research. *Journal of Family Psychology, 11*, 11-22.

Paikoff, R.L., Traube, D.E., and McKay, M.M. (2007). Overview of community collaborative partnerships and empirical findings: The foundation for youth HIV prevention. In M.M. McKay and R.L. Paikoff (Eds.), *Community Collaborative Partnerships: The Foundation for HIV Prevention Research Efforts* (pp. 3-26). Binghamton, NY: Haworth Press.

Palmer, B.A., Pankratz,V.S., and Bostwick, J.M. (2005). The lifetime risk of suicide in schizophrenia: A reexamination. *Archives of General Psychiatry, 62,* 247-253.

Pantin, H., Coatsworth, J.D., Feaster, D.J., Newman, F.L., Briones, E., Prado, G., Schwartz, S.J., and Szapocznik, J. (2003). Familias Unidas: The efficacy of an intervention to promote parental investment in Hispanic immigrant families. *Prevention Sciences, 4,* 189-201.

Pantin, H., Schwartz, S.J., Coatsworth, J.D., Sullivan, S., Briones, E., and Szapocznik, J. (2007). Familias Unidas: A systemic, parent-centered approach to preventing problem behavior in Hispanic adolescents. In P. Tolan, J. Szapocznik, and S. Sambrano (Eds.), *Preventing Youth Substance Abuse: Science-Based Programs for Children and Adolescents* (pp. 211-238). Washington, DC: American Psychological Association.

Pat-Horenczyk, R., Schiff, M., and Doppelt, O. (2006). Maintaining routine despite ongoing exposure to terrorism: A healthy strategy for adolescents? *Journal of Adolescent Health, 39,* 199-205.

Patterson, G.R. (1969). Teaching parents to be behavior modifiers in the classroom. In J. Krumboltz and C.E. Thoresen (Eds.), *Behavioral Counseling: Cases and Techniques* (pp. 155-161). New York: Holt, Rinehart and Winston.

Patterson, G.R. (1974). Retraining of aggressive boys by their parents: Review of recent literature and follow-up evaluation. *Canadian Psychiatric Association Journal, 19,* 142-158.

Patterson, G.R. (1976). The aggressive child: Victim and architect of a coercive system? In E.J. Mash, L.A. Hammerlynck, and L.C. Handy (Eds.), *Behavior Modification and Families* (pp. 267-316). New York: Brunner and Mazel.

Patterson, G.R. (1982). *Coercive Family Process.* Eugene, OR: Castalia.

Patterson, G.R., and Cobb, J.A. (1971). A dyadic analysis of "aggressive" behaviors. In J.P. Hill (Ed.), *Minnesota Symposia on Child Psychology* (vol. 5, pp. 72-129). Minneapolis: University of Minnesota.

Patterson, G.R., and Gullion, M.E. (1968). *Living with Children.* Champaign, IL: Research Press.

Patterson, G.R., DeBaryshe, B.D., and Ramsey, E. (1989). A developmental perspective on antisocial behavior. *American Psychologist, 44,* 329-335.

Patterson, G.R., Reid, J.B., and Eddy, J.M. (2002). A brief history of the Oregon model. In J.B. Reid, G.R. Patterson, and J. Snyder (Eds.), *Antisocial Behavior in Children and Adolescents: A Developmental Analysis and Model for Intervention* (pp. 3-21). Washington, DC: American Psychological Association.

Patterson, G.R., DeGarmo, D.S., and Forgatch, M.S. (2004). Systematic changes in families following prevention trials. *Journal of Abnormal Child Psychology, 32,* 621-633.

Pattison, C., and Lynd-Stevenson, R.M. (2001). The prevention of depressive symptoms in children: The immediate and long-term outcomes of a school-based program. *Behaviour Change, 18,* 92-102.

Paus, T., Zijdenbos, A., Worsley, K., Collins, D.L., Blumenthal, J., Giedd, J.N., Rapoport, J.L., and Evans, A.C. (1999). Structural maturation of neural pathways in children and adolescents: In vivo study. *Science, 283*(5409), 1908-1911.

Paus, T., Collins, D.L., Evans, A.C., Leonard, G., Pike, B., and Zijdenbos, A. (2001). Maturation of white matter in the human brain: A review of magnetic resonance studies. *Brain Research Bulletin, 54*(3), 255-266.

Pearce, B.D. (2001). Schizophrenia and viral infection during neurodevelopment: A focus on mechanisms. *Molecular Psychiatry, 6*(6), 634-646.

Pearson, J.L., and Koretz, D.S. (2001). Opportunities in prevention research at NIMH: Integrating prevention with treatment research. *Prevention and Treatment, 4.* Available: http://journals.apa.org/prevention/volume4/pre0040018.html [accessed February 2009].

Pearson, T.A., and Manolio, T.A. (2008). How to interpret a genome-wide association study. *Journal of the American Medical Association, 299*(11), 1335-1344.

Pedersen, C.B., and Mortensen, P.B. (2001). Evidence of a dose-response relationship between urbanicity during upbringing and schizophrenia risk. *Archives of General Psychiatry, 58,* 1039-1046.

Pedro-Carroll, J.L. (2005). Fostering resilience in the aftermath of divorce: The role of evidence-based programs for children. *Family Court Review, 43,* 52-64.

Pedro-Carroll, J.L., Sutton, J.L., and Wyman, P.A. (1999). A two-year follow-up evaluation of a preventive intervention for young children of divorce. *School Psychology Review, 28,* 467-476.

Pelletier, H., and Abrams, M. (2003, December). *ABCD: Lessons from a Four-State Consortium.* New York: The Commonwealth Fund.

Penner, J.D., and Brown, A.S. (2007). Prenatal infectious and nutritional factors and risk of adult schizophrenia. *Expert Review of Neurotherapeutics, 7*(7), 797-805.

Pennington, B.F., and Ozonoff, S. (1996). Executive functions and developmental psychopathology. *Journal of Child Psychology and Psychiatry, 37*(1), 51-87.

Pentz, M.A. (2003). Anti-drug-abuse policies as prevention strategies. In Z. Sloboda and W.J. Bukoski (Eds.), *Handbook of Drug Abuse Prevention: Theory, Science, and Practice* (Part III, pp. 217-241, Handbook of Sociology and Social Research [Series]). New York: Springer.

Pentz, M.A., MacKinnon, D.P., Dwyer, J.H., Wang, E.Y.I., Hansen, W.B., Flay, B.R., and Johnston, C.L. (1989a). Longitudinal effects of the Midwestern prevention project (MPP) on regular and experimental smoking in adolescents. *Preventive Medicine, 18,* 304-321.

Pentz, M.A., MacKinnon, D.P., Flay, B.R., Hansen, W.B., Johnson, C.A., and Dwyer, J.H. (1989b). Primary prevention of chronic diseases in adolescence: Effects of the Midwestern Prevention Project (MPP) on tobacco use. *American Journal of Epidemiology, 130,* 713-724.

Pentz, M.A., Trebow, E.A., Hansen, W.B., and MacKinnon, D.P. (1990). Effects of program implementation on adolescent drug use behavior: The Midwestern Prevention Project (MPP). *Evaluation Review, 14*(3), 264-289.

Pentz, M.A., Jasuja, G.K., Rohrbach, L.A., Sussman, S., and Bardo, M.T. (2006). Translation in tobacco and drug abuse prevention research. *Evaluation and the Health Professions, 29*(2), 246-271.

Pequegnat, W., and Bray, J. (1997). Families and HIV/AIDS: Introduction to the special sections. *Journal of Family Psychology, 11*(1), 3-10.

Perrin, E., and Stancin, T. (2002). A continuing dilemma: Whether and how to screen for concerns about children's behavior. *Pediatrics in Review, 23,* 264-282.

Perry, C.L., Williams, C.L., Veblen-Mortenson, S., Toomey, T.L., Komro, K.A., Anstine, P.S., McGovern, P.G., Finnegan, J.R., Forster, J.L., Wagenaar, A.C., and Wolfson, M. (1996). Project Northland: Outcomes of a communitywide alcohol use prevention program during early adolescence. *American Journal of Public Health, 86,* 956-965.

Perry, C.L., Williams, C.L., Komro, K.A., Veblen-Mortenson, S., Forster, J.L., Bernstein-Lachter, R., Pratt, L.K., Dudovitz, B., Munson, K.A., Farbakhsh, K., Finnegan, J., and McGovern, P. (2000). Project northland high school interventions: Community action to reduce adolescent alcohol use. *Health Education and Behavior, 27*(1), 29-49.

Perry, C.L., Williams, C.L., Komro, K.A., Veblen-Mortenson, S., Stigler, M.H., Munson, K.A., Farbakhsh, K., Jones, R.M., and Forster, J.L. (2002). Project Northland: Long-term outcomes of community action to reduce adolescent alcohol use. *Health Education Research Theory and Practice, 17,* 117-132.

Perry, C.L., Lee, S., Stigler, M.H., Farbakhsh, K., Komro, K.A., Gewirtz, A.H., and Williams, C. (2007). The impact of Project Northland on selected MMPI-A problem behavior scales. *Journal of Primary Prevention, 28*, 449-465.

Perry, D.F., Dunne, M.C., McFadden, L., and Campbell, D. (2008). Reducing the risk for preschool expulsion: Mental health consultation for young children with challenging behaviors. *Journal of Child and Family Studies, 17*(1), 44-54.

Perry, R.H., Albee, G.W., Bloom, M., and Gullota, T.P. (1996). Training and career pathways in primary prevention. *Journal of Primary Prevention, 16*, 357-371.

Pescosolido, B.A., Jensen, P.S., Martin, J.K., Perry, B.L., Olafsdottir, S., and Fettes, D. (2008). Public knowledge and assessment of child mental health problems: Findings from the national stigma study-children. *Journal of the American Academy of Child and Adolescent Psychiatry, 47*(3), 339-349.

Peterson, B.S. (2003a). Brain imaging studies of the anatomical and functional consequences of preterm birth for human brain development. *Annals of the New York Academy of Sciences, 1008*, 219-237.

Peterson, B.S. (2003b). Conceptual, methodological, and statistical challenges in brain imaging studies of developmentally based psychopathologies. *Development and Psychopathology, 15*, 811-832.

Peterson, B.S. (2004). Habit learning in Tourette syndrome: A translational neuroscience approach to a developmental psychopathology. *Archives of General Psychiatry, 61*(12), 1259-1268.

Peterson, B.S., Skudlarski, P., Anderson, A.W., Zhang, H., Gatenby, J.C., Lacadie, C.M., Leckman, J.F., and Gore, J.C. (1998). A functional magnetic resonance imaging study of tic suppression in Tourette syndrome. *Archives of General Psychiatry, 55*, 326-333.

Peterson, B.S., Skudlarski, P., Zhang, H., Gatenby, J.C., Anderson, A.W., and Gore, J.C. (1999). An fMRI study of Stroop word-color interference: Evidence for cingulate subregions subserving multiple distributed attentional systems. *Biological Psychiatry, 45*, 1237-1258.

Peterson, B.S., Staib, L., Scahill, L., Zhang, H., Anderson, C., Leckman, J.F., Cohen, D.J., Gore, J.C., Albert, J., and Webster, R. (2001). Regional brain and ventricular volumes in Tourette syndrome. *Archives of General Psychiatry, 58*(5), 427-440.

Petras, H., Kellam, S.G., Brown, C.H., Muthén, B.O., Ialongo, N.S., and Poduska, J.M. (2008). Developmental epidemiological courses leading to antisocial personality disorder and violent and criminal behavior: Effects by young adulthood of a universal preventive intervention in first- and second-grade classrooms. *Drug and Alcohol Dependence, 95*(Suppl. 1), S45-S59.

Petrie, J., Bunn, F., and Byrne, G. (2007). Parenting programs for preventing tobacco, alcohol, or drugs misuse in children < 18: A systematic review. *Health Education Research, 22*, 177-191.

Phan, K.L., Fitzgerald, D.A., Nathan, P.J., Moore, G.J., Uhde, T.W., and Tancer, M.E. (2005). Neural substrates for voluntary suppression of negative affect: A functional magnetic resonance imaging study. *Biological Psychiatry, 57*(3), 210-219.

Phillips, S.D., Erkanli, A., Keeler, G., Costello, E.J., and Angold, A. (2006). Disentangling the risks: Parent criminal justice involvement and children's exposure to family risks. *Criminology and Public Policy, 5*, 677-702.

Pignone, M.P., Gaynes, B.N., Rushton, J.L., Burchell, C.M., Orleans, C.T., Mulrow, C.D., and Lohr, K.N. (2002). Screening for depression in adults: A summary of the evidence for the U.S. preventive services task force. *Annals of Internal Medicine, 136*(10), 765-776.

Pigott, T.A. (1999). Gender differences in the epidemiology and treatment of anxiety disorders. *Journal of Clinical Psychiatry, 60*(Suppl. 18), 4-15.

Pilling, S., Bebbington, P., Kuipers, E., Garety, P., Geddes, J., Martindale, B., Orbach, G., and Morgan, C. (2002a). Psychological treatments in schizophrenia: II. Meta-analysis of randomized controlled trials of social skills training and cognitive remediation. *Psychological Medicine, 32*, 783-791.

Pilling, S., Bebbington, P., Kuipers, E., Garety, P., Geddes, J., Orbach, G., and Morgan, C. (2002b). Psychological treatments in schizophrenia: I. Meta-analysis of family intervention and cognitive behavior therapy. *Psychological Medicine, 32*, 763-782.

Pillow, D.R., Sandler, I.N., Braver, S.L., Wolchik, S.A., and Gersten, J.C. (1991). Theory-based screening for prevention: Focusing on mediating processes in children of divorce. *American Journal of Community Psychology, 19*, 809-836.

Pina, A.A., Villalta, I.K., Ortiz, C.D., Gottschall, A.C., Costa, N.M., and Weems, C.F. (2008). Social support, discrimination, and coping as predictors of posttraumatic stress reactions in youth survivors of Hurricane Katrina. *Journal of Clinical Child and Adolescent Psychology, 37*(3), 564-574.

Pine, D.S. (2007). Research review: A neuroscience framework for pediatric anxiety disorders. *Journal of Child Psychology and Psychiatry, 48*(7), 631-648.

Pinto, R.M., McKay, M.M., Baptiste, D., Bell, C.C., Madison-Boyd, S., Paikoff, R., Wilson, M., and Phillips, D. (2007). Motivators and barriers to participation of ethnic minority families in a family-based HIV prevention program. In M.M. McKay and R.L. Paikoff (Eds.), *Community Collaborative Partnerships: The Foundation for HIV Prevention Research Efforts* (pp. 187-201). Binghamton, NY: Haworth Press.

Pitkin, R.M. (2007). Folate and neural tube defects. *American Journal of Clinical Nutrition, 85*(1), 285S-288S.

Pittman, K.J., and Fleming, W.E. (1991, September). *A New Vision: Promoting Youth Development.* Written transcript of live testimony by Karen J. Pittman given before The House Select Committee on Children, Youth and Families. Washington, DC: Center for Youth Development and Policy Research.

Plessen, K.J., and Peterson, B.S. (2008). The neurobiology of impulsivity and self-regulatory control in children with ADHD. In D. Charney and E.J. Nestler (Eds.), *Neurobiology of Mental Illness* (3rd ed.). Oxford, England: Oxford University Press.

Plessen, K.J., Wentzel-Larsen, T., Hugdahl, K., Feineigle, P., Klein, J., Staib, L.H., Leckman, J.F., Bansal, R., and Peterson, B.S. (2004). Altered interhemispheric connectivity in individuals with Tourette's disorder. *American Journal of Psychiatry, 161*(11), 2028-2037.

Plessen, K.J., Bansal, R., Zhu, H., Whiteman, R., Amat, J., Quackenbush, G.A., Martin, L., Durkin, K., Blair, C., Royal, J., Hugdahl, K., and Peterson, B.S. (2006). Hippocampus and amygdala morphology in attention-deficit/hyperactivity disorder. *Archives of General Psychiatry, 63*(7), 795-807.

Podorefsky, D.L., McDonald-Dowdell, M., and Beardslee, W. (2001). Adaptation of preventive interventions for a low-income, culturally diverse community. *Journal of the American Academy of Child and Adolescent Psychiatry, 40*(8), 879-886.

Poduska, J., Kellam, S.G., Wang, W., Brown, C.H., Ialongo, N., and Toyinbo, P. (2008). Impact of the good behavior game, a universal classroom-based behavior intervention, on young adult service use for problems with emotions, behavior, or drugs or alcohol. *Drug and Alcohol Dependence, 95*(Suppl. 1), S29-S44.

Poldrack, R.A., and Packard, M.G. (2003). Competition among multiple memory systems: Converging evidence from animal and human brain studies. *Neuropsychologia, 41*(3), 245-251.

Pollard, J.A., Hawkins, J.D., and Arthur, M.W. (1999). Risk and protection: Are both necessary to understand diverse behavioral outcomes in adolescence. *Social Work Research, 23*, 145-158.

Posner, M.I. (2005). Genes and experience shape brain networks of conscious control. *Progress in Brain Research, 150,* 173-183.

Powell, C.M., and Miyakawa, T. (2006). Schizophrenia-relevant behavioral testing in rodent models: A uniquely human disorder? *Biological Psychiatry, 59*(12), 1198-1207.

Prado, G.J., Pantin, H., Schwartz, S.J., Lupei, N.S., and Szapocznik, J. (2006). Predictors of engagement and retention into a parent-centered, ecodevelopmental HIV prevention intervention for Hispanic adolescents and their families. *Journal of Pediatric Psychology, 31*(9), 874-890.

Prado, G.J., Pantin, H., Briones, E., Schwartz, S.J., Feaster, D., Huang, S., Sullivan, S., Tapia, M.I., Sabillon, E., Lopez, B., and Szapocznik, J. (2007). A randomized controlled trial of a parent-centered intervention in preventing substance use and HIV risk behaviors in Hispanic adolescents. *Journal of Consulting and Clinical Psychology, 75*(6), 914-926.

Prado, G.J., Schwartz, S.J., Maldonado-Molina, M., Huang, S., Pantin, H.M., Lopez, B., and Szapocznik, J. (2009). Ecodevelopmental x intrapersonal risk: Substance use and sexual behavior in Hispanic youth. *Health Education and Behavior, 36*(1), 45-61.

Price, J.M., Chamberlain, P., Landsverk, J., Reid, J., Leve, L., and Laurent, H. (2008). Effects of a foster parent training intervention on placement changes of children in foster care. *Child Maltreatment, 13*(1), 64-75.

Prince, M., Patel, V., Saxena, S., Maj, M., Maselko, J., Phillips, M.R., and Rahman, A. (2007). No health without mental health. *Lancet, 370*(9590), 859-877.

Prinz, R.J., and Dumas, J.E. (2004). Prevention of oppositional defiant disorder and conduct disorder in children and adolescents. In P.M. Barrett and T.H. Ollendick (Eds.), *Handbook of Interventions That Work with Children and Adolescents; Prevention and Treatment* (pp. 475-488). Chichester, West Sussex, England: Hobo.

Prinz, R.J., and Jones, T.L. (2003). Family-based interventions. In C.A. Essau (Ed.). *Conduct and Oppositional Defiant Disorders: Epidemiology, Risk Factors, and Treatment* (pp. 279-298). Mahwah, NJ: Lawrence Erlbaum.

Prinz, R.J., Sanders, M.R., Shapiro, C.J., Whitaker, D.J., and Lutzker, J.R. (2009). Population-based prevention of child maltreatment: The U.S. triple P system population trial. *Prevention Science, 10,* 1-13.

Pruett, M.K., Insabella, G.M., and Gustafson, K. (2005). The collaborative divorce project: A court-based intervention for separating parents with young children. *Family Court Review, 43,* 38-51.

Pryce, C.R., Dettling, A.C., Spengler, M., Schnell, C.R., and Feldon, J. (2004). Deprivation of parenting disrupts development of homeostatic and reward systems in marmoset monkey offspring. *Biological Psychiatry, 56*(2), 72-79.

Pugh, K., Mencl, E.W., Shaywitz, B.A., Shaywitz, S.E., Fulbright, R.K., Skudlarski, P., Constable, R.T., Marchione, K.E., Jenner, A.R., Fletcher, J.M., Liberman, A.M., Shankweiler, D.P., Katz, L., Lacardie, C., and Gore, J.C. (2000). The angular gyrus in developmental dyslexia: Task-specific differences in functional connectivity in posterior cortex. *Psychological Science, 11*(1), 51-56.

Puma, M., Bell, S., Cook, R., Heid, C., and Lopez, M. (2005). *Head Start Impact Study: First Year Findings.* Report Prepared for the U.S. Department of Health and Human Services. Washington, DC: U.S. Administration for Children and Families, Office of Planning, Research and Evaluation.

Pumariega, A.J., and Vance, H.R. (1999). School-based mental health services: The foundation for systems of care for children's mental health. *Psychology in the Schools, 36*(5), 371-378.

Purves, D., Augustine, G.A., Fitzpatrick, D., Katz, L.C., LaMantia, A.-S., and McNamara, J.O. (2000). *Neuroscience* (2nd ed.). Sunderland, MA: Sinauer Associates.

Quayle, D., Dzuirawiec, S., Roberts, C., Kane, R., and Ebsworthy, G. (2001). The effect of an optimism and lifeskillls program on depressive symptoms in preadolescence. *Behaviour Change, 18*, 194-203.

Quirk, G.J., and Mueller, D. (2008). Neural mechanisms of extinction learning and retrieval. *Neuropsychopharmacology, 33*(1), 56-72.

Rakic, P. (2002). Genesis of neocortex in human and nonhuman primates. In M. Lewis (Ed.), *Child and Adolescent Psychiatry. A Comprehensive Textbook* (3rd ed., pp. 25-42). Philadelphia: Lippincott Williams and Williams.

Rakic, P. (2003). Developmental and evolutionary adaptations of cortical radial glia. *Cerebral Cortex, 13*(6), 541-549.

Rakic, P., Bourgeois, J.P., Eckenhoff, M.F., Zecevic, N., and Goldman-Rakic, P.S. (1986). Concurrent overproduction of synapses in diverse regions of the primate cerebral cortex. *Science, 232*(4747), 232-235.

Rakic, P., Bourgeois, J.P., and Goldman-Rakic, P.S. (1994). Synaptic development of the cerebral cortex: Implications for learning, memory, and mental illness. *Progress in Brain Research, 102*, 227-243.

Rakyan, V.K., and Beck, S. (2006). Epigenetic variation and inheritance in mammals. *Current Opinion in Genetics and Development, 16*(6), 573-577.

Ramsey, S.D., McIntosh, M., and Sullivan, S.D. (2001). Design issues for conducting cost-effectiveness analyses alongside clinical trials. *Annual Review of Public Health, 22*, 129-141.

Rapee, R.M. (2001). The development of generalized anxiety. In M.W. Vasey and M.R. Dadds (Eds.), *The Developmental Psychopathology of Anxiety* (pp. 481-504). New York: Oxford University Press.

Rapee, R.M. (2002). The development and modification of temperamental risk for anxiety disorders: Prevention of a lifetime of anxiety. *Biological Psychiatry, 52*, 947-957.

Rapee, R.M., Kennedy, S., Ingram, M., Edwards, S., and Sweeney, L. (2005). Prevention and early intervention of anxiety disorders in inhibited preschool children. *Journal of Consulting and Clinical Psychology, 73*(3), 488-497.

Rash, B.G., and Grove, E.A. (2006). Area and layer patterning in the developing cerebral cortex. *Current Opinion in Neurobiology, 16*(1), 25-34.

Rauch, S.L., Shin, L.M., and Phelps, E.A. (2006). Neurocircuitry models of posttraumatic stress disorder and extinction: Human neuroimaging research—past, present, and future. *Biological Psychiatry, 60*(4), 376-382.

Raudenbush, S.W. (1997). Statistical analysis and optimal design for cluster randomized trials. *Psychological Methods, 2*(2), 173-185.

Raudenbush, S.W., and Bryk, A.S. (2002). *Hierarchical Linear Models: Applications and Data Analysis Methods* (2nd ed.). Thousand Oaks, CA: Sage.

Rauh, V.A., Garfinkel, R., Perera, F.P., Andrews, H.F., Hoepner, L., Barr, D.B., Whitehead, R., Tang, D., and Whyatt, R.W. (2006). Impact of prenatal chlorpyrifos exposure on neurodevelopment in the first 3 years of life among inner-city children. *Pediatrics, 118*(6), e1845-e1859.

Rebok, G.W., Hawkins, W.E., Krener, P., Mayer, L.S., and Kellam, S.G. (1996). Effect of concentration problems on the malleability of children's aggressive and shy behaviors. *Journal of the American Academy of Child and Adolescent Psychiatry, 32*, 193-203.

Reid, J.B., Eddy, J.M., Fetrow, R.A., and Stoolmiller, M. (1999). Description and immediate impacts of a preventive intervention for conduct problems. *American Journal of Community Psychology, 24*(4), 483-517.

Reid, M.J., Webster-Stratton, C., and Beauchaine, T.P. (2001). Parent training in Head Start: A comparison of program response among African American, Asian American, Caucasian, and Hispanic mothers. *Prevention Science, 2*, 209-227.

Reid, M.J., Webster-Stratton, C., and Hammond, M. (2003). Follow-up of children who received the Incredible Years intervention for oppositional-defiant disorder: Maintenance and prediction of a 2-year outcome. *Behavior Therapy, 34*, 471-491.

Reinherz, H.Z., Giaconia, R.M., Hauf, A.M., Wasserman, M.S., and Silverman, A.B. (1999). Major depression in the transition to adulthood: Risks and impairments. *Journal of Abnormal Psychology, 108*(3), 500-510.

Reinherz, H.Z., Tanner, J.L., Paradis, A.D., Beardslee, W.R., Szigethy, E.M., and Bond, A.E. (2006). Depressive disorders. In C.A. Essau (Ed.), *Child and Adolescent Psychopathology: Theoretical and Clinical Implications* (pp. 113-139). London, England: Brunner-Routledge.

Reiss, D. (2001). "Priorities for prevention research at NIMH": Will expanding the definition of prevention research reduce its impact? *Prevention and Treatment, 4*(1), Art. D19C.

Reiss, S. (1991). Expectancy model of fear, anxiety, and panic. *Clinical Psychology Review, 11*, 141-153

Reiss, S., and McNally, R.J. (1985). The expectancy model of fear. In S. Reiss and R.R. Bootzin (Eds.), *Theoretical Issues in Behavior Therapy* (pp. 107-121). New York: Academic Press.

Reiss, S., Silverman, W.K., and Weems, C.F. (2001). Anxiety sensitivity. In M.W. Vasey and M.R. Dadds (Eds.), *The Developmental Psychopathology of Anxiety* (pp. 92-111). London, England: Oxford University Press.

Rescorla, R.A. (1990). The role of information about the response-outcome relation in instrumental discrimination learning. *Journal of Experimental Psychology Animal Behavior Processes, 16*(3), 262-270.

Resnicow, K., Baranowski, T., Ahluwalia, J.S., and Braithwaite, R.L. (1999). Cultural sensitivity in public health: Defined and demystified. *Ethnicity and Disease, 9*(1), 10-21.

Reul, J.M., and Chandramohan, Y. (2007). Epigenetic mechanisms in stress-related memory formation. *Psychoneuroendocrinology, 32*(Suppl. 1), S21-S25.

Reynolds, A., and Ou, S.R. (2003). Promoting resilience through early childhood intervention. In S.S. Luthar (Ed.), *Resilience and Vulnerability: Adaptation in the Context of Childhood Adversities* (pp. 436-462). Cambridge, England: Cambridge University Press.

Reynolds, A.J., Temple, J.A., Robertson, D.L., and Mann, E.A. (2001). Long-term effects of an early childhood intervention on educational achievement and juvenile arrest: A 15-year follow-up of low-income children in public schools. *Journal of the American Medical Association, 285*, 2339-2346.

Rhinn, M., Picker, A., and Brand, M. (2006). Global and local mechanisms of forebrain and midbrain patterning. *Current Opinion in Neurobiology, 16*(1), 5-12.

Richards, A., Barkham, M., Cahill, J., Richards, D., Williams, C., and Heywood, P. (2003). PHASE: A randomized, controlled trial of supervised self-help cognitive behavioral therapy in primary care. *British Journal of General Practice, 53*(495), 764-770.

Richards, E.J. (2006). Inherited epigenetic variation—revisiting soft inheritance. *Nature Reviews Genetics, 7*(5), 395-401.

Richardson, A.J., and Montgomery, P. (2005). The Oxford–Durham study: A randomized controlled trial of dietary supplementation with fatty acids in children with developmental coordination disorder. *Pediatrics, 115*, 1360-1366.

Richardson, A.J., and Puri, B.K. (2002). A randomized double-blind, placebo-controlled study of the effects of supplementation with highly unsaturated fatty acids on ADHD-related symptoms in children with specific learning difficulties. *Progress in Neuropsychopharmacology & Biological Psychiatry, 26*, 233-239.

Richters, J.E., and Martinez, P.E. (1993). Children as victims of and witnesses to violence in a Washington, DC neighborhood. In L.A. Leavitt and N.A. Fox (Eds.), *The Psychological Effects of War and Violence on Children* (pp. 281-301). Mahwah, NJ: Lawrence Erlbaum.

Riggs, D.S., Rothbaum, B.O., and Foa, E.B. (1995). A prospective examination of symptoms of posttraumatic stress disorder in victims of nonsexual assault. *Journal of Interpersonal Violence, 10*, 201-214.

Riggs, N.R., and Greenberg, M.T. (2004). After-school youth development programs: A developmental-ecological model of current research. *Clinical Child and Family Psychology Review, 7*(3), 177-190.

Riley, A.W., Valdez, C.R., Barrueco, S., Mills, C., Beardslee, W., Sandler, I., and Rawal, P. (2008). Development of a family-based program to reduce risk and promote resilience among families affected by maternal depression: Theoretical basis and program description. *Clinical Child Family Psychology Review, 11*, 12-29.

Rimm-Kaufman, S.E., Pianta, R.C., and Cox, M.J. (2000). Teacher's judgments of problems in the transition to kindergarten. *Early Childhood Research Quarterly, 15*(2), 147-166.

Ringel, J.S., and Sturm, R. (2001). National estimates of mental health utilization and expenditures for children in 1998. *The Journal of Behavioral Health Services and Research, 28*(3), 319-333.

Ringwalt, C.L., Ennett, S., Vincus, A., Thorne, J., Rohrbach, L.A., and Simons-Rudolph, A. (2002). The prevalence of effective substance use prevention curricula in U.S. middle schools. *Prevention Science, 3*(4), 257-265.

Ripple, C.H., and Zigler, E. (2003). Research, policy, and the federal role in prevention initiatives for children. *American Psychologist, 58*(6-7), 482-490.

Rizzolatti, G., and Craighero, L. (2004). The mirror-neuron system. *Annual Review of Neuroscience, 27*, 169-192.

Robbins, M.S., Szapocznik, J., Alexandra, J.F., and Miller, J. (1998). Family systems therapy with children and adolescents. In M. Hersen and A.S. Bellack (Series Eds.) and T.H. Ollendick (Ed.), *Comprehensive Clinical Psychology, Children and Adolescents: Clinical Formulation and Treatment* (vol. 5, pp. 149-480). Oxford, England: Elsevier Science.

Roberts, C., Kane, R., Thomson, H., Bishop, B., and Hart, B. (2003). The prevention of depressive symptoms in rural school children: A randomized controlled trial. *Journal of Consulting and Clinical Psychology, 71*(3), 622-628.

Roberts, C., Kane, R., Bishop, B., Matthews, H., and Thomson, H. (2004). Prevention of depressive symptoms in rural school children: A follow-up study. *International Journal of Mental Health Promotion, 6*, 4-16.

Roberts, R.E., Roberts, C.R., and Xing, Y. (2007). Comorbidity of substance use disorders and other psychiatric disorders among adolescents: Evidence from an epidemiologic survey. *Drug and Alcohol Dependence, 88*(Suppl. 1), S4-S13.

Robertson, P.J., Roberts, D.R., and Porras, J.I. (1993). Dynamics of planned organizational change: Assessing empirical support for a theoretical model. *Academy of Management Journal, 36*(3), 619-634.

Robins, L.N., and McEvoy, L. (1990). Conduct problems as predictors of substance abuse. In L.N. Robins and M. Rutter (Eds.), *Straight and Devious Pathways from Childhood to Adulthood* (pp. 182-204). New York: Cambridge University Press.

Robinson, R. (2005). *Illinois Is Testing Ground for Mental Health Plan Targeting Schoolchildren.* Available: http://www.illinoisfamily.org/informed/contentview.asp?c=25661 [accessed February 2009].

Rodgers, B., Power, C., and Hope, S. (1997). Parental divorce and adult psychological distress: Evidence from a national birth cohort, a research note. *Journal of Child Psychology and Psychiatry, 38*(7), 867-872.

Rogers, E.M. (1995). *Diffusion of Innovations* (4th ed). New York: Free Press.

Rogers, P.J., Appleton, K.M., Kessler, D., Peters, T.J., Gunnell, D., Hayward, R.C., Heatherley, S.V, Christian, L.M., McNaughton, S.A., and Ness, A.R. (2008). No effect of n-3 long-chain polyunsaturated fatty acid (EPA and DHA) supplementation on depressed mood and cognitive function: A randomized controlled trial. *British Journal of Nutrition, 99,* 421-431.

Romeo, R.D. (2003). Puberty: A period of both organizational and activational effects of steroid hormones on neurobehavioural development. *Journal of Neuroendocrinology, 15*(12), 1185-1192.

Romeo, R.D., Byford, S., and Knapp, M. (2005). Annotation: Economic evaluations of child and adolescent mental health interventions, a systematic review. *Journal of Child Psychology and Psychiatry, 46*(9), 919-930.

Rooney, B.L., and Murray, D.M. (1996). A meta-analysis of smoking prevention programs after adjustment for errors in the unit of analysis. *Health Education Quarterly, 23,* 48-64.

Roosa, M.W., Sandler, I.N., Gehring, M., Beals, J., and Cappo, L. (1988). The children of alcoholics life events schedule: A stress scale for children of alcohol abusing parents. *Journal of Studies on Alcohol, 49,* 422-429.

Roosa, M.W., Jones, S., Tein, J.Y., and Cree, W. (2003). Prevention science and neighborhood influences on low-income children's development: Theoretical and methodological issues. *American Journal of Community Psychology, 31*(1-2), 55-72.

Roozendaal, B., Okuda, S., de Quervain, D.J., and McGaugh, J.L. (2006). Glucocorticoids interact with emotion-induced noradrenergic activation in influencing different memory functions. *Neuroscience, 138*(3), 901-910.

Rosen, C., Storfer-Isser A., Taylor, G., Kirchner, L., Emancipator, J., and Redline, S. (2004). Increased behavioral morbidity in school-aged children with sleep-disordered breathing. *Pediatrics, 114,* 1640-1648.

Rosenbaum, D.P., and Gordon, H. (1998). Assessing the effects of school-based drug education: A six-year multilevel analysis of project D.A.R.E. *Journal of Research in Crime and Delinquency, 35*(4), 381-412.

Rosenbaum, J.F., Biederman, J., Bolduc-Murphy, B.A., Faraone, S.V., Chaloff, J., and Hirshfeld, D.R. (1993). Behavioral inhibition in childhood: A risk factor for anxiety disorders. *Harvard Review of Psychiatry, 1,* 2-16.

Rosenberg, D.R., and Keshavan, M.S. (1998). Toward a neurodevelopmental model of the obsessive-compulsive disorder. *Biological Psychiatry, 43*(9), 623-640.

Rosvold, H., and Mishkin, M. (1961). Nonsensory effects of frontal lesions on discrimination learning and performance. In J. Delafresnaye (Ed.), *Brain Mechanisms and Learning* (pp. 555-576). Oxford, England: Blackwell.

Roth, T.L., and Sullivan, R.M. (2005). Memory of early maltreatment: Neonatal behavioral and neural correlates of maternal maltreatment within the context of classical conditioning. *Biological Psychiatry, 57*(8), 823-831.

Rothbart, M.K., and Posner, M.I. (2006). Temperament, attention, and developmental psychopathology. In D. Cicchetti (Ed.), *Developmental Psychopathology, Developmental Neuroscience* (2nd ed., vol. 2, pp. 465-501). Hoboken, NJ: Wiley.

Rotheram-Borus, M.J., and Duan, N. (2003). Next generation of preventive interventions. *Journal of the American Academy of Child and Adolescent Psychiatry, 42,* 518-530.

Rotheram-Borus, M.J., Lee, M.B., Gwadz, M., and Draimin, B. (2001). An intervention for parents with AIDS and their adolescent children. *American Journal of Public Health, 91,* 1294-1302.

Rotheram-Borus, M.J., Stein, J.A., and Lin, Y.Y. (2001). Impact of parent death and an intervention on the adjustment of adolescents whose parents have HIV/AIDS. *Journal of Consulting and Clinical Psychology, 69,* 763-773.

Rotheram-Borus, M.J., Lee, M.B., Leonard, N., Lin, Y.Y., Franzke, L., and Lightfoot, M.A. (2003). Four-year behavioral outcomes of an intervention for parents living with HIV and their adolescent children. *AIDS, 17,* 1217-1225.

Rothman, K.J., and Greenland, S. (Eds.). (1998). *Modern Epidemiology* (2nd ed.). Philadelphia: Lippincott-Raven.

Rowland, A.S., Lesesne, C.A., and Abramowitz, A.J. (2002). The epidemiology of attention-deficit/hyperactivity disorder (ADHD): A public health view. *Mental Retardation and Developmental Disabilities Research Reviews, 8*(3), 162-170.

Rubin, D.B. (1974). Estimating causal effects of treatments in randomized and nonrandomized studies. *Journal of Education and Psychology, 66,* 688-701.

Rubin, D.B. (1978). Bayesian inference for causal effects: The role of randomization. *Annals of Statistics, 6,* 34-58.

Rubin, D.B. (1987). *Multiple Imputation for Nonresponse in Surveys.* New York: Wiley.

Rueda, M.R., Posner, M.I., and Rothbart, M.K. (2005). The development of executive attention: Contributions to the emergence of self-regulation. *Developmental Neuropsychology, 28*(2), 573-594.

Rueda, M.R., Rothbart, M.K., McCandliss, B.D., Saccomanno, L., and Posner, M.I. (2005). Training, maturation, and genetic influences on the development of executive attention. *Proceedings of the National Academy of Sciences, 102*(41), 14931-14936.

Rusby, J.C., Smolkowski, K., Marquez, B., and Taylor, T.K. (in press). Proactive approaches for enhancing children's social development in child care homes. Submitted to *Early Childhood Research Quarterly.*

Rutter, M. (1979). Protective factors in children's responses to stress and disadvantage. In M.W. Kent and J.E. Rolf (Eds.), *Primary Prevention of Psychopathology Social Competence in Children* (vol. 3, pp. 49-74). Hanover, NH: University Press of New England.

Rutter, M. (1987). Psychosocial resilience and protective mechanisms. *American Journal of Orthopsychiatry, 57,* 316-331.

Rutter, M. (1996). Transitions and turning points in developmental psychopathology: As applied to the age span between childhood and mid-adulthood. *International Journal of Behavioral Development, 19,* 603-626.

Rutter, M. (2003). Genetic influences on risk and protection: Implications for understanding resilience. In S.S. Luthar (Ed.), *Resilience and Vulnerability: Adaptation in the Context of Childhood Adversities* (pp. 489-509). New York: Cambridge University Press.

Rutter, M., and Silberg, J. (2002). Gene-environment interplay in relation to emotional and behavioral disturbance. *Annual Reviews in Psychology, 53,* 463-490.

Rutter, M., Silberg, J., O'Connor, T., and Simonoff, E. (1999a). Genetics and child psychiatry: I Advances in quantitative and molecular genetics. *Journal of Child Psychology and Psychiatry, 40,* 3-18.

Rutter, M., Silberg, J., O'Connor, T., and Simonoff, E. (1999b). Genetics and child psychiatry: II Empirical research findings. *Journal of Child Psychology and Psychiatry, 40,* 19-55.

Rutter, M., Kreppner, J.M., and O'Connor, T.G. (2001). Specificity and heterogeneity in children's responses to profound institutional privation. *British Journal of Psychiatry, 179,* 97-103.

Rutter, M., Pickles, A., Murray, R., and Eaves, L. (2001). Testing hypotheses on specific environmental causal effects on behavior. *Psychological Bulletin, 127,* 291-324.

Rutter, M., Caspi, A., and Moffitt, T. (2003). Using sex differences in psychopathology to study causal mechanisms: Unifying issues and research strategies. *Journal of Child Psychology and Psychiatry, 44,* 1092-1115.

Rutter, M., Moffitt, T.E., and Caspi, A. (2006). Gene-environment interplay and psychopathology: Multiple varieties but real effects. *Journal of Child Psychology and Psychiatry, 47,* 226-261.

Ryan, A.S., and Zhou, W. (2006). Lower breastfeeding rates persist among the special supplemental nutrition program for women, infants and children participants. *Pediatrics, 117,* 1136-1146.

Ryerson, W.N. (2008). *The Effectiveness of Entertainment Mass Media in Changing Behavior.* Available: http://www.freerangethought.com/index.php?option=com_contentandtask= viewandid=295andItemid=41 [accessed August 2008].

Sabatini, M.J., Ebert, P., Lewis, D.A., Levitt, P., Cameron, J.L., and Mirnics, K. (2007). Amygdala gene expression correlates of social behavior in monkeys experiencing maternal separation. *Journal of Neuroscience, 27*(12), 3295-3304.

Safe Schools/Healthy Students Initiative. (2009). *Information and Application Procedures for Fiscal Year 2009.* Washington, DC: U.S. Departments of Education, Health and Human Services, and Justice. Available: http://www.ed.gov/programs/dvpsafeschools/2009-184l. pdf [accessed April 2009].

Saltzman, W., Babayon, T., Lester, P., Beardslee, W., and Pynoos, R. (2008). Family-based treatment for child traumatic stress: A review and report on current innovations. In D. Brom, R. Pat-Horenczyk, and J.D. Ford (Eds.), *Treating Traumatized Children: Risk, Resilience, and Recovery* (Part III, pp. 240-254). New York: Routledge.

Sameroff, A.J., and Fiese, B.H. (1990). Transactional regulation and early intervention. In S.J. Meisels and J.P. Shonkoff (Eds.), *Handbook of Early Childhood Intervention* (pp. 119-149). New York: Cambridge University Press.

Sameroff, A.J., Bartko W.T., Baldwin, A., Baldwin, C., and Seifer, R. (1998). Family and social influences on the development of child competence. In M. Lewis and C. Feiring (Eds.), *Families, Risk, and Competence* (pp. 161-185). Mahwah, NJ: Lawrence Erlbaum.

Sameroff, A.J., Gutman, L.M., and Peck, S.C. (2003). Adaptation among youth facing multiple risks: Prospective research findings. In S.S. Luthar (Ed.), *Resilience and Vulnerability: Adaptation in the Context of Childhood Adversities* (pp. 364-391). New York: Cambridge University Press.

Sampson, R.J. (2001). How do communities undergird or undermine human development? Relevant contexts and social mechanisms. In A. Booth, and A.C. Crouter (Eds.), *Does It Take a Village? Community Effects on Children, Adolescents, and Families* (pp. 3-30). Mahwah, NJ: Lawrence Erlbaum.

Sampson, R.J., and Laub, J.H. (1993). *Crime in the Making Pathways and Turning Points through Life.* Cambridge, MA: Harvard University Press.

Sampson, R.J., Raudenbush, S.W., and Earls, F. (1997). Neighborhoods and violent crime: A multilevel study of collective efficacy. *Science, 277,* 918-924.

Sanchez, M.M., Ladd, C.O., and Plotsky, P.M. (2001). Early adverse experience as a developmental risk factor for later psychopathology: Evidence from rodent and primate models. *Development and Psychopathology, 13*(3), 419-449.

Sanders, A.R., Duan, J., and Gejman, P.V. (2004). Complexities in psychiatric genetics. *International Review of Psychiatry, 16*(4), 284-293.

Sanders, D., and Haines, A. (2006). Implementation research is needed to achieve international health goals. *PLoS Medicine, 3*(6)e186:719-722.

Sanders, M.R., Markie-Dadds, C., Tully, L.A., and Bor, W. (2000). The Triple P-Positive Parenting Program: A comparison of enhanced, standard, and self-directed behavioral family intervention for parents of children with early onset conduct problems. *Journal of Consulting and Clinical Psychology, 68,* 624-640.

Sanders, M.R., Montgomery, D.T., and Brechman-Toussaint, M.L. (2000). The mass media and the prevention of child behavior problems: The evaluation of a television series to promote positive outcomes for parents and their children. *Journal of Child Psychology and Psychiatry, 41,* 939-948.

Sanders, M.R., Pidgeon, A.M., Gravestock, F., Connors, M.D., Brown, S., and Young, R.W. (2004). Does parental attributional retraining and anger management enhance the effects of the Triple P-Positive Parenting Program with parents at risk of child maltreatment? *Behavior Therapy, 35,* 513-535.

Sanders, M.R., Ralph, A., Sofronoff, K., Gardiner, P., Thompson, R., Dwyer, S., and Bidwell, K. (2008). Every family: A population approach to reducing behavioral and emotional problems in children making the transition to school. *Journal of Primary Prevention, 29,* 197-222.

Sandler, I.N., and Chassin, L. (2002). Training of prevention researchers: Perspectives from the Arizona State University prevention research training program. *Prevention and Treatment, 5,* Art. 6.

Sandler, I.N., Wolchik, S.A., Braver, S.L., and Fogas, B.S. (1986). Significant events of children and divorce: Toward the assessment of a risky situation. In S.M. Auerbach and A. Stolberg (Eds.), *Crisis Intervention with Children and Families* (pp. 65-83). New York: Hemisphere.

Sandler, I.N., Gersten, J.C., Reynolds, K., Kallgren, C.A., and Ramirez, R. (1988). Using theory and data to plan support interventions: Design of a program for bereaved children. In B.H. Gottlieb (Ed.), *Marshaling Social Support: Formats, Processes, and Effects* (pp. 53-83). Thousand Oaks, CA: Sage.

Sandler, I.N., Tein, J.-Y., Mehta, P., Wolchik, S., and Ayers, T. (2000). Coping efficacy and psychological problems of children of divorce. *Child Development, 71*(4), 1099-1118.

Sandler, I.N., Ayers, T.S., and Romer, A.L. (2001). Fostering resilience in families in which a parent has died. *Journal of Palliative Medicine, 5*(6), 945-956.

Sandler, I.N., Ayers, T.S., Wolchik, S.A., Tein, J.-Y., Kwok, O.M., Lin, K., Padgett-Jones, S., Weyer, J.L., Cole, E., Kriege, G., and Griffin, W.A. (2003). Family bereavement program: Efficacy of a theory-based preventive intervention for parentally bereaved children and adolescents. *Journal of Consulting and Clinical Psychology, 71,* 587-600.

Sandler, I.N., Ayers, T.S., Suter, J., Schultz, A.S., and Twohey, J.L. (2004). Adversities, strengths, and public policy. In K. Maton, C. Schellenbach, B. Leadbeater, and A. Solarz (Eds.), *Investing in Children, Youth, Families, and Communities: Strengths-based Public Policies* (pp. 31-49). Washington, DC: American Psychological Association.

Sandler, I.N., Ostrom, A., Bitner, M., Ayers, T., Wolchik, S., and Daniel, V. (2005). Developing effective prevention services for the real world: A prevention service development model. *American Journal of Community Psychology, 35,* 127-142.

Sandler, I.N., Miles, J., Cookston, J.T., and Braver, S.L. (2008). Effects of father and mother parenting on children's mental health in high- and low-conflict divorces. *Family Court Review, 46*(2), 282-296.

Sandler, I.N., Wolchik, S.A., Ayers, T.S., Tein, J.-Y., Coxe, S., and Chow, W. (2008). Linking theory and intervention to promote resilience of children following parental bereavement. In M. Stroebe, M. Hansson, W. Stroebe, and H. Schut (Eds.), *Handbook of Bereavement Research: Consequences, Coping and Care.* Washington, DC: American Psychological Association.

Sandler, J. (2007). Community-based practices: Integrating dissemination theory with critical theories of power and justice. *American Journal of Community Psychology, 40,* 272-289.

Santos, D., Assis, A., Bastos, A., Santos, L., Santos, C., Strina, A., Prado, M.S., Almeida-Fielho, N.M., Rodrigues, L.C., and Barreto, M.L. (2008). Determinants of cognitive function in childhood: A cohort study in a middle income context. *BMC Public Health, 8*(1), 202.

Schafer, J.L. (1997). *Analysis of Incomplete Multivariate Data.* London, England: Chapman and Hall.

Schafer, J.L., and Graham, J.W. (2002). Missing data: Our view of the state of the art. *Psychological Methods*, 7(2), 147-177.

Schechter, R., and Grether, J.K. (2008). Continuing increases in autism reported to California's developmental services system: Mercury in retrograde. *Archives of General Psychiatry*, 65, 19-24.

Scheier, M., and Carver, C. (1992). Effects of optimism on psychological and physical well-being: Theoretical overview and empirical update. *Cognitive Therapy and Research, 16*, 201-228.

Schensul, J.J. (1999). Organizing community research partnerships in the struggle against AIDS. *Health Education and Behavior, 26*(2), 266-283.

Schinke, S.P., Di Noia, J., and Glassman, J.R. (2004). Computer-mediated intervention to prevent drug abuse and violence among high-risk youth. *Addictive Behaviors, 29*(1), 225-229.

Schinke, S.P., Schwinn, T.M., Di Noia, J., and Cole, K.C. (2004). Reducing the risks of alcohol use among urban youth: Three-year effects of a computer-based intervention with and without parent involvement. *Journal of Studies on Alcohol, 65*(4), 443-449.

Schmidt, L.A., Fox, N.A., Rubin, K.H., Hu, S., and Hamer, D.H. (2002). Molecular genetics of shyness and aggression in preschoolers. *Personality and Individual Differences, 33*, 227-238.

Schmidt, N.B., Eggleston, A.M., Woolaway-Bickel, K., Fitzpatrick, K.K., Vasey, M.W., and Richey, J.A. (2007). Anxiety Sensitivity Ameliorating Training (ASAT): A longitudinal primary prevention program targeting cognitive vulnerability. *Journal of Anxiety Disorders, 21*(3), 302-319.

Schmiege, S.J., Khoo, S.T., Sandler, I.N., Ayers, T.S., and Wolchik, S.A. (2006). Impact of intervention and gender on recovery curves of child mental health problems following parental death. *American Journal of Preventive Medicine, 31*, 152-160.

Schneider, J.M., Fuji, M.L., Lamp, C.L., Lonnerdal, B., Dewey, K.G., and Zidenberg-Cherr, S. (2005). Anemia, iron-deficiency, and iron-deficiency anemia in 12-36 month-old children from low-income families. *American Journal of Clinical Nutrition, 82*, 1269-1274.

Schoenwald, S.K., and Hoagwood, K. (2001). Effectiveness, transportability, and dissemination of interventions: What matters when? *Psychiatric Services, 51*, 1190-1197.

Schorr, L., and Marchand, V. (2007). *Pathway to Children Ready for School and Succeeding at Third Grade*. Available: http://www.pathwaystooutcomes.org/_uploads/documents/live/3RDGRADEPATHWAYPDF8-15-07.pdf [accessed May 2009].

Schulenberg, J.E., and Zarrett, N.R. (2006). Mental health during emerging adulthood: Continuity and discontinuity in courses, causes, and functions. In J.J. Arnett and J.L. Tanner (Eds.), *Emerging Adults in America: Coming of Age in the 21st Century* (pp. 135-172). Washington, DC: American Psychological Association.

Scogin, F.R., Hanson, A., and Welsh, D. (2003). Self-administered treatment in stepped-care models of depression treatment. *Journal of Clinical Psychology, 59*, 341-349.

Scott, S., Knapp, M., Henderson, J., and Maughan, B. (2001). Financial costs of social exclusion: Follow-up study of antisocial children into adulthood. *British Medical Journal, 323*(7306), 191.

Scottish Executive. (2003). *National Programme for Improving Mental Health and Well-Being. Action Plan 2003-2006*. Edinburg: The Scottish Government. Available: http://www.scotland.gov.uk/Publications/2003/09/18193/26509 [accessed April 2009].

Sears, L.L., Finn, P.R., and Steinmetz, J.E. (1994). Abnormal classical eye-blink conditioning in autism. *Journal of Autism and Developmental Disorders, 24*(6), 737-751.

Sebastian, L. (1993). *Overcoming Postpartum Depression and Anxiety*. Omaha, NE: Addicus.

Sebat, J., Lakshmi, B., Malhotra, D., Troge, J., Lese-Martin, C., Walsh, T., et al. (2007). Strong association of de novo copy number mutations with autism. *Science, 316*(5823), 445-449.

Secrest, L.A., Lassiter, S.L., Armistead, L.P., Wychoff, S.C., Johnson, J., Williams, W.B., and Kotchick, B.A. (2004). The parents matter program: Building a successful investigator-community partnership. *Journal of Child and Family Studies, 13*, 35-45.

Seehusen, D.A., Baldwin, L.M., Runkle, G.P., and Clark, G. (2005). Are family physicians appropriately screening for postpartum depression? *Journal of the American Board of Family Medicine, 18*(2), 104-112.

Segawa, E., Ngwe, J.E., Li, Y., Flay, B.R., and Aban Aya Coinvestigators. (2005). Evaluation of the effects of the Aban Aya youth project in reducing violence among African American adolescent males using latent class growth mixture modeling techniques. *Evaluation Review, 29*(2), 128-148.

Seidman, E., and Pedersen, S. (2003). Holistic contextual perspectives on risk, protection, and competence among low-income urban adolescents. In S.S. Luthar (Ed.), *Resilience and Vulnerability: Adaptation in the Context of Childhood Adversities* (pp. 318-343). New York: Cambridge University Press.

Seidman, E., Aber, J.L., and French, S.E. (2004). The organization of schooling and adolescent development. In K.I. Maton, C.J. Schellenbach, B.J. Leadbeater, and A.L. Solarz (Eds.), *Investing in Children, Youth, Families, and Communities: Strengths-based Research and Policy* (pp. 233-250). Washington, DC: American Psychological Association.

Seligman, M.E.P., Schulman, P., DeRubies, R.J., and Hollon, S.D. (1999). The prevention of depression and anxiety. *Prevention and Treatment, 2*(8), 1-21.

Semansky, R.M., Koyanagi, C., and Vandivort-Warren, R. (2003). Behavioral health screening policies in Medicaid programs nationwide. *Psychiatric Services, 54*(5). Available: http://psychservices.psychiatryonline.org [accessed February 2009].

Senge, P. (1994). *The Fifth Discipline.* New York: Doubleday.

Serketich, W.J., and Dumas, J.E. (1996). The effectiveness of behavioral parent training to modify antisocial behavior in children: A meta-analysis. *Behavior Therapy, 27*, 171-186.

Serretti, A., and Mandelli, L. (2008). The genetics of bipolar disorder: Genome "hot regions," genes, new potential candidates, and future directions. *Molecular Psychiatry, 13*(8), 742-771.

Seto, B. (2001). History of medical ethics and perspectives on disparities in minority recruitment and involvement in health research. *American Journal of Medical Science, 322*(5), 248-252.

Sevelinges, Y., Moriceau, S., Holman, P., Miner, C., Muzny, K., Gervais, R., Mouly, A.M., and Sullivan, R.M. (2007). Enduring effects of infant memories: Infant odor-shock conditioning attenuates amygdala activity and adult fear conditioning. *Biological Psychiatry, 62*(10), 1070-1079.

Shadish, W.R. (2002). Revisiting field experimentation: Field notes for the future. *Psychological Methods, 7*(1), 3-18.

Shafritz, K.M., Marchione, K.E., Gore, J.C., Shaywitz, S.E., and Shaywitz, B.A. (2004). The effects of methylphenidate on neural systems of attention in attention deficit hyperactivity disorder. *American Journal of Psychiatry, 161*(11), 1990-1997.

Shair, H.N., Brunelli, S.A., Masmela, J.R., Boone, E., and Hofer, M.A. (2003). Social, thermal, and temporal influences on isolation-induced and maternally potentiated ultrasonic vocalizations of rat pups. *Developmental Psychobiology, 42*(2), 206-222.

Shanahan, L., Copeland, W., Costello, E.J., and Angold, A. (2008). Specificity of putative psychosocial risk factors for psychiatric disorders in children and adolescents. *Journal of Child Psychology and Psychiatry, 49*, 32-42.

Shanahan, M.J., and Hofer, S.M. (2005). Social context in gene-environment interactions: Retrospect and prospect. *Journals of Gerontology Series B, Psychological Sciences and Social Sciences, 60,* 65-76.

Shapiro, M.L., and Eichenbaum, H. (1999). Hippocampus as a memory map: Synaptic plasticity and memory encoding by hippocampal neurons. *Hippocampus, 9*(4), 365-384.

Shaw, P., Greenstein, D., Lerch, J., Clasen, L., Lenroot, R., Gogtay, N., Evans, A., Rapoport, J., and Giedd, J. (2006). Intellectual ability and cortical development in children and adolescents. *Nature, 440*(7084), 676-679.

Shaw, P., Lerch, J., Greenstein, D., Sharp, W., Clasen, L., Evans, A., Giedd, J., Castellanos, F.X., and Rapoport, J. (2006). Longitudinal mapping of cortical thickness and clinical outcome in children and adolescents with attention-deficit/hyperactivity disorder. *Archives of General Psychiatry, 63*(5), 540-549.

Sheldon, S.B. (2003). Linking school-family-community partnerships in urban elementary schools to student achievement on state tests. *Urban Review, 35*(2), 149-165.

Sher, K.J., Grekin, E.R., and Williams, N.A. (2005). The development of alcohol use disorders. *Annual Review of Clinical Psychology, 1,* 492-523.

Sherman, L.W., Gottfredson, D., MacKenzie, D., Eck, J., Reuter, P., and Bushway, S. (1997). *Preventing Crime: What Works, What Doesn't, What's Promising.* (NCJ #165366). Washington, DC: U.S. Department of Justice.

Shinn, M., and Toohey, S. (2001). Refocusing on primary prevention. *Prevention and Treatment, 4*(1), Art. 21.

Shohamy, D., Myers, C.E., Kalanithi, J., and Gluck, M.A. (2008). Basal ganglia and dopamine contributions to probabilistic category learning. *Neuroscience & Biobehavioral Reviews, 32*(2), 219-236.

Shrout, P.E., and Bolger, N. (2002). Mediation in experimental and nonexperimental studies: New procedures and recommendations. *Psychological Methods, 7*(4), 422-445.

Shulman, G.L., Fiez, J.A., Corbetta, M., Buckner, R.L., Miezin, F.M., Raichle, M.E., and Petersen, S.E. (1997). Common blood flow changes across visual tasks: II. Decreases in cerebral cortex. *Journal of Cognitive Neuroscience, 9*(5), 648-663.

Silow-Carroll, S. (2008). *Iowa's 1st Five Initiative: Improving Early Childhood Developmental Services Through Public-Private Partnerships.* (Issue brief). New York: The Commonwealth Fund. Available: http://www.commonwealthfund.org/Content/Publications/Issue-Briefs/2008/Sep/Iowas-1st-Five-Initiative—Improving-Early-Childhood-Developmental-Services-Through-Public-Private-P.aspx [accessed February 2009].

Silverman, W.K., and Pina, A.A. (2008). Psychosocial treatments for phobic and anxiety disorders in youth. In R.G. Steele, T.D. Elkin, and M.C. Roberts (Eds.), *Handbook of Evidence-Based Therapies for Children and Adolescents: Bridging Science and Practice* (pp. 65-82). New York: Springer.

Silverman, W.K., Kurtines, W.M., Ginsburg, G.S., Weems, C.F., Lumpkin, P.W., and Carmichael, D.H. (1999). Treating anxiety disorders in children with group cognitive-behavioral therapy: A randomized clinical trial. *Journal of Consulting and Clinical Psychology, 67,* 995-1003.

Simons, R.L., Johnson, C., Beaman, J., Conger, R.D., and Whitbeck, L.B. (1996). Parents and peer groups as mediators of the effect of community structure on adolescent problem behavior. *American Journal of Community Psychology, 24*(1), 145-171.

Singh, S., and Darroch, J.E. (2000). Adolescent pregnancy and childbearing: Levels and trends in developed countries. *Family Planning Perspectives, 32*(1), 14-23.

Singhal, A., Cody, M., Rogers, E.M., and Sabido, M. (2003). *Entertainment-Education and Social Change: History, Research, and Practice.* Mahwah, NJ: Lawrence Erlbaum.

Sinn, N., and Bryan, J. (2007). Effect of supplementation with polyunsaturated fatty acids and micronutrients on ADHD-related problems with attention and behavior. *Journal of Developmental & Behavioral Pediatrics, 28*(2), 82-91.

Skinner, D., Matthews, S.A., and Burton, L.M. (2005). Combining ethnography and GIS technology to examine constructions of developmental opportunities in contexts of poverty and disability. In T.S. Weisner (Ed.), *Discovering Successful Pathways in Children's Development: Mixed Methods in the Study of Childhood and Family Life*. Chicago, IL: MacArthur Foundation and University of Chicago Press.

Smit, F., Cuijpers, P., Oostenbrink, J., Batelaan, N., de Graaf, R., and Beekman, A. (2006). Costs of nine common mental disorders: Implications for curative and preventive psychiatry. *The Journal of Mental Health Policy and Economics, 9*, 193-200.

Smith, E.A., Swisher, J.D., Vicary, J.R., Bechtel, L.J., Minner, D., Henry, K.L., and Palmer, R. (2004). Evaluation of Life Skills Training and infused-life skills training in a rural setting. *Journal of Alcohol and Drug Education, 48*(1), 51-70.

Smith, E.P., Boutte, G.S., Zigler, E., and Finn-Stevenson, M. (2004). Opportunities for schools to promote resilience in children and youth. In K.I. Maton, C.J. Schellenbach, B.J. Leadbeater, and A.L. Solarz (Eds.), *Investing in Children, Youth, Families, and Communities: Strength-Based Research and Policy* (pp. 213-232). Washington, DC: American Psychological Association.

Smyke, A.T., Dumitrescu, A., and Zeanah, C.H. (2002). Attachment disturbances in young children. I: The continuum of caretaking casualty. *Journal of the American Academy of Child Adolescent Psychiatry, 41*(8), 972-982.

Smyke, A.T., Koga, S.F., Johnson, D.E., Fox, N.A., Marshall, P.J., Nelson, C.A., Zeanah, C.H., and the BEIA Core Group. (2007). The caregiving context in institution-reared and family-reared infants and toddlers in Romania. *Journal of Child Psychology and Psychiatry, 48*(2), 210-218.

Snowden, L.R., and Yamada, A. (2005). Cultural differences in access to care. *Annual Review of Psychology, 1*, 143-166.

Snyder, C.R., and Elliott, T.R. (2005). Twenty-first century graduate education in clinical psychology. *Journal of Clinical Psychology, 61*, 1033-1054.

Snyder, H.N. (2006). *Juvenile Arrests 2004*. Office of Juvenile Justice and Delinquency Prevention Juvenile Justice Bulletin. Washington, DC: U.S. Department of Justice. Available: http://www.ncjrs.gov/pdffiles1/ojjdp/214563.pdf [accessed August 2008].

Snyder, J., Reid, J., Stoolmiller, M., Howe, G., Brown, C.H., Dagne, G.A., Cross, W., and Masyn, K. (2006). Measurement systems for randomized intervention trials: The role of behavioral observation in studying treatment mediators and short-term outcomes. *Prevention Science, 7*, 43-56.

Sobolewski, J.M., and King, V. (2005). The importance of the coparental relationship for nonresident fathers' ties to children. *Journal of Marriage and Family, 67*, 1196-1212.

Solantaus, T., and Toikka, S. (2006). The effective family programme: Preventative services for the children of mentally ill parents in Finland. *International Journal of Mental Health Promotion, 8*(3), 37-43.

Sonuga-Barke, E.J., Taylor, E., Sembi, S., and Smith, J. (1992). Hyperactivity and delay aversion-I. The effect of delay on choice. *Journal of Child Psychology and Psychiatry, 33*(2), 387-398.

Sousa, N., Almeida, O.F., and Wotjak, C.T. (2006). A hitchhiker's guide to behavioral analysis in laboratory rodents. *Genes, Brain, and Behavior, 5*(Suppl. 2), 5-24.

Sowell, E.R., Peterson, B.S., Thompson, P.M., Welcome, S.E., Henkenius, A.L., and Toga, A.W. (2003). Mapping cortical change across the human life span. *Nature Neuroscience, 6*(3), 309-315.

Sowell, E.R., Thompson, P.M., Welcome, S.E., Henkenius, A.L., Toga, A.W., and Peterson, B.S. (2003). Cortical abnormalities in children and adolescents with attention-deficit hyperactivity disorder. *Lancet, 362*(9397), 1699-1707.

Sowell, E.R., Peterson, B.S., Kan, E., Woods, R.P., Yoshii, J., Bansal, R., Xu, D., Zhu, H., Thompson, P.M., and Toga, A.W. (2007). Sex differences in cortical thickness mapped in 176 healthy individuals between 7 and 87 years of age. *Cerebral Cortex, 17*(7), 1550-1560.

Spence, S.H., and Shortt, A.L. (2007). Can we justify the widespread dissemination of universal, school-based interventions for the prevention of depression among children and adolescents. *Journal of Child Psychology and Psychiatry, 48*(6), 526-542.

Spessot, A.L., Plessen, K.J., and Peterson, B.S. (2004). Neuroimaging of developmental psychopathologies: The importance of self-regulatory and neuroplastic processes in adolescence. *Annals of the New York Academy of Sciences, 1021*, 86-104.

Spirito, A., Brown, R.T., D'Angelo, E., Delamater, A., Rodriguez, J., and Siegel, L. (2003). Society of Pediatric Psychology Task Force report: Recommendations for the training of pediatric psychologists. *Journal of Pediatric Psychology, 28*(2), 85-98.

Spoth, R.L., and Greenberg, M.T. (2005). Toward a comprehensive strategy for effective practitioner-scientist partnerships and larger-scale community health and well-being. *American Journal of Community Psychology, 35*, 107-126.

Spoth, R.L., and Redmond, C. (2000). Research on family engagement in preventive interventions: Toward improved use of scientific findings in primary prevention practice. *Journal of Primary Prevention, 21*(2), 267-284.

Spoth, R.L., and Redmond, C. (2002). Project family prevention trials based in community-university partnerships: Toward scaled-up preventive interventions. *Prevention Science, 3*(3), 203-221.

Spoth, R.L., Redmond, C., Hockaday, C., and Yoo, S. (1996). Protective factors and young adolescent tendency to abstain from alcohol use: A model using two waves of intervention study data. *American Journal of Community Psychology, 24*, 749-770.

Spoth, R.L., Goldberg, C., and Redmond, C. (1999). Engaging families in longitudinal preventive intervention research: Discrete-time survival analysis of socioeconomic and social-emotional risk factors. *Journal of Consulting and Clinical Psychology, 67*, 157-163.

Spoth, R.L., Redmond, C., and Lepper, H. (1999). Alcohol initiation outcomes of universal family-focused preventive interventions: One- and two-year follow-ups of a controlled study. *Journal of Studies on Alcohol and Drugs, 13*(Suppl. 13), 103-111.

Spoth, R.L., Redmond, C., Shin, C., and Huck, S. (1999). A protective process model of parent-child affective quality and child mastery effects on oppositional behaviors: A test and replication. *Journal of School Psychology, 37,* 49-71.

Spoth, R.L., Redmond, C., and Shin, C. (2000). Reducing adolescents' aggressive and hostile behaviors: Randomized trial effects of a brief family intervention 4 years past baseline. *Archives of Pediatrics and Adolescent Medicine, 154,* 1248-1257.

Spoth, R.L., Kavanagh, K.A., and Dishion, T.J. (2002). Family-centered preventive intervention science: Toward benefits to larger populations of children, youth, and families. *Prevention Science, 3*(3), 145-152.

Spoth, R.L., Redmond, C., Trudeau, L., and Shin, C. (2002). Longitudinal substance initiation outcomes for a universal preventive intervention combining family and school programs. *Psychology of Addictive Behaviors, 16*(2), 129-134.

Spoth, R.L., Greenberg, M., Bierman, K., and Redmond, C. (2004). PROSPER community-university partnership model for public education systems: Capacity-building for evidence-based, competence-building prevention (PROmoting School-community-university Partnerships to Enhance Resilience). *Prevention Science, 5*, 31-40.

Spoth, R.L., Clair, S., Shin, C., and Redmond, C. (2006). Long-term effects of universal preventive interventions on methamphetamine use among adolescents. *Archives of Pediatric and Adolescent Medicine, 160,* 876-882.

Spoth, R.L., Shin, C., Guyll, M., Redmond, C., and Azevedo, K. (2006). Universality of effects: An examination of the comparability of long-term family intervention effects on substance use across risk-related subgroups. *Prevention Science, 7,* 209-224.

Spoth, R.L., Guyll, M., Lillehoj, C.J., Redmond, C., and Greenberg, M.T. (2007). PROSPER study of evidence-based intervention implementation quality by community-university partnerships. *Journal of Community Psychology, 35,* 981-989.

Spoth, R.L., Redmond, C., Shin, C., Clair, S., Greenberg, M.T., and Feinberg M.E. (2007). Toward public health benefits from community-university partnerships: PROSPER effectiveness trial results for substance use at 1½ years past baseline. *American Journal of Preventive Medicine, 32,* 395-402.

Spoth, R.L., Greenberg, M., and Turrisi, R. (2008). Preventive interventions addressing underage drinking: State of the evidence and steps toward public health impact. *Pediatrics, 121*(Suppl. 4), S311-S336.

Spoth, R., Randall, G.K., and Shin, C. (2008). Experimental support for a model of partnership-based family intervention effects on long-term academic success. *School Psychology Quarter, 23*(1), 70-89.

Sroufe, L.A., Egeland, B., and Kreutzer, T. (1990). The fate of early experience following developmental change: Longitudinal approaches to individual adaptation in childhood. *Child Development, 61,* 1363-1373.

St. Pierre, T.L., Osgood, D.W., Mincemoyer, C.C., Kaltreider, D.L., and Kauh, T.J. (2005). Results of an independent evaluation of Project ALERT delivered in schools by cooperative extension. *Prevention Science, 6*(2), 305-317.

Stahmer, A.C., Leslie, L.K., Hurlburt, M., Barth, R.P., Webb, M.B., Landsverk, J., and Zhang, J. (2005). Developmental and behavioral needs and service use for young children in child welfare. *Pediatrics, 116*(4), 891-900.

Stancin, T., and Mizell Palermo, T. (1997). A review of behavioral screening practices in pediatric settings: Do they pass the test? *Developmental and Behavioral Pediatrics, 18*(3), 183-194.

Stanton, B., Romer, D., Ricardo, I., Black, M., Feigelman, S., and Galbraith, J. (1993). Early initiation of sex and its lack of association with risk behaviors among adolescent African-Americans. *Pediatrics, 92*(1), 146-148.

Stead, L.F., and Lancaster, T. (2005). Interventions for preventing tobacco sales to minors. *Cochrane Database of Systematic Reviews, 1,* Art. No. CD001497.pub2.DOI: 10.1002/14651858.CD001497.pub2. Available: http://mrw.interscience.wiley.com/cochrane/clsysrev/articles/CD001497/frame.html [accessed February 2009].

Stefanacci, L., Suzuki, W.A., and Amaral, D.G. (1996). Organization of connections between the amygdaloid complex and the perirhinal and parahippocampal cortices in macaque monkeys. *Journal of Comparative Neurology, 375,* 552-582.

Stefani, G., and Slack, F.J. (2008). Small noncoding RNAs in animal development. *Nature Reviews Molecular Cell Biology, 9*(3), 219-230.

Stefansson, H., Rujescu, D., Cichon, S., Pietilainen, O.P.H., Ingason, A., Steinberg, S., et al. (2008). Large recurrent microdeletions associated with schizophrenia. *Nature, 455*(7210), 232-236.

Steinberg, L.D. (1999). *Adolescence* (5th ed.). New York: McGraw-Hill.

Steinhausen, H.C. (2006). Developmental psychopathology in adolescence: Findings from a Swiss study, the NAPE Lecture 2005. *Acta Psychiatrica Scandinavica, 113,* 6-12.

Stern, C.D. (2001). Initial patterning of the central nervous system: How many organizers? *Nature Reviews Neuroscience, 2*(2), 92-98.

Stevens, J., Ammerman, R.T., Putnam, F.G., and Van Ginkel, J. (2002). Depression and trauma history in first-time mothers receiving home visitation. *Journal of Community Psychology, 30*(5), 551-564.

Stevens, J., Kelleher, K.J., Gardner, W., Chisolm, D., McGeehan, J., Pajer, K., and Buchanan, L. (2008). Trial of computerized screening for adolescent behavioral concerns. *Pediatrics, 121*(6), 1099-1105.

Stevens, L., Zhang, W., Peck, L., Kuczek, T., Grevstad, N., Mahon, A., Zentall, S.S., Arnold, L.E., and Burgess, J.R. (2003). EFA supplementation in children with inattention, hyperactivity, and other disruptive behaviors. *Lipids, 38,* 1007-1021.

Stevenson, H.C., and White, J.J. (1994). AIDS prevention struggles in ethnocultural neighborhoods: Why research partnerships with community-based organizations can't wait. *AIDS Education and Prevention, 6*(2), 126-139.

Stice, E., and Peterson, C. (2007). Assessment of eating disorders. In E.J. Mash and A. Barkley (Eds.), *Assessment of Childhood Disorders* (pp. 751-780). New York: Guilford Press.

Stice, E., and Shaw, H. (2004). Eating disorder prevention programs: A meta-analytic review. *Psychological Bulletin, 130*(2), 206-227.

Stice, E., Burton, E.M., and Shaw, H. (2004). Prospective relations between bulimic pathology, depression, and substance abuse: Unpacking comorbidity in adolescent girls. *Journal of Consulting and Clinical Psychology, 72,* 62-71.

Stigler, M.H., Perry, C.L., Komro, K.A., Cudeck, R., and Williams, C.L. (2006). Tearing apart a multiple component approach to adolescent alcohol prevention: What worked in project northland? *Prevention Science, 7,* 269-280.

Stolberg, A.L., and Mahler, J. (1994). Enhancing treatment gains in a school-based intervention for children of divorce through skill training, parental involvement, and transfer procedures. *Journal of Consulting and Clinical Psychology, 62,* 147-156.

Stolk, M.N., Mesman, J., van Zeijl, J., Alink, L.R.A., Bakermans-Kranenburg, M.J., van Ijzendoorn, M.H., Juffer, F., and Koot, H.M. (2007). Early parenting intervention: Family risk and first-time parenting related to intervention effectiveness. *Journal of Child and Family Studies, 17*(1), 55-83.

Stormshak, E.A., Dishion, T.J., Light, J., and Yasui, M. (2005). Implementing family-centered interventions within the public middle school: Linking service delivery to change in student problem behavior. *Journal of Abnormal Child Psychology, 33*(6), 723-733.

Stouthamer-Loeber, M., Loeber, R., Farrington, D.P., Zhang, Q., van Kammen, W., and Maguin, E. (1993). The double edge of protective and risk factors for delinquency: Interrelations and developmental patterns. *Development and Psychopathology, 5,* 683-701.

Straussner, S.L.A., and Senreich, E. (2002). Educating social workers to work with individuals affected by substance use disorders. In M.R. Haack and A. Hoover (Eds.), *Strategic Plan for Interdisciplinary Faculty Development: Arming the Nation's Health Professional Workforce for a New Approach to Substance Use Disorders* (Chapter 11, pp. 319-340). Providence, RI: Association for Medical Education and Research in Substance Abuse. Available: http://www.projectmainstream.net/newsfiles/1134/SPACdocfinal.pdf [accessed April 2009].

Suarez-Balcazar, Y., Davis, M.I., Ferarri, J., Nyden, P., Olson, B., Alvarez, J., Molloy, P., and Toro, P. (2003). University-community partnerships: A framework and an exemplar. In L.A. Jason, C.B. Keys, Y. Suarez-Balcazar, R.R. Taylor, and M.I. Davis (Eds.), *Participatory Community Research: Theories and Methods in Action* (pp. 105-120). Washington, DC: American Psychological Association.

Substance Abuse and Mental Health Services Administration. (2003). *National Registry of Effective Prevention Programs.* Available: http://modelprograms.samhsa.gov [accessed August 2008].

Substance Abuse and Mental Health Services Administration. (2004). 21 states, 2 territories awarded strategic prevention framework grants. *SAMHSA News, 12*(6), Art. 1. Available: http://www.samhsa.gov/samhsa_news/VolumeXII_6/article1.htm [accessed August 2008].

Substance Abuse and Mental Health Services Administration. (2005). *Center for Mental Health Services' Prevention Initiatives and Priority Programs Development Branch.* Available: http://mentalhealth.samhsa.gov/cmhs/SpecialPopulations/ [accessed August 2008].

Substance Abuse and Mental Health Services Administration. (2007a). *Promotion and Prevention in Mental Health: Strengthening Parenting and Enhancing Child Resilience.* (HHS Pub. No. CMHA-SFP-6-1089). Rockville, MD: U.S. Department of Health and Human Services.

Substance Abuse and Mental Health Services Administration. (2007b). Results from the 2006 National Survey on Drug Use and Health: National Findings. Office of Applied Studies, NSDUH Series H-32, DHHS Pub. No. SMA 07-4293. Rockville, MD: U.S. Department of Health and Human Services.

Sullivan, M., Kone, A., Senturia, K.D., Chrisman, N.J., Ciske, S.J., and Krieger, J.W. (2001). Researcher and researched community perspectives: Toward bridging the gap. *Health Education and Behavior, 28*(2), 130-149.

Susser, E., Neugebauer, R., Hoek, H.W., Brown, A.S., Lin, S., Labovitz, D., and Gorman, J.M. (1996). Schizophrenia after prenatal famine: Further evidence. *Archives of General Psychiatry, 53,* 25-31.

Sutton, J.M. (2007). Prevention of depression in youth: A qualitative review and future suggestions. *Clinical Psychology Review, 27,* 552-571.

Suzuki, W.A., and Amaral, D.G. (1994). Perirhinal and parahippocampal cortices of the macaque monkey: Cortical afferents. *Journal of Comparative Neurology, 350,* 497-533.

Swain, J.E., Lorberbaum, J.P., Kose, S., and Strathearn, L. (2007). Brain basis of early parent-infant interactions: Psychology, physiology, and *in vivo* functional neuroimaging studies. *Journal of Child Psychology and Psychiatry, 48*(3-4), 262-287.

Sweet, M.A., and Appelbaum, M.L. (2004). Is home visiting an effective strategy? A meta-analytic review of home visiting programs for families with young children. *Child Development, 75,* 1435-1456.

Swisher, J.D. (2000). Sustainability of prevention. *Addictive Behaviors, 25,* 965-973.

Szapocznik, J., and Coatsworth, J.D. (1999). An ecodevelopmental framework for organizing the influences on drug abuse: An ecodevelopmental model for risk and prevention. In M. Glantz and C.R. Hartel (Eds.), *Drug Abuse: Origins and Interventions* (pp. 331-366). Washington, DC: American Psychological Association.

Szapocznik, J., and Kurtines, W.M. (1993). Family psychology and cultural diversity: Opportunities for theory, research, and application. *American Psychologist, 48*(1), 400-407.

Szapocznik, J., Perez-Vidal, A., and Brickman, A.L. (1988). Engaging adolescent drug abusers and their families in treatment: A strategic structural systems approach. *Journal of Consulting and Clinical Psychology, 56*(4), 552-557.

Takeuchi, D., Williams, D.R., and Adair, R. (1991). Economic stress and children's emotional and behavioral problems. *Journal of Marriage and the Family, 53*(4), 1031-1041.

Tallal, P. (1991). Hormonal influences in developmental learning disabilities. *Psychoneuroendocrinology, 16*(1-3), 203-211.

Tang, Y.Y., Ma, Y., Wang, J., Fan, Y., Feng, S., Lu, Q., Yu, Q., Sui, D., Rothbart, M.K., Fan, M., and Posner, M.I. (2007). Short-term meditation training improves attention and self-regulation. *Proceedings of the National Academy of Sciences, 104*(43), 17152-17156.

Taylor, R.W., and Wang, M.C. (Eds.). (1997). *Social and Emotional Adjustment of Family Relations in Ethnic Minority Families.* Mahwah, NJ: Lawrence Erlbaum.

Taylor, S.E., Kemeny, M.E., Reed, G.M., Bower, J.E., and Gruenewald, T.L. (2000). Psychological resources, positive illusions, and health. *American Psychologist, 55*, 99-109.

Tein, J.Y., Sandler, I.N., MacKinnon, D.P., and Wolchik, S.A. (2004). How did it work? Who did it work for? Mediation in the context of a moderated prevention effect for children of divorce. *Journal of Consulting and Clinical Psychology, 72*(4), 617-624.

Tein, J.Y., Sandler, I.N., Ayers, T.S., and Wolchik, S.A. (2006). Mediation of the effects of the family bereavement program on mental health problems of bereaved children and adolescents. *Prevention Science, 7*, 179-197.

Temple, J.A., and Reynolds, A.J. (2007). Benefits and costs of investments in preschool education: Evidence from the child-parent centers and related programs. *Economics of Education Review, 26*, 126-144.

Teplin, L.A., Abram, K.M., McClelland, G.M., Dulcan, M.K., and Mericle, A.A. (2002). Psychiatric disorders in youth in juvenile detention. *Archives of General Psychiatry, 59*(12), 1133-1143.

Tessier-Lavigne, M., and Goodman, C.S. (1996). The molecular biology of axon guidance. *Science, 274*(5290), 1123-1133.

Thapar, A., and Stergiakouli, E. (2008). Genetic influences on the development of childhood psychiatric disorders. *Psychiatry, 7*(7), 277-281.

Thapar, A., Harold, G., Rice, F., Langley, K., and O'Donovan, M. (2007). The contribution of gene-environment interaction to psychopathology. *Development and Psychopathology, 19*(4), 989-1004.

Thomas, S.B., and Quinn, S.C. (1991). The Tuskegee syphilis study, 1932 to 1972: Implications for HIV education and AIDS risk education programs in the black community. *American Journal of Public Health, 81*(11), 1498-1505.

Thompson, P.M., Vidal, C., Giedd, J.N., Gochman, P., Blumenthal, J., Nicolson, R., Toga, A.W., and Rapoport, J.L. (2001). Mapping adolescent brain change reveals dynamic wave of accelerated gray matter loss in very early-onset schizophrenia. *Proceedings of the National Academy of Sciences, 98*(20), 11650-11655.

Thompson, R.F. (2005). In search of memory traces. *Annual Review of Psychology, 56*, 1-23.

Tierney, J.P., Grossman, J.B., and Resch, N.L. (1995). *Making a Difference: An Impact Study of Big Brothers/Big Sisters*. Philadelphia: Public/Private Ventures.

Tobler, N.S., Roona, M.R., Ochshorn, P., Marshall, D.G., Streke, A.V., and Stackpole, K.M. (2000). School-based adolescent drug prevention programs: 1998 meta-analysis. *Journal of Primary Prevention, 20*, 275-336.

Togerni, W., and Anderson, S.E. (2003). *Beyond Islands of Excellence: What Districts Can Do to Improve Instruction and Achievement in all Schools*. Washington, DC: Learning First Alliance.

Toikka, S., and Solantaus, T. (2006). The effective family programme II: Preventative services for the children of mentally ill parents in Finland. *International Journal of Mental Health Promotion, 8*(4), 4-10.

Tolan, P., and Dodge, K. (2005). Children's mental health as a primary care and concern. *American Psychologist, 60*(6), 601-614.

Tolou-Shams, M., Paikoff, R., McKirnan, D.J., and Holmbeck, G.N. (2007). Mental health and HIV risk among African American adolescents: The role of parenting. In M.M. McKay and R.L. Paikoff (Eds.), *Community Collaborative Partnerships: The Foundation for HIV Prevention Research Efforts* (pp. 27-58). Binghamton, NY: Haworth Press.

Trasande, L., Schechter, C., Haynes, K.A., and Landrigan, P.J. (2006). Applying cost analyses to drive policy that protects children. *Annals of the New York Academy of Sciences, 1076*, 911-923.

Tremblay, R.E., and Schaal, B. (1996). Physically aggressive boys from age 6 to 12 years. Their biopsychosocial status at puberty. *Annals of the New York Academy of Sciences, 794,* 192-207.

Trickett, E.J., and Espino, S.L.R. (2004). Collaboration and social inquiry: Multiple meanings of a construct and its role in creating useful and valid knowledge. *American Journal of Community Psychology, 34,* 1-69.

Troxel, W.M., and Matthews, K.A. (2004). What are the costs of marital conflict and dissolution on children's physical health? *Clinical Child and Family Psychology Review, 7*(1), 29-57.

Trudeau, L., Spoth, R., Lillehoj, C., Redmond, C., and Wickrama, K.A.S. (2003). Effects of a preventive intervention on adolescent substance use initiation, expectancies, and refusal intentions. *Prevention Science, 4*(2), 109-122.

Trudeau, L., Spoth, R., Randall, G.K., and Azevedo, K. (2007). Longitudinal effects of a universal family-focused intervention on growth patterns of adolescent internalizing symptoms and polysubstance use: Gender comparisons. *Journal of Youth and Adolescence, 36,* 740-745.

Tsankova, N.M., Berton, O., Renthal, W., Kumar, A., Neve, R.L., and Nestler, E.J. (2006). Sustained hippocampal chromatin regulation in a mouse model of depression and antidepressant action. *Nature Neuroscience, 9*(4), 519-525.

Tsankova, N.M., Renthal, W., Kumar, A., and Nestler, E.J. (2007). Epigenetic regulation in psychiatric disorders. *Nature Reviews Neuroscience, 8*(5), 355-367.

Tsuang, M.T., and Faraone, S.V. (1994). Epidemiology and behavioral genetics of schizophrenia. In S.J. Watson (Ed.), *Biology of Schizophrenia and Affective Disease* (pp. 163-195). New York: Raven.

Tsuang, M.T., and Faraone, S.V. (2000). The frustrating search for schizophrenia genes. *American Journal of Medical Genetics, 97,* 1-3.

Tsuang, M.T., and Faraone, S.V. (2002). Diagnostic concepts and the prevention of schizophrenia. *Canadian Journal of Psychiatry, 47,* 515-517.

Tsuang, M.T., Stone, W.S., and Faraone, S.V. (2000). Towards the prevention of schizophrenia. *Biological Psychiatry, 48,* 349-356.

Tsuang, M.T., Stone, W.S., Tarbox, S.I., and Faraone, S.V. (2002). An integration of schizophrenia with schizotypy: Identification of schizotaxia and implications for research on treatment and prevention. *Schizophrenia Research, 54,* 169-175.

Turner, J.E., and Cole, D.A. (1994). Development differences in cognitive diatheses for child depression. *Journal of Abnormal Child Psychology, 22,* 15-32.

Turner, S.M., Beidel, D.C., and Costello, A. (1987). Psychopathology in the offspring of anxiety disorders patients. *Journal of Consulting and Clinical Psychology, 55,* 229-235.

Turrisi, R., Jaccard, J., Taki, R., Dunnam, H., and Grimes, J. (2001). Examination of the short-term efficacy of a parent-based intervention to reduce college student drinking tendencies. *Psychology of Addictive Behaviors: Special Issue on Understanding Binge Drinking, 15,* 366-372.

Ubel, P.A., Hirth, R.A., Chernew, M.E., and Fendrick, A.M. (2003). What is the price of life and why doesn't it increase at the rate of inflation? *Archives of Internal Medicine, 163*(14), 1637-1641.

Ungerleider, L.G., Doyon, J., and Karni, A. (2002). Imaging brain plasticity during motor skill learning. *Neurobiology of Learning and Memory, 78*(3), 553-564.

United Nations Children's Fund. (2001). *Innocenti Report Card 3. A League Table of Teenage Births in Rich Nations.* Florence, Italy: UNICEF Innocenti Research Centre. Available: http://www.unicef-irc.org/cgi-bin/unicef/series_down.sql?SeriesId=16 [accessed February 2009].

University of Akron. (2003). D.A.R.E. curriculum gets high marks. *Akron Update*, February 21. Available: http://www.uakron.edu/aupdate/Feb212003/Feature_58.php [accessed August 2008].

Urani, A., Chourbaji, S., and Gass, P. (2005). Mutant mouse models of depression: Candidate genes and current mouse lines. *Neuroscience and Biobehavioral Reviews, 29*(4-5), 805-828.

U.S. Census Bureau. (2005). *Number, Timing, and Duration of Marriages and Divorces: 2001.* (Report No. P70-97). Washington, DC: U.S. Department of Commerce.

U.S. Department of Education. (n.d.). *Office of Safe and Drug Free Schools: Programs/Initiatives.* Available: http://www.ed.gov/about/offices/list/osdfs/programs.html [accessed August 2008].

U.S. Department of Education. (2001). *Exemplary and Promising Safe, Disciplined and Drug Free Schools Program 2001.* Available: http://www.ed.gov/admins/lead/safety/exemplary01/exemplary01.pdf [accessed August 2008].

U.S. Department of Education. (2007). *The Condition of Education 2007.* (NCES 2007-064). Available: http://eric.ed.gov/ERICDocs/data/ericdocs2sql/content_storage_01/0000019b/80/29/91/8b.pdf [accessed August 2008].

U.S. Department of Education. (2008). *National Center for Education Statistics: Participation in Education.* Available: http://nces.ed.gov/programs/coe/list/index.asp [accessed August 2008].

U.S. Department of Health, Education, and Welfare. (1964). *Smoking and Health Report of the Advisory Committee to the Surgeon General of the Public Health Service.* Washington, DC: Author.

U.S. Environmental Protection Agency. (2004). *What You Need to Know About Mercury in Fish and Shellfish.* Available: http://www.epa.gov/waterscience/fishadvice/advice.html [accessed March 2008].

U.S. Government Accountability Office. (2007, October). *School Mental Health: Role of the Substance Abuse and Mental Health Services Administration and Factors Affecting Service Provision.* (GAO-08-19R). Available http://www.gao.gov/new.items/d0819r.pdf [accessed June 2008].

U.S. Office of Management and Budget. (2003). *Government Performance and Results Act.* Available: http://www.whitehouse.gov/omb/mgmt-gpra/gplaw2m.html [accessed August 2008].

U.S. Preventive Services Task Force. (2002). Screening for depression: Recommendations and rationale. *Annals of Internal Medicine, 136*(10), 760-764.

U.S. Public Health Service. (1999a). *Mental Health: A Report of the Surgeon General.* Rockville, MD: U.S. Department of Health and Human Services.

U.S. Public Health Service. (1999b). *The Surgeon General's Call to Action to Prevent Suicide.* Rockville, MD: U.S. Department of Health and Human Services.

U.S. Public Health Service. (2000). *Report of the Surgeon General's Conference on Children's Mental Health: A National Action Agenda.* Rockville, MD: U.S. Department of Health and Human Services.

U.S. Public Health Service. (2001a). *Mental Health: Culture, Race, and Ethnicity. A Supplement to Mental Health: A Report of the Surgeon General.* Rockville, MD: U.S. Department of Health and Human Services.

U.S. Public Health Service. (2001b). *National Strategy for Suicide Prevention: Goals and Objectives for Action.* Rockville, MD: U.S. Department of Health and Human Services.

U.S. Public Health Service. (2001c). *Youth Violence: A Report of the Surgeon General.* Rockville, MD: U.S. Department of Health and Human Services.

U.S. Public Health Service. (2007). *The Surgeon General's Call to Action to Prevent and Reduce Underage Drinking*. Rockville, MD: U.S. Department of Health and Human Services.

U.S. Social Security Administration. (2000). *Intermediate Assumptions of the 2000 Trustees Report*. Washington, DC: Office of the Chief Actuary of the Social Security Administration.

Vaidya, C.J., Austin, G., Kirkorian, G., Ridlehuber, H.W., Desmond, J.E., Glover, G.H., and Gabrieli, J.D.E. (1998). Selective effects of methylphenidate in attention deficit hyperactivity disorder: A functional magnetic resonance study. *Proceedings of the National Academy of Sciences, 95*(24), 14494-14499.

Valente, T.W. (1996). Social network thresholds in the diffusion of innovations. *Social Network, 18*, 69-89.

van Belzen, M.J., and Heutink, P. (2006). Genetic analysis of psychiatric disorders in humans. *Genes and Behavior, 5*(Suppl. 2), 25-33.

van den Bree, M.B.M., and Owen, M.J. (2003). The future of psychiatric genetics. *Annals of Medicine, 35*(2), 122-134.

van Emmerik, A.A., Kamphuis, J.H., Hulsbosch, A.M., Emmelkamp, P.M. (2002). Single session debriefing after psychological trauma: A meta-analysis. *Lancet, 360*, 766-771.

van Praag, H., Shubert, T., Zhao, C., and Gage, F.H. (2005). Exercise enhances learning and hippocampal neurogenesis in aged mice. *Journal of Neuroscience, 25*(38), 8680-8685.

Vander Stoep, A., Weiss, N.S., Kuo, E.S., Cheney, D., and Cohen, P. (2003). What proportion of failure to complete secondary school in the U.S. population is attributable to adolescent psychiatric disorder? *Journal of Behavioral Health Services and Research, 30*(1), 119-194.

VanVoorhees, B.W., Ellis, J.M., Gollan, J.K., Bell, C.C., Stuart, S.S., Fogel, J., Corrigan, P.W., and Ford, D.E. (2007). Development and process evaluation of a primary care internet-based intervention to prevent depression in emerging adults. *Primary Care Companion to the Journal of Clinical Psychiatry, 9*(5), 346-355.

VanVorhees, B.W., Fogel, J., Reinecke, M.A., Gladstone, T., Stuart, S., Gollan, et al. (2008). Randomized clinical trial of an internet-based depression prevention program for adolescents (Project CATCH-IT) in primary care: 12-week ouitcomes. *Journal of Developmental & Behavioral Pediatrics, 30*(1), 23-37.

Ventura, S.J., Mosher, W.D., Curtin, S.C., Abma, J.C., and Henshaw, S. (2001). Trends in pregnancy rates for the United States, 1976-1997: An update. *National Vital Statistics Reports, 49*(4), 1-10.

Vitaro, F., Brendgen, M., and Tremblay, R.E. (2001). Preventive intervention: Assessing its effects on the trajectories of delinquency and testing for mediational processes. *Applied Developmental Science, 5*, 201-213.

Voigt, R.G., Llorente, A.M., Jensen, C.L., Fraley, J.K., Berretta, M.C., and Heird, W.C. (2001). A randomized, double-blind, placebo-controlled trial of docosahexaenoic acid supplementation in children with attention-deficit/hyperactivity disorder. *The Journal of Pediatrics, 139*(2), 189-196.

Voisin, R., Baptiste, D., Martinez, D., and Henderson, G. (2005). Exporting a U.S.-HIV/AIDS prevention program to a Caribbean-island nation: Lessons from the field. *International Social Work, 49*, 75-86.

Vreeland, B. (2007). Bridging the gap between mental and physical health: A multidisciplinary approach. *Journal of Clinical Psychiatry, 68*(Suppl. 4), 26-33.

Wagenaar, A.C., and Toomey, T.L. (2002). Effects of minimum drinking age laws: Review and analyses of the literature from 1960 to 2000. *Journal of Studies on Alcohol,* Supplement no. 14, 206-225.

Wagenaar, A.C., Murray, D.M., Gehan, J.P., Wolfson, M., Forster, J.L., Toomey, T.L., and Jones-Webb, R. (2000). Communities mobilizing for change on alcohol: Outcomes from a randomized community trials. *Journal of Studies on Alcohol, 61*(1), 85-94.

Waites, C.L., Craig, A.M., and Garner, C.C. (2005). Mechanisms of vertebrate synaptogenesis. *Annual Review of Neuroscience, 28*(1), 251-274.

Wakschlag, L.S., Lahey, B.B., Loeber, R., Green, S.M., Gordon, R.A., and Leventhal, B.L. (1997). Maternal smoking during pregnancy and the risk of conduct disorder in boys. *Archives of General Psychiatry, 54,* 670-676.

Walker, A.E., Grimshaw, J., Johnston, M., Pitts, N., Steen, N., and Eccles, M. (2003). PRIME—PRocess modelling in ImpleMEntation research: Selecting a theoretical basis for interventions to change clinical practice. *BMC Health Services Research, 3.* Available: http://www.biomedcentral.com/content/pdf/1472-6963-3-22.pdf [accessed April 2009].

Walker, E., Kestler, L., Bollni, A., and Hochman, K.M. (2004). Schizophrenia: Etiology and course. *Annual Review of Psychology, 55,* 401-430.

Walker, H.M., and Severson, H.H. (1990). *Systematic Screening for Behavior Disorders.* Longmont, CO: Sopris West.

Walker, H.M., Severson, H.H., and Seeley, J. (2007). *Universal, School-based Screening for the Early Detection of Academic and Behavioral Problems Contributing to Later Destructive Outcomes.* Paper prepared for the Board on Children, Youth, and Families of the Institute of Medicine, November 21. Eugene: University of Oregon, Oregon Research Institute.

Walker, H., Seeley, J., Small, J., Golly, A., Severson, H., and Feil, E. (2008). The First Step to Success Program for Preventing Antisocial Behavior in Young Children: Update on past, current, and planned research. *Report on Emotional & Behavioral Disorders in Youth,* 17-23.

Walker, H.M., Seeley, J.R., Small, J., Severson, H.H., Graham, B., Feil, E.G. Golly, A.M., and Forness, S.R. (in press). A randomized controlled trial of the First Step to Success early intervention: Demonstration of program efficacy outcomes within a diverse, urban school district. Submitted to *Journal of Emotional and Behavioral Disorders.*

Walker, S.P., Wachs, T.D., Gardner, J.M., Lozoff, B., Wasserman, G.A., Pollitt, E., Carter, J.A., and International Child Development Steering Group. (2007). Child development: Risk factors for adverse outcomes in developing countries. *Lancet, 369*(9556), 145-157.

Walsh, T., McClellan, J.M., McCarthy, S.E., Addington, A.M., Pierce, S.B., Cooper, G.M., et al. (2008). Rare structural variants disrupt multiple genes in neurodevelopmental pathways in schizophrenia. *Science, 320*(5875), 539-543.

Walters, P. (2001). Educational access and the state: Historical continuities and discontinuities in racial inequality in American education. *Sociology of Education,* 35-49.

Wandersman, A. (2003). Community science: Bridging the gap between science and practice with community-centered models. *American Journal of Community Psychology, 3,* 227-242.

Wandersman, A., and Florin, P. (2003). Community interventions and effective prevention. *American Psychologist, 58,* 441-448.

Wang, C.P., Brown, C.H., and Bandeen-Roche, K. (2005). Residual diagnostics for growth mixture models: Examining the impact of a preventive intervention on multiple trajectories of aggressive behavior. *Journal of the American Statistical Association, 100,* 1054-1076.

Wang, P.S., Demler, O., Olfson, M., Pincus, H.A., Wells, K.B., and Kessler, R.C. (2006). Changing profiles of service sectors used for mental health care in the United States. *The American Journal of Psychiatry, 163*(7), 1187-1198.

Wang, Z., and Peterson, B.S. (2008). Partner-matching for the automated identification of reproducible ICA components from fMRI datasets: Algorithm and validation. *Human Brain Mapping, 29*(8), 875-893.

Warne, G.L., and Zajac, J.D. (1998). Disorders of sexual differentiation. In H.G. Burger and R.I. McLachlan (Eds.), *Gonadal Disorders* (pp. 945-967). Philadelphia: W.B. Saunders.

Warner, K.E. (1979). Clearing the airwaves: The cigarette ad ban revisited. *Policy Analysis, 5,* 435-450.

Warner, K.E. (2006). Tobacco policy research: Insights and contributions to public health policy. In K.E. Warner (Ed.), *Tobacco Control Policy* (Chapter 1, pp. 3-86). San Francisco: Jossey-Bass.

Warren, S.L., Huston, L., Egeland, B., and Sroufe, L.A. (1997). Child and adolescent anxiety disorders and early attachment. *Journal of the American Academy of Child and Adolescent Psychiatry, 36,* 637-644.

Weaver, I.C. (2007). Epigenetic programming by maternal behavior and pharmacological intervention. Nature versus nurture: Let's call the whole thing off. *Epigenetics, 2*(1), 22-28.

Weaver, I.C., Champagne, F.A., Brown, S.E., Dymov, S., Sharma, S., Meaney, M.J., and Szyf, M. (2005). Reversal of maternal programming of stress responses in adult offspring through methyl supplementation: Altering epigenetic marking later in life. *Journal of Neuroscience, 25*(47), 11045-11054.

Webster-Stratton, C. (1984). A randomized trial of two parent-training programs for families with conduct-disordered children. *Journal of Consulting and Clinical Psychology, 52*(4), 666-678.

Webster-Stratton, C. (1990). *The Incredible Years Parent Training Program Manual: Effective Communication, Anger Management and Problem-Solving (ADVANCE).* Seattle, WA: Incredible Years.

Webster-Stratton, C. (1998). Preventing conduct problems in Head Start children: Strengthening parent competencies. *Journal of Consulting and Clinical Psychology, 66,* 715-730.

Webster-Stratton, C. (2000). Enhancing the effectiveness of self-administered videotape parent training for families with conduct-problem children. *Journal of Abnormal Child Psychology, 18*(5), 479-492.

Webster-Stratton, C., Reid, M.J., and Hammond, M. (2004). Treating children with early-onset conduct problems: Intervention outcomes for parent, child, and teacher training. *Journal of Clinical Child and Adolescent Psychology, 33,* 105-124.

Webster-Stratton, C., Reid, M.J., and Stoolmiller, M. (2006). *Preventing Aggression and Improving Social, Emotional, and Academic Competence: Evaluation of Dina Dinosaur Classroom Curriculum in High-Risk Schools.* Unpublished manuscript, University of Washington. Available: http://www.incredibleyears.com/ [accessed August 2008].

Webster-Stratton, C., Reid, M.J., and Stoolmiller, M. (2008). Preventing conduct problems and improving school readiness: Evaluation of the incredible years teacher and child training programs in high-risk schools. *Journal of Child Psychology and Psychiatry, 49*(5), 471-488.

Weeks, M., Schensul, J., Williams, S., Singer, M., and Grier, M. (1995). AIDS prevention for African American and Latina women: Building culturally and gender-appropriate intervention. *AIDS Education and Prevention, 7*(3), 251-264.

Wegner, D.M. (1992). You can't always think what you want: Problems in the suppression of unwanted thoughts. In M.P. Zanna (Ed.), *Advances in Experimental Social Psychology* (vol. 25, pp. 193-225). San Diego, CA: Academic Press.

Wegner, D.M. (1994). Ironic processes of mental control. *Psychological Review, 101,* 34-52.

Weiser, M., Reichenberg, A., Rabinowitz, J., Kaplan, Z., Mark, M., Bodner, E., Nahon, D., and Davidson, M. (2001). Association between nonpsychotic psychiatric diagnosis in adolescent males and subsequent onset of schizophrenia. *Archives of General Psychiatry, 58*(10), 959-964.

Weissberg, R.P., and Greenberg, M.T. (1998). School and community competence—Enhancement and prevention programs. In W. Damon (Series Ed.), I.E. Siegel and K.A. Renninger (Vol. Eds.), *Handbook of Child Psychology: Child Psychology in Practice* (vol. 4, 5th ed., pp. 877-954). New York: Wiley.

Weissman, M.M., Warner, V., Wickramaratne, P.J., and Kandel, D.B. (1999). Maternal smoking during pregnancy and psychopathology in offspring followed to adulthood. *Journal of the American Academy of Child and Adolescent Psychiatry, 38*, 892-899.

Weissman, M.M., Wickramaratne, P., Nomura, Y., Warner, V., Pilowsky, D.J., and Verdeli, H. (2006). Offspring of depressed parents 20 years later. *American Journal of Psychiatry, 163*, 1001-1008.

Weisz, J.R., Sandler, I.N., Durlak, J.A., and Anton, B.S. (2005). Promoting and protecting youth mental health through evidence-based prevention and treatment. *American Psychologist, 60*(6), 628-648.

Welsh, B.C., and Farrington, D.P. (2001). Toward an evidence-based approach to preventing crime. *Annals of the American Academy of Political and Social Science, 578*, 158-173.

Welsh, B.C., and Farrington, D.P. (Eds.). (2006). *Preventing Crime: What Works for Children, Offenders, Victims, and Places.* Dordrecht, the Netherlands: Springer.

Wen, S.W., Liu, S., Kramer, M.S., Joseph, K., Levitt, C., Marcoux, S., and Liston, R.M. (2000). Impact of prenatal glucose screening on the diagnosis of gestational diabetes and on pregnancy outcomes. *American Journal of Epidemiology, 152*(11), 1009-1014.

Werner, E.E. (1996). Vulnerable but invincible: High-risk children from birth to adulthood. *European Child and Adolescent Psychiatry, 5*(Suppl. 1), 47-51.

Werner, E.E., and Smith, R.S. (1982). *Vulnerable but Invincible: A Study of Resilient Children.* New York: McGraw-Hill.

Werner, E.E., and Smith, R.S. (1992). *Overcoming the Odds: High-risk Children from Birth to Adulthood.* Ithaca, NY: Cornell University Press.

West, M.J. (1999). Stereological methods for estimating the total number of neurons and synapses: Issues of precision and bias. *Trends in Neurosciences, 22*(2), 51-61.

West, S.G., and Aiken, L.S. (1997). Toward understanding individual effects in multicomponent prevention programs: Design and analysis strategies. In K.J. Bryant, M. Windle, and S.G. West (Eds.), *The Science of Prevention: Methodological Advances in Alcohol and Substance Abuse Research* (pp. 167-209). Washington, DC: American Psychological Association.

West, S.G., and Sagarin, B.J. (2000). Subject selection and loss in randomized experiments. In L. Bickman (Ed.), *Research Design: Donald Campbell's Legacy* (pp. 117-154). Thousand Oaks, CA: Sage.

West, S.G., Aiken, L.S., and Todd, M. (1993). Probing the effects of individual components in multiple component prevention programs. *American Journal of Community Psychology, 21*(5), 571-605.

West, S.G., Biesanz, J.C., and Pitts, S.C. (2000). Causal inference and generalization in field settings: Experimental and quasi-experimental designs. In H.T. Reis and C.M. Judd (Eds.), *Handbook of Research Methods in Social and Personality Psychology* (pp. 40-84). New York: Cambridge University Press.

Whisman, M.A. (2007). Marital distress and DSM-IV psychiatric disorders in a population-based national survey. *Journal of Abnormal Psychology, 116*, 638-643.

Whitaker, R.C., Orzol, S.M., and Kahn, R.S. (2006). Maternal mental health, substance use, and domestic violence in the year after delivery and subsequent behavior problems in children at age 3 years. *Archives of General Psychiatry, 63*, 551-560.

White, D., and Pitts, M. (1998). Educating young people about drugs: A systematic review. *Addiction, 93*, 1475-1487.

Whitebeck, L.B., Conger, R.D., and Kao, M. (1993). The influence of parental support, depressed affect, and peers on the sexual behavior of adolescent girls. *Journal of Family Issues, 14,* 261-278.

Whitelaw, N.C., and Whitelaw, E. (2006). How lifetimes shape epigenotype within and across generations. *Human Molecular Genetics Review, 15*(2), R131-R137.

Wiesel, T.N. (1982). Postnatal development of the visual cortex and the influence of environment. *Nature, 299*(5884), 583-591.

Wilcox, H.C., Kellam, S.G., Brown, C.H., Poduska, J.M., Ialongo, N.S., Wang, W., and Anthony, J.C. (2008). The impact of two universal randomized first and second grade classroom interventions on young adult suicide ideation and attempts. *Drug and Alcohol Dependence, 95*(Suppl. 1), S60-S73.

Wiley, C.C., Burke, G.S., Gill, P.A., and Law, N.E. (2004). Pediatricians' views of postpartum depression: A self-administered survey. *Archives of Women's Mental Health, 7*(4), 231-236.

Willemsen, R., Oostra, B.A., Bassell, G.J., and Dictenberg, J. (2004). The fragile X syndrome: From molecular genetics to neurobiology. *Mental Retardation and Developmental Disabilities Research Reviews, 10*(1), 60-67.

Williams, C., and Whitfield, G. (2001). Written and computer-based self-help treatments for depression. *British Medical Bulletin, 57,* 133-144.

Williams, C.L., Perry, C.L., Dudovitz, B., Veblen-Mortenson, S., Anstine, P.S., Komro, K.A., and Toomey, T.L. (1995). A home-based prevention program for sixth-grade alcohol use: Results from Project Northland. *The Journal of Primary Prevention, 16,* 125-147.

Williams, C.L., Grechanaia, T., Romanova, O., Komro, K.A., Perry, C.L., and Farbakhsh, K. (2001). Russian-American partners for prevention: Adaptation of a school-based parent-child programmed for alcohol use prevention. *European Journal of Public Health, 11,* 314-321.

Williams, J., and Ross, L. (2007). Consequences of prenatal toxin exposure for mental health in children and adolescents. *European Child & Adolescent Psychiatry, 16*(4), 243-253.

Williams, J.H., Waiter, G.D., Gilchrist, A., Perrett, D.I., Murray, A.D., and Whiten, A. (2006). Neural mechanisms of imitation and "mirror neuron" functioning in autistic spectrum disorder. *Neuropsychologia, 44*(4), 610-621.

Wills, T.A., Gibbons, F.X., Gerrard, M., Murry, V.M., and Brody, G.H. (2003). Family communication and religiosity related to substance use and sexual behavior in early adolescence: A test for pathways through self-control and prototype perceptions. *Psychology of Addictive Behaviors, 17*(4), 312-323.

Wills, T.A., Murry, V.M., Brody, G.H., Gibbons, F.X., Gerrard, M., Walker, C., and Ainette, M.G. (2007). Ethnic pride and self-control related to protective and risk factors: Test of the theoretical model for the strong African American families program. *Health Psychology, 26*(1), 50-59.

Wilson, D.B., Gottfredson, D.C., and Najaka, S.S. (2001). School-based prevention of problem behaviors: A meta-analysis. *Journal of Quantitative Criminology, 17*(3), 247-272.

Wilson, J.M.G., and Jungner, G. (1968). *Principles and Practice of Screening for Disease.* Geneva, Switzerland: World Health Organization.

Wilson, S.J., and Lipsey, M.W. (2006a). *The Effects of School-Based Social Information Processing Interventions on Aggressive Behavior, Part I: Universal Programs.* A Campbell Collaboration Systematic Review. Available: http://db.c2admin.org/doc-pdf/Wilson_SocInfoProc_UnivProg_review.pdf [accessed April 2009].

Wilson, S.J., and Lipsey, M.W. (2006b). *The Effects of School-Based Social Information Processing Interventions on Aggressive Behavior, Part II: Selected/Indicated Pull-out Programs.* A Campbell Collaboration Systematic Review. Available: http://db.c2admin.org/doc-pdf/Wilson_SocInfoProc_PullOutProg_review.pdf [accessed April 2009].

Wilson, S.J., and Lipsey, M.J. (2007). Effectiveness of school-based intervention programs on aggressive behavior: Update of a meta-analysis. *American Journal of Preventive Medicine, 33*(Suppl. 2), S130-S143.

Wilson, S.J., Lipsey, M.W., and Derzon, J.H. (2003). Effectiveness of school-based intervention program on aggressive behavior: A meta-analysis. *Journal of Consulting and Clinical Psychology, 71*, 136-149.

Wilson, S.J., Lipsey, M.W., and Noser, K.A. (2007). *Meta-Analysis of the Effects of Early Intervention on Risk Factors for Antisocial Behavior.* Falls Church, VA: Society for Prevention Research.

Wittchen, H.U., Essau, C.A., von Zerssen, D., Krieg, J.C., and Zaudig, M. (1992). Lifetime and six-month prevalence of mental disorders in the Munich follow-up study. *European Archives of Psychiatry and Clinical Neuroscience, 241*, 247-258.

Wittchen, H.U., Nelson, C.B., and Lachner, G. (1998). Prevalence of mental disorders and psychosocial impairments in adolescents and young adults. *Psychological Medicine, 28*, 109-126.

Wittchen, H.U., Beesdo, K., Höfler, M., Bittner, A., and Lieb, R. (2004). *How Similar Are Predictors of Onset and Course in Generalised Anxiety Disorders?* Paper presented at the XXXIV Annual EABCT Congress, September 9-11, Manchester, England.

Wojtkowiak, J.W., Fouad, F., LaLonde, D.T., Kleinman, M.D., Gibbs, R.A., Reiners, Jr., J.J., Borch, R.F., and Mattingly, R.R. (2008). Induction of apoptosis in neurofibromatosis type 1 malignant peripheral nerve sheath tumor cell lines by a combination of novel farnesyl transferase inhibitors and lovastatin. *Journal of Pharmacology and Experimental Therapeutics, 326*, 1-11.

Wolchik, S.A., West, S.G., Sandler, I., Tein, J., Coatsworth, D., Lengua, L., Weiss, L., Anderson, E.R., Greene, S.M., and Griffin, W.A. (2000). An experimental evaluation of theory-based mother and mother-child programs for children of divorce. *Journal of Consulting and Clinical Psychology, 68*(5), 843-856.

Wolchik, S.A., Wilcox, K.L., Tein, J.Y., and Sandler, I.N. (2000). Maternal acceptance and consistency of discipline as buffers of divorce stressors on children's psychological adjustment problems. *Journal of Abnormal Child Psychology, 28*(1), 87-102.

Wolchik, S.A., Sandler, I.N., Millsap, R.E., Plummer, B.A., Greene, S.M., Anderson, E.R., Dawson-McClure, S.R., Hipke, K.N., and Haine, R.A. (2002). Six-year follow-up of a randomized, controlled trial of preventive interventions for children of divorce. *Journal of the American Medical Association, 288*, 1874-1881.

Wolchik, S.A., Sandler, I.N., Winslow, E., and Smith-Daniels, V. (2005). Programs for promoting parenting of residential parents: Moving from efficacy to effectiveness. *Family Court Review, 42*, 65-80.

Wolchik, S.A., Tein, J.Y., Sandler, I., and Ayers, R.S. (2006). Self-system beliefs as mediators of the relations between positive parenting and children's adjustment problems after parental death. *Journal of Abnormal Child Psychology, 34*, 221-238.

Wolchik, S.A., Sandler, I.N., Weiss, L., and Winslow, E.B. (2007). New Beginnings: An empirically based program to help divorced mothers promote resilience in their children. In J.M. Briesmeister and C.E. Schaefer (Eds.), *Handbook of Parent Training: Helping Parents Prevent and Solve Problem Behaviors* (pp. 25-62). New York: Wiley.

Wolraich, M. (1998). Attention deficit hyperactivity disorder. *Professional Care of Mother and Child, 8*, 35-37.

Wolraich, M., Drotar, D., Dworkin, P., and Perrin, E. (2008). *Developmental-Behavior Pediatrics: Evidence and Practice.* Philadelphia: Elsevier.

Woods, D.W., Himle, M.B., Miltenberger, R.G., Carr, J.E., Osmon, D.C., Karsten, A.M., Jostad, C., and Bosch, A. (2008). Durability, negative impact, and neuropsychological predictors of tic suppression in children with chronic tic disorder. *Journal of Abnormal Child Psychology, 36*(2), 237-245.

Woods, V.D., Montgomery, S.B., and Herring, R.P. (2004). Recruiting black/African American men for research on prostate cancer prevention. *Cancer, 100*(5), 1017-1025.

Woodward, L.J., and Fergusson, D.M. (1999). Childhood peer relationship problems and psychosocial adjustment in late adolescence. *Journal of Abnormal Child Psychology, 27*, 87-104.

Worden, J.W., and Silverman, P.R. (1996). Parental death and the adjustment of school-age children. *Omega, 33*, 91-102.

World Health Organization. (1986). *Ottawa Charter for Health Promotion.* Geneva, Switzerland: Author.

World Health Organization. (1993). *ICD-10 Classification of Mental and Behavioral Disorders: Diagnostic Criteria for Research.* Geneva, Switzerland: Author.

World Health Organization. (2004). *Prevention of Mental Disorders: Effective Interventions and Policy Options, Summary Report.* A report of the World Health Organization in collaboration with the Prevention Research Centre of the Universities of Nijmegen and Maastricht. Geneva, Switzerland: Author.

World Health Organization. (2005). *Mental Health Action Plan for Europe: Facing the Challenges, Building Solutions.* Copenhagen: Author.

Wright, J.P., Dietrich, K.N., Ris, M.D., Harnung, R.W., Wessel, S.D., Lanphear, B.P., Ho, M., and Rac, M.N. (2008). Association of prenatal and childhood blood lead concentrations with criminal arrests in early adulthood. *PLoS Medicine 5*(5), 732-840.

Wulczyn, F., Barth, R.P., Yuan, Y.Y., Jones-Harden, B., and Landsverk, J. (2005). *Beyond Common Sense: Child Welfare, Child Well-being, and the Evidence for Policy Reform.* Somerset, NJ: Transaction Aldine.

Wyatt, R.J., Apud, J.A., and Potkin, S. (1996). New directions in the prevention and treatment of schizophrenia: A biological perspective. *Psychiatry, 59*, 357-370.

Wyman, P.A. (2003). Emerging perspectives on context-specificity of children's adaptation and resilience: Emergence from a decade of research with urban children in adversity. In S. Luthar (Ed.), *Resilience and Vulnerability: Adaptation in the Context of Childhood Adversity.* New York: Cambridge University Press.

Wyman, P.A., Cowen, E.L., Work, W.C., and Kerley, J.H. (1993). The role of children's future expectations in self-esteem functioning and adjustment to life stress: A prospective study of urban at-risk children. *Development and Psychopathology, 5*, 649-661.

Wyman, P.A., Sandler, I., Wolchik, S.A., and Nelson, K. (2000). Resilience as cumulative competence promotion and stress protection: Theory and intervention. In D. Cicchetti, J. Rappaport, I. Sandler, and R.P. Weissberg (Eds.), *The Promotion of Wellness in Children and Adolescents* (pp. 133-184). Washington, DC: Child Welfare League of America.

Wyman, P.A., Brown, C.H., Inman, J., Cross, W., Schmeelk-Cone, K., Guo, J., and Peña, J. (2008). Randomized trial of a gatekeeper program for suicide prevention: One-year impact on secondary school staff. *Journal of Consulting and Clinical Psychology, 76*, 104-115.

Xu, B., Roos, J.L., Levy, S., van Rensburg, E.J., Gogos, J.A., and Karayiorgou, M. (2008). Strong association of de novo copy number mutations with sporadic schizophrenia. *Nature Genetics, 40*(7), 880-885.

Yakovlev, P.I., and Lecours, A.R. (1967). The myelogenetic cycles of regional maturation of the brain. In A. Minkowski (Ed.), *Regional Development of the Brain in Early Life* (pp. 3-70). Oxford, England: Blackwell Scientific.

Yang, H., Stanton, B., Li, X., Cottrel, L., Galbraith, J., and Kaljee, L. (2007). Dynamic association between parental monitoring and communication and adolescent risk involvement among African-American adolescents. *Journal of the National Medical Association, 99*(5), 517-524.

Yau, L.H.Y., and Little, R.J. (2001). Inference for complier-average causal effect from longitudinal data subject to noncompliance and missing data, with application to a job training assessment for the unemployed. *Journal of the American Statistical Association, 96*, 1232-1244.

Yehuda, R., Flory, J.D., Southwick, S., and Charney, D.S. (2006). Developing an agenda for translational studies of resilience and vulnerability following trauma exposure. *Annals of the New York Academy of Sciences, 1071*, 379-396.

Yoshikawa, H. (1994). Prevention as cumulative protection: Effects of early family support and education on chronic delinquency and its risks. *Psychological Bulletin, 115*, 28-54.

Yoshikawa, H., Schindler, H., and Caronongen, P. (2007). *The Prevention of Mental Health Disorders, Delinquency, and Problem Behaviors Through Intervention in Infancy and Early Childhood: Current Status and Future Directions.* Paper commissioned by the Committee on Prevention of Mental Disorders and Substance Abuse Among Children, Youth, and Young Adults: Research Advances and Promising Interventions. Board on Children, Youth, and Families, National Research Council and Institute of Medicine, Washington, DC.

Young, J.F., Mufson, L., and Davies, M. (2006). Efficacy of interpersonal psychotherapy-adolescent skills training: An indicated preventive intervention for depression. *Journal of Child Psychology and Psychiatry, 47*(12), 1254-1262.

Young, L.J., and Wang, Z. (2004). The neurobiology of pair bonding. *Nature Neuroscience, 7*(10), 1048-1054.

Young, S.E., Smolen, A., Stallings, M.C., Corley, R.P., and Hewitt, J.K. (2003). Sibling-based association analyses of the serotonin transporter polymorphism and internalizing behavior problems in children. *Journal of Child Psychology and Psychiatry, 44*, 961-967.

Yu, D.L., and Seligman, M.E.P. (2002). Preventing depressive symptoms in Chinese children. *Prevention and Treatment, 5*, Art. 9, 1-39.

Yung, A.R., and McGorry, P.D. (1996a). The initial prodrome in psychosis: Descriptive and qualitative aspects. *Australian and New Zealand Journal of Psychiatry, 30*, 587-599.

Yung, A.R., and McGorry, P.D. (1996b). The prodromal phase of first-episode psychosis: Past and current conceptualizations. *Schizophrenia Bulletin, 22*, 353-370.

Yung, A.R., McGorry, P.D., McFarlane, C.A., Jackson, H.J., Patton, G.C., and Rakkar, A. (1996). Monitoring and care of young people at incipient risk of psychosis. *Schizophrenia Bulletin, 22*, 283-303.

Zaff, J.F., and Calkins, J. (2001). *Background for Community-Level Work on Mental Health and Externalizing Disorders in Adolescence: Reviewing the Literature on Contributing Factors.* Washington, DC: Child Trends.

Zahn, R., Moll, J., Krueger, F., Huey, E.D., Garrido, G., and Grafman, J. (2007). Social concepts are represented in the superior anterior temporal cortex. *Proceedings of the National Academy of Sciences, 104*(15), 6430-6435.

Zahn-Waxler, C., Shirtcliff, E.A., and Marceau, K. (2008). Disorders of childhood and adolescence: Gender and psychopathology. *Annual Review of Clinical Psychology, 4*(1), 275-303.

Zeger, S.L., Liang, K.Y., and Albert, P.S. (1988). Models for longitudinal data: A generalized estimating equation approach. *Biometrics, 44*(4), 1049-1060. [Erratum appears in 1989, *Biometrics, 45*(1), 347].

Zeichmeister, I., Kilian, R., McDaid, D., and the Mental Health European Economics Network Group. (2008). Is it worth investing in mental health promotion and prevention of mental illness?: A systematic review of the evidence from economic evaluations. *BMC Public Health, 8*(20). Available: http://www.biomedcentral.com/1471-2458/8/20 [accessed April 2009].

Zerhouni, E.A. (2006). The promise of personalized medicine. *NIH Medline Plus*. Available: http://www.nih.gov/about/director/interviews/NLMmagazinewinter2007.pdf [accessed April 2009]

Zhou, Q., Sandler, I., Millsap, R., Wolchik, S., and Dawson-McClure, S. (2008). Mother-child relationship quality and effective discipline as mediators of the six-year effects of the New Beginnings Program for children from divorced families. *Journal of Consulting and Clinical Psychology, 76*(4), 579-594.

Zilbovicius, M., Boddaert, N., Belin, P., Poline, J.B., Remy, P., Mangin, J.F., Thivard, L., Barthélémy, C., and Samson, Y. (2000). Temporal lobe dysfunction in childhood autism: A PET study. *American Journal of Psychiatry, 157*(12), 1988-1993.

Zilbovicius, M., Meresse, I., Chabane, N., Brunelle, F., Samson, Y., and Boddaert, N. (2006). Autism, the superior temporal sulcus and social perception. *Trends in Neurosciences, 29*(7), 359-366.

Zill, N., Morrison, D.R., and Coiro, M.J. (1993). Long-term-effects of parental divorce on parent-child relationships, adjustment, and achievement in young adulthood. *Journal of Family Psychology, 7*(1), 1-13.

Zito, J.M., Safer, D.J., dosReis, S., Magder, L.S., Gardner, J., and Zarin, D.A. (1999). Psychotherapeutic medication patterns for youths with attention deficit hyperactivity disorder. *Archives of Pediatrics & Adolescent Medicine, 153*, 1257-1263.

Zlatanova, J. (2005). MeCP2: The chromatin connection and beyond. *Biochemistry and Cell Biology, 83*(3), 251-262.

Zlotnick, C., Johnson, S.L., Miller, I.W., Pearlstein, T., and Howard, M. (2001). Postpartum depression in women receiving public assistance: Pilot study of an interpersonal-therapy-oriented group intervention. *American Journal of Psychiatry, 158*(4), 638-640.

Zlotnick, C., Miller, I.W., Pearlstein, T., Howard, M., and Sweeney, P. (2006). A preventive intervention for pregnant women on public assistance at risk for postpartum depression. *American Journal of Psychiatry, 163*(8), 1443-1445.

Zoghbi, H.Y. (2003). Postnatal neurodevelopmental disorders: Meeting at the synapse? *Science, 302*(5646), 826-830.

Zucker, R.A., Donovan, J.E., Masten, A.S., Mattson, M.E., and Moss, H.B. (2008). Early developmental processes and the continuity of risk for underage drinking and problem drinking. *Pediatrics, 121*, 252-272.

Zuckerman, B., Amaro, H., Bauchner, H., and Cabral, H. (1989). Depressive symptoms during pregnancy: Relationship to poor health behaviors. *American Journal of Obstetrics and Gynecology, 160*, 1107-1111.

Zuckerman, B., Bachner, H., Parker, S., and Cabral, H. (1990). Maternal depressive symptoms during pregnancy, and newborn irritability. *Journal of Developmental Behavioral Pediatrics, 11*, 190-194.

Appendixes

Appendix A

Biographical Sketches of Committee Members and Staff

Kenneth E. Warner (*Chair*) is dean of the University of Michigan School of Public Health and Avedis Donabedian Distinguished University Professor of Public Health. A faculty member since 1972, he is also director of the university's Tobacco Research Network. His research has focused on economic and policy aspects of disease prevention and health promotion, with a special emphasis on tobacco and health. He served as the World Bank's representative to negotiations on the World Health Organization's first global health treaty, the Framework Convention on Tobacco Control. He also served as the senior scientific editor of the 25th anniversary surgeon general's report on smoking and health. He is on the editorial boards of three journals, chairs the board of *Tobacco Control*, and was a founding member of the board of directors of the American Legacy Foundation. During 2004-2005 he was president of the Society for Research on Nicotine and Tobacco and in 1989 was awarded the Surgeon General's Medallion by C. Everett Koop. In 1996, he was elected to the Institute of Medicine (IOM) and in 1999 to its governing council. In 2003, at the World Conference on Tobacco or Health, he received the inaugural award for outstanding research contribution in the international Luther L. Terry Awards for Exemplary Leadership in Tobacco Control. An economist, he has an A.B. from Dartmouth College and a Ph.D. from Yale University.

Thomas F. Boat (*Vice Chair*) is executive associate dean for the University of Cincinnati College of Medicine. He is immediate past director of the Children's Hospital Research Foundation and past chairman of the University of Cincinnati College of Medicine's Department of Pediatrics. He also was physician-in-chief of Children's Hospital Medical Center of Cincinnati. A current focus is creating high-value systems of care at Cincinnati Children's and the College of Medicine that are more responsive to the individual needs of patients and families. A pediatric pulmonologist by training, he worked early in his career to define the pathophysiology of airway dysfunction and develop more effective therapies for chronic lung diseases of childhood, such as cystic fibrosis. More recently he has worked at local and national levels to improve research efforts, subspecialty training, and clinical care in pediatrics. He has a special interest in issues posed by children's mental health for pediatric care and training. He is a member of the IOM and serves as cochair of the IOM Forum on the Science of Health Care Quality Improvement and Implementation. He has been a member of the Association for the Accreditation of Human Research Protection Programs board of directors since 2004 and is currently board president. He has served as chair of the American Board of Pediatrics and president of the Society for Pediatric Research, as well as the American Pediatric Society. He has an M.D. from the University of Iowa.

William R. Beardslee is director of the Baer Prevention Initiatives in the Department of Psychiatry at Children's Hospital Boston and Gardner Monks professor of child psychiatry at Harvard Medical School. He is interested in the protective effects of self-understanding in enabling youngsters and adults to cope with adversity and has studied self-understanding in civil rights workers, survivors of cancer, and children of parents with affective disorders. He and his colleagues developed preventive interventions designed to enhance resilience and understanding in families with depressed parents and demonstrated long-term positive effects from these approaches. The approach has been implemented in several large-scale projects, including a nationwide program for children of depressed parents in Finland and in programs for low-income families. He received the Blanche F. Ittleson Award of the American Psychiatric Association, a Faculty Scholar Award from the William T. Grant Foundation, and, in 1999, received the Irving Philips Award for Prevention and the Catcher in the Rye Award for Advocacy for Children from the American Academy of Child and Adolescent Psychiatry. In 2003, he received the Agnes Purcell McGavin Award for Prevention of Mental Disorder in Children from the American Psychiatric Association. He serves on the Carter Center Mental Health Task Force and on the Board of Mental Health America. He is an active member of the IOM Board on Children, Youth, and Families (BCYF) and served on the Committee on Adolescent Health and Development. He currently serves on the IOM Committee on Depression, Parenting Practices, and the Healthy Development of Young Children. He has an M.D. from Case Western Reserve University.

Carl C. Bell is president and chief executive officer of the Community Mental Health Council and Foundation, Inc., in Chicago. He is also the director of public and community psychiatry and a clinical professor of psychiatry and public health at the University of Illinois at Chicago. He is principal investigator of Using CHAMP to Prevent Youth HIV Risk in a South African Township. He is a member and former chairman of the National Medical Association's section on psychiatry, a fellow of the American College of Psychiatrists, a distinguished life fellow of the American Psychiatric Association, and a founding member and past board chairman of the National Commission on Correctional Health Care. He has published numerous articles and book chapters on mental health and African Americans. He is editor of *Psychiatric Perspectives on Violence: Understanding Causes and Issues in Prevention and Treatment* and author of *The Sanity of Survival: Reflections of Community Mental Health and Wellness*. He was a member of the IOM Committee on the Pathophysiology and Prevention of Adolescent and Adult Suicide. He serves on the National Mental Health Advisory Council of the National Institute of Mental Health. He has a B.S from the University of Illinois and an M.D. from Meharry Medical College.

Anthony Biglan is a senior scientist at Oregon Research Institute and director of the Center on Early Adolescence. He has been doing research for the past 25 years on the prevention of adolescent problem behaviors. His work has included studies of the risk and protective factors associated with tobacco, alcohol, and other drug use; high-risk sexual behavior; and anti-social behavior. He has conducted numerous experimental evaluations of interventions to prevent tobacco use through both school-based programs and community-wide interventions. He has also experimentally evaluated interventions to prevent adolescent substance use and high-risk sexual behavior, as well as to prevent reading failure and aggressive social behavior in children. He and colleagues at the Center for Advanced Study in the Behavioral Sciences published *Helping Adolescents at Risk: Prevention of Multiple Problem Behaviors*, a book summarizing the epidemiology, cost, etiology, prevention, and treatment of youth with multiple problems. He also coauthored the monograph *Community-Monitoring Systems: Tracking and Improving the Well-Being of America's Children and Adolescents* and the 1995 book, *Changing Cultural Practices: A Contextualist Framework for Intervention Research*. He has a Ph.D. in social psychology from the University of Illinois in Urbana and took postdoctoral training in clinical psychology at the University of Washington.

C. Hendricks Brown is distinguished university health professor of epidemiology and biostatistics in the College of Public Health at the University of South Florida. He holds adjunct professor positions in the Department of Biostatistics and the Department of Mental Health at the Johns Hopkins University Bloomberg School of Public Health. He is also a senior research scholar at the American Institutes for Research and a collaborating senior scientist at the Oregon Center for Research to Practice. For the past 20 years, he has received support from the National Institute of Mental Health and more recently from the National Institute on Drug Abuse and the Centers for Disease Control and Prevention to develop statistical methods for the design and analysis of preventive and early intervention field trials. As director of the Prevention Science and Methodology Group, Brown leads a national network of methodologists who are working on the design of preventive field trials and their analysis, particularly with advanced techniques for growth analysis, multilevel modeling, and designs for implementation research. He is the codirector of the multisite Center for Integrating Education and Prevention in Schools, which is now planning a large-scale randomized field trial in Baltimore. He is codirector of the Center for Prevention of Suicide Research at the University of Rochester and coleads randomized trials in youth prevention research. He has a Ph.D. in statistics from the University of Chicago.

Elizabeth Jane Costello is professor of medical psychology in the Department of Psychiatry and Behavioral Sciences at Duke University Medical Center and has been a faculty member of the department since 1988. She has served as director for the Psychiatric Epidemiology Training Program at the University of Pittsburgh School of Medicine. She is a member of the American College of Epidemiology and has served as council member and chair in the mental health section of the American Public Health Association. In 2007 she was president of the International Society for Research in Child and Adolescent Psychopathology and a recipient of a distinguished investigator award from the National Alliance for Research on Schizophrenia and Depression. Costello's areas of research interest include developmental epidemiology, life-span developmental psychopathology, mental health services for children and adolescents, and clinical decision making. She has also published numerous works in refereed journals on developmental psychology and epidemiology. At the National Research Council (NRC), Costello served on the Panel on Prevention, Treatment and Control of Juvenile Crime. She has a Ph.D. in psychology from the University of London, M.Phil. and B.Sci. degrees from the London School of Economics, and an M.A. from Oxford University.

Wendy E. Keenan (*Program Associate*) provides administrative and research support for BCYF and its various program committees. She also helps organize planning meetings and workshops that cover current issues related to children, youth, and families. Ms. Keenan has been on the National

Academies' staff for 10 years and worked on studies for both the NRC and the IOM. As senior program assistant, she worked with the NRC's Board on Behavioral, Cognitive, and Sensory Sciences. Prior to joining the National Academies, Ms. Keenan taught English as a second language for Washington, DC, public schools. She received a B.A. in sociology from The Pennsylvania State University and took graduate courses in liberal studies from Georgetown University.

Bridget B. Kelly (*Senior Program Associate*) first came to the National Academies in September 2007 as a Christine Mirzayan Science and Technology Policy Graduate Fellow. She then joined BCYF as staff for the Committee on the Prevention of Mental Disorders and Substance Abuse Among Children, Youth, and Young Adults as well as the Committee on Depression, Parenting Practices, and the Healthy Development of Children. She has since also worked as project director for the Workshop on Strengthening Benefit-Cost Methodology for the Evaluation of Early Childhood Interventions and in IOM's Board on Gobal Health as study director for the Committee on Preventing the Global Epidemic of Cardiovascular Disease: Meeting the Challenge in Developing Countries. She received an M.D. and a Ph.D. in neurobiology as part of the Medical Scientist Training Program at Duke University and a B.A. from Williams College.

Teresa D. LaFromboise is associate professor of counseling psychology in the School of Education and chair of Native American Studies at Stanford University. She is most concerned about stress-related problems of ethnic minority youth. She has developed school- and community-based preventive interventions with adolescents and is a recognized contributor to American Indian mental health initiatives. Her current research investigates the effectiveness of a culturally tailored suicide prevention intervention for American Indian middle school students. In addition to this outcome study, she is exploring the role of cumulative stress, acculturation, cultural identity, depression, and substance use in American Indian adolescent mental health. LaFromboise has received many professional awards for the book *American Indian Life Skills Development Curriculum*, including recognition from the Carter Center for Public Policy, the Department of Health and Human Services as a Substance Abuse and Mental Health Services Administration Program of Excellence, the First Nations Behavioral Health Association, and the Mental Health/Social Service Program of the Indian Health Service as an Outstanding Contribution to American Indian Mental Health. This intervention has been included in the National Registry of Effective Programs. LaFromboise lectures and teaches courses in counseling psychology, adolescent development, and American Indian mental health and serves on the Board of Family and Children Services in Palo Alto, California. She has a B.A. from Butler University, an M.Ed. from the University of North Dakota, Grand Forks, and a Ph.D. in counseling psychology from the University of Oklahoma.

Ricardo F. Muñoz is professor of psychology at the University of California, San Francisco (UCSF), chief psychologist at San Francisco General Hospital (SFGH), and director of the Clinical Psychology Training Program there. He directs the UCSF/SFGH Latino Mental Health Research Program, which develops Spanish- and English-language interventions designed to prevent and treat major depression and makes the resulting manuals available for download at http://www.medschool.ucsf.edu/latino/. To expand the reach of this work, he founded the UCSF/SFGH Internet World Health Research Center, which has as its mission developing and testing evidence-based Internet interventions for several health problems (such as smoking and depression) in several languages so that participants can use them worldwide (see http://www.health.ucsf.edu). He is coauthor of *The Prevention of Depression: Research and Practice* (1993) and editor of *Depression Prevention: Research Directions* (1987). He received the 1994 Lela Rowland Prevention Award from the National Mental Health Association for the San Francisco Depression Prevention Research Project. Muñoz was a member of the IOM committee that produced the report *Reducing Risks for Mental Disorders: Frontiers for Preventive Intervention Research*. He also served on the IOM Board on Health Promotion and Disease Prevention. He has an A.B. from Stanford University and a Ph.D. from the University of Oregon.

Mary Ellen O'Connell (*Study Director*) is a senior program officer in the Division of Behavioral and Social Sciences and Education (DBASSE) of the NRC. She has served as study director for four previous consensus studies: on international education and foreign languages, ethical considerations for research on housing-related health hazards involving children, reducing underage drinking, and assessing and improving children's health. She also served as study director for the Committee on Standards of Evidence and the Quality of Behavioral and Social Science Research, a DBASSE-wide strategic planning effort; developed standalone workshops on welfare reform and children and gun violence; and facilitated meetings of the national coordinating committee of the Key National Indicators Initiative. She came to DBASSE from the U.S. Department of Health and Human Services (HHS), where she spent eight years in the Office of the Assistant Secretary for Planning and Evaluation, most recently as director of state and local initiatives. Prior to HHS, she worked at the U.S. Department of Housing and Urban Development on homeless policy and program design issues and for the Commonwealth of Massachusetts as the director of field services. She has a B.A. (with distinction) from Cornell University and an

M.A. in the management of human services from the Heller School for Social Policy and Management at Brandeis University.

Peter J. Pecora has a joint appointment as the senior director of research services for Casey Family Programs and professor in the School of Social Work at the University of Washington. He was a line worker and later a program coordinator in a number of child welfare service agencies. He has worked with the state departments of social services to implement intensive home-based services, child welfare training, and risk assessment systems for child protective services. He has provided training to program leaders and staff in the United States, Australia, Canada, Italy, Great Britain, and Portugal. He has served as an expert witness for the states of Arizona, Florida, New Mexico, Washington, and Wisconsin. His coauthored books and articles focus on child welfare program design, administration, and research. He has provided consultation regarding evaluation of child and family services to HHS and a number of foundations, including the Annie E. Casey Foundation, the Colorado Trust, the Edna McConnell Clark Foundation, the McKnight Foundation, and the Stuart Foundation. In 2002 he was awarded a J. William Fulbright scholarship in Australia. He has a Ph.D. from the University of Washington.

Bradley S. Peterson is director of child and adolescent psychiatry, director of MRI research, and Suzanne Crosby Murphy professor in pediatric neuropsychiatry at Columbia University and the New York State Psychiatric Institute. His research interests lie primarily in the applications of neuroimaging to the study of brain-behavior associations in normal development and in serious childhood neuropsychiatric disorders, such as autism, Tourette syndrome, obsessive-compulsive disorder, attention deficit hyperactivity disorder, and affective disorders. He also is actively involved in studying the long-term effects of premature birth on brain development and neurobehavioral outcomes. His imaging studies typically aim to integrate anatomical and functional magnetic resonance imaging data with behavioral, neuropsychological, biological, and symptom measures in large samples of participating children. He has an M.D. from the University of Wisconsin-Madison Medical School.

Linda A. Randolph is president and chief executive officer of the Developing Families Center, Inc., an innovative, nonprofit, one-stop service center for childbearing and childrearing families in northeast Washington, DC. She has spent her career working to make things happen at the community level that promote the health and well-being of mothers, children, and families and working to make needed changes in public policy. This has included work in public health at the federal, state, and local government levels and in academia. She served as clinical professor of community medicine, pediatrics, and psychiatry at the Mt. Sinai School of Medicine and is currently visiting professor at the Georgetown University School of Nursing and Health Studies. She serves on the board of directors of Children's Futures, a multimillion-dollar city-wide initiative in Trenton, New Jersey, focusing on the healthy growth and development of children from birth to age 3. She is also a member of the national advisory committee to the Kellogg Health Scholars Program. Randolph has served on two previous IOM study committees: the Committee on Nutritional Status during Pregnancy and Lactation and the Committee on Improving the Disability Decision Process of the Social Security Administration. She has a B.S. from Howard University, an M.P.H. from the School of Public Health at the University of California, Berkeley, and an M.D. from the Howard University College of Medicine.

Irwin Sandler is Regent's Professor of Psychology at Arizona State University. He is the principal investigator of the Prevention Research Center for Families in Stress and of the Family Bereavement Program. For over 20 years, he has been involved in the development, evaluation, and dissemination of programs to promote resilience for children experiencing stressful life situations. His current interests focus on the transition of prevention programs from successful efficacy trials to studies of effectiveness and implementation in community organizations. His research focuses on preventive interventions for children in high-stress situations, including the study of mechanisms of resilience, and the longitudinal evaluation of the effects of preventive interventions for children who have experienced parental divorce and bereavement. He has written extensively on evidence-based prevention and treatment, particularly the development and evaluation of prevention programs based on models of resilience in response to serious stressful life events for children. He is coauthor of the *Handbook of Children's Coping* and coeditor of *The Promotion of Wellness in Children and Adolescents*. He has a B.A. from Brooklyn College and a Ph.D. in clinical psychology from the University of Rochester.

Appendixes B-F are available online.
Go to htttp://www.nap.edu and search for *Preventing Mental, Emotional, and Behavioral Disorders Among Young People.*

Index

D

Dads for Life, 173
Defining prevention
 cost-benefit perspective, 60-61; *see also*
  Indicated interventions; Selective
  interventions; Universal interventions
 current approach, 64-65
 debates, 62-64
 developmental perspective, 60
 early frameworks, 60-61
 IOM 1994 framework, xiv, 59-60, 61-
  62, 65
 issues in, 59-64
 mental health promotion component,
  65-69
 NAMHC approach, 62-63, 65
 personalized medicine (preemptive
  psychiatry) concept, 63-64
 public health perspective, 60, 61, 64
 recommendations, 14, 69
 treatment distinguished from prevention,
  xiii, xiv, 1, 2, 19, 29-30, 59, 60, 61,
  62, 65, 69
Delinquency. *See also* Deviant peers
 comorbidities, 183
 design of interventions, 267
 efficacy/effectiveness of interventions, 68,
  90-91, 168, 169, 170, 172-173, 183-
  184, 300, 301
 grant programs, 348, 349
 implementation of interventions, 187,
  270, 289, 300, 301, 308, 316
 opportunities for intervention, 390
 rates, 54, 78
 risk factors, 78, 89, 109, 167, 181, 183,
  248, 267
 screening for interventions, 223, 224
Delivery systems for services
 clearinghouses, 356
 identifying effective interventions, 22,
  352-355
 linking research and services, 355-356
 recommendations, 371-374
 technical assistance, 356
Department of Education. *See* U.S.
 Department of Education
Department of Health and Human Services.
 See U.S. Department of Health and
 Human Services
Department of Justice. *See* U.S. Department
 of Justice

Department of Labor. *See* U.S. Department
 of Labor
Depression
 age at onset, 49, 50, 92, 106, 191
 antidepressants, 120, 129
 children and adolescents, 4, 46, 48, 55,
  65, 91, 92, 152-153, 167, 195-196,
  197, 225, 228, 238-239, 303-304,
  379, 384, 390, 515, 524
 comorbidities, 48, 96, 99, 153, 192, 528
 cost and health burdens, 15, 181, 247,
  248
 cost-effectiveness of interventions, 253,
  256
 cultural adaptation of programs, 303
 data sources, 511, 512, 513, 516, 517
 efficacy/effectiveness of interventions, 4,
  91, 152-153, 155, 176, 178, 180,
  182, 184, 193-194, 195-197, 216,
  225, 311, 377, 391-392
 epidemiology, 30, 42-50, 54, 92, 103,
  379, 384
 genetic component, 52, 115, 117, 118,
  120
 gender and, 54, 92, 140
 major depressive episode rates, 40, 46,
  153, 195, 197
 meta-analyses, 515
 neurodevelopmental factors and, 129,
  140
 parental, 3, 4, 9, 52, 53, 87, 92, 93, 101,
  104, 105, 161-162, 167, 172, 176,
  178, 180, 196-197, 199, 209, 221,
  222, 225, 226, 233, 237, 247, 256,
  350, 389, 393
 pathways to, 106, 512
 peripartum, 161-162, 350
 preventive interventions, 2, 25, 66, 92-93,
  138, 172, 188, 195-197, 198, 199,
  311, 312, 316, 389, 393, 394, 515
 protective factors, 76, 89, 109-110, 214,
  215, 225
 research, 25, 38, 178, 344, 363, 385,
  420
 risk factors, 18, 52, 76, 91, 92-93, 99-
  100, 102, 103, 105, 106, 107, 109-
  110, 115, 117, 118, 167-168, 177,
  178, 213-214, 225, 231, 238-239,
  247, 522-525
 screening for, 9, 38, 39, 40, 41, 46, 65,
  161-162, 221, 226, 228, 234, 237,
  238-239, 350, 389